2012
Essential Med Notes
Clinical Handbook

Handbook Editors
Jonathan Hong
Kamini Raghuram

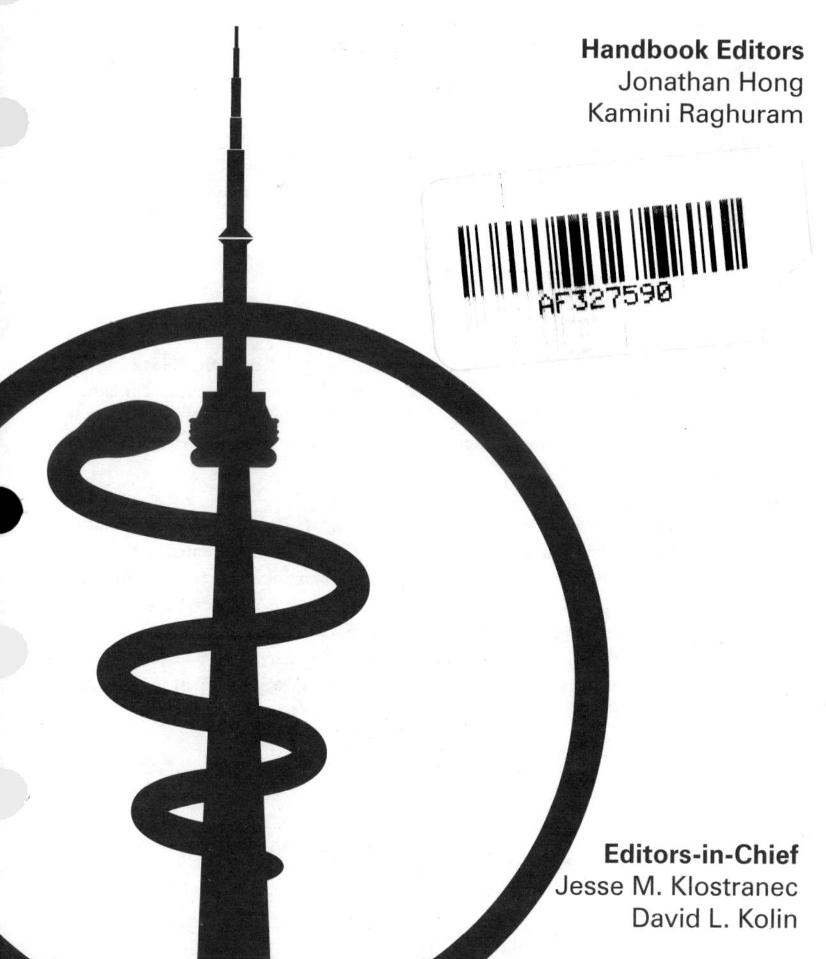

Editors-in-Chief
Jesse M. Klostranec
David L. Kolin

First Edition

Copyright © 2012
Toronto Notes for Medical Students, Inc.
Toronto, Ontario, Canada

ISBN 978-1-927363-00-3

Handbook Editors:
Jonathan Hong
Kamini Raghuram

Editors-in-Chief:
Jesse M. Klostranec
David L. Kolin

Typeset and production by Type & Graphics Inc.

Notice

The editors of this edition have taken every effort to ensure the information contained herein is accurate and conforms to the standards accepted at the time of publication. However, due to the constantly changing nature of the medical sciences and the possibility of human error, the reader is encouraged to exercise clinical judgement and consult with other sources of information that may become available with continuing research. Furthermore, the *Essential Med Notes Clinical Handbook* is a clinical tool and should not replace clinical judgement in the direct care of individual patients.

Library of Congress Cataloging-in-Publication Data is available upon request

Dear Readers,

We are happy to bring you the 2012 Essential Med Notes Clinical Handbook! This handbook is the result of a collaborative effort by University of Toronto medical students, and is intended to be a quick reference for your senior medical school clinical rotations. The Clinical Handbook was designed to include the most essential, evidenced-based, and up-to-date information for the clinical clerk. For more detailed information on the topics presented in the handbook, we suggest that you refer to your Essential Med Notes 2012 textbook.

As a result of feedback from last year's patrons, we have rigorously edited the content in the handbook and streamlined it to fit into a single, convenient, portable binder. As always, all the content in the handbook was updated by our chapter editors and reviewed by our Faculty to include the most current, evidence-based information. The first few chapters of the handbook are put together to serve as an overall guide for your clinical rotations, and now includes an entire chapter dedicated to Medical Imaging for your reference. We have also added more procedures in the *Common Procedures* chapter, and provided you with New England Journal of Medicine (NEJM) clinical video references for these procedures. Finally, this year's handbook includes the ACLS Protocol for cardiac arrest, adult bradycardia, and adult tachycardia.

This handbook would not have been possible without all the hard work of our Faculty Reviewers and our classmates in the University of Toronto Class of 2012. We would like to thank Jesse Klostranec and Dave Kolin, our Essential Med Notes Editors-in-Chief for all their support and efforts in coordinating so many aspects of this handbook. We would also like to thank all the Faculty Reviewers, Associate Editors, Chapter Editors, Production Managers, and Copy Editors for their irreplaceable contributions to the content and production of the handbook. Finally, we would like to thank T&G Inc. for their invaluable time and effort in formatting, re-formatting, and ultimately helping to create the final product.

We are also very grateful to the 2011 Handbook editors, Dr. Reema Shah and Dr. Alon Vaisman, for their guidance and foresight in shaping this year's handbook as well as future editions of the handbook.

It has been a privilege to be part of producing the 2012 Essential Med Notes Clinical Handbook this year. We hope you enjoy using this handbook as much as we have enjoyed creating it.

Sincerely,

Jonathan Hong and *Kamini Raghuram*
Clinical Handbook Editors
Essential Med Notes 2012

Contributors

Handbook Editors
Jonathan Hong
Kamini Raghuram

Editors-in-Chief
Jesse Klostranec
David Kolin

Production Managers
Jeffrey Alfonsi
Josh Levitz

Past Handbook Editors
Reema Shah
Alon Vaisman

Chapter Editors

Ethics, Legal and Organizational Medicine
Rami Shoucri

Anesthesia
Lei Du
Keerat Grewal
Alexander White

Cardiology and Cardiovascular Surgery
Gur Chandhoke
Colleen Parker
Darwin Yeung

Clinical Pharmacology
Andrew Gao
Kapil Goela

Dermatology
Adam Durbin
Jonathan Levy
Jane Ridley
Jessica Woolfson

Emergency Medicine
Nelab Alingary
Michael Misch
Brodie Nolan

Endocrinology
Priyanka Hansraj
Subhani Ragunathan
Tina Zhu

Family Medicine
Sarah Basma
Karen Dobkin
Vanessa Rambihar
Ashley Zaretsky

Gastroenterology
Mihan Han
Hanna Lee
Jenny Wang

General Surgery
Daniel Kagedan
Rachel Rae
Kenneth Van Dewark
Phil Zhang

Geriatric Medicine
Jillian Alston
Andrea Kirou-Mauro
Melinda Li

Gynecology
Anca Matei
Eva Seto
Yimeng Zhang

Hematology
Cheryl Foster
Christe Henshaw
Larissa Liontos

Infectious Disease
Marcus Barron
Melanie Finkbeiner
Stephen Gauthier
Laura Wagner

Medical Imaging
Kevin Lian
Peter Yang

Nephrology
Anna Holland
Michael Li
Julie Wright

Neurology
Matthew Burke
Kristen Krysko
Melissa Mackenzie
Janice Wong

Neurosurgery
Stephano Chang
Daipayan Guha
Amparo Wolf

Obstetrics
Kim Lazare
Lynn Sterling
Jennifer Sy

Ophthalmology
Corey Boimer
Raageen Kanjee
Zaid Mammo

Orthopedics
Joshua Bennitz
Andrea Chan
Eric Crawford

Otolaryngology
Lisa Caulley
Lara Gotha
Gavin le Nobel
Cheryl Volling

Pediatrics
Navneet Binepal
Bryan Li
Amber Makino
Anjali Rastogi

Plastic Surgery
Ashley Guttman
James Jung
Maria-Alexandra Petre
Dale Podolsky

Population and Community Health
Jennifer Loo
Nikita Patel
Arielle Rochman

Psychiatry
Melanie Beswick
Tara McGregor
Chris Zroback

Respirology
Calvin Ke
Marcus Miller
Terence Yung

Rheumatology
Meghan Ho
Danielle Rodin
Alexandra Saltman

Urology
Dhiraj Dhanjani
Mohammad Hajiha
Nobuhiko Okubo

Copy Editors
Erin Boyd
Carl Bradley
Erica Burry
Jessica Chin
Alexandra Cristian
Chris Gilchrist
Sofia Khan
Alex Koculym
Kapilan Kugathasan
Caeser Lim
Kate Querengesser
Tiffany Lo
Gavinn Niroopan
Matthew Orava
Jessica Page
Craig Peters
Tal Platzker
Lauren Willoughby
Savio Yu

Table of Contents

Table of Contents

Table of Contents

Table of Contents

Table of Contents

Guide to Clerkship

Admission Note

Identifying Data (ID)
- Patient's name, age, sex, relationship status, living arrangement (at home, in nursing home, etc.), occupation, and ethnicity

Chief Complaint/Reason for Referral (CC/RFR)
- Brief statement of why patient sought medical attention, duration of complaint

History of Presenting Illness (HPI)
- Use **OPQRSTUVW** mnemonic → **O**nset (chronology of symptoms, frequency, duration, progression, pattern), **P**rovoking and **P**alliative (alleviating) factors, **Q**uality of pain, **R**adiation of pain, **S**everity, **T**iming and progression, How does it affect '**U**' in your daily life?, déjà **V**u? (Has it happened before?), **W**hat do you think it is?
- Associated symptoms (from the relevant system)
- Severity of chronic disease (e.g. CCS Class in Coronary Artery Disease)
- Include any information relevant to patient's current medical problem
- Always include constitutional symptoms in HPI (appetite, diet, energy, fatigue, weight loss, fever, chills, night sweats)

Past Medical History (PMHx)
- General state of health, past illnesses (including childhood if relevant), injuries (type and date), hospitalizations (reasons for admission and dates), surgeries (type of procedure, date, hospital, and surgeon's name), psychological history, immunization history, sexual history, gynecological history, obstetrical history
- Risk factors relevant to CC and DDx

Medications (MEDS)
- Prescription drugs (name, dosage, route, frequency), compliance/adherence, over-the-counter (OTC), complementary and alternative, vitamins, herbs, supplements

Allergies (ALL)
- Drug-related allergies (reaction and timing), environmental and ingestible (food)

Smoking
- Pack-years (PY) = number of years a patient has smoked cigarettes multiplied by the number of packs per day

Alcohol (EtOH)
- Type, weekly consumption amount; if alcohol abuse is suspected, complete CAGE questionnaire
- Time of last drink (relevant for withdrawal)

Drugs
- Type, quantity, frequency, date of most recent use

Family History (FHx)
- In pedigree format document immediate family members age and health status, cause of death if deceased
- General screen for FHx of cancer, diabetes mellitus, hypertension, heart disease, high cholesterol, stroke

Social History (SocHx)
- Education, occupation, marital status and offspring, home structure, finances, religious beliefs, effect of the patient's illness on daily life, patient attitude, outlook and insight, social support network, travel history, sick contacts

Review of Systems/Functional Inquiry (ROS/FI)
- **Head, Eyes, Ears, Nose, Throat (HEENT):** masses, lymphadenopathy, epistaxis, sinus pain, dental disease, hoarseness, rhinorrhea, sore throat
- **Cardiovascular (CVS):** chest pain, dyspnea on exertion, orthopnea, paroxysymal nocturnal dyspnea (PND), dependent edema, palpitations, claudication, palpitations
- **Respiratory (RESP):** cough, sputum, hemoptysis, shortness of breath, pleuritic chest pain
- **Gastrointestinal (GI):** nausea, vomiting, dysphagia, abdominal pain, bowel habits, diarrhea, constipation, melena, hematochezia
- **Genitourinary (GU):** urination habits, frequency, urgency, nocturia, dysuria, hematuria, discharge, polyuria, flank pain
- **Gynecological (OBGYN):** menarche, GTPAL, contraception, LMP, menopause, pelvic pain, sexual history
- **Musculoskeletal (MSK):** joint pain, swelling, arthritis, myalgias
- **Endocrine (ENDO):** heat/cold intolerance, polydypsia, polyphagia, tremor, sweating, hair/skin changes
- **Neurological (Neuro):** headaches, seizures, memory loss, aphasia, visual changes, tinnitus, vertigo, hearing loss, weakness, paresthesias, ataxia
- **Psychiatric (PSYCH, ψ):** mood changes, anxiety, hallucinations, sleep disturbances, drug dependency/abuse, MSE
- **Dermatology (DERM):** rashes, skin discolourations, pruritus, hair changes, nail changes

Physical Examination (P/E)

Principles of Inspection Palpation Percussion Auscultation (IPPA)
- **GENERAL (GEN)**
  - Level of Consciousness: awake, drowsy, unconscious
  - Appearance: well, ill/toxic, acute distress
  - Age: appears stated age, older than stated age, younger than stated age
  - Physical Appearance: tall/short, underweight/obese, malnourished/well-nourished, skin colour, BMI
  - Gross Behaviour: eye contact, speech pattern, articulation, fluency, tremor, cooperation with exam, mood, affect
- **VITALS (VS)**
  - Heart rate/pulse and blood pressure (both arms, orthostatic changes), respiratory rate and % O_2 saturation on amount of oxygen, temperature and where on body it was taken
- **Head, Eyes, Ears, Nose, Throat (HEENT)**
  - HEAD: bruising, masses; check fontanelles in infants/young children
  - EYES: proptosis, ptosis, periorbital edema, conjunctivitis, scleritis, episcleritis, icterus, fundoscopy
  - EARS: external ear, auditory acuity, tympanic membranes (shiny, dull, intact, injected, bulging), tenderness
  - NOSE: nasal discharge (coryza, rhinorrhea), polyps, bleeding mucosa
  - MOUTH & THROAT: mucous membrane colour and moisture, oral lesions, dentition, pharynx, tonsils, tongue, palate, uvula
  - NECK: thyroid (size, masses, tenderness, bruit, special maneuvers), lymphadenopathy, carotid bruits
- **CARDIOVASCULAR SYSTEM (CVS)**
  - Inspect: JVP including waveform, hepatojugular reflux, height
  - Palpate: carotid pulse, parasternal lifts, thrills, point of maximal impulse (PMI or apex beat) noting size, location, and character
  - Percuss: cardiac dullness
  - Auscultate (over all four areas): first and second heart sounds (S1, S2, splitting), extra sounds (S3, S4), murmurs (graded I-VI) and their location, clicks

- **RESPIRATORY (RESP)**
  - Inspect: tachypnea, accessory muscle use, intercostals/subcostal indrawing, central/peripheral cyanosis, clubbing, chest wall shape/size
  - Palpate: chest expansion, tactile fremitus, trachea mobility and location
  - Percuss: diaphragmatic excursion, dullness in lung fields
  - Auscultate: adventitious sounds, wheezing, crackles, prolonged expiratory phase, egophony, whispered pectoriloquy
- **PERIPHERAL VASCULAR SYSTEM (PVS)**
  - Inspect: chronic vascular changes, skin/muscle/hair/nail atrophy, edema, pallor
  - Palpate: edema, temperature, pulses (radial, femoral, popliteal, posterior tibial, dorsalis pedis)
  - Auscultate: bruits at carotid, femoral, renal arteries
  - Special Tests: capillary refill, Allen's, Berger's, ankle-brachial index
- **ABDOMEN (ABDO)**
  - Inspect: contour (flat, obese, distended), scars, bulging flanks
  - Auscultate: bowel sounds, bruits (abdominal, renal, hepatic, splenic)
  - Palpate/Percuss: tenderness, rebound, guarding, masses, liver and spleen size, ascites, costovertebral angle tenderness
  - All abdominal exams should include a digital rectal exam, where appropriate
- **MUSCULOSKELETAL (MSK)**
  - Look (Inspect): asymmetry in SEADS (swelling, erythema, atrophy, deformity, skin changes)
  - Feel (Palpate): warmth, tenderness, crepitus, effusion, synovial thickening
  - Move (Range of Motion, ROM): active, passive, stress pain
  - Special Tests: as appropriate (e.g. ligament, tendon stability/pathology)
- **NEUROLOGICAL (NEURO)**
  - Cognition: level of consciousness (LOC), orientation, mini-mental status examination, consider more in-depth cognitive testing if deficits found or expected
  - Cranial Nerves (CN):
    - I:　　　　smell – vinegar, coffee
    - II:　　　pupils (size, symmetry, reaction, accommodation)
      　　　　visual acuity (Snellen chart)
      　　　　visual fields (confrontation, counting fingers)
      　　　　pupillary light reflex (afferent)
      　　　　fundoscopy
    - III, IV, VI: extraocular movements (EOM), ptosis, diplopia, miosis
    - V:　　　sensory – all 3 branches (pain, light touch)
      　　　　motor – mastication
      　　　　reflex – corneal (afferent)
    - VII:　　sensory – taste to anterior 2/3 of tongue, anterior part of external ear (vesicles)
      　　　　motor – facial expression, above and below eye
    - VIII:　auditory acuity, Weber and Rinne tests, nystagmus
    - IX:　　taste/sensation to posterior 1/3 of tongue + soft palate
    - X:　　sensory – oropharynx
      　　　　motor – gag reflex, throat sounds
    - XI:　　motor – sternocleidomastoid (SCM), trapezius
    - XII:　motor – tongue strength, deviation
  - Motor:
    - Central – pronator drift
    - Peripheral – muscle bulk, posture, fasiculations, tone (rigidity, spasticity) power 0-5
  - Reflexes:
    - Deep Tendon Reflexes – biceps, brachialis, triceps, patellar, achilles (graded 0-4+, clonus)
    - Upper Motor Neuron – plantar (Babinski), Hoffman
  - Sensory:
    - 1° modalities – light touch, pain (sharp vs. dull), temperature, vibration, proprioception
    - 2° modalities – stereognosis, graphesthesia, 2-pt discrimination

- Coordination:
  - Axial stability, rapid alternating movements (upper and lower limb), finger-nose, dysarthria
- Stance and Gait:
  - Romberg, tandem gait, postural stability
- **PSYCHIATRIC (PSYCH, ψ) (Mental Status Examination)**
  - Affect, abnormal thought process (e.g. circumstantiality, tangentiality, incoherence, neologism, perseveration), insight, judgment, suicidality, homocidality, previous attempts, hallucinations, delusions
- **UROLOGICAL (URO)**
  - Erythema, swelling, masses, tenderness in penis/scrotum, testicular masses/nodules, varicocele, inguinal masses/hernias
- **BREAST**
  - Dimpling, tenderness, lumps, nipple discharge, axillary masses, asymmetry
- **GYNECOLOGICAL**
  - External genitalia, vaginal mucosa, cervical discharge and colour, lesions, uterine size and shape, masses, adnexal masses, ovaries, cervical motion tenderness (CMT)

Investigations (Ix):
- Bloodwork
- Microbiology
- Imaging

Impression (Imp):
- Differential Diagnosis (DDx):
- Assessment and Plan (A&P):
- Issues: list in order of priority

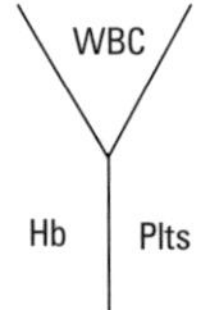

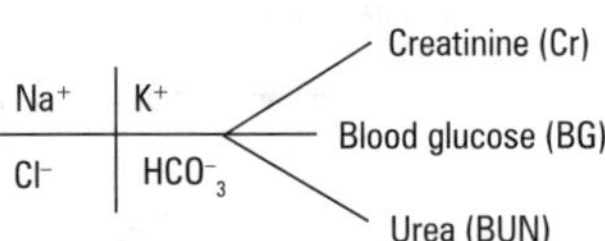

Admission Orders: ADDAVID

Admit, **D**iagnosis, **D**iet, **A**ctivity, **V**ital Signs (and monitoring), **I**nvestigations, **IV** Fluids, **D**rugs

Admit
- Admit to (your service) under (your attending physician)

Diagnosis
- What you suspect is the primary reason for admission (e.g. acute renal failure, congestive heart failure)

Diet
- **DAT** (diet as tolerated), **NPO** (nil per os/by mouth; if going for surgery or procedures, or if aspiration risk) **Sips Only, CF** (Clear Fluids), **FF** (Full Fluids), **Thickened Fluids** (dysphagia diet with thickened fluids), **Advancing Diet** (NPO to sips to clear fluids to full fluids to DAT), **Diabetic Diet** (indicate calories e.g. 1800 Kcal, 2200 Kcal), **Cardiac Diet, Renal Diet**, assessments by dietitian or SLP

Activity
- **AAT** (Activity as Tolerated), **NWB** (Non-Weight bearing), **FWB** (Full Weight bearing), **BR** (Bed Rest), **BR** with **BRP** (Bed Rest with Bathroom Privileges), **Ambulation** (Up in Chair tid, Ambulate bid), **Head of Bed elevated**

Vital Signs
- **VSR** [Vital Signs Routine] (HR, RR, BP, O₂ sat, temp. q8-12h, q shift), **VS q4h** (particularly sick patient requiring more frequent vitals), **Special parameters** (e.g. postural vitals, neuro vitals)

- Monitor
    - Accurate Ins and Outs (surgery, volume status pts.)
    - Daily weights (e.g. renal failure, edematous/CHF, infants)
    - Telemetry or continuous cardiac monitoring
- Capillary glucose monitoring (qid or with sliding scale) call MD if blood glucose <4.0 or >20.0 mmol/L

Investigations
- Hematology
    - Daily CBC + diff, PTT/INR
- Biochemistry
    - Daily electrolytes (Na^+, K^+, Cl^-, HCO_3^-), daily urea, daily creatinine, Ca^{2+}, Mg^{2+}, PO_4^{3-}, glucose, CSF cell count, CSF protein and glucose
- Microbiology
    - Urine R&M/C&S, blood cultures (take multiple and before administering antibiotics if suspicious)
    - Culturable entities: CSF, sputum, urine, feces, pus from wounds, blood, ascitic/pleuritic fluid
- Imaging
    - CT head, CXR, EKG
- Consults: social work, PT, OT, speech and language pathology, wound care, etc.

IV Fluids
- Specify a solution and a maintenance rate. Maintenance fluids are usually only needed if the patient is NPO. Note that the patient may need fluid for volume repletion [large amount over a short and defined amount of time (e.g. 250 cc/h NS IV 8 h) or for maintenance (follow 4-2-1 rule)]
- See <u>Nephrology</u>

Drugs
- Past: all the medications the patient is already on. Exercise judgment as to which ones the patient still needs
- Present: what the patient needs right now. They will likely need an IV but may also need antibiotics, diuretics, anti-arrhythmics etc.
- Future: anticipate what the patient might need. Think about DVT prophylaxis, sleeplessness, nausea and pain, bowel routine

"5 A's"
Analgesics
Anti-emetics
Anticoagulants
Antibiotics
All other meds (i.e. home meds and meds applicable to the specific case)

Progress (SOAP) Note

(Specialty Service) Progress Note (Ward #)
Date________   Time _________

****For Surgery, include post-operative day (POD)****
****For Obstetrics, include post-partum day (PPD)****

ID
- Age, sex with a history of (non-active/chronic issues) admitted with (list active/acute issues for why the patient is admitted). May also include a list of recent events that occurred since the most recent note.

Subjective
- How patient's night was (overnight) and how they feel that day and any new concerns they have
- What has changed since the previous note. Does the patient have any new symptoms?
- How is the patient coping with active issues: symptoms, progression, better/worse
- If patient is non-verbal, ask the parents, caregiver or patient's nurse
- Remember to ask about: behaviour, activity, sleep, appetite, bowel/bladder routine, pain control

Objective
- **Vitals**: HR, BP, RR, SaO_2, temp, daily weights, inputs (diet, IVF), output (U/O, BM/diarrhea, Vx, drains, e.g. JP)
- **General**: what the patient is doing, appearance, behaviour, cognition, cooperation, disposition
- **Focused P/E of system involved plus CVS, RESP, ABDO, EXT/MSK** as it is common for hospitalized patients to develop problems in these regions. In surgery include incision/wound status, commonly clean/dry/intact (CDI)
- **Ix**: new lab results, imaging or diagnostic tests/interventions

Medications
- Review daily for changes regarding those that are new/held/discontinued/restarted/modified

Assessment/Impression (A/P or IMP)
- Summarize what the new findings mean, what progress is being made. Improved? Stable? Waiting investigations/consult? Differential diagnosis if anything has been ruled in/out

Plan (A/P or I/P)
- Issue (1) → plan (e.g. UTI on day 2 of empiric abx, likely 14 d course required, await urine C&S)
- Issue (2) → plan...

Name, designation (CC\PGY), pager number

Discussed with Dr. ________________

Dictation/Discharge Summary Template

Type of Note: hospital name, department, type (admission, consult, discharge)
Your name, Designation
Attending MD
Patient Identification: name, patient identification #, DOB
Copies of this report to:
attending MD, family doctor, consultants, medical records including addresses
Date of Admission: under which service + consultant
Date of Discharge, length of stay
Admitting Diagnosis / Reason for Admission
Discharge Diagnosis
Other (non-active) Diagnoses
History of Presenting Illness: admitting history (pertinent details only)
Physical Examination: admitting physical (pertinent details only)
Course in Hospital: include treatment, response, new issues procedures, complications
Investigations and Results
Disposition: to home, nursing home, with or without home care
Discharge Medications
Follow-up and other special medical instructions
Thank you,
Your name, designation and attending MD name
End of dictation

Consultation Request

- Consults are arranged when your team needs an expert opinion to assist with diagnosis or management, or to perform a surgical procedure
- The details of requesting a consult will vary slightly but here is a quick general approach. Remember to write the order for the consult in the chart and contact the consultant directly (must be done for dietitians, physiotherapy, occupational therapy, speech pathology, and homecare, and medical/surgical consults)
- Have the chart in front of you so that you can answer questions regarding blood work, specific dates, hospital number, etc.
- Page the RESIDENT on-call that day for the specialty service you need
- Be concise!

1. Hello, Dr. ___________ this is (Name, CC or PGY) from (service), I have a patient we would like you to see
2. (Pause for acknowledgement by consultant)
3. (Name) is a (age, sex) (admitted under, floor, bed #) who presented (date) complaining of/admitted with
    ____
4. I'd like you to evaluate our patient for (clearly state why the consultation is beingrequested). Reason for Consult:
    (1) To answer the following questions
    (2) To help manage the following medical conditions or findings
5. Give relevant history and data. (Note: some services may not require a detailed history over the phone)
    PMHx: list of the relevant history
    HPI: include all relevant details
    FHx, SocHx: If relevant to the consult
6. I think the most likely diagnosis is ___________
7. This is what we've done for him already ___________
8. His condition right now is ___________
    (express urgency of consult e.g. stable, emergent, urgent, non-urgent)
9. Thank you and please page me once you have seen the patient

OR Note

Date:
Time:
Surgeon: Dr. (staff)
Assistants: Dr. (staff/resident/clerk), (PGY/CC)
Anesthesia: general anesthesia by ETT, Dr. (anesthetist)
Pre-op Dx:
Post-op Dx: same
Procedure:
Estimated Blood
Loss (EBL):   minimal/250 cc/500 cc
Findings: none
Specimens:
Complications: none
Drains: none
Counts: counts correct, complete/incomplete
Disposition: to recovery room (PACU) in stable/unstable condition
Name, Designation (CC\PGY), Pager Number

Post-Op Orders

• Use "**ADDAVID**" mnemonic – ask your resident for specifics regarding orders for their specialty

Common Medication Abbreviations

Type		Route		Freq	
app	applicator	AAA	apply to affected areas	ac	before meals
aq	water	AD	right ear	AM	morning
cap	capsule	AS	left ear	bid	twice a day
cmpd	compound	AU	both ears	d	day/daily
cr, crm	cream	ETT	endotracheal tube	f	for
elix	elixir	ID	intradermal	f3d	for 3 days
gtt(s)	drop(s)	IM	intramuscular	h	hour
inj	injection	inh	inhale	hs	at bedtime
liq	liquid	IP	intraperitoneal	mo, m	month
lot	lotion	IV	intravenous	p	after
MDI	metered dose inhaler	OD	right eye	pc	after meals
neb	nebulizer	OS	left eye	pc breakfast	after breakfast
sol	solution	OU	both eyes	PM	evening or nighttime
supp	suppository	PO	by mouth/orally	prn	as needed
susp	suspension	pr, rec, r	by rectum	q	every
syr	syrup	pv, vag	vaginally	qam	every morning
sys	spray	SC, subq, sub q	subcutaneous	qd	once daily
tab	tablet	SL	sublingual	qh	every hour
tbsp	tablespoon	top	topical	qid	four times a day
tsp	teaspoon			qod	every other day
ung, oint	ointment			qpm	every evening
				qXh	every X hours
				tid	three times a day
				ud	as directed
				wk	week

Amount					
mEq, meq	milliequivalent	ml, cc	milliliter, cubic centimetre	M:	mitte/send/give
µg, mcg	microgram	l	litre	w, c	with
mg	milligram	IU	international units	w/o	without
gm	gram	max	maximum	d/c	discontinue
oz	ounce (~30 grams)	min	minimum	kg	kilogram

Frequently Used Lab Values and Conversions

To convert from the conventional unit to the SI unit, multiply by conversion factor
To convert from the SI unit to the conventional unit, divide by conversion factor

	Conventional Unit	Conversion Factor	SI Unit
ACTH	pg/mL	0.22	pmol/L
Albumin	g/dL	10	g/L
Bilirubin	mg/dL	17.1	μmol/L
Calcium	mg/dL	0.25	mmol/L
Cholesterol	mg/dL	0.0259	mmol/L
Cortisol	μg/dL	7.59	nmol/L
Creatinine	mg/dL	88.4	μmol/L
Creatinine clearance	mL/min	0.0167	mL/s
Ethanol	mg/dL	0.217	mmol/L
Ferritin	ng/mL	2.247	pmol/L
Glucose	mg/dL	0.0555	mmol/L
HbA1c	%	0.01	proportion of 1.0
Hemoglobin	g/dL	10	g/L
HDL cholesterol	mg/dL	0.0259	mmol/L
Iron, total	μg/dL	0.179	μmol/L
Lactate (lactic acid)	mg/dL	0.111	mmol/L
LDL cholesterol	mg/dL	0.0259	mmol/L
Leukocytes	x 10^3 cells/mm^3	1	x 10^9 cells/L
Magnesium	mg/dL	0.411	mmol/L
MCV	μm^3	1	fL
Platelets	x 10^3 cells/mm^3	1	x 10^9 cells/L
Reticulocytes	% of RBCs	0.01	proportion of 1.0
Salicylate	mg/L	0.00724	mmol/L
Testosterone	ng/dL	0.0347	nmol/L
Thyroxine (T$_4$)	ng/dL	12.87	pmol/L
Total Iron Binding Capacity	μg/dL	0.179	μmol/L
Triiodothyronine (T$_3$)	pg/dL	0.0154	pmol/L
Triglycerides	mg/dL	0.0113	mmol/L
Urea nitrogen	mg/dL	0.357	mmol/L
Uric acid	mg/dL	59.48	μmol/L

Celsius → Fahrenheit	F = (C x 1.8) + 32
Fahrenheit → Celsius	C = (F – 32) x 0.5555
Kilograms → Pounds	1 kg = 2.2 lbs
Pounds → Ounces	1 lb = 16 oz
Ounces → Grams	1 oz = 28.3 g
Inches → Centimetres	1 in = 2.54 cm

Common Procedures

Procedure Note

Procedure Notes should be added to the chart after anything significant is done to the patient (e.g. LP, bone marrow aspiration, thoracentesis). The format is similar to that of the operative note, but not as detailed. The note should include the name of the procedure, your name and position, patient consent status, indications for the procedure (including risks quoted to patient) and relevant labs, (e.g. INR/PTT, platelet count), pre-procedure examination (if applicable), procedure description: technique, sterile prep, anesthetic, amount of fluid obtained, character of fluid, estimated blood loss, complications, procedure was/was not well tolerated, post-procedure vital signs and any tests ordered (e.g. chest x-ray post thoracentesis), sign-off

Arterial Blood Gas (ABG)

Indications: *Diagnostic*: assess ventilatory status, oxygenation and acid base status, assess the response to an intervention, rapid measurement of serum electrolytes in a critically ill patient, assessment for home O_2
Measures: arterial partial pressures of oxygen (PaO_2), carbon dioxide ($PaCO_2$), pH (acid-base status), and oxygen saturation of hemoglobin. Bicarbonate level is calculated from these numbers. Many analyzers will also measure electrolytes, lactate, glucose, hematocrit, and levels of carboxyhemoglobin and methemoglobin

Contraindications: Infection over puncture site, absence of palpable radial artery pulse or severe PVD, positive modified Allen's test (see below), coagulation defects (relative), AV fistula

Pulse Oximetry
Advantages: Uses light absorption at two wavelengths to determine hemoglobin saturation, non-invasive, immediate and continuous data
Disadvantages: Does not assess ventilation (pCO_2) or acid-base status, unreliable when saturations fall below 70-80%, Technical sources of error (ambient or fluorescent light, hypoperfusion, nail polish, skin pigmentation), cannot detect methemoglobin or carboxyhemoglobin

Equipment: Personal protective equipment (gloves), materials for skin cleansing and bandaging (alcohol, cotton, gauze, tape), pre-heparinised 3 to 5 mL syringe with 23- to 25-gauge needle, specimen bag filled with ice for transport
Optional: Syringe with 3 to 5 mL of 1% lidocaine and a 23- to 25-gauge needle

Procedure
1) Gather equipment and explain procedure to patient (obtain consent)
2) Wash your hands and put on disposable clean gloves (not necessarily sterile gloves)
3) Locate approximate position of artery using your index and middle fingers
    Radial artery runs along lateral aspect of volar forearm deep to superficial fascia, between styloid process of radius and flexor carpi radialis tendon
    Point of maximum pulsation usually palpated just proximal to wrist
    Why radial artery? It is superficial, has collaterals and is easily compressed
    Alternatives: femoral, dorsalis pedis, brachial can all be used, usually only in emergencies
4) Perform modified Allen's test to assess patency of ulnar artery and adequacy of collateral flow
    While hand is supinated, compress both radial and ulnar arteries simultaneously with your fingers around patient's wrist
    Allow for blood to drain from hand while patient opens and closes fist several times
    Release pressure on ulnar artery while keeping the radial artery occluded

    Negative test: normal skin colour should return to ulnar side then radial side of palm within 3-5 sec
    Positive test: hand remains white indicating either absence or occlusion of ulnar artery (do not draw ABG on that side) or inadequate collateral flow

5) Position the wrist volar side up on a firm surface and slightly extended. You may hold the hand steady using a long piece of tape stuck to the table. Clean skin over site of puncture.

6) Anesthetize the skin over the proposed site of puncture with 1% lidocaine (note: do not infuse a large volume, as the anatomy will distort and make the artery difficult to palpable). Make sure not to inject into a vessel

7) Palpate again the point of maximal pulsation of radial artery using index and middle fingers with a separation in between that will be the site of puncture

8) With your dominant hand hold the syringe like a pencil with the plunger set to collect a 0.5-1 ml sample. The syringe is "vented" at the plunger (i.e. the plunger should be set at 0.5-1.0 cc prior to puncturing the skin). It is not necessary to draw the sample up into the syringe – arterial pressure is adequate to fill the syringe

9) Rest dominant hand on patient's thenar eminence to steady syringe

10) Hold syringe at a 30- to 45-degree angle and insert needle bevel-up between your 2 fingers palpating the artery

11) Slowly advance the needle until you get a "flash" of blood in the hub of the needle, then "freeze" needle and syringe in that position. Wait until the blood level rises to the plunger. If the blood does not rise briskly, or if the blood is dark, you may have hit a vein. Achieve hemostasis with direct pressure then try again with another syringe

12) If no blood is obtained, withdraw the needle slowly (you may have gone through the artery, in which case you'll find the lumen while withdrawing) to a position just under the skin, check the position of the artery, and try again. Do not move or "sweep" the needle when it is inside the patient – only advance or withdraw. Moving the needle in any other direction will only cause pain and damage, with NO prospect of hitting the artery

13) Once you have the sample remove the needle and apply direct pressure (get the patient or an assistant to do this) with a 2"x2" gauze for 5 min

14) Expel all air bubbles from the sample by holding the syringe upright and allowing the bubbles to collect near the hub, then pushing gently on the plunger until only blood remains in the tube (Air in syringe can affect the results by raising the PO_2)

15) Carefully cap the syringe with a rubber stopper

16) Label the tube with patient's name and/or Medical Record Number, according to your institution)

17) Place the sample in the bag containing ice and send to the lab

18) Document the reason for the ABG and remainder of the procedure note

Complications: Hematoma formation (recheck hand within 20 min), hand ischemia (rare), radial artery aneurysm (rare)

Clinical Video: Dev, SP, Hillmer, MD, Ferri, M. Arterial Puncture for Blood Gas Analysis. *NEJM* 2011; 364:e7

Nasogastric (NG) Tube Insertion

Indications: The function of an NG tube is to remove stomach contents. *Diagnostic*: GI bleeding, penetrating/ blunt trauma. *Therapeutic*: paralytic ileus, gastric dilatation, intestinal obstruction, drainage and/or lavage in drug overdose or poisoning, heating or cooling for temperature abnormalities. *Prophylactic*: decompression prior to surgery, prevention of vomiting and aspiration in trauma. Other: instillation of materials, such as medications, enteral feeding, contrast, charcoal

Contraindications: Loss of integrity of cribriform plate (midface fracture, can use orogastric tube), esophageal stricture, comatose patients without airway protection, penetrating neck trauma (Note: varices are not a contraindication)

Equipment: personal protective equipment (gloves, consider face, eye protection and a gown), NG/OG tube (typically 12 or 14 French – smaller tubes are easier to insert but become blocked more easily), catheter tip 60 ml syringe, water-soluble lubricant, preferably 2% lidocaine jelly, adhesive tape, low powered suction device OR drainage bag, stethoscope, cup of water with straw (if necessary)/ice chips, emesis basin, pH indicator strips, lidocaine spray (optional)

Procedure
1) Gather equipment and explain procedure to patient (obtain consent)
2) Wash your hands and put on disposable clean gloves (not necessarily sterile gloves)
3) If possible, sit patient upright for optimal neck/stomach alignment
4) Examine nostrils for deformity/obstructions to determine best side for insertion
5) Measure tubing from bridge of nose to earlobe, then to the point halfway between the end of the sternum and the navel
6) Mark measured length with a marker or note the distance on the NG tube
7) Lubricate the first 2-4 inches of tube (2% lidocaine) and spray lidocaine to the back of the throat if available
8) Position the patient fully sitting or completely supine, with as much neck flexion as possible
9) Pass tube via either nare along the floor of the nose posteriorly (not upwards), past the pharynx into the esophagus
10) When you feel resistance ask the patient to swallow (offer water via straw if patient is sitting) and advance tube as patient swallows
11) If resistance is met, ask the patient to try to force their chin into their chest, rotate tube slowly with downward advancement toward closest ear. Do not force. Withdraw tube immediately if changes occur in patient's respiratory status, if tube coils in mouth, or if the patient begins to cough or become cyanotic
12) Advance tube until mark is reached
13) Check for placement by attaching syringe to free end of tube and aspirate sample of gastric contents or auscultate over stomach while inserting a quick puff of air. The pH of the aspirated contents can be checked to ensure that the contents are acidic (pH <6). Obtain an x-ray to verify placement before instilling any feedings/medications or if you have concerns about the placement of the tube
14) Secure tube with tape or commercially prepared tube holder (most difficult and important step!)
15) If placed for suction, remove syringe from free end of tube; connect to suction; set machine suction and pressure as prescribed
16) Document the reason for the NG tube insertion and remainder of the procedure note

Complications: Epistaxis, sinusitis, sore throat, esophageal perforation (rare), pneumothorax (rare), aspiration (rare), intracranial placement (very rare)

Clinical Video: Thomsen TW, Shaffer RW, Setnik GS. Nasogastric Intubation. *NEJM* 2006; 354:e16.

Urethral Catheterization (Foley Insertion)

Indications: *Diagnostic*: collect uncontaminated urine specimen, study anatomy of urinary tract, urine output monitoring (sensitive indicator of volume status and renal perfusion). *Therapeutic*: acute urinary retention, chronic bladder outlet obstruction causing hydronephrosis, intermittent bladder decompression for neurogenic bladder, chronically bed-ridden patients for hygiene

Contraindications: *Urethral injury*: in patients with multisystem trauma or pelvic fractures consider urethral injury if blood at meatus of the urethra, scrotal hematoma, pelvic fracture or a high-riding prostate on DRE

Equipment: Personal protective equipment (sterile gloves, consider universal precautions), sterile drapes, cleansing solution e.g. betadine, cotton swabs, forceps, sterile water (usually 10 cc), Foley catheter (usually 16-18 French for adults, 5-12 F for children, 5 F feeding tube for infants <6 months), syringe (usually 10 cc), transurethral topical lidocaine jelly (Uro-jet® or other lidocaine or water-based jelly), collection bag and tubing, catheter tray

COMMON PROCEDURES

Procedure
1) Gather equipment and explain procedure to patient (obtain consent)
2) Wash your hands
3) Assist patient into supine position with legs spread and feet together (frog leg)
4) Use pair of disposable/non-sterile gloves to localize urethral meatus and place a sheet under the patient's buttocks
5) Put on sterile gloves, open catheterization kit and catheter
6) Check balloon for patency and generously coat the distal portion (2-5 cm) of the catheter with lubricant
7) Prepare sterile field with cleansing solution
8) Apply sterile drapes
9) If female, separate labia using non-dominant hand. If male, hold the penis with the non-dominant hand. Maintain hand position until preparing to inflate balloon. This hand is considered non-sterile or contaminated
10) In the male, lift the penis to a position perpendicular to patient's body and apply light upward traction with non-dominant, contaminated hand
11) Using dominant hand to handle forceps, cleanse peri-urethral mucosa with cleansing solution. Cleanse anterior to posterior, inner to outer, one swipe per swab, discard swab away from sterile field
12) Insert intraurethral anesthetic
13) Pick up catheter with gloved (and still sterile) dominant hand. Hold end of catheter loosely coiled in palm of dominant hand
14) Identify the urinary meatus and gently insert lubricated catheter until urine is obtained, then insert a further 1 to 2 inches. Make sure the draining end of the catheter is placed into the basin accompanying the Foley kit. Once inserted you may release labia or penis
15) Inflate balloon using correct amount of sterile liquid (usually 10 cc but check actual balloon size)
16) Gently pull catheter until inflation balloon is snug against bladder neck
17) Connect catheter to drainage system
18) Secure catheter to abdomen or thigh using tape without tension on tubing
19) Place drainage bag below level of bladder
20) Evaluate catheter function and amount, colour, odour, and quality of urine

Note: Consider prophylactic antibiotics for acute prostatitis

Complications: Inability to locate urethra, vaginal catheterization, paraphimosis, urethral stricture, enlarged prostate, UTI, inability to deflate, renal inflammation, nephro-cysto-lithiasis, pyelonephritis

Clinical Videos: Ortega R, Ng L, Sekhar P, Song, M. "Female Urethral Catheterization" *NEJM* 2008; 358:e15; Thomsen TW, Setnik GS. "Male Urethral Catheterization" NEJM 2006; 354:e22;

Lumbar Puncture (LP)

Indications: *Diagnostic*: suspected CNS infection, suspected subarachnoid hemorrhage, other reasons (Guillain-Barré syndrome, carcinomatous meningitis), *Therapeutic*: removal of CSF (e.g. pseudotumor cerebri, normal pressure hydrocephalus), placement of intrathecal chemotherapy

Contraindications: *Absolute*: unequal pressures between the supratentorial and infratentorial compartments, usually inferred by characteristic findings of SOL on the brain CT scan (e.g. midline shift, loss of suprachiasmatic and basilar cisterns, posterior fossa mass, loss of the superior cerebellar cistern, loss of the quadrigeminal plate cistern), local skin infection over the needle entry site, raised intracranial pressure (ICP) (exception is pseudotumor cerebri). *Relative*: increased intracranial pressure, coagulopathy/uncontrolled bleeding diathesis, brain abscess, spinal column deformities, suspected spinal cord mass or intracranial mass lesion based on lateralizing neurological findings or papilledema, lack of patient cooperation

Indications for CT head scan prior to LP: older than 60 yrs, immunocompromised, known CNS lesions, seizure within 1 wk of presentation, abnormal level of consciousness, focal findings on neurological examination

Equipment

Personal protective equipment (sterile gloves, consider universal precautions); sterile drapes, spinal or lumbar puncture tray (antiseptic solution with skin swabs (Chlorhexidine), sterile drape, sponge sticks, gauze, lidocaine 1% without epinephrine, syringe (3 mL), needles 20- and 25-gauge, spinal needles, 20- and 22-gauge, three-way stopcock, manometer with extension, four plastic test tubes, numbered 1-4 with cap, sterile dressing). *Optional*: syringe, 10 mL

Procedure

1) Gather equipment and explain procedure to patient (obtain consent)
2) Wash your hands
3) Provide necessary analgesia and/or sedation as required
4) Position patient: lateral decubitus position with "fetal ball" (curling up with the hips, knees and chin flexed towards chest with a pillow to support the head) OR seated and leaning over a bedside table with neck flexed; both positions will open up the lumbar interspinous spaces
5) Wearing non-sterile gloves identify the L4-L5 interspace (L4 usually lies at the level between iliac crests) as well as the interspaces above (L3-4) and below (L5-S1) to find the widest space. Do not use above L2-3 because the conus medullaris terminates at L2. You will aim the needle towards the navel (i.e. slightly cephalad)
6) Mark the entry site with a thumbnail or marker or use the end of a needle cap to make a circle mark on the skin. To help open the interlaminar spaces, the patient can be asked to practice pushing the entry site area out toward the practitioner
7) Open the spinal tray, change to sterile gloves, and prepare the equipment. Open the numbered plastic tubes and place them upright, assemble the stopcock on the manometer, and draw the lidocaine into the 10 mL syringe
8) Use the skin swabs and antiseptic solution to clean the skin in a circular fashion starting at the L3-L4 interspace and moving outwards to include at least 1 interspace above and below. Just before applying the skin swabs, warn the patient that the solution is very cold since this can be unnerving to the patient
9) Apply sterile drapes
10) Administer local anesthesia by raising a skin wheal using 25 gauge needle and then switch to the longer 20 gauge needle to anesthetize the deeper tissue. Gradually insert the needle all the way to the hub, periodically aspirating to confirm that the needle is not in a blood vessel, and then injecting a small amount. Continue this process above, below, and to the sides very slightly (using the same puncture site). If you can identify and anesthetize the bony landmarks in the process, this will help you find the path for the spinal needle. A 10 mL syringe may be more useful than the usual 3 mL syringe supplied with the standard lumbar puncture kit
11) Insert the spinal needle with stylet (20 or 22 gauge) at 10-15 degrees cephalad (aim for umbilicus) bevel parallel to the longitudinal dural fibers to increase the chances of the needle separating the fibers rather than cutting them (bevel facing up in the lateral recumbent position and facing to either side in the sitting position; this reduces the incidence of post-LP headache). Advance the needle slowly but smoothly using your index fingers while using your non-dominant hand to landmark
12) When the needle is in the ligamentum flavum you will feel more resistance, as if the needle were advancing through cork. When the needle passes into the subarachnoid space, you will often feel a very light "pop", at which point the stylet can be removed to see if CSF drains. Otherwise, the stylet should be withdrawn after approximately 4-5 cm (or 1 cm of ligamentum flavum) and observed for fluid return. If no fluid returns, replace the stylet, advance or withdraw the needle a few millimeters, and recheck for fluid return. Continue this process until fluid is successfully returned
13) To measure the opening pressure, the patient must be in the lateral recumbent position. After fluid returns from the needle, attach the manometer through the stopcock and note the height of the fluid column (should be 20 cm or less). The patient's legs should be straightened when measuring open pressure or a falsely elevated pressure will be obtained
14) Collect at least 10 drops of CSF in each of the 4 plastic tubes (1-2 mL of CSF each), starting with Tube 1. The CSF that is in the manometer should be used (if possible) for Tube 1
　　Tube 1: cell count and differential
　　Tube 2: Gram stain, bacterial and viral cultures
　　Tube 3: glucose, protein, protein electrophoresis
　　Tube 4: reserve tube for any special tests or send for another cell count and differential

15) Replace the stylet and remove the needle. Clean off the skin prep solution. Apply a sterile dressing and place the patient in the supine position for 1-2 h. Order neurovital signs to be examined after the procedure is finished

Notes: If patient is dehydrated, a falsely negative dry tap may be obtained (very low CSF volume and pressure), if dehydration is suspected, attempt to rehydrate the patient prior to the procedure. If procedure is performed in sitting position and an opening pressure is required (e.g. pseudotumor cerebri), replace stylet and patient can be repositioned in left lateral recumbent position carefully with assistance. No evidence of increased complications associated with position change. Amount of lidocaine provided in most kits is often inadequate, but can be supplemented with 10 cc syringe, but must not exceed maximal recommended dose of 4.5 mg/kg of lidocaine. If CSF flow is too slow, ask patient to cough or bear down (Valsalva maneuver), or ask an assistant to intermittently press on patient's abdomen to increase the flow, or rotate needle 90 degrees. Never delay IV antibiotics more than 30-60 min for a CT scan or LP. Smaller needles lower the risk of developing a post-lumbar puncture headache. If you only obtain a small amount of fluid, you can send even 1 drop for microbiology, then the priority is for the cell count/differential and finally biochemistry in that order.

Complications: Post-spinal puncture headache, bloody tap, dry tap, bleeding from puncture site, infection, hemorrhage, dysesthesia, cerebral herniation, hematoma

Clinical Video: Ellenby MS, Tegtmeyer K, Lai S, Braner DAV. Lumbar Puncture. *NEJM* 2006; 355:e12.

Paracentesis

Indications: *Diagnostic*: Evaluate evaluate new-onset ascitic fluid ascites to help determine etiology (i.e. to differentiate transudate vs. exudate, detect the presence of cancerous cells, rule out spontaneous or secondary bacterial peritonitis), *Therapeutic*: relief of respiratory distress, abdominal pain or pressure secondary to ascites drain a large-volume ascites to relieve abdominal pain or pressure, or respiratory distress

Contraindications: *Absolute*: acute abdomen requiring surgery. *Relative*: Severe thrombocytopenia (platelet $<20 \times 10^3$/pL) and/or severe coagulopathy (INR >2.0) (platelets and/or fresh frozen plasma (FFP) generally not recommended prior to performing the procedure), pregnancy, distended urinary bladder, abdominal wall cellulitis, distended bowel, intra-abdominal adhesions

Equipment
- Personal protective equipment (sterile gloves, consider use universal precautions)
- Sterile drapes
- Disposable paracentesis/thoracentesis kit:
1) Antiseptic swab sticks
2) Fenestrated drape
3) Lidocaine 1%, 5 mL ampule
4) Syringe, 10 mL
5) Two injection needles, 22 gauge (ga)
6) Injection needle, 25 ga
7) Scalpel, #11 blade
8) Angiocatheter needle, 18 ga
9) Needle with 3-way stopcock, self-sealing valve, and a 5 mL LuerLock syringe
10) Syringe, 60 mL
11) Tubing set with roller clamp
12) Drainage bag or vacuum container
13) Specimen vials or collection bottles (3)
- Gauze, 4"x4". Adhesive dressing
- 1-liter vacuum bottles

Landmarking
• 5 cm superior and medial to the anterior superior iliac spines on either side, avoid previous surgical incisions

Procedure
1) Gather equipment and explain procedure to patient (obtain consent)
2) Wash your hands
3) Obtain relevant patient history, and perform a physical exam to document and localize ascitic fluid
4) Ask patient to empty bladder or empty bladder with catheter
5) Provide necessary analgesia and/or sedation as required
6) If ultrasound machine is available, scan patient to localize fluid collections and perform the procedure under real-time ultrasound guidance
7) Place patient in supine position, with head elevated 45-60 degrees
8) Position patient: if severe ascites then supine but if mild ascites then lateral decubitus with skin entry site near bed. This position is also advantageous because bowel loops tend to float in a distended abdominal cavity
9) Open paracentesis tray, change to sterile gloves, and prepare equipment
10) Clean paracentesis site with antiseptic solution in a circular fashion from the centre out and apply sterile drapes
11) Administer local anesthesia using 5 mL syringe and 25 ga needle by raising a small lidocaine skin wheal at entry site
12) Switch to angiocatheter needle and begin to introduce needle in a perpendicular to the skin. Pull down the skin as you enter in order to create a discontinuous tract ("Z" technique) to stop ascitic fluid from leaking out after the procedure is complete. Continuously apply negative pressure (aspirate) to the syringe as the needle is advanced
13) Progress the needle at 5 mm increments. As the needle progresses, aspirate contents and watch for blood flashback. Inject lidocaine if no blood flashback. Continue to progress along track with continual aspiration and injection of lidocaine
14) Upon entry to the peritoneal cavity, loss of resistance is felt and ascitic fluid can be seen filling the syringe. At this point, advance the device 2-4 mm into the peritoneal cavity to assure correct placement. Avoid advancing the needle any deeper than necessary
15) Use one hand to firmly hold the needle and syringe, and use the other hand to disengage the syringe. Use your finger to block the ascitic fluid from flowing freely from the open end of the angiocatheter needle
16) If performing a diagnostic paracentesis, attach the 60 mL syringe to the catheter and aspirate to obtain ascitic fluid and distribute it to the specimen vials, with the help of an assistant who is not under sterile conditions
17) If performing a therapeutic paracentesis, connect the other end of the fluid collection tubing to a vacuum bottle or a drainage bag. The tubing must be blocked using a stopping device before insertion into a vaccum bottle; this will maintain the difference in pressure between the abdomen and the bottle. Once the tubing is inserted into the bottle, the stopping device is disengaged and the fluid should start to flow into the bottles. This step must be performed by an assistant who is not under sterile conditions. The person who inserted the needle must continue to be under sterile conditions in order to hold the needle in place and prevent displacement of the catheter
18) The catheter can become occluded by a loop of bowel or omentum; reposition as necessary
19) Remove the catheter after the desired amount of ascitic fluid has been drained. Apply firm pressure, as necessary, to stop bleeding. Clean off skin prep solution. Place a bandage over the skin puncture site
20) Alternatively, you may leave the catheter in place and attach a stopcock to the open end in order to perform a repeat paracentesis in the near future (i.e. within the next day or two)
21) After the procedure, ask the patient to lie supine for 4 h and ensure vital signs checked q1h for 4 h to avoid hypotension
22) If large volume paracentesis then must give albumin to avoid intravascular fluid shift and renal failure. Give 25 cc of 25% albumin for every 2 litres of ascitic fluid removed (e.g. If 4L paracentesis then give 50 mL of albumin IV)
23) Send for cell count, Gram stain, cultures, AFB, fungal, protein, albumin, LDH, specific gravity, glucose, triglycerides, bilirubin

Notes
- If no fluid is drawn, try different angles or sites.
- If fluid is draining well into a vacuum then stops, detach from vacuum and hold drainage bag below the site. This allows gravity to draw the fluid out by positive pressure. The bowel may be stuck up against the catheter due to the vacuum's negative pressure
- After proper antiseptic preparation and local anesthesia, diagnostic tap can be performed with a 10 to 20 mL syringe and an 18 ga needle or a therapeutic tap can be performed with an IV catheter over the needle connected to drainage tubing
- In patients who are afebrile, alert, and have no other signs of bacterial peritonitis or decompensated cirrhosis, ascitic fluid labs are often not necessary to rule out spontaneous bacterial peritonitis (SBP)
- To minimize the risk of persistent leak from the puncture site, use a small gauge needle or take a "Z" track during insertion of the needle as suggested above
- Be wary with large-volume paracentesis in end-stage cirrhosis with impaired renal function. A maximum of 6 L should be removed

Complications
- Failed attempt to collect peritoneal fluid, persistent leak from puncture site (try a suture or apply an ostomy bag around site until it seals off), wound infection, abdominal wall hematoma, spontaneous hemoperitoneum (rare, due to mesenteric variceal bleeding post large paracentesis), hollow viscous perforation, catheter laceration and loss in abdominal cavity, laceration of major blood vessel, post-paracentesis hypotension (may be delayed by up to 12 h), dilutional hyponatremia, hepatorenal syndrome

Clinical Video: Thomsen TW, Shaffer, RW, White, B, Setnik, GS. Paracentesis. *NEJM* 2006; 355:e21

Thoracentesis

Indications: *Diagnostic*: determine cause of new-onset pleural effusion (transudate vs. exudate, isolation of cancerous cells), rule out empyema
Therapeutic: relieve symptoms of respiratory distress. In patients with definite CHF (bilateral pleural effusion without fever), a trial of diuresis may be given.

Contraindications: Uncooperative patient, uncorrected bleeding diathesis/coagulopathy, chest wall cellulitis at site of puncture, bullous disease (e.g. emphysema), positive end-expiratory pressure (PEEP) mechanical ventilation, only one functioning lung, small volume of fluid (less than 1 cm thickness on a lateral decubitus film)

Equipment
- Personal protective equipment (sterile gloves, consider universal precautions)
- Disposable thoracentesis/paracentesis kit:
1) Antiseptic swab sticks
2) Fenestrated drape
3) Lidocaine 1% or 2% with epinephrine
4) Syringes, 10 mL
5) Two injection needles, 22 gauge (ga)
6) Injection needle, 25 ga for anesthetic
7) Scalpel, #11 blade
8) Eight-French catheter over 18 ga x 7½"
9) Needle with 3-way stopcock, self-sealing valve, and a 5 mL LuerLock syringe
10) Syringe, 60 mL
11) Introducer needle, 20 ga
12) Tubing set with roller clamp
13) Drainage bag or vacuum container
14) Specimen vials or collection bottles (3)
15) Gauze, 4"x4"
16) Adhesive dressing

- 2 x 1-litre vacuum bottles for fluid collection
- Optional: 60-mL syringe with 3-way stopcock

Procedure
1) Gather equipment and explain procedure to patient (obtain consent)
2) Wash your hands
3) Obtain relevant patient history, and perform a physical exam to document and localize effusion
4) Obtain a lateral decubitus film ipsilateral to side of effusion
5) If the effusion is small (<1 cm on lateral decubitus film) or not free flowing, ultrasound to mark effusion and/or look for loculation. Have ultrasound quantify the amount of fluid. If ultrasound machine is available, scan patient to localize fluid collections and perform the procedure under real-time ultrasound guidance
6) Provide necessary analgesia and/or sedation as required
7) Have the patient seated upright comfortably on the side of the bed and leaning forward slightly on the bedside table with back fully exposed. If possible and especially for therapeutic taps, place the patient on a pulse oximeter
8) Auscultate chest to confirm site and size of pleural effusion. Percuss chest to determine upper border of effusion. Entry site is 1-2 intercostal spaces (1-2 cm) below fluid level but above diaphragm
9) Identify midscapular line posteriorly. Entry site must be at least 2 inches below scapular tip
10) Identify entry point directly above the closest corresponding rib to avoid hitting neurovascular structures. Mark the spot with a pen or syringe cap or something that won't be erased by antiseptic
11) Open thoracentesis tray, change to sterile gloves, and prepare equipment
12) Clean thoracentesis entry site with antiseptic solution in a circular fashion from the centre out and apply sterile drapes
13) Administer local anesthesia using 5 mL syringe and 25 ga needle by raising a small lidocaine skin wheal at entry site. Switch to longer 20 ga needle and anesthetize the rib, marching up until you are just above the rib and into the pleural space. Be sure to aspirate as you advance and to anesthetize the pleura, which is quite pain-sensitive. If lidocaine enters the pleural space, it will simply mix with the effusion and be of little concern. If you obtain fluid at this point, note the depth of the needle
14) For a diagnostic tap, use an 18-20 ga needle attached to a 20-30 cc syringe
15) Remove thoracentesis or blood tubing from its packaging, and close the midpoint clamp securely. Attach the 18 ga needle to the free end of the tubing and other end of stop cock to vacuum container
16) With the free 18 ga needle, puncture the skin at the marked intercostal space. Advance the needle up rib, marching up until you are just above the rib and until you feel a slight give and enter the pleural space. If you are in the right location, you will aspirate fluid into the syringe. Advance the catheter without advancing the needle, and aspirate again to make sure that the fluid is still flowing freely. Remove the needle (being careful to cover the catheter opening to prevent air from entering), and connect the tubing to the catheter. Open the clamp/stop cock. This will provide negative pressure from the evacuated bottle and fluid will drain spontaneously into the bottle. If flow stops then slightly withdraw or turn the flexible catheter. Having the patient Valsalva or cough can also increase fluid flow. If you cannot restore fluid flow, close the clamp and try reinserting a new needle and catheter
    Do not remove more than 1.5 litres, otherwise there is an increased risk of re-expansion pulmonary edema
17) If frank blood returns, lungs may have been punctured. Withdraw needle slowly until fluid flows. If no fluid flows at all, withdraw needle until it is just under the skin and reinsert
18) If you aspirate air (air bubbles in syringe) or patient develops hypotension, desaturation, or respiratory distress, stop immediately and obtain CXR or perform immediate needle decompression for tension pneumothorax
17) Before withdrawing, clamp tubing or stop flow to the vacuum container by closing the stop cock and then withdraw the needle completely from the patient while asking them to Valsalva
18) Dress puncture site with an occlusive dressing and clean off antiseptic
19) Re-examine the patient to correlate the location of the effusion (Step 8)
20) Send fluid for cell count, Gram stain, cultures, LDH, glucose, pH, cytology, total protein, AFB
21) Obtain a post procedure radiograph to check for iatrogenic pneumothorax

Complications
- Pneumothorax, hemopneumothorax, hemorrhage, hypotension due to a vasovagal response, pulmonary edema due to lung reexpansion, spleen or liver puncture, air embolism, infection

Clinical Video: Thomsen TW, DeLaPena, J, Setnik, GS. Thoracentesis. *NEJM* 2006; 355:e16

Chest Tube Insertion (Thoracostomy Tube Placement)

Indications:*Therapeutic*: drainage of hemothorax or large pleural effusion of any cause, drainage of large pneumothorax (greater than 25%), drainage of an empyema or loculated effusion, unilateral air entry or hypotension in a patient with chest trauma

Contraindications
- Infection over insertion site, uncontrolled bleeding diathesis/coagulopathy

Equipment
- Personal protective equipment (sterile gloves, gown, mask)
- Sterile prep solution
- Chest tube with or without trocar OR Fuhrman catheter
- Chest tube suction unit (Pleurevac® or Sahara®), tubing, wall suction hookup
- Chest tube (thoracostomy) tray to include scalpel blade and handle, large Kelly clamps, needle driver, scissors
- Packet of 0 or 1-0 silk suture on a curved needle
- Tape, gauze
- 2% lidocaine with epinephrine, 20 cc syringe, 23-gauge needle for infiltration
- Size of chest tube:
  - Adult or teen male: 28-32 Fr
  - Adult or teen female: 28 Fr
  - Child: 18 Fr
  - Newborn: 12-14 Fr

Landmarking
- Mid-axillary line, between 4th and 5th ribs

Procedure
1) Gather equipment and explain procedure to patient (obtain consent)
2) Wash your hands
3) Obtain relevant patient history and perform a physical exam to document and localize pathology
4) Obtain a pre-procedure x-ray
5) Provide necessary analgesia and/or conscious sedation as required (if patient stable)
6) Place the patient on a pulse oximeter and have them lying supine on the bed with their ipsilateral arm over their head to "open up" ribs, if possible
7) Auscultate chest to confirm site and size of pleural pathology (effusion, hemothorax, pneumothorax). Percuss chest to determine upper border of pleural pathology. Site for chest tube insertion is typically mid-axillary line, between 4th and 5th ribs, parallel to the rib margins and lateral to the nipple on the ipsilateral side of pathology. Mark the spot with a pen or syringe cap
8) Open thoracostomy tray, change to sterile gloves, and prepare equipment
9) Clean thoracostomy entry site with antiseptic solution in a circular fashion from the centre out and apply sterile drapes (prepare a large field)
10) Administer local anesthesia using 20 mL syringe and 23 ga needle by raising a small lidocaine skin wheal at entry site, anesthetizing at least 2 inches of skin at the site of insertion, the underlying tissues and intercostal muscles, the inferior rib and the pleura. Be sure to aspirate as you advance and to anesthetize the pleura which is quite pain-sensitive. If lidocaine enters the pleural space, it will simply mix with the effusion and be of little concern. If you obtain fluid at this point, note the depth of the needle

11) After infiltrating insertion site with local anesthetic, make a 3-4 cm incision through skin and subcutaneous tissues between the 4th and 5th ribs, parallel to the rib margins
12) Continue incision through the intercostal muscles, and right down to the pleura
13) Insert Kelly clamp through the pleura and open the jaws widely, again parallel to the direction of the ribs (this "creates" a pneumothorax, and allows the lung to fall away from the chest wall somewhat)
14) Insert finger through your incision and into the thoracic cavity. Make sure you are feeling lung (or empty space) and not liver or spleen
15) Clamp outer tube end, then grasp end of chest tube with the Kelly forcep (convex angle towards ribs with tips inside drainage holes in tubing) and insert chest tube through the hole you have made in the pleura. After tube has entered thoracic cavity, remove Kelly, and manually advance the tube. Direct the tube anterior/superiorly for a pneumothorax and posterior/interiorly for an effusion/hemothorax
16) Attach tube to suction unit and remove clamp
17) Suture and tape tube in place
18) Obtain post procedure chest x-ray for placement; tube may need to be advanced or withdrawn slightly
19) Re-examine the patient to correlate the location of the pathology (Step 7)
20) Send fluid for cell count, Gram stain, cultures, LDH, glucose, pH, cytology, total protein, AFB
21) Obtain a post-procedure radiograph to check for iatrogenic pneumothorax or other complications

Complications
• Puncture of liver or spleen or heart, hemothorax, hemorrhage, passage of tube along chest wall instead of into chest cavity, hypotension due to a vasovagal response, pulmonary edema due to lung re-expansion, air embolism, infection

Clinical Video: Dev SP, Nascimiento, B, Simone, C, Chien, V. Chest-Tube Insertion. *NEJM* 2007; 357:e15

Arthrocentesis (Knee Joint)

Indications: *Diagnostic*: crystal-induced arthritis/arthropathy, septic arthritis, hemarthrosis, unexplained joint effusion or monoarthritis, *Therapeutic*: symptomatic relief of a large effusion, complete drainage of a known septic arthritis

Contraindications
• Bacteremia, clinician unfamiliar with anatomy of or approach to the joint, inaccessible joint, joint prosthesis, overlying soft tissues infection, severe coagulopathy, severe overlying dermatitis, uncooperative patient

Equipment
• Personal protective equipment (sterile gloves, gown, mask)
• Sterile tray for procedure with the following items placed on a sterile sheet:
1) Sterile gloves
2) Sterile fenestrated drape
3) Syringes (2 mL, 10 mL, and 20 mL)
4) Needles 2 x 21-G (or 18, 20, 22 and 25-G) with 1-inch length
5) 2 x 21-gauge, 1-inch needles
6) Sterile solution (betadine)
7) Sterile gauze 4" x 4" dressings
8) Hemostat (for stabilizing the needle when exchanging the medication syringe for the aspiration syringe)
9) Local anesthetic
10) Sterile basin cup and/or test tubes
11) Green-top tube with liquid anticoagulant (to examine for crystals)
12) Sterile saline
13) Sterile bandage
14) Microscope slides and cover slips
15) Culture media (if looking for infection)

Landmarking
- Medial or lateral approach: one finger breadth from 1/3 of the way down from the lateral or medial aspect of the patella

Procedure
1) Gather equipment and explain procedure to patient (obtain consent)
2) Wash your hands
3) Obtain relevant patient history
4) Provide necessary analgesia
5) Position patient: supine on table with knee extended OR flexed to 15 degrees
6) Examine knee to determine the amount of joint fluid present, check for overlying cellulitis or coexisting pathology in the joint or surrounding tissues
7) The joint can be aspirated by the medial or lateral approach. Palpate the superior 1/3 of the medial or lateral aspect of the patella and mark the skin one fingerbreadth lateral or medial to this site. This location provides the most direct access to the synovium
8) Change to sterile gloves and prepare equipment. Attach the needle (e.g. 21 ga, 1-inch) to a 5-20 mL syringe (depending on the anticipated amount of fluid present for removal)
9) Clean the arthrocentesis site as marked with antiseptic solution in a circular fashion from the centre out and apply sterile drapes
10) Insert needle angled slightly posteriorly through stretched skin, as stretching the pain fibers in the skin with the non-dominant hand can also reduce discomfort. Some physicians administer lidocaine into the skin prior to needle insertion. Always aspirate while advancing needle
11) Once needle has entered the joint space, aspiration is performed and syringe should fill with fluid. Using the non-dominant hand to compress the opposite side of the joint or the patella may aid in arthrocentesis
12) Once syringe has filled, a hemostat can be placed on the hub of the needle. With the needle stabilized with the hemostat, the syringe can be disconnected and the fluid sent for studies
13) Consider using a 3-way stopcock to help to drain large effusions. This will help you to avoid having to change the syringe, which can cause the needle to move or become dislodged after you have already entered the joint space
14) If the fluid stops flowing, the joint space has been drained, or the needle tip has moved/become dislodged, or there are debris or clot obstructing the tip
15) If you suspect the needle has moved, slightly advance or retract the needle, rotate the bevel, or try using less pressure to aspirate
16) Care should be taken not to touch the needle tip against the joint surfaces when removing the syringe
17) Clean the skin and apply a bandage over the puncture site. Warn the patient to avoid forceful activity on the joint while it is anesthetized
18) Send fluid for cell count, Gram stain, cytology, microscopy

Complications
- Infection, bleeding, local allergic reaction, rapid re-accumulation of joint effusion

Clinical Video: Thomsen TW, Shen, S, Shaffer, RW, Setnik, GS. Thoracentesis. *NEJM* 2006; 354:e19

Abscess Incision and Drainage

Indications: *Therapeutic*: cutaneous abscess

Contraindications: Extremely large or deep abscess in a difficult area of body (consider OR), abscesses in palms, soles or nasolabial folds, cutaneous cellulitis without abscess, abnormal/artificial heart valves (consider prophylactic antibiotics)

Equipment: Personal protective equipment (sterile gloves, gown, mask), sterile tray for procedure with the following items placed on a sterile sheet (local anesthetic (e.g. 1% lidocaine with or without epinephrine depending on location), sterile gauze, sterile cleansing agent (e.g. betadine), 5-10mL syringe and large syringe with splash guard, 25- to 30-gauge needle, scalpel blade with handle, curved hemostat, normal saline with sterile bowl, swabs for bacterial culture, packing material), scissors, gauze, and tape

Procedure
1 Gather equipment and explain procedure to patient (obtain consent). Make sure to ask about tetanus immunization!
2) Wash your hands and wear personal protective equipment
3) Position patient so that area of drainage is fully exposed
4) Apply sterile cleansing agent by spreading in a circular motion moving outward from the peak of the abscess
5) Inject anesthetic agent intradermally with 25- or 30-gauge needle
6) Use scalpel to puncture the skin and make an incision in the direction of the long-axis of the abscess, in the same direction it is to be drained (you should see purulent discharge once the cavity has been successfully incised). Do not puncture too deeply as this may result in a puncture deeper than the abscess and cause purulent drainage into the underlying tissue. Use the hemostat to break up loculations and place internal wound packing
7) Obtain swabs for culture from inside the wound. These may be useful later if an infection ensues
8) After allowing the abscess to drain spontaneously, express as much as possible manually. You may need to use more anesthetic at this time. Use the hemostat for blunt dissection in a circular motion to cover the entire wound and make sure that all loculations are broken and completely drained
9) Irrigate the wound with normal saline until the effluent from the wound is clear
10) Pack the wound with packing material, and ensure that all areas of the cavity are packed to allow for further drainage and to keep the walls of the abscess separated. Appropriate packing will allow healing by secondary intention. Packing should be removed 2-3 d after the procedure

Complications: Pain, surrounding cellulitis, fever, other signs of clinical worsening (may need systemic antibiotics)

Clinical Video: Fitch, MT, Manthey DE, McGinnis HD, Nicks BA, Pariyadath M. Abscess Incision and Drainage. *NEJM* 2007; 357:e20

Peripheral Intravenous Access (IV)

Indications: Gaining access to the peripheral circulation to obtain a blood sample, infuse fluids or medications.

Contraindications: Difficult anatomy that increases the risks for fluid extravasation or inadequate flow, including areas of edema, burns, injury or indwelling fistula. Areas of cellulitis should also be avoided

Equipment
- Appropriate size catheter 20G-30mm IV catheter
- Tourniquet
- Alcohol swab
- Non-sterile 2x2 cm gauze
- 6x7 cm Tegaderm™ transparent dressing
- Tape
- IV bag with solution set (tubing)

Procedure
1) Gather equipment and obtain consent
2) Choose a site that is most peripheral and appropriate to the situation. More proximal veins can be used if the attempt fails. The veins on the dorsum of the hand are most accessible
3) Apply a tourniquet proximal to the IV site
4) Visualize and palpate the veins
5) Clean the area with an alcohol swab in an expanding circular motion
6) In non-dominant hand, stabilize the vein and apply countertension to the skin
7) In dominant hand, insert stylet bevel-up through the skin and observe for flashback
8) Reduce the angle of the needle and advance approximately 2-3 mm further into the vein (far enough to include the catheter in the vein, but not far enough to puncture the back wall of the vein)
9) Slowly advance the catheter over the needle and into the vein with non-dominant hand (flexible and dull end of the catheter should not puncture the back wall of the vein)
10) Remove the tourniquet
11) Withdrawal the needle and place into sharps container
12) Use a Tegaderm™ transparent dressing to hold IV in place
13) Connect IV tubing

Notes
- Choose the straightest and largest vein suitable to the situation
- Most mistakes are in the failure to advance the stylet far enough to include the catheter
- The most painful step is the skin puncture, the vein puncture is less painful. You can gently explore and manipulate in the subcutaneous area without any obvious discomfort. It will be painful if there is probing into muscle, tendon, or non-vascular structures

Complications
- Infection, thrombophlebitis and extravasation

Antibiotic Quick Reference

Organisms

BACTERIAL

	Gram positive (GP)		Gram negative (GN)	
	Cocci	**Bacilli**	**Cocci**	**Bacilli**
Aerobes	Staph Strep Enterococcus	Bacillus Listeria Corynebacterium Nocardia	Neisseria Moraxella	Enterobacteriaceae Pseudomonas Hemophilus Legionella
Anaerobes	Peptostreptococcus	Clostridium Propionebacterium Lactobacillus	Veionella	Bacteroides Fusobacterium

Acid-Fast	M. TB, Non-TB mycobacteria, Nocardia
Intracellular	Chlamydia, Rickettsia, Coxiella Spirochetes (Treponema, Borrelia, Leptospira)
NON-BACTERIAL	
Fungal	Endemic mycoses: Histoplasmosis, Blastomycoses, Coccidiomycoses Opportunistic fungi: Candida, Aspergillus, Zygomycetes, Cryptococcus
Viral/Parasitic	

Antimicrobial Classes

Class/Drug Name	Coverage	Common Indications
Penicillins		
Benzyl Penicillin - PenG (IV/IM) - PenV (PO)	GP except staphlycoccal and enterococcal species Oral anaerobes except *Bacteroides*	Actinomycosis, streptococcal pharyngitis, streptococcal skin/soft tissue infections, syphilis
Aminopenicillin - ampicillin (IV) - amoxicillin (PO)	Same as penicillin + *Enterococcus*	Meningitis, endocarditis, AOM, pharyngitis, sinusitis, *H. pylori* treatment, Lyme disease, UTI
Isoxozoyl penicillin - cloxacillin - oxacillin - nafcillin	Same as penicillin + *Staphylococcus*	Skin/soft tissue infections
Ureidopenicillin - piperacillin	Broad spectrum coverage including anerobes and Pseudomonas	Pip-tazo used for wide ranges of infectious including abdominal, skin, gyne and pneumonia
Lactamase Inhibitor - amoxicillin-clavulinate	Same as penicillin + *Staphylococcus* + *H. influenzae*	Infections caused by β-lactamase producing strains, commonly skin/soft tissue, AOM, UTI, RTI

Antimicrobial Classes (continued)

Class/Drug Name	Coverage	Common Indications
Cephalosporins		
1° Generation - cephalexin (PO) - cefazolin (IV)	GP except *Enterococcus*, some GN	Skin/soft tissue, prevention of surgical infections
2° Generation - cefuroxime (PO/IV) - cefprozil (PO)	Some GP, some GN, some anaerobes	RTIs, soft tissue
3° Generation - ceftriaxone (IV) - cefixime (PO) - ceftazidime	Generally broad spectrum of GP and GN, (*Pseudomonas* coverage)	RTI, gonorrhea, meningitis, pyelonephritis, soft tissue infections, abdominal infections
Carbepenems - imipenem - meropenem - ertapenem	Broad spectrum + *Pseudomonas* + anaerobes, except MRSA	Serious infections caused by susceptible organisms, frequently used in critically ill patients
Vancomycin	GP including MRSA	MRSA, severe GP infections, PO version for *C. diff.* infections
Macrolides - erythromycin - clarithromycin - azithromycin	GP except *Enterococcus*, MRSA; atypical coverage	RTI, sinusitis, pneumonia, pharyngitis/tonsillitis, AOM, chlamydia
Clindamycin	GP including most MRSA, anaerobes	Skin/soft tissue, abdominal infections, some pneumonias, susceptible organisms
Chloramphenical	Broad spectrum	Serious infections
Linezolid	GP including MRSA and VRE	Serious GP infections
Aminoglycosides - gentamicin - tobramycin - neomycin - streptomycin - amikacin	GN including *Pseudomonas*	UTIs, pyelonephritis infective endocarditis, neonatal sepsis/infections
Tetracyclines - tetracyline - minocycline - doxycycline	GP, anaerobes, atypicals, malaria prophylaxis	Rickettsial infections, brucellosis, bartonellosis, acne
Fluoroquinolones - ciprofloxacin - ofloxacin - levofloxacin - moxifloxacin	Good GN including *Pseudomonas* "respiratory quinolones", better GP coverage + GN + atypicals	RTI, pneumonia, sinusitis (not cipro), UTI (not respiratory quinolones), prostatitis, joint/soft tissue infections, infectious diarrhea, intra-abdominal infections
Metronidazole	Anaerobes, protozoa	Anaerobic coverage (intra-abdominal, bacterial vaginosis), protozoa (trichomonas, amebiasis, giardiasis)
TMP/SMX	GP, GN enteric, Nocardia, Pneumocystis, Toxoplasmosis	UTI, RTI, GI infections, skin/soft tissue, PCP
Nitrofurantoin	UTI organisms	Cystitis (safe in pregnancy)

Antimicrobial Classes (continued)

Class/Drug Name	Coverage	Common Indications
Anti-Herpesvirus - acyclovir - valacyclovir - famciclovir - ganciclovirF	HSV-1,2 VZV CMV	
Triazoles - fluconazole - itraconazole - voriconazole	Candidiasis + systemic mycoses + aspergillosis	
Imidazoles - clotrimazole - miconazole - ketoconazole	Vulvovaginal candidiasis, dermatomycoses	

Antibiotics for Common Adult Infections

Infection	Causative Organisms	Empiric Antibiotics of Choice
RESPIRATORY		
Pneumonia		
Community-acquired (CAP)	Healthy: *S. pneumo, H. flu, M. catarrhalis, Mycoplasma, Chlamydia, Viral* Elderly: same, plus *S. aureus, Legionella, GN*	CAP Outpatient: Macrolide, or Resp FLQ, or β-lactam+inhibitor, or β-lactam+Macrolide CAP Inpatient: Resp FLQ, or -lactam+Macrolide, or Cephalosporin+Azithro (ICU)
Hospital-acquired (HAP)	*GN, Pseudomonas, S.aureus*	HAP: Ceftriaxone, or Resp FLQ, or Amp/Sulbactam, or Ertapenem HAP with multi-drug resistant risk factors: anti-pseudomonal Cephalosporin, or anti-pseudomonal Carbapenem, or PipTazo PLUS double coverage for pseudomonas if necessary (with FLQ, Aminoglycoside), or coverage for MRSA (Vanco), or coverage for Legionella (Macrolide or FLQ)
HIV (pneumonia)	*P. jiroveci* (PCP)	
Alcoholic	*Klebsiella, GN, S.aureus, anaerobes* (aspiration)	Rifampin + Isoniazid + Pyrazinamide + Ethambutol
Tuberculosis (active)	*Mycobacterium tuberculosis*	
Bronchitis	Viral: Rhinovirus, Coronavirus, Adenovirus, RSV, Influenza, Parainfluenza Bacterial: *S. pneumonia, H. influenza, M. pneumonia, C. pneumoniae*	Abx not recommended for acute bronchitis

Antibiotics for Common Adult Infections (continued)

Infection	Causative Organisms	Empiric Antibiotics of Choice
OTOLOGIC		
Acute Rhinitis (common cold)	Viral: Rhinovirus, Adeno, RSV, Influenza etc.	None
Pharyngitis	Viral: Adeno, Rhinovirus	None
Strep Pharyngitis	Group A β-Hemolytic Strep	Adults: Pen V 300 mg PO tid or 600 mg bid x 10 d, Cefuroxime 250 mg PO bid x 4 d, Clarithromycin 250 mg PO bid x 10 d, Azithromycin 500 mg PO once, then 250 mg daily x 4 d Penicillin allergy: Erythromycin 1000 mg PO div bid-qid
Sinusitis	S. pneumonia, H. influenza, M. catarrhalis, Group A Strep, Anaerobes, S. aureus	1st line: Amoxicillin 1 g PO tid x 10 d (if penicillin allergy: TMP/SMX DS 1 tab PO bid) 2nd line: Amox/Clavulin 2000/125 mg PO tid x 10 d, 3rd line: Clarithromycin XL 1000 mg PO OD x 14 d
OTOLOGIC		
Acute Otitis Media	Viral, S. pneumoniae, H. influenzae, M. catarrhalis	Treat if under 2 yrs for 7 d If >2 yrs, treat if worsens after 48-72 h >2 yrs: 1st line: Amoxicillin 75-80 mg/kg/d PO bid x 5 d, 2nd line: Amoxicillin 90 mg/kg/d + Clavulinic acid 6.4 mg/kg/d PO TID x 10d <2 yrs, complicated or recurrent.: Amoxicillin 75-80 mg/kg/d PO bid x 10 d Penicillin allergy: Cefprozil, Cefuroxime, Azithromycin, Clarithromycin
Otitis Externa	Pseudomonas, S. aureus Fungal	Diabetic: Ciprofloxacin 500 mg PO bid x 14 d Non-diabetic: 1st line: Buro-sol® 2-3 drops tid 2nd line: Cortisporin® otic solution 4 drops tid
UTI		
Cystitis	Klebsiella, E.coli, Enterococcus, Proteus, S.saprophyticus (KEEPS)	Keflex, or Macrobid, or Septra, or Cipro x 3-5 d
Pyelonephritis	KEEPS	3rd Gen Cephalosporin, or Septra, or Cipro, or PipTazo x 7-14 d
Urethritis	Neisseria, Chlamydia	

Antibiotics for Common Adult Infections (continued)

Infection	Causative Organisms	Empiric Antibiotics of Choice
SOFT TISSUE		
Necrotizing Fasciitis	Type I: polymicrobial	Carbapenem OR (3rd gen. Ceph + Ampicillin + Metronidazole)
	Type II: β-hemolytic Strep	Penicillin + Clindamycin
Mastitis	S. aureus, S. pyogenes	Cloxacillin 500 mg PO qid x 7 d, Cephalexin 500 mg PO qid x 7 d
Tinea Cruris/Pedis (Jock Itch/Athlete's Foot)	Trichophyton spp.	Clotrimazole 1% cream – apply bid Ketoconazole 2% cream – apply bid
Cellulitis (uncomplicated)	β-Hemolytic Strep sp. Staphylococcus	1st line: Cephalexin 500 mg PO qid x 10-14 d, 2nd line: Cloxacillin 500 mg PO qid x 10-14 d, Clindamycin 300 mg PO qid x 10-14 d, total <1.8 g/d
Diabetic Foot Ulcer		
Mild	S. aureus	1st gen. Ceph.
Chronic non-limb/Life-threatening	polymicrobial (aerobes + anaerobes)	Fluoroquinolone + Clindamycin or PipTazo or Meropenem
Life-threatening	polymicrobial	Carbapenem + Vanco
BONE		
Osteomyelitis	Staph aureus Elderly: above, plus GN	Vanco + Ceftriaxone Alternative: PipTazo
SEPTIC ARTHRITIS	Young, sexually active: N. gonorrheae S. aureus; Elderly: S. aureus, S. pyogenes, GN	Elderly, simple: Vanco Elderly, traumatic/severe: Vanco + Ceftriaxone
MENINGITIS	S. pneumo, N. meningitidis, H. flu Elderly: same, plus Listeria Non-bacterial: HIV, HSV-2	Ceftriaxone, Vanco (for pen-resistant S. pneumo), ± Ampicillin (for listeria) Acyclovir (IV) (for HSV-2)
BACTERIAL ENDOCARDITIS		
Native valve	S. viridans, S. aureus, enterococcus	pen G + Cloxacillin + Gentamicin
Prosthetic valve	S. epidermidis, S. aureus, S. viridans	Vanco + Gentamicin + Rifampin
Prophylaxis		Amoxicillin OR Clindamycin
OPHTHALMOLOGIC		
Conjunctivitis (viral)	Adenovirus	None (note: very contagious)
Conjunctivitis (bacterial)	S. aureus, S. pneumonia, E. coli, H. influenzae	Sulfacetamide 1-2 gtts q2-6h x 7-10 d, Gentamicin 1-2 gtts q4h x 7-10 d, Erythromycin ointment: apply to lid margins, bid-qid
Blepharitis	Etiology unclear S. aureus, S. epidermidis	Erythromycin ophthalmic ointment of no proven benefit if associated with rosacea: doxycycline 100 mg PO bid x14 d

Antibiotics for Common Pediatric Infections

Disease	Causative Organisms	Empiric Antibiotics of Choice
MENINGITIS/SEPSIS		
Neonatal (birth up to 6 wks)	*GBS, E. coli, Listeria* Other: Gram-negative bacilli	Ampicillin + Aminoglycoside (Gentamicin OR Tobramycin) (sepsis) Ampicillin + Cefotaxime ± Vancomycin (meningitis)
6 wks-3 months	Same pathogens as above and below	Ampicillin + Cefotaxime ± Cloxacillin if risk of *S. aureus* (sepsis) Ampicillin + Cefotaxime ± Vancomycin (meningitis)
>3 months	*S. pneumococcus, N. meningitidis, H. influenzae* type b (>5 yrs)	Cefotaxime + Vanco (sepsis) Ceftriaxone + Vanco (meningitis)
Otitis Media	*S. pneumoniae, H. influenzae, M. catarrhalis, S. pyogenes*	1st line: Amoxicillin 2nd line: high dose Amoxicillin OR Clavulin 3rd line: high dose Clavulin OR Cefuroxime OR Ceftriaxone
Strep Pharyngitis	Group A β-hemolytic *Streptococcus*	Penicillin/amoxicillin OR erythromycin (penicillin allergy) Penicillin V 25-50 mg/kg/d PO div. q6h x10d Amox/Clav 45 mg/kg/d PO div. q12h x10d Azithromycin 12 mg/kg/d PO x5d
UTI	*E. coli, Klebsiella, Proteus, Pseudomonas, S. saprophyticus, Enterococcus, GBS*	Cephalexin, Cefixime (uncomplicated) OR IV Ampicillin and Gentamicin (complicated) OR Ampicillin and Gentamicin (neonates)
Pneumonia (Community Acquired, Bacterial)		
Neonatal	GBS, Gram-negative bacilli (*E. coli*), *C. trachomatis, S. aureus, Listeria*	Ampicillin + Gentamicin, add Erythromycin if Chlamydia suspected
1-3 months	*S. pneumoniae, C. trachomatis, B. pertussis, S. aureus, H. influenzae*	Cefuroxime ± Macrolide (Erythromycin) OR Ampicillin ± Macrolide
3 mos-5 yrs	*S. pneumoniae, S. aureus, H. influenzae, C. pneumoniae, Mycoplasma pneumoniae*	Ampicillin/Amoxicillin OR Clavulin OR Cefuroxime
>5 yrs	As above	Macrolide (1st line) OR Cefuroxime OR Ampicillin/Amoxicillin OR Clavulin

Medical Imaging

Common Approaches

Approach to the Chest X-Ray

- PA and left lateral views (portable AP if unable to do PA)
- Obtain previous CXR for comparison

Chest X-Ray Interpretation

Basics ABCDEF	Analysis ABCDEF
AP, PA or other view	Airways, and hilar Adenopathy
Body position/rotation	Bones and Breast shadows
Confirm name	Cardiac silhouette and Costophrenic angle
Date	Diaphragm and Digestive tract
Exposure/quality	Edges of pleura
Films for comparison	Fields (lung fields)

TECHNICAL FACTORS
- Patient ID: name, MRN, date
- Side markers: left vs. right
- Rotation: medial ends of clavicles should be equidistant from spinous process at midline
- Penetration: thoracic disc spaces should be just visible through heart
- Degree of inspiration: right hemidiaphragm at 6th anterior interspace or 10th posteriorly on good inspiration
- Previous films available

BONES AND SOFT TISSUES
- Neck, axillae, pectoral muscles, breast shadows/nipples, fat, ribs, spine, shoulder, sternum
- Evaluate for: soft tissue masses, amount of soft tissue present, subcutaneous emphysema, scoliosis, kyphosis, fractures, lesions (e.g. metastases), decreased bone density

PLEURA AND DIAPHRAGM
- Identify: parietal and visceral pleura, costophrenic sulcus
- Evaluate for
  - Appearance: thickening, calcifications
  - Mass/effusion: meniscus, blunted angles/thickening, fluid pooling, mediastinal shift
  - Pneumothorax: lung/air contrast, sulcus sign, double diaphragm, mediastinal shift
  - Diaphragm: elevation, depression, free air

CARDIAC
- Identify: structures (PA and lateral view), heart size (cardiothoracic ratio >0.5 is abnormal; may be difficult to assess on portable AP view)
- Evaluate for
  - Pericardial effusion; globular heart, loss of border/indentation, separation of fat pad
  - RA enlargement: curvature increase, SVC enlargement, **right heart border displaced to right**
  - LA enlargement: left border straightening, double heart border, elevated left main bronchus, **splaying of carina**
  - RV enlargement: cardiac apex elevation, loss of retrosternal air space
  - LV enlargement: cardiac apex displacement, boot shaped heart, Rigler's sign (**on lateral film**)
  - Calcifications: vessels, valves, chamber walls

MEDIASTINUM
- Identify: trachea, lymph nodes, ± thymus, great vessels
- Evaluate for
  - Shift, abnormal widening, masses
  - Cervicothoracic sign – anterior mediastinal masses have blurred margins above clavicle

DDx Anterior Mediastinal Mass: The 4 T's
- **Thyroid**
- **Thymus** (thymoma)
- **Teratoma**
- **"Terrible"** lymphoma

LUNG PARENCHYMA

Affected Lung Parenchyma	Findings	Differential
Consolidation (air space disease)	**Air bronchograms**: lucent branching bronchi visible through opacification **Airspace nodules**: fluffy, patchy, poorly marginated appearance with later tendency to coalesce, may take on lobar or segmental distribution	Pus (e.g. pneumonia) Fluid (e.g. pulmonary edema) Blood (e.g. pulmonary hemorrhage) Cells (e.g. bronchoalveolar carcinoma, lymphoma) Protein (e.g. alveolar proteinosis)

Interstitial Disease	**Linear**: fine lines caused by thickened connective tissue septae
	Nodular: 1-5 mm well-defined nodules distributed evenly throughout the lung
	Reticular (Honeycomb): parenchyma replaced by thin walled cysts suggesting extensive destruction of pulmonary tissue and fibrosis
	Reticulonodular: combination of reticular and nodular patterns
	May also see signs of airspace disease (atelectasis and consolidation)
		Occupational/environmental exposure:
		  Inorganic (e.g. asbestosis, silicosis, coal miner's pneumoconiosis)
		  Organic (e.g. Bird fancier's lung, Farmer's lung)
		Autoimmune: CVD, IBD, Celiac disease, vascultitis
		Drug-related: antibiotics (cephalosporins, nitrofurantoin), NSAIDs, phenytoin
		Idiopathic: hypersensitivity pneumonitis, IPF, BOOP

Pulmonary Edema	**General**: Vascular redistribution, pleural effusion, cardiomegaly (if cardiogenic edema/ fluid overload)
	Early (fluid collects in interstitium):
	  Loss of definition of pulmonary vasculature
	  Peribronchial cuffing
	  Kerley B lines: horizontal lines at base of lungs that extend laterally to edge
	  Reticulonodular pattern
	  Thickening of interlobar fissures
	With progression: fluid accumulates in the alveoli causing diffuse airspace disease
	  "Bat wing"/ "butterfly" pattern in perihilar regions with tendency to spare the outermost lung fields
		Cardiogenic (CHF)
		Renal failure
		Volume overload
		Non-cardiogenic (ARDS)

Affected Lung Parenchyma	Findings	Differential
Atelectasis (alveolar collapse)	Increased opacity of involved segment/lobe, silhouette sign Volume loss: fissure deviation, hilar/mediastinal displacement, diaphragm elevation Vascular crowding Compensatory hyperinflation of remaining normal lung Air bronchograms	**Obstructive**: air distal to obstruction is reabsorbed causing alveolar collapse Endobronchial lesion, foreign body, inflammation (granulomatous infections, pneumoconiosis, sarcoidosis, radiation injury), mucous plug (CF) **Compressive** Tumour, bulla, effusion, enlarged heart, lymphadenopathy **Traction**: due to scarring **Adhesive**: due to lack of surfactant e.g. hyaline membrane disease, prematurity **Passive**: due to air or fluid in the pleural space e.g. pleural effusion, pneumothorax
Pulmonary Embolism	**Westermark sign**: localized pulmonary oligemia **Hampton's hump**: triangular peripheral infarct **Other**: enlarged RV and RA, pulmonary edema, atelectasis, pleural effusion	

SILHOUETTE SIGN: Localization of Pathology

Interface Lost	Location of Lung Pathology
Superior vena cava / right superior mediastinum	Right upper lobe
Right heart border	Right middle lobe
Right hemidiaphragm	Right lower lobe
Aortic knob / left superior mediastinum	Left upper lobe
Left heart border	Lingula
Left hemidiaphragm	Left lower lobe

Differential Diagnosis: "CAVITY"

Cancer	Infection
Autoimmune	Trauma
Vascular	Youth (Congenital)

Characteristics of Benign and Malignant Pulmonary Nodules

	Malignant	Benign
Margin	Ill-defined/spiculated ("corona radiata")	Well-defined
Contour	Lobulated	Smooth
Calcification	Eccentric or stippled	Diffuse, central, popcorn, concentric
Doubling Time	20-460 d	<20 d or >460 d
Other Features	Cavitation, collapse, adenopathy, pleural effusion, lytic bone lesions, smoking history	

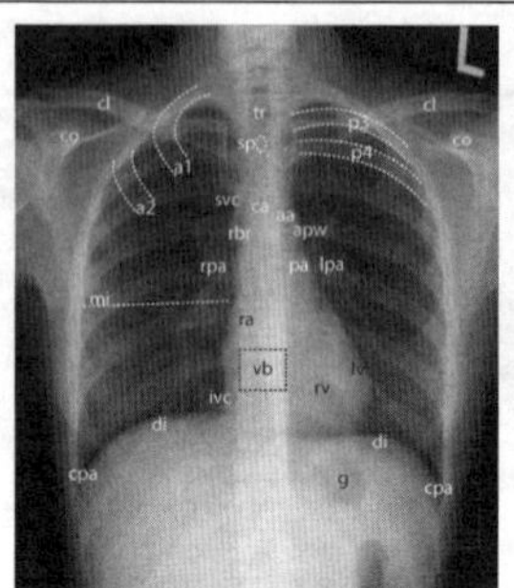
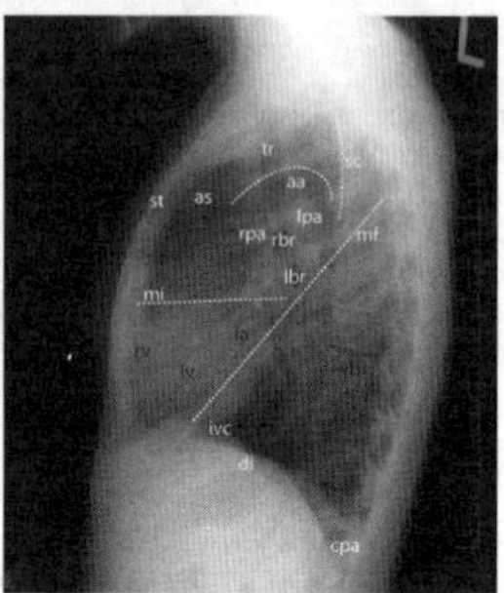

PA View   **Lateral View**

Legend					
a1	anterior 1st rib	co	coracoid process	mf	major fissure
a2	anterior 2nd rib	cpa	costophrenic angle	mi	minor fissure
aa	aortic arch	di	diaphragm	p3	posterior 3rd rib
apw	aorto-pulmonary window	g	gastric bubble	p4	posterior 4th rib
as	anterior airspace	ivc	inferior vena cava	pa	main pulmonary artery
ca	carina	la	left atrium	ra	right atrium
cl	clavicle	lbr	left mainstem bronchus	rbr	right mainstem bronchus
		lpa	left pulmonary artery	rpa	right pulmonary artery
		lv	left ventricle		

rv	right ventricle
sc	scapula
sp	spinous process
st	sternum
svc	superior vena cava
tr	trachea
vb	vertebral body

MEDICAL IMAGING

Approach to the Abdominal X-Ray (AXR)

Approach to the AXR: "IT Free ABDO"	
Identification	**A**ir
Technical factors	**B**owel wall thickening
Free fluid	**D**ensities (bones, calcifications)
	Organs

IDENTIFICATION
- Date, name, age of patient, type of study

TECHNICAL FACTORS
- Good coverage, appropriate penetration, identify view

FREE FLUID
- Assess distance between lateral fat stripes and adjacent colon for evidence of free peritoneal fluid in the paracolic gutters
- Pooling of the bowel to the centre of the supine film
- Ascites (free fluid in the peritoneal cavity) and blood (hemoperitoneum) are the same density on the radiograph, therefore, cannot be differentiated
- Large amounts of fluid, diffuse increased opacification on supine film; bowel floats to centre of anterior abdominal wall

AIR – see Table next page

BOWEL WALL THICKENING
- Increased soft-tissue density in bowel wall, thumb-like indentations in bowel wall "thumb-printing", or a picket-fence appearance of the valvulae conniventes ("stacked coin" appearance)
- Encountered in IBD, infection, ischemia, hypoproteinemic states, and submucosal hemorrhage

DENSITIES
- Bones – look for gross abnormalities of lower ribs, vertebral column and bony pelvis
- Abnormal calcifications – approach by location
  - RUQ: renal stone, adrenal calcification, gallstone, porcelain gallbladder
  - RLQ: ureteral stone, appendicolith, gallstone ileus
  - LUQ: renal stone, adrenal calcification, tail of pancreas
  - LLQ: ureteral stone
  - Central: aorta/aortic aneurysm, pancreas, lymph nodes; pelvis: phleboliths (calcified veins), uterine fibroids, bladder stones

ORGANS
- Kidney, liver, gallbladder, spleen, pancreas, urinary bladder, psoas shadow
- Outlines can occasionally be identified because they are surrounded by more lucent fat, but all are best visualized with other imaging modalities (CT, MRI)
- Ultrasonographic Murphy's Sign (elicited by pressure from ultrasound probe)

Differentiating Small and Large Bowel

Property	Small Bowel	Large Bowel
Mucosal Folds	Uninterrupted valvulae conniventes (or plicae circularis)	Interrupted haustra extend only partway across lumen
Location	Central	Peripheral (picture frame)
Maximum Diameter	3 cm	6 cm (9 cm at cecum)
Maximum Fold Thickness	3 mm	5 mm
Other	Rarely contains solid fecal material	Commonly contains solid fecal material

Abnormal Air on AXR

Air	Appearance	Common Etiologies
Extraluminal intraperitoneal (pneumoperitoneum)	Upright film: air under diaphragm LLD film: air between liver and abdominal wall Supine film: gas outlines of structures not normally seen: Inner and outer bowel wall (Rigler's sign) Falciform ligament Peritoneal cavity ("football" sign)	Perforated viscus Postoperative (up to 10 d to be resorbed)
Extraluminal retroperitoneal	Gas outlining retroperitoneal structures allowing increased visualization: Psoas shadows Renal shadows	Perforation of retroperitoneal segments of bowel: duodenal ulcer, post-colonoscopy
Intramural (pneumatosis intestinalis)	Lucent air streaks in bowel wall, 2 types: 1. Linear 2. Rounded (cystoides type)	Linear: ischemia, necrotizing enterocolitis Rounded/cystoides: Primary (idiopathic) Secondary to COPD
Intraluminal	Dilated loops of bowel, air-fluid levels	Adynamic (paralytic) ileus, mechanical bowel obstruction (see Table below)
Loculated	Mottled, localized in abnormal position without normal bowel features	Abscess (evaluate with CT)
Biliary	Air centrally over liver Cholangitis, emphysematous cholecystitis	Sphincterotomy, gallstone ileus, erosive peptic ulcer
Portal Venous	Air peripherally over liver in branching pattern	Bowel ischemia/infarction

Adynamic Ileus vs. Mechanical Obstruction

Feature	Adynamic Ileus	Mechanical Obstruction
Calibre of Bowel Loops	Normal or dilated	Usually dilated
Air-Fluid Levels	Same level in a single loop	Multiple air fluid levels giving "step ladder" appearance, (erect and LLD films only) Dynamic (indicating peristalsis present) "String of pearls" (row of small gas accumulations in the dilated valvulae conniventes)
Other	Air throughout GI tract generalized or localized In a localized ileus (e.g. pancreatitis, appendicitis): dilated loop "sentinel loop" remains in the same location on serial films, usually adjacent to the area of inflammation	Dilated bowel up to the point of obstruction ("transition point") No air distal to obstructed segment "Hairpin" (180°) turns in bowel Ileocecal valve (ICV) function in large bowel obstruction: Competent ICV: bowel distention from site of obstruction to valve; cecal distention >10 cm represents increased risk for perforation Incompetent ICV: small and large bowel distended; radiographic appearance more similar to paralytic ileus

Approach to Bone X-Rays

Identification
• Name, age of patient, type of study, region of investigation

Soft Tissues
• Swelling, calcification/ossification

Joints
• Alignment, joint space, presence of effusion, osteophytes, erosions, bone density, overall pattern and symmetry of affected joint

Bone
• Periosteum, cortex, medulla, trabeculae, density, articular ends, bone destruction, bone production, appearance of the edges or borders of any lesions

Approach to Fractures
1. Look for fracture lines (abnormal black lines)
2. Look for discontinuation/disruption of cortex border
3. Look for joint space narrowing/widening
4. Look for soft tissue involvement (swelling, calcification)

Characteristics of Benign and Malignant Bone Lesions
Note: for specific bone tumours see Orthopedics

Benign	Malignant
Sharp area of delineation	Poor delineation of lesion – wide zone of transition
Overlying cortex intact	Loss of overlying cortex/bony destruction
No or simple periosteal reaction	Periosteal reaction – aggressive
Sclerotic margins with sharp zone of transition	Wide zone of transition
No soft tissue mass	Soft tissue mass

Characteristic Bone Metastases of Common Cancers

Lytic	Sclerotic	Expansile	Peripheral
Breast	Prostate	Thyroid	Lung
Lung	Breast	Renal	Kidney
Thyroid	Bowel	Melanoma	
Kidney	Lung		
Multiple myeloma	Lymphoma		
	Medulloblastoma		
	Treated tumours		

Approach to CT Chest

- **Soft tissue window**
  - Thyroid, chest wall, pleura
  - Heart: chambers, coronary artery calcifications, pericardium
  - Vessels: aorta, pulmonary artery, smaller vasculature
  - Lymph nodes: mediastinal, axillary
- **Bone window**
  - Look at vertebrae, sternum, manubrium, ribs for fractures, lytic lesions, sclerosis
- **Lung window**
  - Central-trachea: patency, secretions
  - Bronchial trees: anatomic variants, mucus plugs, airway collapse
  - Lung parenchyma: fissures, nodules

Approach to CT Abdomen

1. Look through all images in gestalt fashion to identify any obvious abnormalities
2. Look at each organ/structure individually, from top to bottom evaluating size and shape of each area of increased or decreased density
3. Evaluate the following:
   - Visible lung (bases), liver, gallbladder, spleen, pancreas
   - Adrenals, kidneys, ureters, and bladder
   - Stomach, duodenum, small bowel mesentery, and colon/appendix
   - Retroperitoneum: aorta, vena cava, and mesenteric vessels; look for adenopathy in vicinity of vessels
   - Peritoneal cavity for fluid or masses
   - Vertebrae, spinal cord and bony pelvis
   - Abdominal wall and adjacent soft tissue

Imaging of Liver Masses

Mass	U/S	CT
Metastases	Multiple masses of variable echotexture	Usually low attenuation on contrast enhanced scan
HCC	Single/multiple masses, or diffuse infiltration	Small: hypervascular enhances in arterial phase Large: low-attenuation
Simple Cyst	Well-defined, anechoic, acoustic enhancement	Well-defined, low attenuation, homogenous
Abscess	Poorly defined, irregular margin, hypoechoic contents	Low-attenuation lesion with an irregular enhancing wall
Hydatid Cyst	Simple/multiloculated cyst	Low-attenuation simple or multiloculated cyst; calcification
Hemangioma	Homogenous hyperechoic mass	Peripheral globular enhancement in arterial phase scans; central-filling and persistent enhancement on delayed scans

Imaging of Liver Masses (continued)

Mass	U/S	CT
Focal Nodular	Well-defined mass, central scar seen in 50%	Equal attenuation to liver in portal venous phase, hyperplasia enhancement in arterial phase
Hepatic Adenoma	Most common in young women taking oral contraceptives. Well-defined mass with areas due to hemorrhage hyperechoic	Well-defined margin with heterogeneous texture due to hemorrhage or fat

Approach to CT Head

- Think anatomically, work from superficial to deep
- **Scan** – confirm that the imaging is of the patient of interest, whether contrast was used, if the patient is aligned properly, if there is artifact present
- **Skin/soft tissue** – examine the soft-tissue superficial to the skull, looking for thickening suggestive of hematoma or edema; also evaluate: ear, orbital contents (globe, fat, muscles), parotid, muscles of mastication (masseter, temporalis, pterygoids), visualized pharynx
- **Bone and airspace** (use the bone window) – check calvarium, visualized mandible, visualized c-spine (usually C1 and maybe part of C2) for fractures, absent bone, lytic/sclerotic lesions; inspect sinuses and mastoid air cells for opacity that may suggest fluid, pus, blood, tumour, or fracture
- **Dura and subdural space** – look for crescent-shaped hyperdensity in the subdural space as evidence of subdural hematoma; look for a lentiform hyperdensity in epidural space as evidence of epidural hematoma; check symmetry of dural thickness, where increased thickness may suggest the presence of blood
- **Parenchyma** – look for symmetry of the parenchyma for evidence of midline shift; look for poor contrast between grey and white matter as evidence of possible infarction, tumour, edema, infection, or contusion; look for hyperdensities in the parenchyma suggestive of an enchancing lesions(if contrast was given), intracerebral hemorrhage, or calcification; central grey matter nuclei should be visible, including globus palladus, putamen, and internal capsule, otherwise suspect infarct, tumour, or infection
- **Ventricles/sulci/cisterns** – examine position of ventricles for evidence of midline compression/shift; look for hyperdensities in the ventricles indicative of ventricular/subdural hemorrhage; look at ventricular size for evidence of hydrocephalus; obliteration of sulci may suggest presence of edema causing effacement, possible blood filling in the sulci, or tumour; cistern hyperdensities may suggest blood, pus, or tumour

Common Imaging Modalities

GU Diagnositic Modalities

Imaging Modality Based on Presentation

- Acute testicular pain = Doppler, U/S
- Amenorrhea = U/S, MRI (brain)
- Bloating = U/S, CT
- Flank pain = U/S, CT
- Hematuria = U/S, cystoscopy, CT
- Infertility = hysterosalpingogram, MRI
- Lower abdominal mass = U/S, CT
- Lower abdominal pain = U/S, CT
- Renal colic = U/S, KUB, CT
- Testicular mass = U/S
- Urethral stricture = urethrogram

CT UROGRAPHY

- Historically, intravenous urography (IVU) provided anatomical and functional information about the urogenital system; this has largely been replaced by CT urography

Excretory-phase CT

- The new imaging technique of choice exclusively to assess the renal collecting systems. It has a high sensitivity (95%) in detecting upper urinary tract uroepithelial malignancies, and is also useful for detecting renal calculi

Indications
- Hematuria (with negative cystoscopy and U/S studies ruling out parenchymal causes), unexplained hydronephrosis on U/S, evaluation of the renal collecting system post-trauma (e.g. post pelvic surgery)

CT Features
- Renal cysts: fluid filled lesions with smooth, well-defined borders, low density, no enhancement with contrast (smooth-walled, bright lesions on non-contrast CT may suggest hyperdense cysts consisting of debris from proteinaceous material or previous hemorrhage into a benign cyst)
- Complex renal cysts: thick-walled, may contain calcifications, some may be septated, walls may enhance with contrast
- Renal cell carcinoma: less-defined borders, same density as kidney, enhancement with contrast (characterizing vascularity) ± areas of necrosis
- Angiomyolipoma (a benign renal neoplasm composed of fat, vascular, and smooth muscle elements): fat density seen on non-contrast CT, some enhancement with contrast (less intense than renal cell carcinoma), association with tuberous sclerosis and lymphangioleiomyomatosis

U/S
- Initial study for evaluation of kidney size and nature of renal masses (solid vs. cystic renal masses vs. complicated cysts)
- Technique of choice for screening patients with suspected hydronephrosis (no intravenous contrast injection, no radiation to patient, and can be used in patients in renal failure)
- Solid renal masses: echogenic (bright on U/S)
- Cystic renal masses: smooth well-defined walls with anechoic interior (dark on U/S)
- Complicated cysts: internal echoes within a thickened, irregular-walled cyst
- Transrectal U/S (TRUS) useful to evaluate prostate gland and guide biopsies
- Doppler U/S to assess renal vasculature

Neurologic Diagnostic Modalities

Modality Based on Presentation
- Cognitive decline = CT
- Cord compression = MRI
- Decreased LOC = CT
- Fish bone/other ingested foreign body = CT
- LBP, radiculopathy = MRI
- Multiple sclerosis = MRI
- Neck infection = CT
- Orbital infection = CT
- R/O bleed = CT
- R/O aneurysm = CTA, MRA
- Seizure = CT
- Sinusitis = CT
- Stroke = CT, MRI
- Trauma = CT
- Weakness, systemically unwell = CT

CT
- The modality of choice for most neuropathology; even under circumstances when MRI is preferred, CT is frequently the initial study because of its speed, availability and lower cost
- Often done first without and then with intravenous contrast to show vascular structures or anomalies
- Vascular structures and areas of blood-brain barrier impairment are hyperattenuating (white/show enhancement) with contrast injection
- When in doubt, look for circle of Willis or confluence of dural venous sinuses to determine presence of contrast enhancement
- Posterior fossa can be obscured by bone streak artifact
- Used to rule out skull fracture, epidural hematoma (lenticular shape), subdural hematoma (crescentic shape), subarachnoid hemorrhage, space occupying lesion, hydrocephalus, and cerebral edema

- CT is preferred for:
  - Acute head trauma: CT is best for visualizing "bone and blood." MRI is used in this setting only when CT fails to detect an abnormality in the presence of strong clinical suspicion
  - Acute stroke: MRI would be ideal test but CT is a good substitute, can also do CT perfusion imaging
  - Suspected subarachnoid or intracranial hemorrhage
  - Meningitis: rule out mass lesion (e.g. abscess) prior to lumbar puncture
  - Tinnitus and vertigo: CT and MRI are used in combination to detect bony abnormalities and CN VIII tumours, respectively

---

DDx for Ring-enhancing Lesion on CT with Contrast: "MAGICAL DR"
Metastases*
Abscess*
Glioblastoma (high grade astrocytoma)*
Infarct
Contusion
AIDS (*Toxoplasma gondii* encephalitis, primary CNS lymphoma, cryptococcomas, TB, CMV, neurosyphilis)
Lymphoma
Demyelination
Resolving hematoma

[* by far the 3 most common Dx's]

SKULL FILMS
- Rarely performed; CT is modality of choice
- Indications include:
  - Facial fracture, sinus disease, penetrating trauma, destructive bony lesions (e.g. metastases), metabolic disease, skull anomalies, post-operative changes
  - Generally not indicated for non-penetrating head trauma
- Standard views (each designed to demonstrate a particular area of the skull)
  - PA (frontal bones, frontal/ethmoid sinuses, nasal cavity, superior orbital rims, and mandible)
  - Lateral (frontal, parietal, temporal, and occipital bones, mastoid region, sella turcica, orbital roofs, and lateral aspects of facial bones)
  - Towne's view/occipital; "half-axial" (occipital bone, mastoid and middle ear regions, foramen magnum, and zygomatic arches)
  - Base view (basal structures of skull, including major foramina)
  - Water's view/occipitomental (facial bones and sinuses)
  - Panoramic view (mandible)

MRI (see under *Comparison of Imaging Modalities*)
- Shows brain anatomy in fine detail
- Clearly distinguishes white from grey matter (especially T1-weighted series)
- Multiplanar reconstruction helpful in pre-op assessment

CEREBRAL ANGIOGRAPHY
- Evaluation of vascular lesions such as atherosclerotic disease, aneurysms, vascular malformations: **still gold standard test to evaluate the arterial and venous system in the brain**
- Digital subtraction angiography (DSA) commonly used to create images of vessels

Nuclear Medicine

THYROID

Radioactive Iodine Uptake (see Endocrinology)
- Index of thyroid function (trapping and organification of iodine)
- Radioactive ^{131}I or ^{123}I PO in fasting patient
- Measured as a percentage of administered iodide taken up by thyroid
- Increased RAIU: toxic multinodular goiter, toxic adenoma, Graves' (although may be normal)
- Decreased RAIU: subacute thyroiditis, late Hashimoto's disease, hormone suppression
- Falsely decreased in patient with recent radiographic contrast studies, high dietary iodine (i.e. seaweed)
- Contraindicated in pregnancy

Thyroid Imaging (Scintiscan)
- ^{99m}Tc pertechnetate IV or radioactive iodine (^{123}I)
- Provides functional anatomic detail
- Hot (hyperfunctioning) lesions
    - Adenoma, toxic multinodular goiter
    - Usually benign, cancer very unlikely (less than 1%)
- Cold (hypofunctioning) lesions
    - Cancer must be considered until biopsy negative even though only 6-10% are cancerous
- Cool lesions
    - Cancer must be considered as a cool lesion may represent cold nodules superimposed on normal tissue
    - If cyst suspected, correlate with U/S
- Serum thyroglobulin to detect recurrent thyroid cancer post treatment

Radioiodine Ablation
- ^{131}I for Graves, multinodular goiter, thyroid cancer

BONE

Bone Scan

Indications for a Bone Scan
- Bone pain of unknown origin, AVN, suspected malignancy, staging malignancy (cancer of breast, prostate, kidney, thyroid or lung), follow up after treatment, detection and follow-up of primary bone disease, assessment of skeletal trauma, detection of soft tissue calcification, suspected infection

Isotopes
- ^{99m}Tc-MDP:
    - Triphasic bone scan: perfusion → blood pool → delayed bone images
    - Uptake can distinguish bone vs. soft tissue infection and septic arthritis vs. osteomyelitis vs. peripheral cellulitis
    - Acute osteomyelitis: increased activity in blood pool and delayed bone images, usually does not cross joint
    - Septic arthritis and cellulitis: increased activity in blood pool and normal or slightly increased activity in delayed images, may cross joint
- ^{111}In WBC: tracks the active migration of the WBC – more specific for infection
- ^{67}Ga citrate: may see uptake in some tumours e.g. lymphoma, also more specific for infection
- Radioactive tracer binds to hydroxyapatite of bone matrix
- Increased binding when increased blood supply to bone and/or high bone turnover (active osteoblasts)

Findings
- Positive bone scan: bone metastases from breast, prostate, lung, thyroid, primary bone tumour, arthritis, fracture, infection, anemia, Paget's disease
- Multiple myeloma: typically normal or cold (false negative); need a skeletal survey
- Superscan: good visualization of bone, but not kidneys, due to diffuse metastases

RESPIRATORY

V/Q Scan
- Examine areas of lung in which ventilation and perfusion do not match
- Ventilation scan
  - Patient breathes radioactive gas through a closed system, filling alveoli proportional to ventilation
  - Ventilation scan defects indicate: airway obstruction, chronic lung disease, bronchospasm, tumour mass obstruction
- Perfusion scan
  - Radiotracer injected IV → trapped in pulmonary capillaries (1 in 1500 arterioles occluded) according to blood flow
  - Gives a map of pulmonary circulation
- Relatively contraindicated in severe pulmonary HTN and right-to-left shunt
- PE areas of lung are well ventilated but not perfused (unmatched defect)
- PE is wedge-shaped, extend to periphery, usually bilateral and multiple
- Reported as high probability, intermediate, low, very low or normal
- V/Q scans for PE have been largely replaced by **multidetector** CT scan with contrast (see <u>Respirology</u>)

VQ Scanning for PE
- For PE investigation: normal scan makes PE unlikely
- Probability of PE: High 80-100%, intermediate 20-80%, low <20%, very low <10%

Ventilation scan defects indicate: Airway obstruction, chronic lung disease, bronchospasm, tumour mass obstruction.

Perfusion scan defects indicate: reduced blood flow due to PE, COPD, asthma, bronchogenic carcinoma, inflammatory lung diseases (pneumonia, sarcoidosis), mediastinitis, mucus plug, vasculitis.

ABDOMEN

HIDA (Hepatobiliary IminoDiacetic Acid) Scan
- IV injection of ^{99m}Tc-disofenin (DISIDA) or ^{99m}Tc-mebrofenin (BRIDA) which is bound to protein, taken up, and excreted by hepatocytes into biliary system
- Can be performed in non-fasting state but prefer NPO after midnight
- Gallbladder visualized when cystic duct is patent, usually seen by 30 min to 1 h
- If gallbladder is not visualized, suspect obstructed cystic duct (acute or chronic cholecystitis)
- Acute cholecystitis: no visualization of gallbladder at 4 h or after administration of morphine at 30 min
- Chronic cholecystitis: no visualization of gallbladder at 1 h but seen at 4 h or after morphine administration
- Differential diagnosis of obstructed cystic duct: acute cholecystitis, decreased hepatobiliary function (commonly due to alcoholism), bile duct obstruction, parenteral nutrition, fasting less than 4 h or more than 24 h
- Filling of gallbladder rules out cholecystitis (<1% probability)
- Assess bile leaks post-operatively

RBC Scan
- IV injection of radiotracer with sequential images of the abdomen (99mTc RBCs)
- GI bleed
  - If bleeding acutely at <0.5 mL/min, the focus of activity in the images generally indicates the site of the acute bleed, look for a change in shape and location on sequential image
  - If bleeding acutely at >0.5 mL/min, use angiography (more specific)
  - RBC scan is more sensitive for lower GI bleed
- Liver lesion evaluation
  - Hemangioma has characteristic appearance: cold early, fills in later

Comparison of Imaging Modalities

Modality	Positives and Negatives	Indications and Contraindications
PLAIN FILM High attenuation structures appear white (metal > bone > water > fat > air)	**Positives** Inexpensive, non-invasive, readily available **Negatives** Radiation exposure Poor at distinguishing soft tissue	**Indications** Initial imaging study in suspected thoracic, MSK disease, penetrating head trauma **Contraindications** Pregnancy (relative)
CT Multiple x-rays producing cross-sectional reconstruction of anatomy	**Positives** Fast data acquisition Delineates surrounding soft tissues, bones Excellent for identifying nodules, metastases Can be used for guided biopsies **Negatives** High radiation exposure IV contrast injection Relatively expensive Claustrophobia: rare, much less so than with MRI	**Indications** Evaluation of CXR abnormality Staging malignancy, metastatic disease Detecting PE, aortic dissection, renal stones Evaluation of bone cortex, soft tissue calcification, acute head trauma, acute stroke **Contraindications** Pregnancy (relative) Renal failure Dehydration *DM (relative) *Severe CHF *Multiple myeloma *These three conditions require careful consideration before giving the patient intravenous contrast. Non-contrast CT is not an issue for these conditions.
X-RAY IMAGING **with contrast agents** Used to examine structures without inherent contrast differences Given by mouth, rectum, or injection	**Positives** Delineates intraluminal anatomy Demonstrates patency, lumen integrity, filling defects With fluoroscopy can provide info re: function of organ **Negatives** Risk of contrast reaction Intravenous contrast may cause renal failure in dehydrated DM pts, myeloma, or pre-existing renal disease	**Indications** IV contrast to determine lesion vascularity **Contraindications** Previous adverse reaction to contrast Renal failure Multiple myeloma Dehydration DM Severe heart failure
ULTRASOUND High freq. sound waves transmitted from transducer and passed through tissue Sound wave reflections picked up by transducer and transformed to images Doppler – determines vascularity of structures Duplex scan – Doppler and visual images	**Positives** Relatively low cost Non-invasive No radiation Real time imaging Used for guided biopsies **Negatives** Highly operator dependant Air in bowel may prevent imaging of midline structures in abdomen Limited by patient habitus	**Indications** Identify and tap pleural effusions Soft tissue masses identified for biopsy Determines cystic vs. solid Pregnancy **Contraindications** None
MRI Patient is placed in magnetic field Radio-frequency pulse applied to manipulate protons to provide MR images Note: water is white on T2	**Positives** Excellent soft tissue contrast Multiple plane capability Visualize vascular structures without contrast use **Negatives** Expensive Poor availability	**Indications** Neuropathology (shows brain anatomy in fine detail) Image soft tissues including nerves (i.e. brachial plexus), tumours, ligaments, tendons Determines cystic vs. solid Pregnancy **Contraindications** Metal implants (i.e. aneurysm clips or shrapnel), pacemaker, neurostimulators, cochlear implant, claustrophobia

MR Signal Intensities

Tissue or Body Fluid	T1-weighted	T2-weighted
Gas	Nil i.e. signal void	Nil i.e. signal void
Mineral-rich tissue (e.g. cortical bone, calculi)	Nil i.e. signal void	Nil i.e. signal void
Collagenous tissue (e.g. ligaments, tendons, scars)	Low	Low
Hemosiderin	Low	Low
Fat	High	Medium to high
Protein-containing fluid (e.g. abscess, complex cyst)	Intermediate-high	High
Synovium	Low	Intermediate
Nucleus pulposus	Medium	High
High bound-water tissues:		
Muscle	Low	Low-intermediate
Hyaline cartilage	Low	Intermediate
Liver	Intermed-high	Low
Pancreas	High	Intermediate
Adrenal	High	Intermediate
High free-water tissues: CSF, urine, bile, edema, simple cysts	Low	High
Kidney	Intermediate-high	Intermediate
Thyroid	Intermediate-low	High
Hemorrhage:		
Hyperacute (<6 h): intracellular oxyHb	Low-intermediate	High
Acute (2-3 d): intracellular deoxy Hb	Low-intermediate	Low
Chronic (>7 d)		
• Intracellular met Hb (several days)	High	Low
• Extracellular met Hb (week-months)	High	High
Late: hemosiderin	Low-intermediate	Low
Neuropathology:	Low	High
Ischemia		
Edema		
Demyelination		
Most malignant tumours		
Meningioma	Intermediate	Variable Intermediate-high

Ethical, Legal & Organizational Aspects of Medicine

Consent

Elements of Valid Consent
- Honest: truth-telling is required for valid consent
  - Exceptions to truth-telling: patient may waive their right to know the truth about their situation
- Patient must be capable: must understand choices and consequences
- Informed: what a "reasonable person" would want to know regarding risks and benefits
- Not coerced or under undue influence (e.g. money, addiction)
- If the patient is not capable, Substitute Decision Maker must provide consent (see below)

Age of Consent to Treatment
- Province-specific: some provinces have an Age of Consent (PEI, NB, QC, SK, BC), but "capable persons" under the age of consent may have the right to make decisions
- In provinces without an Age of Consent, a minor deemed capable may provide consent (ON)

Situations in which Consent is NOT Required
- Emergencies, so long as treatment doesn't violate known previous wishes (e.g. Jehovah's Witness)
- When the patient has been placed on a Form under the *Mental Health Act*
- When Public Health legislation allows for detention or mandatory treatment

Assessing Capacity

Capacity: The ability to
- Understand the problem, proposed actions, alternatives, option of refusal
- Appreciate the consequences of treatment or refusal of treatment
- Make a decision not based on delusions or depression

With a Finding of Incapacity
- Substitute Decision Maker must be determined and provide consent
- Further assessment may be required (e.g. psychiatry, legal review boards, etc.)

Substitute Decision Makers (SDMs)

SDM Must Act
- First: according to patient's previously expressed wishes
- Second: in the patient's best interests

SDM Hierarchy is Province-Specific
- In Ontario, the SDM is the highest ranking person on this list who is available, capable, and willing to make these decisions:
  - Power of Attorney for personal care (if one is designated); spouse, common-law spouse or partner; child (if they are 16 yrs of age or older) or parent with right of access only (custodial parents rank ahead of non-custodial parents); sibling; any other relative by blood, marriage or adoption; the Office of the Public Guardian and Trustee (the provincial Public Guardian and Trustee is the SDM of last resort)

Instructional Advance Directives

- Made while a patient is capable and only takes effect once the patient is incapable
- Directives include:
  - Living Will: documents patient's wishes
  - Proxy Directive: specifies who is to become patient's decision-maker
  - Instructional Directive: specifies what care the patient would want their proxy to make in particular situations
  - DNR Order: no artificial resuscitation (CPR/intubation/ICU) but can include comfort measures and active treatment for disease

Confidentiality

Disclosure of Health Information is Ethically and Legally Permissible
- With the patient's consent
- Without the patient's express consent, if sharing with health care team members within the "circle of care"
- Without the patient's consent in cases where:
  - The patient poses a threat to others (Duty to Warn)
  - Disclosure of health records is required by a court order/warrant/subpoena
  - A birth or death has occurred
  - The coroner is involved
  - There are statutory reporting obligations (see below)

Statutory Reporting Obligations
- Child abuse and neglect; patient unfit to drive/fly; reportable diseases; sexual misconduct by health professional
- Situations to notify coroner if death occurs include violence, negligence, misconduct, pregnancy, sudden or unexpected disease NOT treated, infants, cause other than the known disease, suspicious circumstances

Approach to Breaking Bad News (SPIKES)

S   **SETTING** and **LISTENING SKILLS** (don't underestimate the value of listening)

P   Patient's **PERCEPTION** of condition and seriousness

I   **INVITATION** from patient to give information

K   **KNOWLEDGE** – giving medical facts

E   **EXPLORE EMOTIONS AND EMPATHIZE** as patient responds

S   **STRATEGY** and **SUMMARY**

Strategy	Summary
Consider best medical options	Summarize the discussion
Assess patient's expectations of condition, treatment and outcome	Invite and answer patient's questions
	Assess patient's response
Propose a strategy for care	Acknowledge their concerns; if you don't
Agree on a plan	know answers, explain how you will obtain them
A clear contract for the next contact	

Anesthesia and Perioperative Medicine

Essential History, Physical Exam and Guidelines

History

ANESTHESIA PRE-OP ASSESSMENT
* Any patient undergoing surgery requires an assessment prior to induction
  The pre-operative assessment may change how the anesthesiologist manages the patient during surgery, including the type of airway and which medications to use/avoid for induction and pain control
* Hx: Head-to-toe approach
* CNS: seizures, strokes, other neurological problems including neuromuscular (i.e. myasthemia gravis)
* CVS: CAD, MI, CHF, HTN, valvular disease, exercise tolerance (NYHA score), need for endocarditis prophylaxis
* Respiratory: asthma, COPD, smoking, restrictive disease
* GI: GERD, hiatus hernia, liver disease
* Renal: kidney problems, CRF, dialysis
* MSK: arthritis, joint problems, especially TMJ, neck mobility, RA
* Metabolic and Endocrine: DM, thyroid disease, obesity, any other endocrine disorders
* Hematologic: coagulopathies e.g. von Willebrands disease, hemophilia
* Other: any recent infections (fever, cough), smoking history
* Past Surgical Hx: dates and any anesthetic related complications (e.g. post-op nausea and vomiting, difficulty waking, bronchospasm on extubation), opioid exposure
* FHx of Anesthetic Problems: pseudocholinesterase deficiency, malignant hyperthermia
* Meds: current meds and those that were stopped/continued prior to surgery, time of last dosage
* Allergies: all drug allergies and reactions, specifically ask anaphylaxis to eggs, latex allergy, tape sensitivity
* Time of last meal and contents

Physical Exam

OROPHARYNX AND AIRWAY ASSESSMENT: Factors for easier intubation
* Mouth opening: 2 fingerbreadths
* Thyromental distance: 3 fingerbreadths
* Mallampati score: Mallampati I or II
* Neck range of motion: better flexion/extension
* TMJ subluxation: 1 fingerbreadth
* Greater subluxation in thinner patient
* Dentition

Mallampati Classification of Upper Airway Visualization

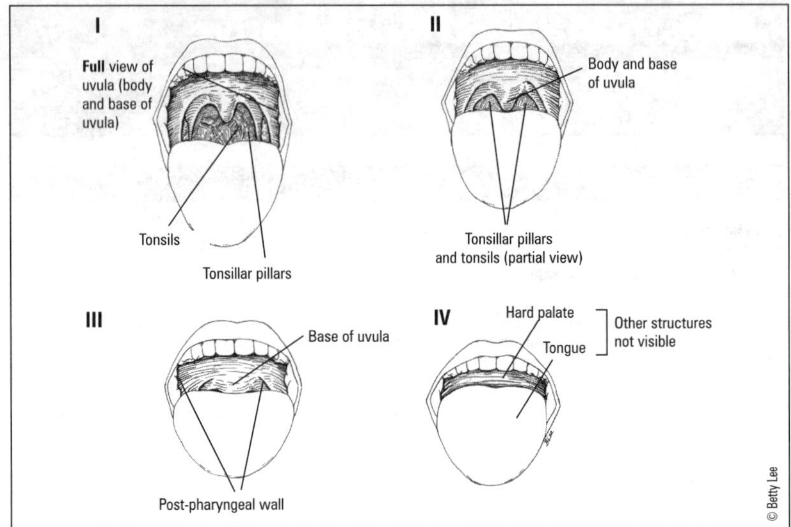

Guidelines

American Society of Anesthesiology (ASA) Classification
- **ASA 1**: healthy, fit patient
- **ASA 2**: patient with mild systemic disease, e.g. controlled type 2 diabetes, controlled essential HTN, obesity, smoker
- **ASA 3**: patient with severe systemic disease that limits activity, e.g. angina, prior MI, COPD, DM, obesity
- **ASA 4**: patient with incapacitating disease that is at constant threat to life, e.g. CHF, renal failure, acute respiratory failure
- **ASA 5**: moribund patient not expected to survive 24 h with/without surgery, e.g. ruptured abdominal aortic aneurysm (AAA), head trauma with increased ICP
- **ASA 6**: declared brain dead, a patient whose organs are being removed for donation purposes
- For emergency operations, add the letter **E** after classification (e.g. ASA 3E)

Fasting Guidelines (Canadian Anesthesiologists' Society)
- 8 h after a meal that includes meat, fried or fatty foods
- 6 h after a light meal (toast, crackers and clear fluid) or infant formula
- 4 h after breastmilk or Jello
- 2 h after clear fluids (water, black coffee, tea, carbonated beverage, juice)

Common Concepts

Methods of Supporting the Airway

	Bag and Mask ± Oral Airway	Laryngeal Mask Airway (LMA)	Endotracheal Tube (ETT)
Advantages/ Indications	Basic Non-invasive Readily available	Easy to insert; Less airway trauma/irritation than ETT; Less chance of Laryngospasm; Frees hands (vs. face mask)	"The **5 P's**" **P**atent airway **P**rotects against aspiration **P**ositive pressure ventilation **P**ulmonary toilet **P**harmacological administration
Disadvantages	Risk of aspiration if decreased LOC Cannot ensure airway patency Imprecise tidal volume Operator fatigue	Risk of gastric aspiration PPV <20 cm H_2O needed Limited TMJ mobility	Insertion can be difficult Muscle relaxant needed Laryngospasm may occur Sympathetic stress
Contraindications	Complete upper airway obstruction	C-spine or laryngeal cartilage fracture; oropharyngeal, retropharyngeal pathology or FB	
Other	Facilitate patency with jaw thrust and chin lift	Does NOT protect against laryngospasm or gastric aspiration Primarily used in spontaneously ventilating patient Sizing (approx): Male: 4.0-5.0; Female: 3.0-4.0	Necessary for rapid sequence induction Auscultate to avoid endobronchial intubation

Endotracheal Tube Size based on Age and Weight

Age	Weight (kg)	ETT Size
Premature	<1.5 kg	2.5
Premature	1.5-2.5 kg	3.0
Newborn	3.5 kg	3.5
1 yr old	10 kg	4.0
2-3 yrs old	15 kg	4.5
4-6 yrs old	20 kg	5.0
7-9 yrs old	30 kg	5.5
10-12 yrs old	40 kg	6.0
13-15 yrs old	50 kg	6.5
>16 yrs old and women (in general)	>60 kg	7.0 or 7.5
Men (in general)		8.0 or 8.5

Pediatric ETT, internal diameter: (Age/4) + 4

General Guidelines to Ensure Safe Extubation

- Ensure face mask for O_2 delivery available
- Patient has normal neuromuscular function and hemodynamic status
- Patient is breathing spontaneously with adequate rate and tidal volume
- Allow ventilation (spontaneous or controlled) with 100% O_2 for 3-5 min
- Suction secretions from pharynx
- Deflate cuff, remove ETT on inspiration (vocal cords are abducted)
- Ensure patient breathing adequately after extubation
- Proper positioning of patient during transfer to recovery room (e.g. lateral decubitus, head elevated)

Epidural and Spinal Anesthesia

ANATOMY OF SPINAL/EPIDURAL AREA
- Spinal cord extends to L2, dural sac to S2 in adults
- Nerve roots (cauda equina) from L2 to S2
- Needle inserted below L2 should not encounter cord, thus L3-L4, L4-L5 interspace commonly used

Epidural vs. Spinal Anesthesia

	Epidural	Spinal
Onset	Significant blockade requires 10-15 min Slower onset of side effects	Rapid blockade (onset in 2-5 min)
Effectiveness	Effectiveness of blockade can be variable	Very effective blockade
Deposition Site	LA deposited in epidural space (potential space between ligamentum flavum and dura) Initial blockade is at the spinal roots followed by some degree of spinal cord anesthesia as LA diffuses into the subarachnoid space through the dura	LA injected into subarachnoid space in the dural sac surrounding the spinal cord and nerve roots
Dosage	Larger volume/dose of LA (usually > toxic IV dose)	Smaller dose of LA required (usually < toxic IV dose)
Specific Gravity/Spread	Solutions injected here spread throughout the potential space; specific gravity of solution does not affect spread	LA solution may be made hyperbaric (of greater specific gravity than the cerebrospinal fluid by mixing with 10% dextrose, thus increasing spread of LA to the dependent areas of the subarachnoid space)
Continuous Infusion	Use of catheter allows for continuous infusion or repeat injections	None
Complications	Failure of technique Hypotension Bradycardia if cardiac sympathetics blocked (only if ~T2-4 block) Epidural or subarachnoid hematoma Accidental subarachnoid injection can produce spinal anesthesia (and any of the above complications) Systemic toxicity of LA (accidental intravenous) Catheter complications (shearing, kinking, vascular or subarachnoid placement) Infection Dural puncture headache	Failure of technique Hypotension Bradycardia if cardiac sympathetics blocked (only if ~T2-4 block), i.e. "high spinal" Epidural or subarachnoid hematoma Post-spinal headache (CSF leak) Persistent paresthesias (usually transient) Spinal cord trauma, infection
Combined Spinal-Epidural	Combines the benefits of rapid, reliable, intense blockade of spinal anesthesia together with the flexibility of an epidural catheter	

Fluid Balance

- Total requirement = maintenance + deficit + ongoing loss
- In surgical settings, this formula must take into account multiple factors including pre-op fasting/decreased fluid intake, increased losses during or before surgery, fluid shifting during surgery, fluids given with blood products and medications

What Is The Maintenance?
- Average healthy adult requires approximately 2,500 mL water/d
  - 200 mL/d GI losses
  - 800 mL/d insensible losses (respiration, perspiration)
  - 1,500 mL/d urine (beware of renal failure)

- Increased requirements with fever, sweating, GI losses (vomiting, diarrhea, NG suction), adrenal insufficiency, hyperventilation and polyuric renal disease
- Decreased requirements with anuria/oliguria, SIADH, highly humidified atmospheres and CHF
- **4:2:1 rule** to calculate maintenance requirements
  - 4 mL/kg/h first 10 kg
  - 2 mL/kg/h second 10 kg
  - 1 mL/kg/h for remaining weight >20 kg
- Maintenance electrolytes
  - Na^+: $\geq$3 mEq/kg/d
  - K^+: $\geq$1 mEq/kg/d
- e.g. 50 kg patient maintenance requirements
  - fluid: 40 + 20 + 30 = 90 mL/h = 2,160 mL/d
  - Na^+: 150 mEq/d (therefore 66 mEq/L)
  - K^+: 50 mEq/d (therefore 22 mEq/L)
- Above patient's requirements roughly met with 2/3 D5W, 1/3 NS
  - e.g. 2/3 + 1/3 at 100 mL/h with 20 mEq KCl per litre

What Is The Deficit?
- Patients should be adequately hydrated prior to anesthesia
- TBW = 60% total body weight (e.g. for a 70 kg adult TBW = 70 x 0.6 = 42 L)
- Total Na^+ content determines ECF volume, $[Na^+]$ determines ICF volume
- Hypovolemia due to volume contraction
  - Extra-renal Na^+ loss
    - GI: vomiting, NG suction, drainage, fistulae, diarrhea
    - Skin/resp: insensible losses (fever), sweating, burns
    - Vascular: hemorrhage
  - Renal Na^+ and H_2O loss
    - Diuretics, osmotic diuresis, hypoaldosteronism, salt-wasting nephropathies
  - Renal H_2O loss
    - Diabetes insipidus (central or nephrogenic)
- Hypovolemia with normal or expanded ECF volume
  - Decreased cardiac output
  - Redistribution
    - Hypoalbuminemia: cirrhosis, nephrotic syndrome
    - Capillary leaking: acute pancreatitis, rhabdomyolysis, ischemic bowel
- Replace water and electrolytes as determined by patient needs
- With chronic hyponatremia correction must be done gradually over >48 h to avoid CNS central pontine myelinolysis

Signs and Symptoms of Dehydration

Percentage of Body Water Loss	Severity	Signs and Symptoms
3%	Mild	Decreased skin turgor, sunken eyes, dry mucous membranes, dry tongue, reduced sweating
6%	Moderate	Oliguria, orthostatic hypotension, tachycardia, low volume pulse, cool peripheries, reduced filling of peripheral veins and CVP, hemoconcentration
9%	Severe	Profound oliguria or anuria and compromised CNS function with or without altered sensorium

What Are the Ongoing Losses?
- Tubes – Foley catheter, NG, surgical drains
- Third spacing – pleura, GI, retroperitoneal, peritoneal, evaporation via exposed viscera, burns
- Blood loss
- Ongoing loss due to type of surgery
  - Minor surgery   4 cc/kg/h
  - Internal surgery   6 cc/kg/h
  - Major surgery   8 cc/kg/h

IV Fluid Solutions

- Improves perfusion but not O_2 carrying capacity of blood

Crystalloid Infusion
- Salt-containing solutions that distribute within ECF
- Maintain euvolemia in patient with blood loss: 3 mL crystalloid infusion per 1 mL of blood loss for volume replacement (i.e. 3:1 replacement)
- If large volumes required, use balanced fluid such as Ringer's lactate or Plasmalyte® as too much normal saline (NS) may lead to hyperchloremic metabolic acidosis

IV Fluid Solutions

		ECF	Ringer's Lactate	0.9 NS	0.45 NS	D5W	2/3 + 1/3	Plasmalyte
mEq/L	Na+	142	130	154	77	–	51	140
	K+	4	4	–	–	–	–	5
	Ca²⁺	4	3	–	–	–	–	–
	Mg²⁺	3	–	–	–	–	–	3
	Cl⁻	103	109	154	77	–	51	98
	HCO₃⁻	27	28*	–	–	–	–	27
mOsm/L		280-310	273	308	407	253	269	294

* converted from lactate

Colloid Infusion
- Collected from donor blood (fresh frozen plasma, albumin, RBCs) or synthetics (e.g. starch products)
- Distributes within intravascular volume
- 1:1 ratio (infusion:blood loss) only in terms of replacing volume

Blood Products

Red Blood Cells (RBCs) (U = unit)
- 1 U RBCs = approx. 300 mL; increases Hb by approx. 10 g/L in a 70 kg patient
- Decision to transfuse based on initial blood volume, premorbid Hb level, present volume status, expected further blood loss, patient health status
- Massive transfusion → 1 x blood volume/24 h

Autologous RBCs
- Replacement of blood volume with one's own RBCs
- Marked decrease in complications (infectious, febrile, etc.)
- Alternative to homologous transfusion in elective procedures, but only if adequate Hb and no infection
- Pre-op phlebotomy with hemodilution prior to elective surgery (up to 4 U collected >2 d before surgery)
- Intraoperative salvage and filtration (cell saver)

Non-RBC Products
- Fresh frozen plasma (FFP)
    - Contains all plasma clotting factors and fibrinogen close to normal plasma levels
    - To prevent/treat bleeding due to coagulation factor depletion/deficiencies, liver failure, massive transfusions
- Cryoprecipitate: contains Factors VIII and XIII, vWF, fibrinogen
- Platelets: used in thrombocytopenia, massive transfusions, impaired platelet function
- Albumin: selective intravascular volume expander
- Erythropoietin: can be used preoperatively to stimulate erythropoiesis

Transfusion Reactions
- Infectious risks: HIV, hepatitis B/C, Epstein-Barr virus (EBV), cytomegalovirus (CMV), brucellosis, malaria, salmonellosis, measles, syphilis
- Hypervolemia, electrolyte changes (increased K^+ in stored blood), coagulopathy, hypothermia, citrate toxicity, hypocalcemia
- Transfusion-related immunosuppression: peri-operative transfusion may be associated with increased risk of post-operative infection, increased short-term mortality and earlier cancer recurrence

Common Medications

Intravenous Induction Agents

	Propofol (Diprivan®)	Thiopental	Ketamine	Benzodiazepine (Midazolam, Diazepam, Lorazepam)
Class Action	Hypnotic Inhibitory at GABA synapse ↓ ICP, SVR, BP and SV	Hypnotic ↓ duration of Cl⁻ channel opening ↓ cerebral metabolism, CPP, CO and respiration	Dissociative May act on NMDA ↑ HR, BP, SVR	Anxiolytic Causes ↑ glycine inhibitory neurotransmitter, facilitates GABA Minimal cardiorespiratory depression
Indications	Induction Maintenance	Induction Control of convulsive states	Major trauma Severe asthma, hypovolemia	Used for sedation, amnesia and anxiolysis
Contraindication/ Cautions	Egg/soy allergy, may cause hypotension Orapnea	Hypotension, shock, cardiac failure, liver disease, status asthmaticus, myxedema, porphyria	Concomitant TCA use, Hx of psychosis, may cause HTN and increased ICP	May cause resp. depression
Dose	1-2 mg/kg	3-6 mg/kg	1-2 mg/kg	Depends on use

Volatile Inhalational Anesthetics

	Sevoflurane	Desflurane	Isoflurane	Enflurane	Halothane	Nitrous Oxide (N_2O)*
MAC (% gas in O_2)	2.0	6.0	1.2	1.7	0.8	104
CNS	↑ ICP	↑ ICP	↓ cerebral metabolic rate, ↑ ICP	EEG seizure-like activity, ↑ ICP	↑ ICP and CBF	
Resp	Respiratory depression (↓↓ TV, ↑ RR), iresponse to respiratory CO_2 reflexes, bronchodilation					
CVS	Less ↓ of contractility, conduction	Tachycardia with rapid ↑ in cases	↓ BP and CO, ↑ HR, chance of coronary steal**	Stable HR ↓ contractility	↓ BP, CO, and sensitizes myocardium to epinephrine arrhythmias	Can cause ↓ HR in pediatric Myocardial depression in those with heart disease
MSK	Muscle relaxation, potentiation of other muscle relaxants, uterine relaxation					

*Properties and Adverse Effects of N_2O
Due to its high MAC, nitrous oxide is combined with other agents to attain surgical anesthesia. A MAC of 104% is possible in a pressurized chamber only.
Expansion of closed spaces: closed spaces such as a pneumothorax, the middle ear, bowel lumen and ETT cuff will markedly enlarge if N_2O is administered.
Diffusion hypoxia: During anesthesia, the washout of N_2O from body stores into alveoli can dilute the alveolar [O_2], creating a hypoxic mixture if the original [O_2] is low.
**Coronary Steal: N_2O causes small vessel dilation which may compromise blood flow to poorly perfused areas of heart.

Sample MAC Value Calculation
35% Nitrous Oxide (MAC = 104%): MAC Value = 35/104 = 0.33 MAC
1.8% Sevoflurane (MAC = 2%): MAC Value = 1.8/2 = 0.9 MAC
Total MAC Value: 0.33 MAC + 0.9 MAC = 1.23 MAC

Muscle Relaxants

Depolarizing Neuromuscular Relaxant (Non-competitive): succinylcholine (SCh)

Mechanism of Action	Mimics ACh and binds to ACh receptors causing depolarization followed by paralysis
Intubating Dose	1-2 mg/kg
Onset	30-60 s – RAPID
Duration	5-10 min – SHORT. There is NO reversal agent for SCh
Metabolism	Plasma cholinesterase

Non-Depolarizing Neuromuscular Relaxants (Competitive)

Mechanism of Action	Competitive blockade of postsynaptic ACh receptors preventing depolarization		
Classification	**Short Acting** mivacuronium	**Intermediate Acting** rocuronium	**Long Acting** pancuronium
Intubating Dose (mg/kg)	0.2	0.6	0.1
Onset (min)	2-3	1.5	3-5
Duration (min)	15-25	30-45	90-120
Metabolism	Plasma cholinesterase	Liver (major) Renal (minor)	Renal (major) Liver (minor)

Reversal Agents for Non-Depolarizing Relaxants
• Atropine and glycopyrrolate are anticholinergic agents administered during the administration of reversal agents to minimize muscarinic effects

Cholinesterase Inhibitor	Neostigmine	Pyridostigmine	Edrophonium
Onset and Duration	Intermediate	Longest	Shortest
Mechanism of Action	Acetylcholinesterase inhibitors: inhibits enzymatic degredation of ACh thus increasing ACh at nicotinic and muscarinic receptors, displacing non-depolarizing muscle relaxants. Muscarinic effects of reversing agents include unwanted bradycardia, salivation and increased bowel peristalsis; countered by anticholinergics		
Dose	0.04-0.08 mg/kg	0.1-0.4mg/kg	0.5-1mg/kg
Recommended Anticholinergic	Glycopyrrolate	Glycopyrrolate	Atropine
Dose of Anticholinergic per mg of Cholinesterase Inhibitor	0.2 mg	0.05 mg	0.014 mg

Opioids

Agent	Infusion Rate	PCA Dose	PCA Lockout Interval
morphine	0.3-0.9 mg/h	0.2-0.3 mg	30 min
fentanyl	25-50 ug/h	20-30 ug	15 min
hydromorphone	0.1-0.2 mg/h	0.15 ug	30 min

Agent	Moderate Dose	Onset	Duration	Special Considerations
morphine	0.2-0.3 mg/kg	Moderate	Moderate	Histamine release leading to decrease in BP
meperidine (Demerol®)	2-3 mg/kg	Moderate	Moderate	Anticholinergic, hallucinations, less pupillary constriction than morphine, metabolite build up may cause seizures
codeine	0.5-1 mg/kg	Moderate	Moderate	Primarily postoperative use, not for IV use
hydromorphone (Dilaudid®)	30-80 µg/kg	Moderate	Moderate	
fentanyl	3-10 µg/kg	Rapid	Short	Transient muscle rigidity in very high doses
remifentanil	0.5-1.5 µg/kg	Rapid	Ultra-short	Only use during induction and maintenance of anesthesia

Opioid Equivalent Doses in Pain Management
• Note: usual starting therapeutic doses are lower than those listed below

Generic Name	Proprietary Name	Route		Comments
		Oral	IV	
Codeine	Tylenol® #1, #2, #3 Codeine Contin	200 mg	120 mg	Metabolized to morphine (~7-10% of whites are non-metabolizers due to CYP2D6 genetic Limited by potential toxicities of acetaminophen with which it is often combined No additional benefit at doses >200 mg
Morphine	MSIR®; MS Contin®; M-Eslon® (controlled release PO); various names for oral IV form	30-60 mg	10 mg	Parenteral 10 mg morphine is (immediate release usual standard for comparison Morphine PO:IV = 60:10 for opioid naïve patient, 30:10 for others Do not crush, break, or chew controlled release morphine
Oxycodone	OxyContin®; Oxy IR®; Endocone®, Percocet, Percodan (with ASA/Acetaminophen)	30 mg	15 mg	Use caution if administering additional acetaminophen or ASA
Hydrocodone	Vicodin®, Lortab®	20 mg	Not available	Quick onset of action and thus highly addictive Limited by potential toxicities of the acetaminophen or ibuprofen with which it is combined
Hydromorphone	Dilaudid	7.5 mg	1.5 mg	PO especially useful for initial dose titration and pm supplementation IV form often used subcutaneously

Opioid Equivalent Doses in Pain Management

Generic Name	Proprietary Name	Route		Comments
		Oral	IV	
Meperidine	Demerol®	300 mg	75 mg	Rarely used May cause seizures due to the accumulation of metabolite normeperidine Should not be used longer than 48h and no more than 600 μg/24h Contraindicated with MAOIs
Fentanyl	Sublimaze®	Not available	0.1 mg	Minimal use in outpatient setting
Fentanyl	Duragesic® (transdermal)	Transdermal 50 μg/h patch = Morphine 100 mg PO/24h = 16 mg PO q4h = 1.4 mg/h IV		Usually for stable pain, especially in patients with GI dysfunction
Methadone	Dolophine®	20 mg	10 mg	Long variable half-life, which may complicate titration
Levorphanol	Levodromoran®	4 mg	2 mg	Long half-life with relatively, short dosing interval

- Opioids are constipating and can induce nausea/vomiting (the latter only at initiation) – do not forget to compensate with stool softeners (e.g. sennekot or lactulose) and antiemetics (e.g. dimenhydrinate)
- Mild to moderate pain: codeine, hydrocodone and oxycodone
- Moderate to severe pain: morphine, hydromorphone, oxycodone, fentanyl, methadone or levophanol
- When converting from one opioid to another, use 50-70% of the equivalent dose to allow for incomplete cross-tolerance. Rapid titration and breakthrough use may be required to ensure effective analgesia for the first 24 h

Local Anesthetic Agents

	Max. Dose	Max. Dose with Epinephrine	Potency	Duration
chlorprocaine	11 mg/kg	14 mg/kg	low	15-30 min
lidocaine	5 mg/kg	7 mg/kg	medium	1-2 h
bupivicaine	2.5 mg/kg	3 mg/kg	high	3-8 h

Conscious Sedation

Adults

Sedation
Midazolam (Versed®): the total dose in adults is 0.02-0.1 mg/kg
Propofol: 10-20 mg increments, titrating to adequate sedation

Analgesia
Morphine sulfate: the dose is 0.1-0.15 mg/kg (5-10 mg initially for adults), with additional doses as needed
Or
Fentanyl (Sublimaze®): the intravenous dose is 2-3 μg/kg (50-200 μg in adults), titrated in 50-100 μg increments

Precautions
Supply supplemental oxygen to patient with saturation monitoring – Prepare for intubation if necessary. Naloxone at bedside
The patient should be observed for at least 1h before being discharged in the care of family or friends

Cardiology and Cardiovascular Surgery

Essential History, Physical Exam and Investigations

History

Signs and Symptoms	Risk Factors and Other Key Questions
Chest pain (OPQRST)	Previous cardiac history (chest pain angina, MI, diagnostic tests, GERD, PUD)
Palpitations	Hospitalizations/ICU admissions)
SOB on exertion/at rest, orthopnea, PND	Cardiac risk factors
Dizziness, pre-syncope, syncope	• **Major**: smoking, DM, HTN, hyperlipidemia, family history (1° male relative
Ankle swelling, increasing abdominal girth	before age 55 and 1° female relatives before age 65)
Cough (pulmonary edema vs. S/E of ACEI)	• **Minor**: male or post-menopausal female, obesity, sedentary lifestyle,
Melena	hyperhomocysteinemia
N&V	Ability to perform ADLs; most vigorous exercise daily/weekly
Diaphoresis	Medications
Fever	EtOH history

SOB: Shortness of breath; PND: Paroxysmal Nocturnal Dyspnea; HTN: hypertension; ADLs: Activities of Daily Living; EtOH: Alcohol; DM: Diabetes Melitus

Physical Exam

Precordial	Other
Inspection	Vitals (including orthostatic if sx of dizziness/presyncope/syncope)
Palpation (PMI, heaves, thrills, lifts, palpable S2)	Chest – auscultation for crackles/wheezes
Percussion (consolidation, changes in cardiac dullness)	JVP, AJR
	Kussmaul's Sign (paradoxical rise in JVP with inspiration, seen in RV dysfunction)
Auscultation (S1, S2, extra heart sounds, murmurs, irregular rhythms, pericardial rubs, crackles, wheezes, reduced breath sounds)	Ankle swelling
	Bruits (carotid, renal)
	Hepatomegaly, ascites, ankle edema
	Capillary refill
	Abdominal tenderness
	Costochondral tenderness

JVP: Jugular Venous Pressure; AJR: Abdominojugular Reflex

JUGULAR VENOUS PRESSURE (JVP)

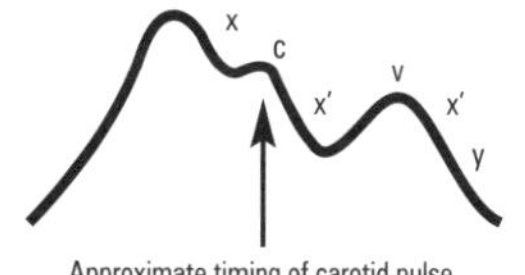

"a" wave   = atrial contraction
"x" descent = atrial relaxation
"c" wave   = bulging of tricuspid valve during RV systole
"x'" descent = descent of base of heart during ventricular systole
"v" wave   = passive atrial filling against closed aortic valve
"y" descent = early rapid atrial emptying following opening of aortic valve

CARDIAC MURMURS

Description of Murmurs

Characteristic	Description
Intensity	**Grade 1-6** Grade 1: the faintest sound (with difficulty) that can be heard with a stethoscope Grade 2: faint but with immediate identification Grade 3: moderately loud Grade 4: loud and associated with a palpable thrill Grade 5: very loud, can be heard with stethoscope slightly off the skin Grade 6: can be heard without the aid of a stethoscope
Pitch	High or low frequency, described as harsh, musical, blowing, or rumbling
Shape	Rising in intensity (crescendo), diminishing (decrescendo), combination of both, or unchanged
Location	Site where murmur is best auscultated
Timing	Grossly divided into continuous, systolic, or diastolic Further subdivided into complete (i.e. holosystolic), early, middle, or late phases of each cardiac cycle component
Radiation	Site outside of the major four zones of auscultation where a murmur is heard (i.e. axilla, clavicle, carotid)

Murmurs in Valvular Disease

Aortic Stenosis
Crescendo-decrescendo systolic ejection murmur
Best heard at base
Radiates to right clavicle and carotid
May be associated with pulsus tardus et parvus
Soft S2 with paradoxical splitting, may hear S4
Distinguished from aortic sclerosis which does not radiate to the clavicle

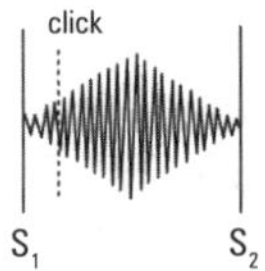

© Anas Nader 2009

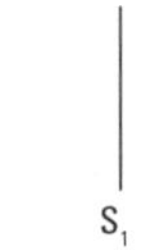

Aortic Regurgitation/Insufficiency
Early decrescendo, high-pitched blowing diastolic
Soft S1, absent S2
Best heard at the lower left sternal border
Accentuated when sitting forward and in full expiration
May radiate to apex and right sternal border
May have mid-systolic flow murmur or Austin Flint murmur (i.e. diastolic rumble)

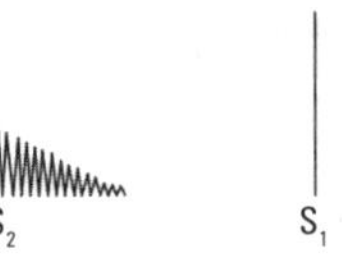

© Anas Nader 2009

Mitral Stenosis
Low-pitched mid-diastolic rumbling murmur
Loud S1, opening snap after S2
Best heard at apex with bell, accentuated in left lateral decubitus position
Little or no radiation

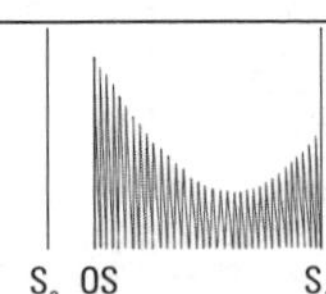

© Anas Nader 2011

Mitral Regurgitation
Holosystolic, high-pitched blowing murmur
Decreased S1, may hear S3
Best heard with diaphragm at the apex
Radiates to the left axilla

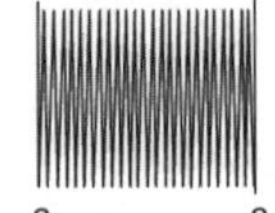

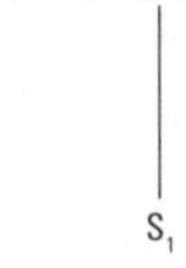
© Anas Nader 2009

Reference: http://www.andrewjohnpublishing.com/CGJIM/CJGIM%20volume%202%20issue%202/cjgim22thephysicalbasisofheartmurmurs.html

Investigations

ECG Waveforms and Normal Values

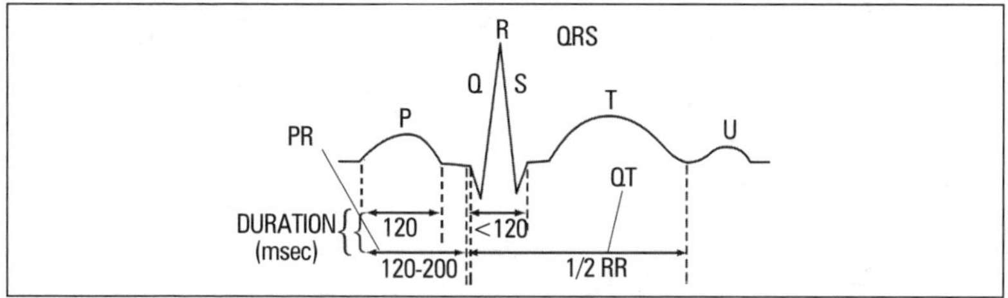

Approach to the ECG

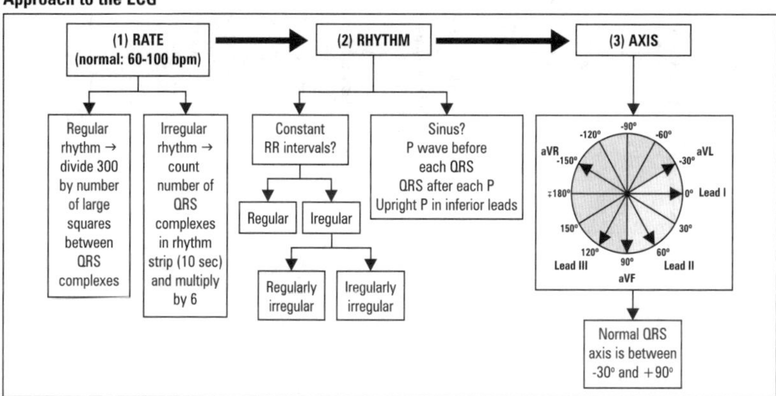

• See next page for Approach to the ECG continued

Approach to the ECG (continued)

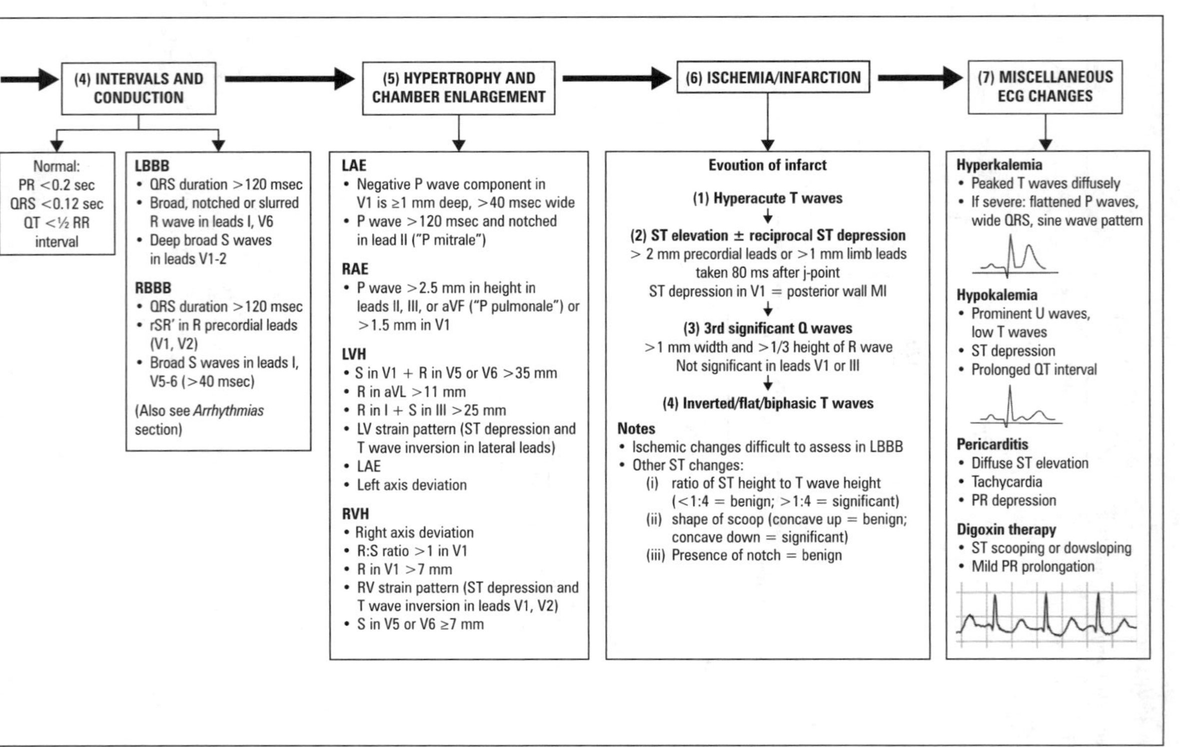

Approach to MI

Anatomic Area of Infarct	Leads with STE	Vessel
Septal	V1, V2	Proximal LAD
Anterior	V3, V4	LAD
Apical	V5, V6	Distal LAD, circumflex, RCA
Anterolateral	I, aVL, V1-V6	LAD
Lateral	I, aVL, V5-V6	Circumflex
Posterior	ST depression in V1, V2	RCA/circumflex
Inferior	II, III, aVF	RCA, rarely circumflex
Right Ventricle	V1, V2, V3R, V4R	RCA

STE – ST segment elevation; LAD – Left anterior descending artery; RCA – right coronary artery

CAUSES OF ST SEGMENT CHANGES
- ST elevation
  - Benign: normal variant "early repolarization" (correlate with old ECGs)
  - Ischemia/infarction: acute MI (STEMI), ischemia with reciprocal change, Prinzmetal's angina (coronary artery spasm), tight coronary stenosis
  - Structural abnormalities: LVH, ventricular aneurysm
  - Other conditions: cardiac [LBBB, acute pericarditis (diffuse ST changes)], systemic [advanced hyperkalemia, hypothermia (Osborne waves)]
- ST depression
  - Ischemia/infarction: NSTEMI or ischemia, STEMI with reciprocal changes, post-MI
  - Structural abnormalities: LVH or RVH with strain
  - Conduction abnormalities: left or right BBB, WPW
  - Digitalis effect ("scooping")

CAUSES OF TALL R-WAVE IN LEAD V1
  - Benign: dextrocardia
  - Ischemic changes: posterior wall MI
  - Structural abnormalties: RVH
  - Conduction abnormalities: RBBB, WPW
  - Other: Duchenne's muscular dystrophy

Stress Testing

Approach to Stress Tests

Test	Indication
Exercise ECG	To diagnose CAD with possible ACS and negative serum biomarkers. Initial evaluation in patients without difficult-to-interpret ECGs who are able to exercise
Exercise Stress Echo	ECG is difficult to interpret (e.g. resting LBBB, resting ST abnormalities, LV strain pattern, patient on digoxin or estrogen) Intermediate pre-test probability with normal/equivocal exercise ECG Post-ACS: used to decide on potential efficacy of revascularization
Dobutamine Stress Echo	In patients unable to exercise and same indications as exercise echo
Exercise Myocardial Perfusion Imaging (MPI)	When ECG is difficult to interpret (e.g. resting LBBB, resting ST abnormalities, LV strain pattern, patient on digoxin or estrogen) Intermediate pre-test probability with normal/equivocal exercise ECG In patients with previous imaging whose symptoms have changed
Dipyridamole/Adenosine MPI	In patients unable to exercise and same indications as exercise echo

Contraindications to Exercise Testing

Acute MI
Aortic dissection
Pericarditis
PE
Severe aortic stenosis
Severe HTN
Inability to exercise adequately

Stress Testing: Sensitivity and Specificity

Test	Sensitivity	Specificity
Exercise ECG	68	77
Stress Echo	76	88
PET scanning	91	82
Myocardial Perfusion Imaging (MPI)	88	77

Common Presentations

Chest Pain

Differential Diagnoses of Chest Pain

Non-pleuritic		Pleuritic	
Pulmonary	**Subdiaphragmatic**	**Pulmonary**	**GI**
Pneumonia	PUD	Pneumonia	Pancreatitis
PE	Gastritis	PE	Subphrenic abscess
Neoplastic	Biliary colic	Pneumothorax	
	Pancreatic	Hemothorax	**MSK**
Cardiac	Achalasia	Bronchiectasis	Costochondritis
MI		Neoplasm	Fractured Rib
Myocarditis	**Vascular**	TB	Myositis
Pericarditis	Dissecting aortic aneurysm	Empyema	Herpes zoster
			Dressler's syndrome
Esophageal	**MSK**	**Cardiac**	
GERD	Costochondritis	Pericarditis	
Spasm	Skin		
Esophagitis	Breast		
Ulceration	Ribs		
Achalasia			
Neoplasm			
Mediastinal			
Lymphoma			
Thymoma			

6 Chest Pains that Kill
- MI
- Tension pneumothorax
- Aortic dissection
- Tamponade
- Massive PE
- Esophageal rupture

Canadian Cardiovascular Society (CCS) Functional Classification of Angina

Class I: Ordinary physical activity (walking, climbing stairs) does not cause angina; angina with strenuous, rapid, or prolonged activity

Class II: Slight limitation of ordinary activity; angina at >2 blocks on level or climbing >1 flight of stairs or by emotional stress

Class III: Marked limitation of ordinary activity; angina at ≤2 blocks on level or climbing ≤1 flight of stairs

Class IV: Inability to carry out any physical activity without discomfort; angina may be present at rest

Campeau L. Grading of angina pectoris(Letter). *Circulation*. 1976; 54:522-523.

Palpitations

- **Cardiac**: arrhythmias (PAB, PVB, SVT, VT), mitral valve prolapse, valvular heart disease, HCM
- **Endocrine**: thyrotoxicosis, pheochromocytoma, hypoglycemia
- **Systemic**: fever, anemia
- **Drugs**: tobacco, caffeine, EtOH, epinephrine, ephedrine, aminophylline, atropine
- **Psychiatric**: panic attack

Syncope

- **Cardiac**
  - **Structural or obstructive causes**: myocardial disease (e.g. ACS), aortic stenosis, HCM with outflow tract obstruction, cardiac tamponade/constrictive pericarditis
  - **Arrhythmias**: bradyarrythmias (sick sinus syndrome, sinus node ischemia, AV block, pacemaker dysfunction); tachyarrhythmias (SVT, ventricular tachycardia/fibrillation, Torsades de Pointes)
- **Non-cardiac**
  - **Hypovolemia/Orthostatic**: blood loss, decreased fluid intake, increased fluid losses, third spacing
  - **Respiratory**: massive PE, pulmonary HTN (exertional), hypoxia, hypercapnia
  - **Neurologic**: stroke/TIA (esp. vertebrobasilar insufficiency), migraine, seizure, neurocardiogenic (vasovagal)
  - **Neurocardiogenic**: i.e. vasovagal
  - **Metabolic**: anemia, hypoglycemia
  - **Drugs**: antihypertensives, antiarrhythmics, β-blockers, CCBs
  - **Psychiatric**: panic attack

Common Conditions

Coronary Artery Disease and Acute Coronary Syndromes

Definitions

Chronic Stable Angina
- Angina reproducible with exertion; relieved with nitroglycerin and rest; no changes in quality or quantity of exertion for pain threshold; and no pain at rest
- Due to narrowed coronary arteries secondary to plaque and atherosclerosis producing reduced coronary blood flow

Unstable Angina
- New onset angina or angina at rest or increasing frequency of angina with reduced thresholds of exertion or angina following MI, PCI or CABG; no ECG changes and no changes in myocardial biomarkers
- Due to plaque rupture or embolism leading to transient myocardial ischemia without evidence of myocardial necrosis

Non ST-elevation Myocardial Infarction (NSTEMI)
- Defined by symptoms of angina or ischemia, rise of myocardial biomarkers (e.g. troponins) and evolution of ischemic ECG changes (not ST-elevation or new BBB)
- Due to plaque rupture or embolism leading to transient myocardial ischemia with evidence of myocardial necrosis

ST-elevation Myocardial Infarction (STEMI)
- Defined by symptoms of ischemia, rise of myocardial biomarkers (e.g. troponins) and ischemic ECG changes demonstrating ST-elevation in 2 contiguous leads (>1 mm in limb leads and >2 mm in precordial leads) or new LBBB
- Due to acute plaque rupture and thrombosis leading to complete coronary occlusion and myocardial necrosis

MANAGEMENT OF ACS (unstable angina, NSTEMI, STEMI)

Risk stratification

TIMI Risk Score for UA/NSTEMI

Characteristics	Points	Characteristics	Points
Historical		**Presentation**	
Age ≥65 yrs	1	Recent (≤24 h) severe angina	1
≥3 risk factors for CAD	1	ST-segment deviation ≥0.5 mm	1
Known CAD (stenosis ≥50%)	1	Increased cardiac markers	1
Aspirin use in past 7 d	1		
		Risk Score = Total Points	(0-7)

Score of 0-1=4.7% risk, 2=8.3%, 3=13.2%, 4=19.9%,, 5=26.2%, 6-7=>40.9%
CAD = coronary artery disease   NSTEMI = non ST-segment elevation myocardial infarction
TIMI = thrombolysis in myocardial infarction   UA = unstable angina   *JAMA* 2000;284:835-842

Contraindications for Thrombolysis in STEMI

Absolute	Relative
Prior intracranial hemorrhage	Chronic, severe, poorly controlled HTN
Known structural cerebral vascular lesion	Uncontrolled HTN (sBP >180, dBP >110)
Known malignant intracranial neoplasm	Current anticoagulation
Significant closed-head or facial trauma (≤3 months)	Noncompressible vascular punctures (i.e. subclavian line site)
Ischemic stroke (≤3 months)	Ischemic stroke (≥3 months)
Active bleeding	Recent internal bleeding (≤2-4 wks)
Suspected aortic dissection	Prolonged CPR or major surgery (≤3 wks)
	Pregnancy
	Active peptic ulcer

Inpatient Management
- Investigations: frequent ECG; 2D echo; consider coronary angiography, stress ECG test and/or stress imaging tests (stress echo or myocardial perfusion imaging)
- Medications: β-blocker to titrate heart rate to 50-60 bpm or non-dihydropyridine calcium channel blocker (e.g. diltiazem, verapamil) if severe reactive airways or bronchospasm and ongoing ischemia; ACEI after initial stabilization; statin regardless of serum cholesterol level; ASA 81 mg; nitroglycerin; clopidrogrel 300 mg unless likely to proceed to CABG; heparin (LMWH or unfractionated), GPIIb/IIIa inhibitor OR clopidogrel if PCI planned or high risk
- Other: CCU observation for 2-3 d

Discharge
- Cardiac rehabilitation program; risk factor evaluation including fasting lipids, blood glucose, smoking cessation program, driving recommendations ± Ministry of Transportantion (MOT) notification. (See CCS Driving Guidelines 2004 for details (mobile Apps available on iOS & BB))

Treatment Algorithm for Chest Pain

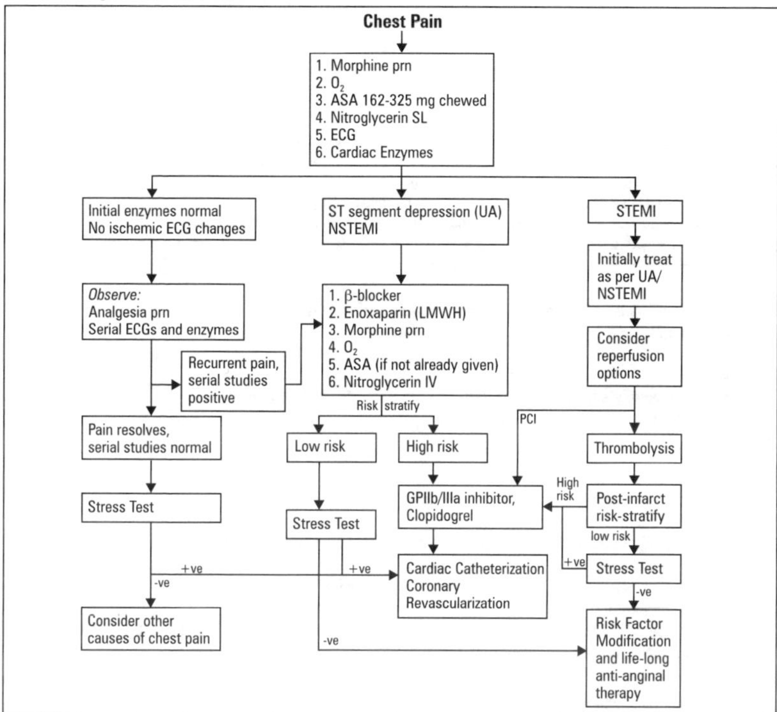

Adapted from *Cecil Essentials of Medicine* 6th Ed. Andreoli and Carpenter. p.101 (2004) with permission from Elsevier

Congestive Heart Failure

Classification
- **Direction**: systolic dysfunction (forward): unable to match cardiac output to meet demands vs. diastolic dysfunction (backward): decreased compliance leading to upstream venous congestion
- **Structural**: left-sided vs. right-sided
- **Output**: low-output vs. high-output: caused by demand for increased cardiac output

Etiologies
- CAD, HTN, idiopathic, valvular disease, EtOH, toxic (e.g. doxorubicin, radiation, uremia), infectious (e.g. Coxsackie virus, Chagas disease, HIV), endocrine (e.g. hyperthyroidism, DM, acromegaly), infiltrative (e.g. amyloidosis, sarcoidosis, hemochromatosis), genetic (e.g. cardiomyopathies, muscular dystrophy), metabolic (e.g. thiamine deficiency)

Precipitants
- **"HEART FAILED"**: **H**ypertension, **E**nvironment/Endocarditis, **A**nemia, **R**heumatic heart disease and other valve disease, **T**hyrotoxicosis, **F**ailure to take medications, **A**rrhythmia, **I**nfection/Ischemia/Infarction, **L**ung problems (e.g. PE, pneumonia, COPD), **E**ndocrine (e.g. pheo, hyperaldosteronism), **D**ietary indiscretions

Differential Diagnoses
• Pneumonia, pneumothorax, pleural effusion, PE, empyema, MI, COPD exacerbation, pulmonary HTN

Symptoms
• SOB with or without exertion, PND, orthopnea, weight gain, ankle swelling, fatigue, nocturnal cough, RUQ discomfort, anorexia

---

New York Heart Association (NYHA) Functional Classification of Heart Failure

Class I: Patients with cardiac disease but ordinary physical activity does not cause undue fatigue, palpitations, dyspnea or angina
Class II: Comfortable at rest, ordinary physical activity results in symptoms
Class III: Marked limitation of activity; less than ordinary physical activity results in symptoms
Class IV: Inability to carry out any physical activity without discomfort; symptoms may be present at rest

---

Signs
• Distended neck veins, increased JVP, abdominojugular reflex, S3 gallop, rales/crackles, wheezing, pleural effusions, peripheral edema, ascites, hepatic congestion

Investigations
• Blood: CBC, electrolytes, TSH, brain natriuretic peptide (BNP), serum transaminases, Cr, fasting blood glucose
• Urine: urinalysis, urine electrolytes, urine output
• Radiologic: ECG, chest x-ray, 2D echo
• Other: daily weights

Management (Inpatient/Outpatient)
• Chronic
  ▪ Mortality benefit for NYHA class III or IV: ACEI/ARB, β-blocker (e.g. carvedilol, bisoprolol), aldosterone antagonists (e.g. spironolactone, epleronone)
  ▪ Morbidity and selective benefit: loop diuretics (e.g. furosemide), inotropes (e.g. digoxin), calcium channel blockers, anti-arrhythmics
  ▪ Contraindicated or cautioned: NSAIDs, metformin, thiazolidinediones, class I and III anti-arrhythmics, PDE5 inhibitors with low blood pressure (e.g. sildenafil)
• Acute
  ▪ Symptomatic relief
  ▪ Lasix
  ▪ Morphine (improves SOB, venodilator, ↓ afterload)
  ▪ Nitrates (venodilator)
  ▪ O_2
  ▪ Position (sit up) and positive pressure ventilation

Pericarditis

Etiology
• Idiopathic (most common), infection (Coxsackie virus, echovirus, *S. pneumoniae*, *S. aureus*, TB, histoplasmosis, blastomycosis), post-MI (Dressler's syndrome if 2-8 wks, direct extension if earlier), metabolic (uremia, hypothyroidism), neoplastic (Hodgkin's disease, breast, lung, renal cell, melanoma), collagen vascular disease (SLE, scleroderma, RA), medications (hydralazine), radiation, infiltrative disease (sarcoidosis)

Signs and Symptoms
• **Diagnostic triad:** pleuritic chest pain (often alleviated by leaning forward), pericardial friction rub (in atrial/ventricular systole ± rapid ventricular filling phase), and characteristic ECG changes (diffuse ST elevation initially that resolves to flattened and inverted T waves over days, PR depression)

Investigations
- Bloodwork: may see increased cardiac markers (e.g. troponin and CK-MB), increased CRP (suggestive)
- ECG changes (above), CXR (normal heart size with pulmonary infiltrates), echo (pericardial effusion)

Treatment
- Treat the underlying cause, high-dose NSAIDs for idiopathic/viral, consider addition of colchicine $\pm$ glucocorticoids if refractory

Arrhythmias

Approach to Arrhythmias

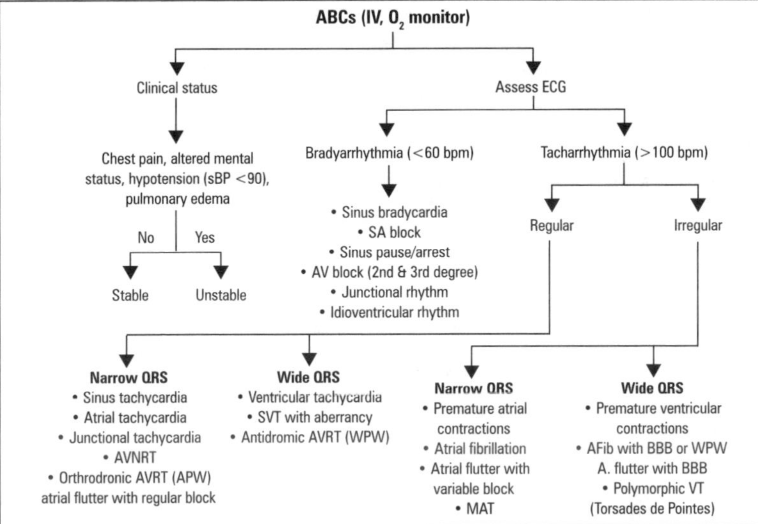

Atrial Fibrillation

Definition
- An irregularly irregular arrhythmia characterized by disordered atrial activity and decrease in cardiac output

Etiology
- HTN, CAD, valvular disease, pericarditis, cardiomyopathy, myocarditis, structural heart defect, PE, COPD, thyrotoxicosis, sick sinus syndrome, EtOH (i.e. holiday heart)

Symptoms
- May be asymptomatic
- Cardiac: chest pain, palpitations, dyspnea, presyncope/syncope
- Neurology: embolic stroke

Investigations
- Bloodwork to investigate possible etiologies/precipitants
- ECG: absence of organized P waves, chaotic baseline with fibrillatory waves, irregular ventricular response >100/min, generally narrow QRS

Atrial Fibrillation (AFib)

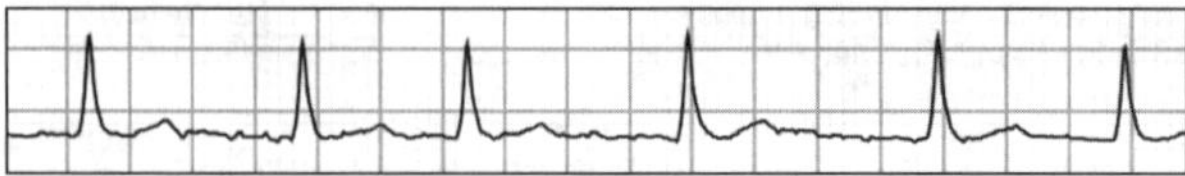

Management

CHADS2 Risk Prediction for Non-Valvular AF

Risk Factor	Points	CHADS Score	Stroke Risk (%/Yr)	Anticoagulation Recommendation
Congestive Heart Failure	1	0	1.9 (low)	ASA 81-325 mg daily
Hypertension	1	1	2.8 (low-mod)	Dabigitran or Warfarin (INR 2-3) or ASA 81-325 mg daily
Age >75	1	2-3	4.0-5.9 (mod)	Dabigitran or Warfarin (INR 2-3)
Diabetes	1	4-6	8.5-18.2 (high)	Dabigitran or Warfarin (INR 2-3)
Stroke/TIA (prior)	2			

JAMA 2001; 285(22):2864-70); Canadian Journal of Cardiology 27 (2011) 74–90.

Management of New-Onset AF

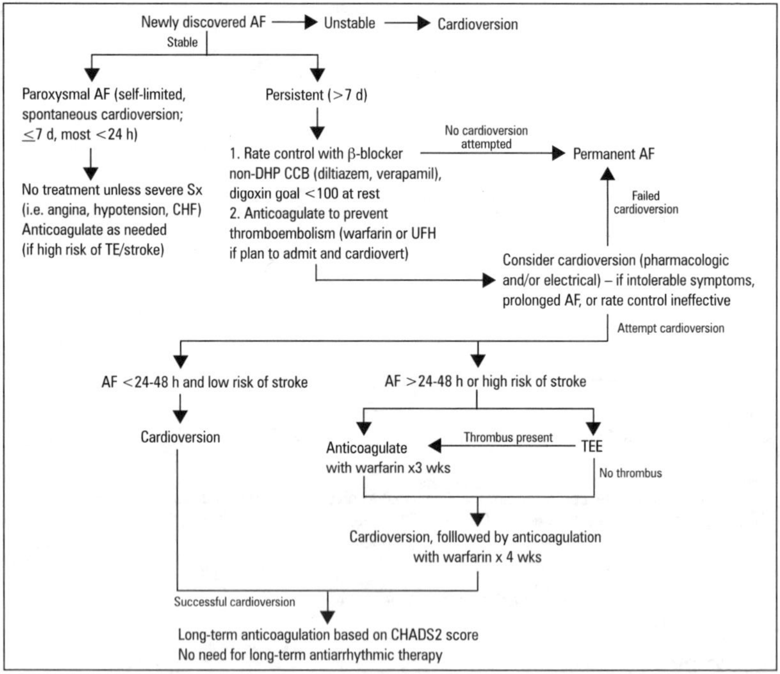

Newly discovered AF ⟶ Unstable ⟶ Cardioversion

Stable

Paroxysmal AF (self-limited, spontaneous cardioversion; ≤7 d, most <24 h)
↓
No treatment unless severe Sx (i.e. angina, hypotension, CHF) Anticoagulate as needed (if high risk of TE/stroke)

Persistent (>7 d)
↓
1. Rate control with β-blocker non-DHP CCB (diltiazem, verapamil), digoxin goal <100 at rest
2. Anticoagulate to prevent thromboembolism (warfarin or UFH if plan to admit and cardiovert)

No cardioversion attempted ⟶ **Permanent AF**

Failed cardioversion

Consider cardioversion (pharmacologic and/or electrical) – if intolerable symptoms, prolonged AF, or rate control ineffective

Attempt cardioversion

AF <24-48 h and low risk of stroke
↓
Cardioversion

AF >24-48 h or high risk of stroke
↓
Anticoagulate with warfarin x3 wks ⟵ Thrombus present ⟵ TEE
No thrombus
↓
Cardioversion, folllowed by anticoagulation with warfarin x 4 wks

Successful cardioversion
↓
Long-term anticoagulation based on CHADS2 score
No need for long-term antiarrhythmic therapy

From ACC/AHA/ESC Guideline for the Management of Patients With Atrial Fibrillation: Executive Summary, *Circulation* 2006; 114:700-52, http://www.americanheart.org

See CCS Atrial Fibrillation Guidelines 2010 for details (mobile apps available on iOS & BB)

Valvular Disease

Mechanical Valve vs. Bioprosthetic Valve

Mechanical Valve	Bioprosthetic Valve
Good durability	Limited long-term durability (mitral<aortic)
Less preferred in small aortic root sizes	Good flow in small aortic root sizes
Increased risk of thromboembolism (1-3%/yr) requiring long-term anticoagulation with coumadin	Decreased risk of thromboembolism: long-term anticoagulation not needed for aortic valves
Target INR • 2.0-3.0 – aortic valves • 2.5-3.5 – mitral valves	Anticoagulation for first three months for AVR and MVR Decreased risk of hemorrhage
Increased risk of hemorrhage: 1-2%/yr	

Vascular Disease

ACUTE ARTERIAL OCCLUSION/INSUFFICIENCY

Signs and Symptoms
• 6 P's: **P**ain, **P**allor, **P**aresthesia, **P**aralysis, **P**olar, **P**ulselessness

Management
• Immediate heparinization (5000 U IV bolus with continuous infusion until PTT >60 sec)
• Embolectomy vs. thrombectomy ± graft/bypass vs. amputation
• Overlap heparin post-op with warfarin; continue warfarin for 3 months

CHRONIC ARTERIAL OCCLUSION/INSUFFICIENCY

Signs and Symptoms
• Claudication: pain with exertion (usually in calves); relieved by short rest; reproducible
• Pulses may be absent at some locations, bruits may be present
• Signs of poor perfusion: hair loss, hypertrophic nails, atrophic muscle, skin ulcerations and infections, slow capillary refill, prolonged pallor with elevation and rubor on dependency, venous troughing (collapse of superficial veins of foot)
• Other manifestations of atherosclerosis: CVD, CAD, impotence, splanchnic ischemia

Management
• Conservative: exercise, weight loss, stop smoking, treat HTN, control/prevent DM
• Medication: antiplatelet (ASA or clopidogrel), cilostazol (for symptoms), pentoxyfilline (second-line)
• Invasive: endovascular angioplasty/stent, surgical bypass graft

Aortic Dissection

Signs and Symptoms
• Sudden onset tearing chest pain that radiates to back; may also have HTN, BP/pulse difference between arms

Classification of Aortic Dissection

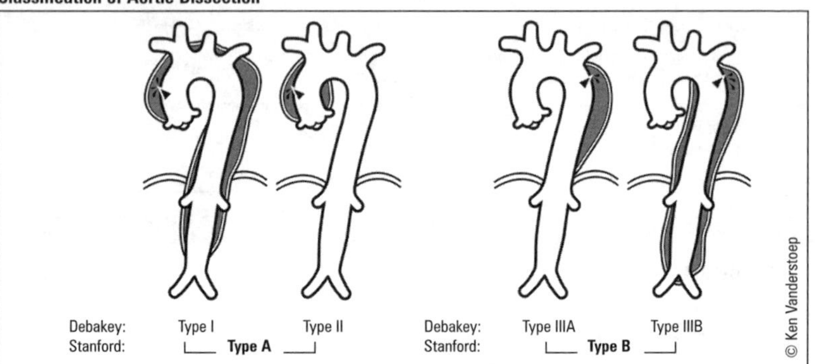

Management
• Type A (i.e. involvement of ascending aorta) requires emergency surgery with cardiopulmonary bypass
• Type B can be initially managed medically (lower BP)

Aortic Aneurysm

• CCS PAD Guidelines 2006 recommend AAA screening among:
  1. Men aged 65-74
  2. Women aged 65 with cardiovascular disease and positive family history of AAA
  3. Men aged 50 and above with a positive family history

• CCS PAD Guidelines 2006 recommend AAA follow-up based on initial size:

<3.0 cm	Repeat ultrasound follow-up in 3-5 yrs
3.1-3.4 cm	Repeat ultrasound in 3 yrs
3.5-3.9 cm	Repeat ultrasound in 2 yrs
4.0-4.5 cm	Repeat ultrasound in 1 yr
>=4.5 cm	Referral to vascular surgeon and repeat ultrasound q6months
If >1 cm growth in one yr	Referral to vascular surgeon for consideration of repair

Signs and Symptoms
• **Classic Triad of Ruptured AAA**: pain, hypotension, pulsatile abdominal mass

Management of Ruptured AAA
• No imaging, straight to OR (confirm diagnosis by laparotomy), crossmatch 10 units PRBCs, start IV if possible
• Repair of asymptomatic AAA is generally not justified if <5.0 cm and growth <0.5 cm over 6 months

Common Medications

Anti-Hypertensive Agents

Classification	Examples	Site of Action	Mechanism of Action (Secondary Effect)	Indication	Dosing	Adverse Effects
Loop diuretics	furosemide (Lasix®) bumetanide (Bumex®/Buinex®) ethacrynate (Edecrin®) torsemide (Demadex®)	Thick ascending of Loop of Henle	$\downarrow$ Na$^+$/K$^+$/2Cl transport $\pm$ renal and peripheral vasodilatory effects (K$^+$ loss; $\uparrow$ H$^+$ secretion; $\uparrow$ Ca^{2+} excretion)	Management of edema secondary to CHF, nephrotic syndrome, cirrhotic ascites; $\uparrow$ free water clearance (e.g. in SIADH-induced hyponatremia), HTN (less effective due to short action)	furosemide: edema – 20-80 mg IV/IM/ PO q6-8h (max 600 mg/d) until desired response HTN – 20-80 mg/d PO OD/ bid dosing	Allergy in sulfa-sensitive individuals Electrolyte abnormalities; hypokalemia, hyponatremia, hypocalcemia, hypercalciuria (with stone formation) Volume depletion with metabolic alkalosis Precipitates gouty attacks
Thiazide diuretics	hydrochlorothiazide (HCTZ) chlorothiazide (Diuril®) indapamide (Lozol®, Lozide®) metolazone (Zaroxolyn®) chlorthalidone (Hygroton®)	Distal convoluted tubule	Inhibit Na$^+$/Cl$^-$ transporter (K$^+$ loss; $\uparrow$ H$^+$ secretion; $\downarrow$ Ca^{2+} excretion)	1st line for essential HTN Treatment of edema Idiopathic hypercalciuria and stones Diabetes Insipidus (nephrogenic)	HCTZ: edema – 25-100 mg PO OD HTN – 12.5-25 PO OD (max 50 mg/d) nephrolithiasis/hypercalciuria – 25-100 mg od	Hypokalemia, hypotension Increased serum urate levels Precipitates gouty attacks, hypercalcemia Elevated lipids Glucose intolerance
Potassium-sparing diuretics	spironolactone (Aldactone®) triamterene (Dyrenium®) amiloride (Midamor®)	Cortical collecting duct ($\downarrow$ Na$^+$ reabsorption)	Aldosterone antagonist Closes apical Na$^+$ channels directly	Reduces K$^+$ loss caused by other diuretics Edema/hypervolemia Severe CHF, ascites (spironolactone), cystic fibrosis (amiloride $\downarrow$ viscosity of secretions)	spironolactone: 25-200 mg/d OD/bid dosing HTN: 50-200 mg/d OD/bid dosing Hyperaldosteronism – 100-400 mg/d OD/bid dosing amiloride: edema/HTN: 5-10 mg PO OD	Hyperkalemia (caution with ACE inhibitor) Triamterene can be nephrotoxic (rare) Nephrolithiasis Gynecomastia (estrogenic effect of spironolactone)
Combination agents	Dyazide® (triamterene + HCTZ) Aldactazide® (spironolactone + HCTZ) Moduretic® (amiloride + HCTZ) Vaseretic® (enalapril + HCTZ) Zestoretic® (lisinopril + HCTZ)		Combine ACE-inhibitor with thiazide for synergistic effect	Combine K$^+$-sparing drug with thiazide to reduce hypokalemia		

Anti-Hypertensive Agents

Classification	Examples	Site of Action	Mechanism of Action (Secondary Effect)	Indication	Dosing	Adverse Effects
ACEI	ramipril (Altace®) enalapril (Vasotec®) lisinopril (Prinivil®) trandolapril (Mavik®) captopril (Capoten®)	Lungs Tissues diffusely	Prevents angiotensin II vasoconstricting vascular smooth muscle → net vasodilation → $\downarrow$ BP Prevents angiotensin II mediated aldosterone release from adrenal cortex and action on proximal renal tubules → $\uparrow$ Na^+ and H_2O excretion → $\downarrow$ BP Reduces fibrosis and atherogenesis	HTN Cardioprotective effects (e.g. CAD, CHF, post MI) Renoprotective effects DM	ramipril: HTN – 2.5-20 mg PO OD/bid dosing renoprotective use – 10 mg PO OD trandolapril: HTN – 1-4 mg PO OD	Cough (10%) Hyperkalemia Angioedema Agranulocytosis (captopril) Acute kidney injury Teratogenic
ARB	losartan (Cozaar®) candesartan (Atacand®) irbesartan (Avapro®) valsartan (Diovan®) telmisartan (Micardis®) eprosartan (Teveten®) olmesartan (Olmetec®)	Vascular smooth muscle, adrenal cortex, proximal tubules	Competitive inhibitor at the angiotensin II receptor: prevents angiotensin II vasoconstricting action on vascular smooth muscle → $\downarrow$ BP Prevents angiotensin II mediated aldosterone release from adrenal cortex and action on proximal renal tubules → $\uparrow$ Na^+ and H_2O excretion	HTN Cardioprotective effects (same as ACEI) Renoprotective effects when ACEI are not tolerated	HTN: losartan 25-100 mg PO OD candesartan 8-32 mg PO OD irbesartan 150-300 mg PO OD valsartan 80-320 mg PO OD telmisartan 20-80 mg PO OD eprosartan 400-800 mg PO OD olmesartan 20-40 mg PO OD	Hyperkalemia Caution – reduce dose in hepatic impairment Acute kidney injury Teratogenic
Renin antagonists	aliskiren (Rasilez®)	Direct renin antagonist	Inhibits renin production and activity Cardioprotective and renoprotective abilities being evaluated	HTN	aliskiren 150-300 mg PO OD	Hyperkalemia

Drug Class	Indications	Examples	Dose	Side Effects	Contraindications
β-BLOCKERS					
β1 antagonists	HTN, CAD, acute MI, post-MI, CHF, AF, SVT	Metoprolol	HTN: start 25-100 mg daily (ER), up to 400 mg/d CHF: start 12.5-25 mg daily, double dose q2wks as tolerated up to 300 mg/d Acute MI: 5 mg increments IV q5-15min up to 15 mg, followed by oral therapy	Hypotension, fatigue, light-headedness, depression, bradycardia, hyperkalemia, bronchospasm, impotence, depression of counter-regulatory response to hypoglycemia, exacerbation of Raynaud's phenomenon and claudication	Sinus bradycardia, 2nd or 3rd degree heart block, hypotension, WPW Caution in asthma, claudication, Raynaud's phenomenon, and CHF (in CHF, start low and go slow)
		Atenolol	Acute MI: 5 mg IV over 5 min, repeat in 10 min HTN: start 25-50 mg daily or divided bid Max 100 mg/d		
		Bisoprolol	HTN: start 2.5-5 mg daily Max 20 mg/d		
β1/β2 antagonists		Labetolol	HTN: start 100 mg bid Max 2400 mg/d HTN emergency: start 20 mg IV slow injection, then 40-80 mg IV q10 min prn up to 300 mg or IV infusion 0.5-2 mg/min		
		Propranolol	HTN: start 20-40 mg bid or 60-80 mg daily Max 640 mg/d		
		Carvedilol	HTN: start 6.25 mg bid Max 50 mg/d		

Drug Class	Indications	Examples	Dose	Side Effects	Contraindications
CALCIUM CHANNEL BLOCKERS (CCBs)					
Benzothiazepines Phenylalkylamines (non-dihydropyridines)	HTN, CAD, SVT, diastolic dysfunction	Diltiazem	AF/flutter/PSVT: bolus 20 mg IV over 2 min; rebolus with 25 mg 15 min later as needed; infusion 5-15 mg/h Angina: start 30 mg qid (IR), max 360 mg/d divided tid-qid HTN: start 120-240 mg daily (ER), Max 540 mg/d	Hypotension, bradycardia, edema Negative inotrope	Sinus bradycardia, 2nd or 3rd degree heart block, hypotension, WPW, CHF
		Verapamil	SVT: 5-10 mg IV over 2 min, Max 5 mg Angina: start 40-80 mg tid-qid (IR), Max 480 mg/d HTN: same as for angina		
Dihydropyridines	HTN	Amlodipine (Norvasc®)	HTN: start 2.5-5 mg daily Max 10 mg daily	Hypotension, edema, flushing, headache, light-headedness	Severe aortic stenosis and liver failure
		Nifedipine (Adalat®)	HTN: 30-60 mg daily (ER) Max 120 mg/d		
		Felodipine (Plendil®)	HTN: start 2.5-5 mg daily Max 10 mg/d		
Inotropes	CHF, AF	Digoxin (Lanoxin®)	CHF, rate control of AF: 0.125-0.25 mg daily (use 0.0625-0.125 mg daily if renal impairment)	AV block, tachyarrhythmias, bradyarrhythmias, blurred or yellow vision (van Gogh syndrome), anorexia, nausea and vomiting	2nd or 3rd degree AV block, hypokalemia, WPW

Anti-Coagulants

Drug Class	Indications	Examples	Dose	Side Effects	Contraindications
Coumadin	AF, LV dysfunction, prosthetic valves	Warfarin (Coumadin®)	Start 2-5 mg daily x 1-2 d, then adjust dose to maintain therapeutic PT/INR	Bleeding (by far the most important side effect), paradoxical thrombosis, skin necrosis	Recent surgery or bleeding, bleeding diathesis, pregnancy
Heparins	Acute MI; when immediate anticoagulant effect needed	Dalteparin (LMWH)	Unstable angina, non-Q-wave MI: 120 units/kg up to 10,000 units SC q12h with aspirin (75-165 mg/d PO) until clinically stable	Bleeding, osteoporosis, heparin-induced thrombocytopenia (less in LMWHs)	Recent surgery or bleeding, bleeding diathesis, thrombocytopenia, renal insufficiency (for LMWHs)
		Enoxaparin (LMWH)	Unstable angina, non-Q-wave MI: 1 mg/kg SC q12h with ASA (100-325 mg PO daily) for ≥2 d and until clinically stable Acute STEMI: if ≤75 yrs: 30 mg IV bolus + 1mg/kg SC dose then 1 mg/kg (Max 100 mg for the 1st two doses) SC q12h; if >75 yrs: 0.75 mg/kg (Max 75 mg for the 1st two doses, no bolus) SC q12h		

Antiplatelet Agents

Drug Class	Indications	Examples	Dose	Side Effects	Contraindications
Salicylates	CAD, acute MI, post-MI, post-PCI and CABG	ASA (Aspirin®)	Acute MI: 160-325 mg/d (have patient chew tablet if not taking ASA before presentation) MI prophylaxis: 75-325 mg/d CABG: 75-325 mg/d starting at 6 h after procedure	Bleeding, GI upset, GI ulceration, impaired renal perfusion	Active bleeding or peptic ulcer disease (PUD)
Thienopyridines	Acute MI, post-MI, post-PCI and CABG	Clopidogrel (Plavix®)	Recent MI/stroke, PVD: 75 mg daily NSTEMI: 300 mg loading dose, then 75 mg daily in combination with ASA STEMI: start with/without 300 mg loading dose, then 75 mg daily in combination with ASA	Bleeding, thrombotic thrombocytopenic purpura, neutropenia (ticlopidine)	Active bleeding or PUD
		Ticlopidine (Ticlid®)	250 mg bid (try to avoid)		
Aggrenox®	Prevention of stroke after TIA/stroke	ASA + dipyridamole	1 cap bid (25 mg ASA/200 mg ER dipyridamole)	Headache, dyspepsia, abdominal pain, nausea, diarrhea, vomiting, GI bleeding, arthralgia	Hypersensitivity to dipyridamole, ASA; allergy to NSAIDs; asthma, rhinitis, and nasal polyps; bleeding disorders (factor VII or IX deficiencies); children <16 yrs of age with viral infections; pregnancy (ASA)
GpIIb/IIIa inhibitors	Acute MI, particularly if PCI is planned	Abciximab	0.25 mg/kg IV bolus via separte infusion line before procedure, then 0.125 mcg/kg/min IV infusion for 12 h; Max 10 mcg/min	Bleeding	Recent surgery or bleeding, bleeding diathesis
Nitrates	CAD, MI, CHF (isosorbide dinitrate plus hydralazine)	Nitroglycerin	IV – for perioperative HTN, acute MI/CHF, acute angina: start 10-20 mcg/min, titrate up by 10-20 mcg/min as needed Spray – for acute angina: 1-2 sprays under the tongue prn, max 3 sprays in 15 min SL – for acute angina: 0.4 mg SL, repeat q5min as needed upto 3 doses in 15 min Transdermal – for angina prophylaxis: 1 patch 12-14 h each day, with nitrate-free period of 10-14 h each day to prevent nitrate tolerance	Headache, dizziness, weakness, postural hypotension	Concurrent use of cGMP phosphodiesterase inhibitors, angle closure glaucoma, increased ICP

Dermatology

Essential History, Physical Exam and Lesion Characterization

History

- Onset, site, number of lesions, spread of lesion, change in lesion
- Aggravating and relieving factors
- Past/current therapy (topical, systemic)
- Associated symptoms (sensation, pain, pruritus, bleeding)
- Constitutional symptoms
- Inquire about skin phototypes (see Table *Skin Phototypes p88*)
- **PMHx**: past derm Hx, illnesses, hospitalizations, surgeries, meds, allergies
- **SocHx**: occupation, hobbies, travel, exposures, IV drug use, sexual Hx
- **FHx**: derm Dx (e.g. psoriasis, melanoma, atopy), relevant systemic diseases
- **ROS**: depends on clinical situation

Physical Exam

Describe Lesions using SCALDA
- **S**ize and **S**urface Area: mm/cm and % body surface area involved
- **C**olour: hyperpigmented, hypopigmented, erythematous
- **A**rrangement: solitary, linear, reticulated, grouped, herpetiform
- **L**esion Morphology (see *Lesion Characteristics*)
- **D**istribution: generalized vs. localized, dermatomal, intertriginous, symmetrical/asymmetrical, follicular
- **A**lways check: hair, nails, mucous membranes and intertriginous areas

Lesion Characteristics

TYPES OF MORPHOLOGICAL LESIONS

Primary Morphological Lesion: initial lesion that has not been altered by trauma or manipulation and has not regressed

Types of Lesions

Profile	<1 cm Diameter	≥1 cm Diameter
Flat Lesion	Macule (e.g. freckle)	Patch (e.g. vitiligo)
Raised Superficial Lesion	Papule (e.g. wart)	Plaque (e.g. psoriasis)
Deep Palpable (dermal or subcutaneous)	Nodule (e.g. dermatofibroma)	Tumour (e.g. lipoma)
Elevated Fluid-filled Lesions	Vesicle [e.g. herpes simplex virus (HSV)]	Bulla (e.g. bullous pemphigoid)

- **Cyst**: a epithelial-lined collection, containing semi-solid or fluid material
- **Pustule**: an elevated lesion containing purulent fluid (white, grey, yellow, green)
- **Erosion**: a disruption of the skin involving the epidermis alone, heals without scarring
- **Ulcer**: a disruption of the skin that extends into the dermis or deeper; heals with scarring
- **Indurated**: descriptive term for a lesion that is hard or firm
- **Scar**: replacement fibrosis of dermis and subcutaneous tissue (hypertrophic or atrophic)
- **Wheal**: a special form of papule or plaque that is blanchable and transient, formed by edema in the dermis (e.g. urticaria)

Secondary Morphological Lesion: a lesion which develops during the evolutionary process of skin disease, or is created by manipulation, or due to complication of primary lesion (e.g. rubbing, scratching, infection)
- **Crust:** dried fluid (serum, blood, or purulent exudate) originating from a lesion (e.g. impetigo)
- **Scale:** excess keratin (e.g. seborrheic dermatitis)
- **Fissure:** a linear slit-like cleavage of the skin
- **Excoriation:** a scratch mark
- **Lichenification:** thickening of the skin and accentuation of normal skin markings (e.g. chronic atopic dermatitis)
- **Xerosis:** pathologic dryness of skin (xeroderma), conjunctiva (xerophthalmia), or mucous membranes
- **Atrophy:** histological decrease in size and number of cells or tissues resulting in thinning or depression of the skin

Other Types of Morphological Lesions
- **Comedones:** collection of sebum and keratin [open comedone (blackhead), closed comedone (whitehead)]
- **Purpura:** extravasation of blood into dermis resulting in hemorrhagic lesions, non-blanchable
- **Petechiae:** small pinpoint purpura
- **Ecchymoses:** large flat purpura (bruise)
- **Telangiectasia:** dilated superficial blood vessels, blanchable

PATTERNS AND DISTRIBUTION
- **Acral:** relating to the hands and feet (e.g. hand foot and mouth disease)
- **Annular:** ring shaped (e.g. granuloma annulare)
- **Follicular:** involving hair follicles
- **Guttate:** lesions following a "drop like" pattern (e.g. guttate psoriasis)
- **Koebner phenomenon:** isomorphic reaction that develops in areas of trauma, after the traumatic event
- **Morbilliform:** maculopapular rash resembling measles
- **Reticulate:** lesions following a net-like pattern (e.g. livedo reticularis)
- **Satellite:** lesions scattered outside of primary lesion (e.g. candida diaper dermatitis)
- **Serpiginous:** lesions following a snake-like pattern (e.g. cutaneous larva migrans)
- **Target/Targetoid:** concentric ring lesions like a dartboard (e.g. erythema multiforme)
- **Other descriptive terms used:** discrete, clustered, linear, confluent, dermatitic

SKIN PHOTOTYPES (FITZPATRICK)

Phototypes	Colour of Skin	Skin's Response to Sun Exposure
I	White	Always burns, never tans
II	White	Always burns, little tan
III	White	Slight burn, slow tan
IV	Pale brown	Slight burn, faster tan
V	Brown	Rarely burns, dark tan
VI	Dark brown/black	Never burns, dark tan

Common Presentations

Differential Diagnosis of Common Presentations

Lesion	Infectious	Inflammatory	Drug/Toxin	Miscellaneous
Brown Macule		Post-inflammatory hypo/hyperpigmentation	UV radiation, actinic/ solar lentigo, freckle (ephelide)	Congenital: café-au-lait spots, congenital nevus, epidermal/junctional nevus Neoplasia: lentigo maligna, malignant melanoma, pigmented Other: melasma/chloasma (pregnancy)
Discrete Red Papule	Folliculitis Furuncle Scabies	Acne vulgaris Lichen planus Rosacea Psoriasis Urticaria	Bite/stings	Vascular: hemangioma, pyogenic granuloma Other: dermatofibroma, milaria rubra
Red Scales	Pityriasis rosea Secondary syphilis Tinea	Dermatitis (atopic, contact, nummular, seborrheic) Discoid lupus Lichen planus Psoriasis	Gold	Neoplastic: mycosis fungoides
Vesicle	Cat-Scratch disease Impetigo Viral: HSV, HZV, VZV, molluscum, Coxsackie Scabies	Acute contact dermatitis Dyshidrotic dermatitis		Other: dermatitis herpetiformis, porphyria cutanea tarda
Bullae	Bullous impetigo	Acute dermatitis EM/SJS/TEN Lupus erythematosus	Drug eruption	Autoimmune: bullous pemphigoid, pemphigus vulgaris Other: dermatitis herpetiformis, porphyria cutanea tarda
Pustule	Candida Dermatophyte Impetigo Sepsis Varicella	Acne vulgaris Rosacea Dyshidrotic dermatitis Pustular folliculitis Pustular psoriasis	Acute generalized exanthematous pustulosis (usually secondary to drug reaction)	Other: hidradenitis suppurativa
Oral Ulcer	Aspergillosis CMV Coxsackie Cryptococcosis HSV/HZ HIV TB Syphilis	Allergic stomatitis EM/SJS/TEN Lichen planus Seronegatives SLE Recurrent aphthous stomatitis Behçet's	Chemotherapy Radiation therapy	Autoimmune: pemphigus vulgaris Congenital: XXY (Klinefelter syndrome) Hematologic: sickle cell disease Neoplasia: BCC, SCC
Skin Ulcer	Plague Syphilis TB Tularemia	RA, SLE, vasculitis Ulcerative colitis (pyoderma gangrenosum)		Autoimmune: diabeticorum (e.g. DM) necrobiosis lipoidica Congenital: XXY Hematologic: sickle cell disease Neoplasia: SCC Vascular: arterial, neurotropic, pressure, venous, aphthous, leukoplakia, traumatic

Cysts

	Epidermal Cyst (Sebaceous)	Pilar Cyst (Trichilemmal)	Dermoid Cyst	Ganglion Cyst	Milium
Clinical Presentation	Round, yellow/flesh coloured, slow growing, mobile, firm, fluctuant	Multiple, hard, varying sized, most of them on scalp, lacks central punctum	Most commonly found at lateral third of eyebrow or midline under nose	Usually solitary, rubbery, translucent; a clear gelatinous viscous fluid may be extruded	1-2 mm superficial, white to yellow subepidermal papules occuring on eyelids, cheeks, and forehead Within pilosebaceous follicles
Pathophysiology	Epithelial cells displaced into dermis, epidermal lining becomes filled with keratin and lipid-rich debris May be post-traumatic, rarely syndromic	Thick walled cyst lined with stratified squamous epithelium and filled with dense keratin Idiopathic Post-trauma, often familial	Rare, congenital hamartomas, which arise from inclusion of epidermis along embryonal cleft closure lines, creating a thick walled cyst filled with dense keratin	Cystic lesion that originates from joint or tendon sheath, called a digital mucous cyst when found on fingertip Associated with osteoarthritis	Small epidermoid cyst, primarily arising from pluripotential cells in epidermal or adnexal epithelium Secondary to blistering, ulceration, trauma, topical corticosteroid atrophy, or cosmetic procedures
Epidemiology	Most common cutaneous cyst in youth – mid age	2nd most common cutaneous cyst F>M	Rare	Older age	Any age and 40-50% of infants
Clinical Course	Central punctum may rupture (foul, cheesy odour, creamy colour) and produce inflammatory reaction Increase in size and number over time, especially in pregnancy	Rupture causes pain and inflammation	If nasal or midline, risk of extension into CNS	Stable	In newborns, spontaneously resolves in first 4 wks of life
Management	Excise completely before it becomes infected	Excision	Excision	Drainage ± steroid injection if painful Compression daily for 6 wks Excision if bothersome	Incision and expression of contents Laser ablation and electrodesiccation Multiple facial milia responds to topical retinoid therapy

Pigmented Lesions

Melanocytic Nevi Classification

Type	Age of Onset	Clinical Presentation	Histology	Management
Congenital NMN	Birth and early infancy	Sharply demarcated pigmented brown plaque with regular/irregular contours ± coarse hairs Rule out leptomeningeal involvement if on head/neck	Nevomelanocytes in epidermis (clusters) and dermis (strands)	Surgical excision if suspicious, due to increased risk of developing melanoma
Acquired NMN	Early childhood to age 40 Involute by age 60	Benign neoplasm of pigment-forming nevus cell Well circumscribed, round, uniformly pigmented macules/papules <1.5 cm Can be classified according to site of nevus cells		Excisional biopsy required if on scalp, soles, mucous membranes, anogenital area, or if varied colours, irregular borders, pruritic, bleeding, exposed to trauma
Junctional NMN	Childhood Majority progress to compound nevus	Flat, irregularly bordered, uniformly tan-dark brown, sharply demarcated smooth macule	Melanocytes at dermal-epidermal junction above basement membrane	Same as above
Compound NMN	Any age	Domed, regularly bordered, smooth, round, tan-dark brown papule Face, trunk, extremities, scalp NOT found on palms or soles	Melanocytes at dermal-epidermal junction; migration into dermis	Same as above
Dermal NMN	Adults	Soft, dome-shaped, skin-coloured to tan/brown papules or nodules, often with telangiectasia Sites: face, neck	Melanocytes exclusively in dermis	Same as above
Dysplastic NMN	Childhood	Variegated macule/papule with irregular indistinct melanocytes in the basal cell layer >6 mm Risk factors: positive family history	Hyperplasia and proliferation of melanocytes extending beyond dermal compartment of the nevus Often with region of adjacent nests	Follow q2-6 months with colour photographs for changes Excisional biopsy if lesion changing or highly atypical
Halo NMN	First 3 decades	Brown oval/round papules surrounded by hypomelanosis Same sites as neocellular nevus (NCN) Spontaneous involution with regression of centrally located pigmented nevus	Dermal or compound NCN surrounded by hypomelanosis, lymphocytes, histocytes	None required Excision if colour variegated or irregular borders Associated with vitiligo, metastatic melanoma
Blue NMN	Childhood and late adolescence	Uniformly blue to blue-black macule/papule with smooth border <6 mm	Pigmented melanocytes and melanophages in dermis	Remove if sudden onset or has changed

NMN: nevamelanocytic nevus

Nail Changes in Systemic and Dermatological Conditions

Nail Abnormalities

Nail Abnormality	Definition/Etiology	Associated Disease(s)
NAIL CHANGES		
Clubbing	Proximal nail plate has greater than 180 degree angle to nail fold, watch-glass nails, bulbous digits	Cyanotic heart disease, bacterial endocarditis, pulmonary disorders, GI disorders, etc.
Koilonychia	Spoon shaped nails	Iron deficiency, malnutrition, DM
Onycholysis	Separation of nail plate from nail bed	Psoriasis, dermatophytes, thyroid disease
Onychogryphosis	Hypertrophy of the nail plate	Poor circulation, chronic inflammation, tinea hyperkeratosis
Onychohemia	Subungual hematoma	Trauma to nail bed
Onychocryptosis (ingrown toenail)	Often hallux with congenital malalignment, painful inflammation, granulation tissue	Tight fitting shoes, excessive nail clipping
Onychomycosis	Fungal infection of nail (dermatophytes, yeasts, moulds)	HIV, DM, peripheral arterial disease
SURFACE CHANGES		
Wedge shaped	Distal margin has v-shaped indentation	Darier's disease (follicular dyskeratosis)
Pterygium inversus unguium	Distal nail plate does not separate from underlying nail bed	Scleroderma
Pitting	Punctate depressions that migrate distally with growth	Psoriasis, alopecia areata, eczema
Transverse ridging	Transverse depressions often more in central portion of nail plate	Serious acute illness slows nail growth (Beau's line's), eczema, chronic paronychia, trauma
Transverse white lines	Bands of white discolouration	Poisons, hypoalbuminemia (Muherke's lines)
COLOUR CHANGES		
Yellow		Tinea, jaundice, tetracycline, pityriasis rubra pilaris, yellow nail syndrome
Green		Pseudomonas
Black		Melanoma, hematoma
Brown		Nicotine use, psoriasis, poisons
Splinter hemorrhage	Extravasation of blood from longitudinal vessels of nail bed, blood attaches to overlying nail plate and moves distally as it grows	Trauma, bacterial endocarditis, blood dyscrasias, psoriasis
Oil spots	Brown-yellow discolouration	Psoriasis
LOCAL CHANGES		
Paronychia	Local inflammation of the nail fold around the nail bed	Acute: painful infection Chronic: constant wetting (e.g. dishwashing, thumbsucking)
Nail fold telangiectasias	Cuticular hemorrhages, roughness, capillary changes	Scleroderma, SLE, dermatomyositis
Herpetic whitlow	HSV infection of distal phalanx	HSV infection

Alopecia

NON-SCARRING (intact hair follicles present)
- **Physiological** (androgenic/male pattern alopecia): fronto-temporal areas progressing to vertex, entire scalp may be bald
- **Physical**: trichotillomania, traumatic (e.g. tight "corn-row" braiding of hair)
- **Telogen Effluvium**: uniform decrease in hair density due to an increased number of hairs in resting stage (impaired mitotic activity)
- **Anagen Effluvium**: hair loss due to insult to hair follicle impairing its mitotic activity
- **Metabolic Alopecia**:
  - Drugs: chemotherapy, danazol, vit. A, retinoids, anticoagulants, antithyroid drugs, OCP, allopurinol, propanolol, salicylates, gentamicin, levodopa
  - Toxins: heavy metals
  - Endocrine: hypothyroidism
- **Alopecia Areata**: autoimmune d/o characterized by patches of complete hair loss
  - Totalis: loss of all scalp hair + eyebrows
  - Universalis: loss of all body hair
  - Associated signs: nail stippling, "exclamation mark" pattern (hairs fractured with tapered shafts)
  - Associated conditions: pernicious anemia, vitiligo, thyroid disease, Addison's disease

SCARRING (irreversible loss of hair follicles + fibrosis)
- **Physical**: radiation, burns
- **Infections**: fungal, bacterial, TB leprosy, viral (HZV)
- **Inflammatory**: lichen planus (lichen planopilaris), discoid lupus (but SLE can also cause non-scarring alopecia), morphea ("coup de sabre" with involvement of central scalp)
- **NOTE**: scarring alopecia requires a biopsy from the active border

Common Conditions

Acne Vulgaris

Clinical Presentation
- Type I: comedonal
- Type II: papular
- Type III: pustular
- Type IV: nodulocystic

Acne Treatments

Drug Name	Mechanism of Action	Notes
MILD ACNE: Topical Therapies		
clindamycin phosphate (e.g. Dalacin T®)	Lincosamide antibiotic; inhibits protein synthesis	Generally regarded as unsafe in lactation
erythromycin	Macrolide antibiotic; inhibits protein synthesis	Local skin reactions (burning, peeling, dryness, pruritus, erythema)
benzoyl peroxide	Protein oxidant with bactericidal effect	Dry skin, contact dermatitis Apply to the point of dryness and erythema, but not discomfort
BenzaClin® gel	1% clindamycin and 5% benzoyl peroxide	See above
erythromycin + benzoyl peroxide (Benzamycin®)	3% erythromycin and 5% benzoyl peroxide	See above
adapalene (e.g. Differin®)	Comedolytic	Less irritating than tretinoin. No interaction with sun
tretinoin (e.g. Retin-A®)	Comedolytic	Sun sensitivity and irritation

Acne Treatments (continued)

MODERATE ACNE: After topical treatments have failed, add oral antibiotics, such as tetracycline (500 mg PO OD to bid), or erythromycin (500 mg PO bid). Antibiotics require 3-6 months of use before assessing efficacy. Consider hormonal therapy, including antiandrogens

tetracycline	Systemic antibiotic	Caution with regard to drug interactions: do not use with isotretinoin
cyproterone acetate-ethinyl estradiol (Diane-35®)	Cyproterone: potent anti-androgenic, progestogenic and antigonadatrophic activity Ethinyl estradiol: increases level of sex hormone binding globulin (SHBG), reducing circulating plasma levels of androgens	After 35 yrs of age, estrogen/progesterone should only be considered in exceptional circumstances, carefully weighing the risk/benefit ratio with physician guidance

SEVERE ACNE: Consider systemic retinoids after above treatments have failed

isotretinoin (Accutane®, Clarus®)	Retinoid that inhibits sebaceous gland function and regluates keratinization	Teratogenic: contraindicated during pregnancy, unsafe in lactation; reliable contraception is necessary Required signed informed consent Baseline lipid profile, hepatic enzymes, β-hCG May transiently exacerbate acne May cause depression D/C at 16-20 wks when nodule count has dropped by >70% May initiate a second course after 2 months PRN Refractory cases may require 3 or more courses of isotretinoin

Atopic Dermatitis

Clinical Presentation

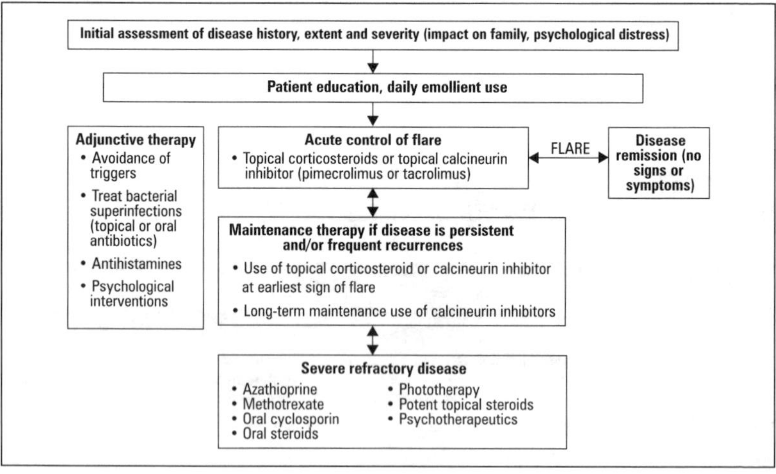

- Subacute and chronic eczematous reaction associated with prolonged severe pruritis
- Distribution is age-dependent
  - Infant: face, scalp, extensor surfaces
  - Childhood: flexural
  - Adult: flexures, wrists, hands, feet, face, forehead, eyelids, neck

Investigations
- None for diagnosis, based on clinical morphology
- May consider: skin biopsy, serum Ig levels, patch testing, skin prick test for allergies

Contact Dermatitis

Contact Dermatitis

	Irritant Contact Dermatitis	Allergic Contact Dermatitis
Mechanism of Reaction	Toxic injury to skin; non-immune mechanism	Cell-mediated delayed (Type IV) hypersensitivity reaction
Type of Reaction	Erythema, dryness, fine scale, burning Acute: quick reaction, sharp margins (e.g. from acid/alkali exposure) Cumulative insult: slow to appear, poorly defined margins (e.g. from soap), more common	Erythema with a papulovesicular eruption, swelling, pruritus
Frequency of Contact Dermatitis	Majority; will occur in anyone given sufficient concentration of irritants	Minority; patient acquires susceptibility to allergen that persists indefinitely
Distribution	Not often helpful in differentiating the two, as both are due to exposure	Dorsum of hand usually involved; often discrete area of skin involvement
Examples	Soaps, weak alkali, detergents, organic solvents, alcohol, oils	Occasionally more linear
Management	Avoidance of irritants Compresses Barrier moisturizers Topical/oral steroids	Patch testing to determine specific allergen Avoid allergen and its cross-reactants Wet compresses soaked in Burow's solution (drying agent) Steroid cream (hydrocortisone 1%, betamethasone valerate 0.05% or 0.1% cream; bid) Systemic steroids prn (prednisone 1 mg/kg, taper over 2 wks)

Psoriasis

Classification
- Psoriasis vulgaris: plaque psoriasis, guttate psoriasis
- Psoratic erythrodermic
- Pustular psoriasis
- Psoriatic arthritis

Differential Diagnosis
- Atopic dermatitis, mycosis fungoides (cutaneous T-cell lymphoma), seborrheic dermatitis, tinea

Diagnosis
- Often clinical, biopsy to confirm
- Psoriasis Area and Severity Index (PASI)
  - Score is based on percentage of surface area involved and symptom severity (including erythema, infiltrations, desquamation)

1. PLAQUE PSORIASIS

Clinical Presentation
- Chronic and recurrent disease characterized by well-circumscribed erythematous papules/plaques with silvery-white scales
- Worse in winter (lack of sun and humidity)
- Koebner phenomenon: induction of new lesion by injury
- Auspitz sign: bleeds from minute points when scale is removed
- Usually non-pruritic
- Exacerbating factors: drugs (lithium, ethanol, chloroquine, β-blockers), stress
- Sites: scalp, extensor surfaces of elbows and knees, trunk, nails, pressure areas

Pathophysiology
- Decreased epidermal transit time from stratum basale to stratum corneum
- Shortened cell cycle of psoriatic compared to normal skin
- TH1-mediated inflammatory response

Epidemiology
- Multifactorial inheritance

Management
- Preventative measures
  - Avoid sunburns
  - Avoid drugs that exacerbate the condition (e.g. β-blockers, lithium, corticosteroid rebound phenomenon, interferon)
- First-line treatment
  - Mainly topical, usually prescribed if less than 5-10% of total body surface area is involved
  - First-line topical treatments include moderate to potent steroids, vitamin D analogues, retinoids, anthralin, coal tar, salicylic acid
  - If the affected area is >10%, use topical medications as adjuncts to phototherapy or systemic drugs
- Second-line treatment
  - Include cyclosporin, methotrexate, acitretin, as well as phototherapy
  - Biologics including alefacept, etanercept, infliximab, adalimumab, ustekinumab
- Systemic treatments should be considered if:
  - Psoriatic lesions cover >10% of TBSA
  - Unsuccessful topical therapies
  - Disease is causing psychological distress
  - Involvement of face, hands or genitalia

Topical Treatment of Psoriasis

Treatment	Mechanism	Comments
Lubricants	Reduce fissure formation	Petrolatum is effective
Salicylic acid 1-12%	Remove scales	
Tar (LCD: Liquor carbonis detergens) 20% coal tar solution	Inhibits DNA synthesis, increases cell turnover	Poor long term compliance
Calcipotriene (Dovonex®, Dovobet®)	Binds to skin 1,25-dihydroxyvitamin D3 to inhibit keratinocyte proliferation	Not to be used on face or skin folds
Corticosteroid ointment	Reduce scaling and thickness	Use appropriate potency steroid in different areas for degree of psoriasis
Tazarotene (Tazorac®) (gel/cream)	Retinoid derivative	Use on nails

Systemic Treatment of Psoriasis

Treatment	Adverse Effects
Methotrexate	Bone marrow toxicity, hepatic cirrhosis
PUVA	Pruritus, burning, cataracts, skin cancer
Acitretin	Alopecia, cheilitis, teratogenicity, epistaxis, xerosis, hypertriglyeridemia
Cyclosporine	Renal toxicity, hypertension, immunosuppression
UVB and "Narrow band" UVB (311-312 nm)	Well tolerated

"Biologics" approved in Canada

Treatment	Route	Dosing Schedule	Effectiveness	Action
alefacept (Amevive®)	IM	Weekly	+	T-cell
etanercept (Enbrel®)*	SC	Twice weekly initially	+++	Anti-TNF
adalimumab (Humira®)*	SC	Once every 2 wks	++++	Anti-TNF
infliximab (Remicade®)*	IV	~Every 2 months	+++++	Anti-TNF
ustekinumab (Stelara®)	SC	Every 12 wks during maintenance	++++	Anti IL 12/23

*Can also be used to treat Psoriatic Arthritis

Infections

BACTERIAL

Comparison of Superficial Folliculitis, Furuncles and Carbuncles

	Superficial Folliculitis	Furuncles (Boils)	Carbuncles
Clinical Presentation	Superficial infection of the hair follicle (versus pseudofolliculitis: inflammation of follicle due to friction, irritation, or occlusion) Acute lesion consists of a dome-shaped pustule at the mouth of hair follicle Pustule ruptures to form a small crust Sites: primarily scalp, shoulders, anterior chest, upper back, other hairbearing areas	Red, hot, tender, inflammatory nodules with central yellowish point, which forms over summit and ruptures Involves subcutaneous tissue that arises from a hair follicle Sites: hair-bearing skin (thigh, neck, face, axillae, perineum, buttocks)	Deep-seated abscess formed by multiple coalescing furuncles Usually in areas of thicker skin Occasionally ulcerates Lesions drain through multiple openings to the surface Systemic symptoms may be associated
Etiology	Normal non-pathogenic bacteria (*Staphylococcus* – most common; *Pseudomonas* – hot tub) *Pityrosporum*	*S. aureus*	*S. aureus*
Management	Antiseptic (Hibitane®) Topical antibacterial (fusidic acid, mupirocin, or erythromycin) Oral cloxacillin for 7-10 d	Incise and drain large carbuncles to relieve pressure and pain If afebrile: hot wet packs, topical antibiotic If febrile/cellulitis: culture blood and aspirate pustules (Gram stain and C&S) Cloxacillin for 1-2 wks (especially for lesions near external auditory canal/nose, with surrounding cellulitis, and not responsive to topical therapy)	Same as for furuncles

VIRAL

Different Manifestations of HPV Infection

	Definition and Clinical Features	Differential Diagnosis	Distribution	HPV Type
Verruca Vulgaris (Common Warts)	Hyperkeratotic, elevated discrete epithelial growths with papillated surface caused by HPV Paring of surface reveals punctate, red-brown specks (dilated capillaries)	*Molluscum contagiosum*, seborrheic keratosis	Located at trauma sites: fingers, hands, knees of children and teens	At least 80 types are known
Verruca Plantaris (Plantar Warts) and Verruca Palmaris (Palmar Warts)	Hyperkeratotic, shiny, sharply marginated growths Paring of surface reveals red-brown specks (capillaries), interruption of epidermal ridges	Need to scrape ("pare") lesions to differentiate wart from callus and corn	Located at pressure sites: heads of metatarsal, heels, toes	Commonly HPV 1, 2, 4, 10
Verruca Planae (Flat Warts)	Multiple discrete, skin coloured, flat topped papules grouped or in linear configuration Common in children	Syringoma, seborrheic keratosis, *Molluscum contagiosum*, lichen planus	Sites: face, dorsa of hands, shins, knees	Commonly HPV 3, 10
Condyloma Acuminata (Genital Warts)	Skin-coloured pinhead papules to soft cauliflower like masses in clusters Often occurs in young adults, infants, children Can be asymptomatic, lasting months to years Highly contagious, transmitted sexually and non-sexually (e.g. Koebner phenomenon via scratching, shaving), and can spread without clinically apparent lesions Investigations: acetowhitening (subclinical lesions seen with 5% acetic acid x 5 min and hand lens) Complications: fairy-ring warts (satellite warts at periphery of treated area of original warts)	Condyloma lata (secondary syphilitic lesion, dark field strongly +ve), *Molluscum contagiosum*	Sites: genitalia and perianal areas	Commonly HPV 6 and 11 HPV 16, 18, 31, 33 cause cervical dysplasia, SCC, and invasive cancer

Malignant Skin Tumours

Comparison of Common Skin Malignancies

	Malignant Melanoma	Squamous Cell Carcinoma	Basal Cell Carcinoma
Definition	Malignant neoplasm of melanocytes and nevus cells	Malignant neoplasm of keratinocytes	Malignant neoplasia of basal cells of the epidermis
Epidemiology	Lifetime risk, all comers 1:55 Risk factors: numerous moles, blistering sunburn, fair skin, red hair, PMHx/FHx, large congenital nevi, dysplastic nevus syndrome (100% lifetime risk) Most common sites: back (M), calves (F) Worse prognosis if: M, on scalp, hands, feet, late lesion, no pre-existing nevus present	Primarily on sun exposed skin in the elderly, M>F, skin phototypes I and II, chronic sun exposure Predisposing factors: UV radiation, ionizing radiation therapy/exposure, PUVA, immunosuppression, actinic keratoses, atrophic skin lesions, chemical carcinogens such as arsenic, tar, nitrogen mustards	75% of all malignant skin tumours, onset usually >40 yrs, increased prevalence in the elderly Predisposing factors: M>F, skin phototypes I and II cumulative sun exposure, scar formation, radiation, trauma, arsenic exposure, genetic predisposition (Gorlin syndrome), nevus sebaceous

Comparison of Common Skin Malignancies (continued)

	Malignant Melanoma	Squamous Cell Carcinoma	Basal Cell Carcinoma
Differential Diagnosis	Pigmented BCC, seborrheic keratosis, irritated nevus, pigmented actinic keratosis	BCC, Bowen's disease, melanoma, nummular eczema, psoriasis, keratoaranthoma	SCC, intradermal melanocytic nevus, nodular malignant melanoma, sebaceous hyperplasia, angiofibroma
Signs and Symptoms	Malignant mole characteristics (**ABCDE**): **A** – Asymmetry **B** – Border irregular **C** – Colour varied **D** – Diameter increasing/>6 mm **E** – Evolution, enlargement, elevation Sites: skin, mucous membranes, eyes, CNS	Indurated erythematous nodule/plaque with surface scale/crust, eventual ulceration More rapid enlargement than BCC Sites: face, ears, scalp, forearms, dorsum of hands	Noduloulcerative (typical): skin-coloured papule/nodule with rolled, translucent ("pearly") telangiectatic border and depressed/eroded/ulcerated centre Sites: face (>80% of cases), scalp, ears, neck
Subtypes	1. Superficial spreading melanoma (60-70% of all melanomas) Irregular, indurated, enlarging plaques with red/white/blue discolouration, focal papules/nodules 2. Lentigo maligna melanoma (15%) Flat, brown, stain-like lesion, enlarges Colour changes to dark brown with black and blue hues 3. Nodular melanoma (30%) Uniformly ulcerated, blue-black, sharply delineated plaque/nodule Rapidly fatal 4. Acrolentiginous melanoma (5%) Ill-defined dark brown, blue-black macule Palmar, plantar, subungual skin Poor prognosis if on mucous membranes		1. Noduloulcerative (typical) 2. Pigmented variant Flecks of pigment in translucent lesion with surface telangiectasia May mimic malignant melanoma 3. Superficial variant Scaly plaque with fine telangiectasia 4. Sclerosing variant Flesh/yellowish-coloured, shiny papule/plaque with indistinct borders
Treatment	Excisional biopsy preferable, otherwise incisional biopsy Remove full depth of dermis and extend beyond edges histologic diagnosis Chemotherapy (cis-platinum, BCG), high-dose interferon gamma for stage II (regional) and stage III (distant) disease Radiotherapy is curative for uveal melanomas, palliative for bone and brain metastases	Surgical excision with primary closure, skin flaps or grafting Lifelong follow-up Radiotherapy if surgery not feasible	Electrodesiccation and curettage Surgical excision ± microscopically controlled Radiotherapy, cryotherapy primary superficial lesions if surgical management is inappropriate
In situ lesions	Lentigo maligna (malignant melanoma in situ) Malignant melanoma in situ: 2-6 cm, tan/brown/black uniformly flat macule or patch with irregular borders Sites: face, sun exposed areas 1/3 evolve into lentigo maligna melanoma	Bowen's Disease (SCC in situ): Erythematous plaque, sharply demarcated red, scaly border 1-3 cm in diameter, found on skin and mucous membranes Evolves to SCC in 10-20% of cutaneous lesions and >20% of mucosal lesions Scaly plaque with fine telangiectasia at margin	

Serious Skin Eruptions

• **Triad**: fever, exanthematous eruption, internal organ involvement

Serious Eruptions

Comparison	Erythema Multiforme (EM)	Stevens-Johnson Syndrome (SJS)	Toxic Epidermal Necrolysis (TEN)
Lesion	Macules/papules with central vesicles Classic bull's-eye pattern of concentric light and dark rings (typical target lesions) Bilateral and symmetric All lesions appear within 72 h Edema Lesion "fixed" for at least 7 d	Similar to EM but with more mucous membrane involvement "Atypical lesions": red circular patch with dark purple centre (aka targetoid) "Sicker" (high fever) Sheet-like epidermal detachment in <10% (Nikolsky sign)	Severe mucous membrane involvement, and blistering "Atypical lesions": 50% have no target lesions Diffuse erythema then necrosis and sheet-like epidermal detachment in >30%
Sites	Dorsa of hands and forearms Mucous membrane involvement (lips, tongue, buccal mucosa) is possible Extremities with face > trunk Involvement of palms and soles	Generalized with prominent face and trunk involvement Palms and soles may be spared	Generalized Nails may also shed
Other Complications	Burning and stinging Recurrences Secondary bacterial infection	Scarring, contractures, eruptive nevomelanocytic nevi, corneal scarring, blindness, phimosis and vaginal synechiae	Tubular necrosis and acute renal failure, epithelial erosions of trachea
Constitutional Symptoms	Weakness, malaise	Prodrome 1-14 d prior to eruption with fever and flu-like illness	High fever >38°C
Etiology	Infection – HSV, or *Mycoplasma pneumoniae*	15% are drug-related (NSAIDs, anticonvulsants, sulfonamides, penicillins) Occurs up to 1-3 wks after drug exposure with more rapid onset upon rechallenge	50% are drug related <5% are due to viral infection, immunization
Differential Diagnosis	Giant urticaria, granuloma annulare, mycosis fungoides, vasculitis	Scarlet fever, phototoxic, eruption, GVHD, SSSS, exfoliative dermatitis, Kawasaki disease, paraneoplastic pemphigus	Scarlet fever, phototoxic eruption, GVHD, SSSS, exfoliative dermatitis
Course and Prognosis	Lesions last 2 wks and heal without complications	4-6 wk course 5% mortality	30% mortality due to fluid loss, regrowth of epidermis by 3 wks, secondary infection
Management	Symptomatic Rx (oral antihistamines, antacids) Corticosteroids in severely ill (controversial) Prophylactic oral acyclovir for 6-12 months for HSV-associated EM with frequent recurrences	Prolonged hospitalization Withdraw suspect drug Intravenous fluids Corticosteroids (controversial) Infection prophylaxis Consider IVIG	As for SJS Admit to burn unit Debride frankly necrotic tissue Consider IVIG

Pediatric Exanthems

Definition
- Exanthem: an eruption on the skin occurring as a symptom of a systemic disease typically with a fever (see also *Pediatric Infectious Diseases*)
- Enanthem: an eruption on a mucous membrane occurring in the context of an exanthem

CHICKEN POX
- **Etiology**
  - Human herpes virus (HHV) 3, incubation 10-21d, communicable 1-2d pre-rash to 5d post-rash
- **Clinical Description**
  - Diffuse vesicular pustular eruption beginning on thorax spreading to extremities, new lesions every 2-3d
  - Enanthems
- **Important Complications**
  - Necrotizing fasciitis, encephalitis, cerebellar ataxia, disseminated intravascular coagulation (DIC), hepatitis
- **Management**
  - Supportive therapy, acyclovir if severe, varicella zoster immunoglobulin (within 96 h of contact)
  - Varicella vaccine

ENTROVIRAL
- **Etiology**
  - Enteroviruses
  - Most common exanthem in summer and fall
- **Clinical Description**
  - Polymorphous rash (macules, papules, vesicles, petechiae, urticaria)
- **Important Complications**
  - None
- **Management**
  - Supportive care for majority
  - Serious cases (immunosuppressed) can be treated with pleconaril

ERYTHEMA INFECTIOSUM
- **Etiology**
  - Parvovirus B19, incubation 4-14d
  - Peaks in winter and spring
- **Clinical Description**
  - Slapped cheeks (red, flushed cheeks) then 1-4 d later lacy/reticular maculo-papular rash of trunk/extremities
- **Important Complications**
  - **STAR** complex (**S**ore **T**hroat, **A**rthritis, **R**ash)
  - Fetal infection (anemia, fetal hydrops or death)
- **Management**
  - No treatment: children often feel well
  - NSAIDs for symptomatic arthropathy

GIANOTTI-CROSTI SYNDROME
- **Etiology**
  - Epstein-Barr virus most common, hepatitis B, coxsackie, parvovirus
  - Spring and early summer
- **Clinical Description**
  - Symmetric papular eruption of face, buttocks, and extremities
- **Important Complications**
  - None
- **Management**
  - Supportive treatment

HAND, FOOT AND MOUTH DISEASE
- **Etiology**
  - Coxsackie A and B viruses
  - Highly contagious virus
- **Clinical Description**
  - Vesicular eruption of palms and soles with an erosive stomatitis
- **Important Complications**
  - Pulmonary neurological death
- **Management**
  - Supportive treatment

KAWASAKI DISEASE
- See Pediatrics pg 404

MEASLES
- **Etiology**
  - Paramyxovirus
  - Incubation 10-14d, communicable 4d before and after rash
- **Clinical Description**
  - Erythematous macular eruption beginning on head and spreading downwards, desquamates, no palm or sole involvement
  - Enanthem: Koplik spots (grey/white papules on buccal mucosa)
- **Important Complications**
  - Otitis media, pneumonia, encephalitis, SJS, glomerular nephritis, myocarditis/pericarditis
- **Management**
  - Vitamin A, immunoglobulin, measles/mumps/rubella (MMR) vaccine

ROSEOLA
- **Etiology**
  - HHV 6, HHV 7, incubation 9-10d
- **Clinical Description**
  - Pink macules and papules on trunk, neck, proximal extremities, and occasionally face
  - Eruption after high fever ends
- **Important Complications**
  - Neurological involvement
  - Viral reactivation in immunosuppressed patients
- **Management**
  - Supportive treatment
  - Antipyretics during the febrile period

RUBELLA
- **Etiology**
  - RNA virus of the Togaviridae family, incubation 16-18 d
- **Clinical Description**
  - 1-5 d following mild prodrome (fever, headache, respiratory symptoms), a pink maculo-papular rash erupts on face spreading in a cephalocaudal direction
  - Occipital and retroauricular nodes
- **Important Complications**
  - STAR complex
  - Congenital rubella (cataract, glaucoma, thrombocytopenia, hepatitis, deafness, congenital heart disease)
- **Management**
  - Supportive treatment
  - MMR vaccine
  - Serologic testing in rubella-exposed pregnant women

SCARLET FEVER

- **Etiology**
  - Group A β-hemolytic streptococci toxin types A, B, and C
  - Late fall, winter, and early spring
- **Clinical Description**
  - Generalized rash, red papules, "sand-paper" texture, desquamation, flexural accentuation
  - Enanthem (strawberry tongue, petechiae on palate)
  - Pastia's lines – linear petechial streaks in axillary, inguinal, and antecubital areas
- **Important Complications**
  - Mastoiditis, otitis, sinusitis, pneumonia, meningitis, myocarditis, arthritis, hepatitis, rheumatic fever, and glomerulonephritis
- **Management**
  - 10-14 d course of penicillin

Skin Manifestations of Systemic Disease

Skin Manifestations of Systemic Illnesses

AUTOIMMUNE DISORDERS	
Behçet disease	Painful aphthous ulcers in oral cavity ± genital mucous membranes, erythema nodosum
Buerger's disese	Superficial migratory thrombophlebitis, pallor, cyanosis, gangrene, ulcerations
Dermatomyositis	Periorbital heliotrope and perioral violaceous erythema with edema, periungual erythema, telangiectasia, calcinosis cutis, Gottron's papules (violaceous flat-topped papules with atrophy over nape of neck, shoulders, IP joints)
Polyarteritis nodosa	Polyarteritic nodules, stellate purpura, erythema, gangrene, splinter hemorrhages, livedo reticularis
Rheumatic fever	Petechiae, urticaria, erythema nodosum, EM, rheumatic nodules
Scleroderma	Raynaud's, nonpitting edema, waxy/shiny/tense atrophic skin (morphea), ulcers, cutaneous calcification, periungual telangiectasia, acrosclerosis
SLE	Malar erythema, discoid rash (erythematous papules or plaques with keratotic scale, follicular plugging, atrophic scarring on face, hands, and arms), hemorrhagic bullae, palpable purpura, patchy/diffuse alopecia, mucosal ulcers, photosensitivity Cutaneous: Sharply marginated annular or psoriaform bright red plaques with scales, telangiectasia, marked scarring, diffuse non-scarring alopecia
Ulcerative colitis (UC)	Pyoderma gangrenosum, erythema nodosum
ENDOCRINE DISORDERS	
Addison's disease	Generalized hyperpigmentation or limited to skin folds, buccal mucosa and scars
Cushing's syndrome	Moon facies, purple striae, acne, hyperpigmentation, hirsutism, atrophic skin with telangiectasia
Diabetes mellitus	Infections (boils, carbuncles, candidiasis, S. aureus, dermatophytoses, tinea pedis and cruris, infectious eczematoid dermatitis), pruritus, eruptive xanthomas, necrobiosis lipoidica diabeticorum (well-demarcated multicoloured plaques on anterior and lateral aspect of lower legs), granuloma annulare, diabetic foot, diabetic bullae, acanthosis nigricans, calciphylaxis
Hyperthyroid	Moist, warm skin, seborrhea, acne, nail atrophy, hyperpigmentation, toxic alopecia, pretibial myxedema, acropachy, onycholysis
Hypothyroid	Cool, dry, scaly, thickened, hyperpigmented skin; toxic alopecia with dry, coarse hair, brittle nails, myxedema, loss of lateral 1/3 eyebrows

Skin Manifestations of Systemic Illnesses (continued)

HIV

Infections	Viral (HSV, VZV, HPV, CMV, molluscum contagiosum, oral hairy leukoplakia), bacterial (impetigo, acneiform folliculitis, dental caries, cellulitis, bacillary epithelioid angiomatosis, syphilis), other (candidiasis)
Inflammatory	Seborrhea, psoriasis, pityriasis rosea, vasculitis
Malignancies	Kaposi's sarcoma, lymphoma, BCC, SCC, malignant melanoma

MALIGNANCY

Adenocarcinoma

Gastrointestinal	Peutz-Jeghers: pigmented macules on lips/oral mucosa
Cervix/anus/rectum	Paget's Disease: eroding scaling plaques of perineum

Carcinoma

Breast	Paget's Disease: eczematous and crusting lesions of breast
GI	Palmoplantar keratoderma: thickened skin of palms/soles
Thyroid	Sipple's Syndrome: multiple mucosal neuromas
Breast/GU/lung/ovary	Dermatomyositis: heliotrope erythema of eyelids and purplish plaques over knuckles

MALIGNANCY

Lymphoma/Leukemia

Hodgkin's	Ataxia Telangiectasia: telangiectasia on pinna, bulbar conjunctiva
Acute Leukemia	Ichthyosis: generalized scaling especially on extremities
Bloom's syndrome	Butterfly erythema on face, associated with short stature
Multiple Myeloma	Amyloidosis: large smooth tongue, waxy papules on eyelids/nasolabial folds/lips, facial petechiae

OTHERS

Liver disease	Pruritus, hyperpigmentation, spider nevi, palmar erythema, white nails (Terry's nails), porphyria cutanea tarda xanthomas, hair loss
Renal disease	Pruritus, pigmentation, half and half nails
Pruritic urticarial papules and plaques of pregnancy	Erythematous papules or urticarial plaques in distribution of striae distensae: buttocks, thighs, upper inner arms and lower backs
Cryoglobulinemia	Palpable purpura in cold-exposed areas, Raynaud's, cold urticaria, acral hemorrhagic necrosis, bleeding disorders, associated with hepatitis C infection

Common Medications

Sunburns and Sunscreens

SUNBURNS
- Erythema 2-6 h post UV exposure often associated with edema, pain and blistering with subsequent desquamation of the dermis, and hyperpigmentation
- Chronic UVB exposure leads to photoaging, immunosuppression, photocarcinogenesis
- Prevention: avoid peak UVR (10 am to 4 pm), wear appropriate clothing, wide- brimmed hat, sunglasses, and broad-spectrum sunscreen
- Clothing with UV protection expressed as UV protection factor (UPV) is analogous to SPF of sunscreen

SUNSCREENS
- Sun protection factor (SPF): under ideal conditions, an SPF of 10 means that a person who normally burns in 20 min will burn in 200 min following the application of the sunscreen

- Chemical blockers: absorbs UV light
  - Requires application at least 15-60 min prior to exposure, should be reapplied every 2 h (more often if sweating, swimming)
  - UVB absorbers: PABA, salicylates, cinnamates, benzylidene camphor derivatives
  - UVA absorbers: benzophenones, anthranilates, dibenzoylmethanes, benzylidene camphor derivatives
- Physical blockers: reflects and scatters UV light
  - Titanium dioxide, zinc oxide, kaolin, talc, ferric chloride and melanin, all are effective against the UVA and UVB spectrum
  - Less risk of sensitization than chemical sunscreens and water proof, but may cause folliculitis or milia
- Some sunscreen ingredients may cause contact or photocontact allergic reactions, but are uncommon

TREATMENT

- Sunburn: if significant blistering present, consider treatment in hospital; otherwise, symptomatic treatment
- Antioxidants, both oral and topical are being studied for their abilities to protect the skin; topical agents are limited by their ability to penetrate the skin

Topical Steroids

Potency Ranking of Topical Steroids

Relative Potency	Relative Strength	Generic Names	Trade Names	Usage
Weak	x1	hydrocortisone 1%	Emo Cort®	Intertriginous areas, children, face, thin skin
Moderate	x3	hydrocortisone 2% 17-valerate – 0.2% desonide mometasone furorate	Westcort® Tridesilon® Elocom®	Arm, leg, trunk
Potent	x6	betamethasone – 0.1% 17-valerate – 0.1% amcinonide	Betnovate® Celestoderm – V® Cyclocort®	Body
Very Potent	x9	betamethasone dipropionate – 0.05% fluocinonide – 0.05%	Diprosone® Lidex, Topsyn gel® Lyderm®	Palms and soles
Extremely Potent	x12	clobetasol propionate (most potent) betamethasone dipropionate ointment halobetasol propionate	Dermovate® Diprolene® Ultravate®	Palms and soles

- Relative ability for a topical steroid to be absorbed:
  - Back < forearm < scalp < forehead < cheeks < axilla < scrotum

When to Use which Kind of Vehicle

- **Ointments:** consist of organic hydrocarbons, alcohols, acids; form a greasy impermeable layer and prevent evaporation
- **Creams:** mixture of ointments and water; better cosmesis
- **Pastes:** mixture of a powder in an ointment; when noxious chemical applied to skin without getting onto surrounding skin
- **Lotions:** liquid; for wet surfaces or hairy areas

Dermatological Therapies

Common Topical Therapies

Drug Name	Dosing Schedule	Indications	Comments
Calcipotriol (Dovonex®)	0.005% cream, ointment, scalp solution, apply BID For maintenance therapy apply OD	Psoriasis	Burning, itching, skin irritation, worsening of psoriasis Avoid face, mucous membranes, eyes; wash hands after application Maximum weekly dosage of cream by age: 2-5 yrs – 25 g/wk 6-10 yrs – 50 g/wk 11-14 yrs – 75 g/wk >14 – 100 g/wk
Imiquimod (Aldara®, Zyclara – 3.75%)	5% cream applied 3x/wk Apply at bedtime, leave on 6-10 h, then wash off with mild soap and water Max. duration 16 wks	Genital Warts Cutaneous warts Actinic keratosis Superficial basal cell carcinoma	Avoid natural/artificial sun exposure Local reactions Erythema, ulceration, edema, flu-like symptoms Works best for warts on mucosal surfaces May induce inflammation and erosion
Permethrin (Kwellada® P Lotion and Nix® Dermal Cream)	5% cream, applied once overnight to all skin areas from neck down	Scabies (Kwellada-P Lotion, Nix® Dermal Cream) Pediculosis (Kwellada-P Crème Rinse®, Nix Crème Rinse®)	Do not use in children <2 yrs old Hypersensitivity to drug, or known sensitivity to chrysanthemums Local reactions resolve rapidly (e.g. burning, pruritis) Low toxicity Consider 2nd application after 7 d, excellent results
Pimecrolimus (Elidel®)	1% cream BID Use for as long as lesions persist and d/c upon resolution of symptoms	Atopic dermatitis (mild to moderate)	Burning Lacks adverse effects of steroids May be used on all skin surfaces including head, neck, and intertriginous areas Expensive
Tacrolimus topical (Protopic®)	0.03% (children) or 0.1% (adults) ointment BID Continue for duration of disease PLUS x 1 wk after clearing and OD 2x weekly to trouble areas as maintenance therapy	Atopic dermatitis (mild to moderate)	Burning Lacks adverse effects of steroids May be used on all skin surfaces, neck, and intertriginous areas. Can't apply to scalp if full head of hair Expensive

Emergency Medicine, Trauma and Toxicology

Rapid Primary Survey

- **A**irway maintenance with cervical spine control
- **B**reathing and ventilation
- **C**irculation (pulses, hemorrhage control)
- **D**isability (neurological status)
- **E**xposure (complete) and **E**nvironment (temperature control)

AIRWAY

- Secure airway and think about future airway patency
- Assume C-spine injury in every trauma patient; immobilize with collar-board
- Assess ability to breathe, speak
- Look for signs of airway obstruction: noisy breathing, dysphonia, agitation, confusion, respiratory distress, cyanosis
- If airway not secure, first try basic airway management: head tilt, chin lift/jaw thrust, nasopharyngeal or oropharyngeal airway
- Indications for definitive airway management (endotracheal intubation):
    - Unable to protect airway
    - Inadequate oxygenation
    - Profound shock
    - Anticipate need for intubation in near future (e.g. in trauma, overdose, CHF, asthma/COPD, for transfer)
- Surgical airway (cricothyroidotomy) if unable to intubate

Approach to Endotracheal Intubation in an Injured Patient

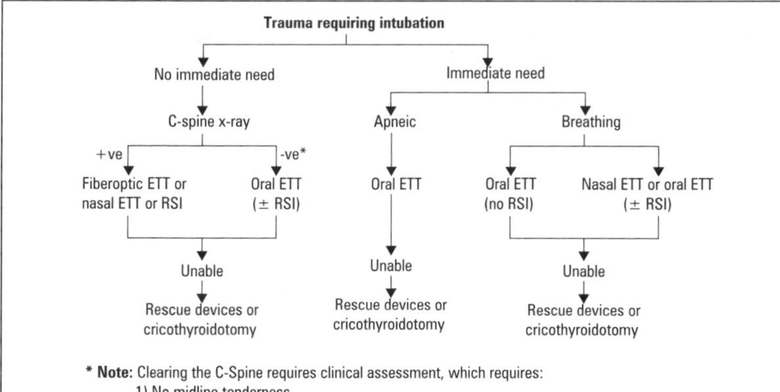

BREATHING AND VENTILATION
- Assess respiratory rate, O_2 sat (pulse oximetry)
- **Look**: mental status (agitation, anxiety), LOC, colour, chest movement
- **Listen**: sounds of obstruction, breath sounds, symmetry of air entry
- **Feel**: flow of air, tracheal shift, crepitus/subcutaneous emphysema, flail segments, sucking chest wounds
- Arterial blood gas (ABG), A-a gradient, peak flow rate (PFR) as indicated
- Manage poor ventilation with nasal prongs, simple face mask, oxygen reservoir mask, CPAP/BiPAP, or mechanical ventilation

CIRCULATION
- Assess for signs of shock – hypotension, weak pulses, shallow/rapid respirations, cool, cyanotic, anxious, unconscious
- Assume shock in trauma patient is hemorrhage until proven otherwise
- Signs of hemorrhage – tachypnea, tachycardia, reduced urine output, delayed capillary refill, cool extremities, mottled extremities, hypotension (late), altered mental status (late)
- Control external bleeding by applying direct pressure
- 2 large bore IVs in place – infuse 1-2 L NS as rapidly as possible
- Group and screen blood, consider transfusion
- If inadequate response to fluids, consider ongoing internal blood loss – may need operative management

Estimation of Degree of Hemorrhagic Shock

Class	I	II	III	IV
Blood loss (% of blood volume)	<750 cc (<15%)	750-1500 cc (15-30%)	1500-2000 cc (30-40%)	>2000 cc (>40%)
Pulse	<100	>100	>120	>140
Blood pressure	Normal	Normal	Decreased	Decreased
Respiratory rate	20	30	35	>45
Capillary refill	Normal	Decreased	Decreased	Decreased
Urinary output	30 cc/h	20 cc/h	10 cc/h	None
Fluid replacement	Crystalloid	Crystalloid	Crystalloid + blood	Crystalloid + blood

Major Types of Shock

Hypovolemic	Cardiogenic	Distributive	Obstructive
Hemorrhage (external and internal)	MI	Septic	Cardiac tamponade
Severe burns	Arrhythmias	Anaphylactic	Tension pneumothorax
High output fistulas	CHF	Neurogenic (spinal cord injury)	Pulmonary embolism
	Cardiomyopathies		Aortic stenosis
	Cardiac valve problems		Constrictive pericarditis

Disability – Neurologic Status
- Assess LOC by Glasgow Coma Score (GCS) or AVPU method:
  - **A** – **A**lert
  - **V** – responds to **V**erbal stimuli
  - **P** – responds to **P**ainful stimuli
  - **U** – **U**nresponsive
- Assess size/reactivity of pupils, assess ability to move all 4 limbs

Glasgow Coma Scale

Eyes Open		Best Verbal Response		Best Motor Response	
Spontaneously	4	Answers questions appropriately	5	Obeys commands	6
To voice	3	Confused, disoriented	4	Localizes to pain	5
To pain	2	Inappropriate words	3	Withdraws from pain	4
No response	1	Incomprehensible sounds	2	Decorticate (flexion)	3
		No verbal response	1	Decerebrate (extension)	2
				No response	1

EXPOSURE AND ENVIRONMENT
- Undress patient completely to assess all areas for possible injury
- Avoid hypothermia by warming patient with blanket ± radiant heaters

Detailed Secondary Survey

History

"SAMPLE"
Signs and **S**ymptoms
Allergies
Medications
Past medical history
Last meal
Events related to injury

Physical Exam

HEAD AND NECK
- Pupils
  - Assess equality, size, symmetry, reactivity to light – inequality suggests local eye problem or lateralizing CNS lesion
- Reactivity/level of consciousness (LOC)
  - Reactive pupils + decreased LOC → ? metabolic or structural cause
  - Non-reactive pupils + decreased LOC → ? structural cause (especially if asymmetric)
- Extraocular movements and nystagmus
- Fundoscopy (papilledema, hemorrhages)
- Palpation of facial bones, scalp
- Tympanic membranes, fluid in ear canal, hemotympanum, Battle's sign (mastoid bruising), neck tenderness
- Relative afferent pupillary defect – optic nerve damage

CHEST
- Inspect for flail segment, contusion
- Palpate for subcutaneous emphysema
- Auscultate lung fields

ABDOMEN
- Assess for peritonitis, abdominal distention, and evidence of intra-abdominal bleeding
- FAST (**F**ocused **A**ssessment with **S**onography for **T**rauma), diagnostic peritoneal lavage (DPL) or CT
- Rectal exam for GI bleed, high riding prostate and anal tone (best to do during the log roll)
- Bimanual exam in females as appropriate

MSK
- Examine all extremities for swelling, deformity, contusion, tenderness
- Log roll and palpate thoracic and lumbar spines
- Palpate iliac crests and pubic symphysis, pelvic stability (lateral, AP, vertical)

NEUROLOGICAL
- GCS
- Alterations of rate and rhythm of breathing are signs of structural or metabolic abnormalities
    - Progressive deterioration of breathing pattern implies a failing CNS
- Full cranial nerve exam
- Assessment of spinal cord integrity
    - Conscious patient: assess distal sensation and motor ability
    - Unconscious patient: response to painful or noxious stimulus applied to extremities

Detailed Secondary Survey

- Done after rapid primary survey problems have been addressed
- Identifies major injuries or areas of concern
- Full physical exam and x-rays (C-spine, chest, pelvis – required in blunt trauma, consider T-spine and L-spine)
- CT may replace screening spine x-rays

Management of Specific Traumas

Head Trauma

CANADIAN CT HEAD RULE
- **CT Head is only required for patients with minor head injuries with any one of the following**:
    - High risk (for neurological intervention)
        - GCS <15 at 2 h after injury
        - Suspected open or depressed skull fracture
        - Any sign of basal skull fracture (hemotympanum, "raccoon" eyes, cerebrospinal fluid otorrhea/rhinorrhoea, Battle's sign)
        - Vomiting ≥2 episodes
        - Age ≥65 yrs
    - Medium risk (for brain injury on CT)
        - Amnesia before impact >30 min
        - Dangerous mechanism (pedestrian struck by motor vehicle, occupant ejected from motor vehicle, fall from height >3 feet or five stairs)
- Minor head injury is defined as witnessed loss of consciousness, definite amnesia, or witnessed disorientation in a patient with a GCS 13-15

The Lancet 2001; 357:9266;1391-1396.

Spine Trauma

CANADIAN C-SPINE RULES
- For alert and stable patients where cervical spine injury is a concern:
    - Any high risk factor that mandates radiography? IF YES, patient needs radiograph:
        - Age >65 yrs
        - Dangerous mechanism
        - Fall from >1 meter/5 stairs
        - Axial load to head
        - MVC high speed (>100 km/h), rollover, ejection
        - Motorized recreational vehicles
        - Bicycle collision
        - Paraesthesias in extremities

- Any low risk factor that allows safe assessment of range of motion?
  IF NO, patient needs radiograph:
  - Simple rear end MVC (excludes being pushed into oncoming traffic, hit by a large bus/truck, rollover, or collision at high speed)
  - Sitting position in ED
  - Ambulatory at any time
  - Delayed onset of neck pain
  - Absence of midline C-spine tenderness
- Able to actively rotate neck? IF NO, patient needs radiograph

In brief: Can clear the C-spine if
- No posterior midline cervical tenderness
- No evidence of intoxication
- Oriented to person, place, time and event
- No focal neurological deficits
- No painful distracting injuries (e.g. long bone fracture)

Approach to Clearing the C-spine

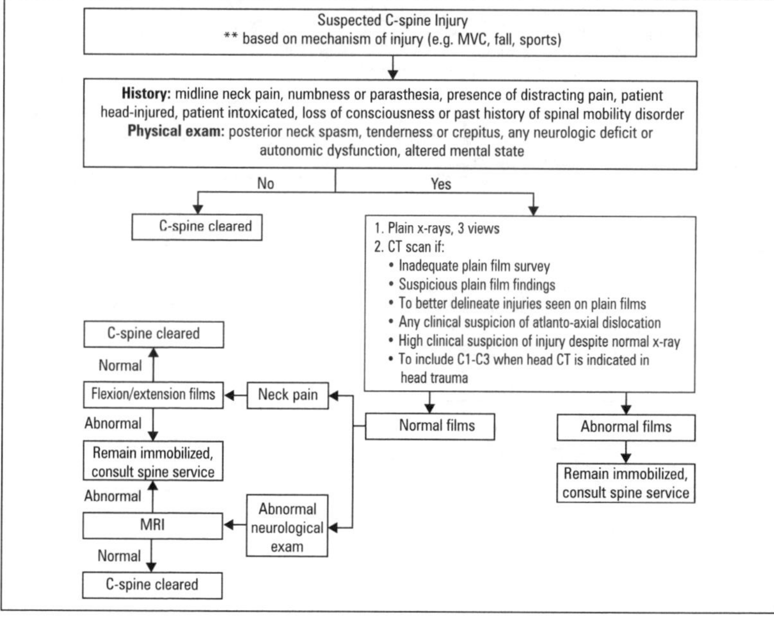

Chest Trauma

Life-Threatening Chest Injuries Found in 1° Survey

	Physical Exam	Investigations	Management
Airway Obstruction	Anxiety, stridor, hoarseness, altered mental status, apnea, cyanosis	Do not wait for ABG to intubate	Definitive airway Intubate early Remove FB if visible with laryngoscope prior to intubation
Tension Pneumothorax Clinical diagnosis One-way valve causing accumulation of air in pleural space	Respiratory distress, tachycardia, distended neck veins, cyanosis, asymmetry of chest wall motion Tracheal deviation away from pneumothorax Percussion hyperresonance Unilateral absence of breath sounds	Non-radiographic diagnosis	Needle thoracostomy – large bore needle, 2nd ICS mid clavicular line above 3rd rib, followed by chest tube in 5th ICS, anterior axillary line
Open Pneumothorax Air entering chest from wound rather than trachea	Gunshot or other wound (hole >2/3 tracheal diameter) ± exit wound Unequal breath sounds	ABG: decreased pO_2	Air-tight dressing sealed on 3 sides Chest tube Surgery
Massive Hemothorax >1500 cc blood loss in chest cavity	Pallor, flat neck veins, shock Unilateral dullness Absent breath sounds, hypotension	Usually only able to do supine CXR – entire lung appears radioopaque as blood spreads out over posterior thoracic cavity	Restore blood volume Chest tube Thoracotomy if: >1500 cc total blood loss ≥200 cc/h continued drainage
Flail Chest Free-floating segment of chest wall due to >2 rib fractures, each at 2 sites Underlying lung contusion (cause of morbidity and mortality)	Paradoxical movement of flail segment Palpable crepitus of ribs Decreased air entry on affected side	ABG: decreased pO_2, increased pCO_2 CXR: rib fractures, lung contusion	O_2 + fluid therapy + pain control Judicious fluid therapy in absence of systemic hypotension Positive pressure ventilation ± intubation and ventilation
Cardiac Tamponade Clinical diagnosis Pericardial fluid accumulation impairing ventricular function	Penetrating wound (usually) Beck's triad: hypotension, distended neck veins, muffled heart sounds Tachycardia, tachypnea Pulsus paradoxus Kussmaul's sign	Echocardiogram Bedside ultrasound (FAST)	IV fluids Pericardiocentesis Open thoracotomy

Potentially Life-Threatening Chest Injuries Found in 2° Survey

	Physical Exam	Investigations	Management
Pulmonary Contusion	Blunt trauma to chest Interstitial edema impairs compliance and gas exchange	CXR: areas of opacification of lung within 6 h of trauma	Maintain adequate ventilation Monitor with ABG, pulse oximeter and ECG Chest physiotherapy Positive pressure ventilation if severe
Ruptured Diaphragm	Blunt trauma to chest or abdomen (e.g. high lap belt in MVC)	CXR: abnormality of diaphragm/ lower lung fields/NG tube placement CT scan and endoscopy – sometimes helpful for diagnosis	Laparotomy for diaphragm repair and because of associated intra-abdominal injuries
Esophageal Injury	Usually penetrating trauma (pain out of proportion to degree of injury)	CXR: mediastinal air (not always) Esophagram (Gastrograffin) Flexible esophagoscopy	Early repair (within 24 h) improves outcome but all require repair

Potentially Life-Threatening Chest Injuries Found in 2° Survey (continued)

	Physical Exam	Investigations	Management
Aortic Tear 90% tear at subclavian (near ligamentum arteriosum), most die at scene Salvageable if diagnosis made rapidly	Sudden high speed deceleration (e.g. MVC, fall, airplane crash), complaints of chest pain, dyspnea, hoarseness frequently absent) Decreased femoral pulses, differential arm BP (arch tear)	CXR, CT scan, transesophageal echo (TEE), aortography (gold standard)	Thoracotomy (may treat other severe injuries first)
Blunt Myocardial Injury (Rare)	Blunt trauma to chest (usually in setting of multi-system trauma and therefore difficult to diagnose Physical examination: overlying injury, i.e. fractures, chest wall contusion	ECG: arrhythmias, ST changes Patients with a normal ECG and normal hemodynamics never get dysrhythmias	O_2 Antiarrhythmic agents Analgesia

Abdominal Trauma

Imaging must be done if:
- Equivocal abdominal examination, suspected intra-abdominal injury or distracting injuries
- Patient with multiple injuries resulting in unreliable physical exam
- Unexplained shock/hypotension
- Patient must undergo anesthesia
- Fractures to lower ribs, pelvis, spine
- Positive FAST

Orthopedic Emergency

UPPER EXTREMITY INJURIES
- Anterior shoulder dislocation
  - Axillary nerve (lateral aspect of shoulder) and musculocutaneous nerve (extensor aspect of forearm) at risk
  - Seen on lateral view: humeral head anterior to glenoid
    - Reduce (traction, scapular manipulation), immobilize in internal rotation, re-x-ray, out-patient appointment with ortho
    - With forceful injury, look for fracture
- Colles' fracture
  - Distal radius fracture with dorsal displacement
  - From fall on an outstretched hand (FOOSH)
  - AP film: shortening, radial deviation, radial displacement
  - Lateral film: dorsal displacement, volar angulation
  - Reduce, immobilize with splint, out-patient with ortho or immediate ortho referral if complicated fracture
  - If involvement of articular surface, emergent ortho referral
- Scaphoid fracture
  - Tenderness in anatomical snuff box, pain on scaphoid tubercle, pain on axial loading of thumb
  - Negative x-ray: thumb spica splint, re-x-ray in 1 wk ± bone scan
  - Positive x-ray: thumb spica splint x 6-8 wks
  - Risk of AVN of scaphoid if not immobilized
  - Outpatient ortho appointment

LOWER EXTREMITY INJURIES
- Ankle and foot fractures
  - See Ottawa Ankle and Foot Rules (see Figure below)
- Knee injuries
  - See Ottawa Knee Rules (see Figure below)
- Avulsion of the base of 5th metatarsal
  - Occurs with inversion injury
  - Supportive tensor or below knee walking cast for 3 wks
- Calcaneal fracture
  - Associated with fall from height
  - Associated injuries may involve ankles, knees, hips, pelvis, lumbar spine

Ottawa Ankle Rules

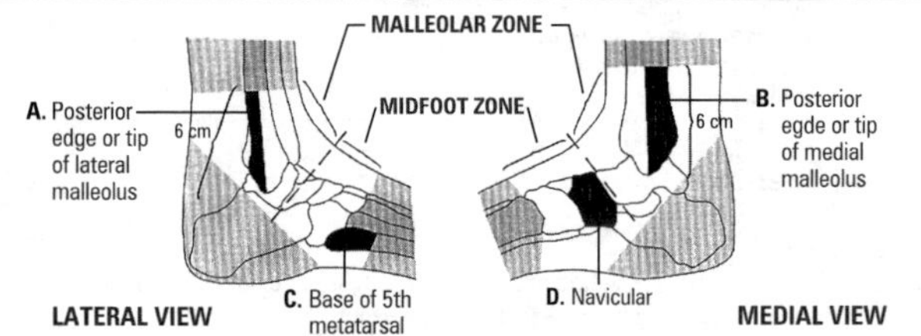

An ankle radiographic series is required only if there is any pain in malleolar zone and any of these findings:
1. bone tenderness at A

or

2. bone tenderness at B

or

3. inability to bear weight both immediately and in emergency department

A foot radiographic series is required only if there is any pain in midfoot zone and any of these findings:
1. bone tenderness at C

or

2. bone tenderness at D

or

3. inability to bear weight both immediately and in emergency department

Reprinted with permission from Stiell et. al. *JAMA* 1994; 271(11):827-832. © 1994, American Medical Association.

Ottawa Knee Rules

- A knee x-ray examination is required only for acute injury patients with one or more of:
  - Age 55 yrs or older
  - Tenderness at head of fibula
  - Isolated tenderness of patella*
  - Inability to flex to 90°
  - Inability to bear weight both immediately and in the emergency department (four steps)**

* No bony tenderness of knee other than patella
**Unable to transfer weight twice onto each lower limb regardless of limping

Reprinted with permission from: Stiell et. al. *JAMA* 1997; 278(23):611-615. © 1997, American Medical Association.

Common Presentations

Abdominal Pain

Life-Threatening Causes
- CVS: MI, aortic dissection, ruptured AAA (tearing pain)
- GI: perforated viscus, hepatic/splenic injury, ischemic bowel (diffuse pain)
- Gynecologic: ectopic pregnancy

Additional Differential Diagnosis
- GI: appendicitis, diverticulitis, bowel obstruction, hepatitis, cholecystitis, pancreatitis
- Urinary: cystitis, pyelonephritis, ureteral calculi
- Genital
    - Female: pelvic inflammatory disease (PID)/salpingitis/tubo-ovarian abscess, ovarian torsion/cyst, endometriosis
    - Male: testicular torsion, epididymitis

History and Physical Examination
- Determine onset, course, location and character of pain: **OPQRST**
- Broad differential, including GU, Gyne, GI, respiratory and CV systems

Investigations
- CBC, electrolytes, glucose, LFTs, amylase, BUN/creat, U/A, + others if indicated: β-hCG, ECG, troponins
- AXR: look for calcifications, free air, gas pattern, air fluid levels
- CXR upright: look for pneumoperitoneum (free air under diaphragm)
- U/S: biliary tract, ectopic pregnancy, AAA, free fluid
- CT: trauma, AAA, pancreatitis, nephro/urolithiasis, appendicitis and diverticulitis

Management
- NPO, IV, NG tube, analgesics – treat as appropriate
- Consult as necessary: general surgery, vascular, gynecology, etc.

Acute Pelvic Pain

- Ruptured ovarian cysts – most common cause of pelvic pain
- Ovarian torsion – rare, 50% will have ovarian mass
- Leiomyomas (uterine fibroids) – especially with torsion of a pedunculated fibroid or in pregnant patient (degeneration)
- Ectopic pregnancy – ruptured/expanding/leaking
- Spontaneous abortion – threatened or incomplete
- Infection – PID, endometritis, tubo-ovarian abscess, retained products of conception
- Dysmenorrhea and endometriosis – rarely cause new onset acute pelvic pain
- Non-gynecological: appendicitis, constipation, diverticulitis, IBD, IBS, cystitis, pyelonephritis, ureteric stone
- Other – porphyria, abdominal angina, aneurysm, hernia, zoster

History and Physical Exam
- Associated symptoms: vaginal bleeding, bowel or bladder symptoms, radiation
- Vitals, gynecological exam, abdominal exam

Investigations
- β-hCG, CBC and differential, PTT, INR
- Pelvic and abdominal U/S – evaluate adnexa, look for free fluid in the pelvis or masses, evaluate thickness of endometrium
- Doppler flow studies for ovarian torsion

Management
- General: analgesia, determine if admission and consults needed
  - Gynecology consult if history and physical suggestive of serious cause
  - Other consults as indicated – general surgery, urology, etc.
- Specific:
  - Ovarian cysts
    - Unruptured or ruptured and hemodynamically stable – analgesia and follow-up
    - Ruptured with significant hemoperitoneum – may require surgery
  - Ovarian torsion – surgical detorsion or removal of ovary
  - Uncomplicated leiomyomas, endometriosis and secondary dysmenorrhea can usually be treated on an outpatient basis, discharge with gynecology follow-up
  - PID: requires broad spectrum antibiotics

Altered Level of Consciousness (LOC)

Etiology of Coma

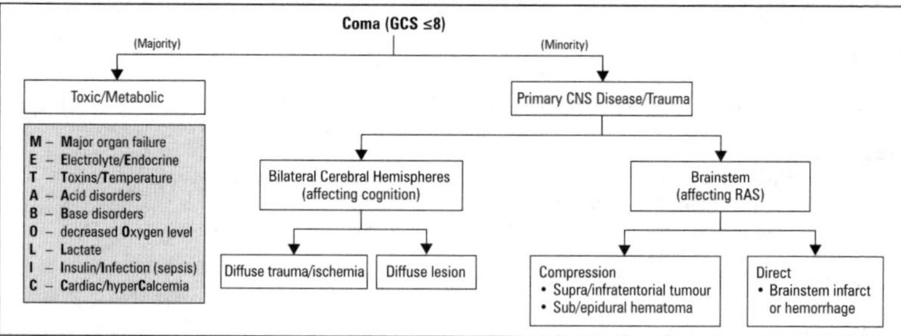

Management
- Administer appropriate universal antidotes
  - Thiamine 100 mg IV if history of EtOH or patient looks malnourished
  - One ampule D50W IV if low blood sugar on finger-stick
  - Naloxone 0.4-2 mg IV or IM if opiate overdose suspected
- Distinguish between structural and toxic-metabolic coma
  - Structural coma
    - Pupils, extraocular movements and motor findings are asymmetric or absent
  - Toxic-metabolic coma
    - Dysfunction at lower levels of the brainstem (e.g. caloric unresponsiveness)
    - Respiratory depression in association with an intact upper brainstem (e.g. equal and reactive pupils; see exceptions in Table)
    - Extraocular movements and motor findings are symmetric or absent

Toxic – Metabolic Causes of Fixed Pupils

Dilated	Dilated to Normal	Constricted
Anoxia	Hypothermia	Cholinergic agents (e.g. organophosphates)
Anticholinergic agents (e.g. atropine, TCAs)	Barbiturates	Opiates (e.g. heroin), except meperidine
Cocaine		
Opioid withdrawal		

- Essential to re-examine frequently – status can change rapidly
- Diagnosis may become apparent only with the passage of time
  - Delayed deficit after head trauma suggestive of epidural hematoma (characteristic "lucid interval")

Anaphylaxis

Anaphylaxis Immediate Treatment
- ABC's
- Very low threshold for intubation – beware of oropharyngeal edema!
- O_2, IV access
- Drugs
  - Epinephrine 0.3-0.5 mL (1:1000) IM in anterolateral thigh q3-5 mins PRN (adult); 0.01 mL/kg/dose up to 0.4 mL/dose 1:1000 epinephrine (children)
  - Diphenhydramine 25-50 mg IV q4-6 h
  - Ranitidine 50 mg IV
  - Methylprednisolone 125 mg IV
  - Albuterol 2.5-5 mg in 3 mL saline via nebuliser (if refractory to epi)
  - Glucagon 1-2 mg IV for patients on β-blockers (inadequate response to epi)

Bites

INSECTS
- Bee stings
  - ABC management, epinephrine 0.1 mg IV over 5 min if shock, antihistamines, cimetidine 300 mg IV/IM/PO, steroids, β-agonists for SOB/wheezing 3 mg in 5 mL NS via nebulizer, local site management
- West Nile Virus (see <u>Infectious Diseases</u>)
  - General symptoms: fever, malaise, anorexia, headache, altered mental status, motor weakness, ataxia, extrapyramidal signs, GI signs, myalgias, lymphadenopathy, rash, myocarditis, optic neuritis
  - Diagnosis: CSF and serum for serology
  - Management: ABCs, IV fluids for dehydration, antibiotics if signs of meningitis (based on CSF analysis), analgesia, antipyretics, interferon-α 2b, ribavirin

MAMMALIAN BITES
- Initial management
  - Wound cleansing and copious irrigation as soon as possible
  - Irrigate/debride puncture wounds if feasible, but not if sealed or very small openings; avoid hydrodissection along tissue planes
  - Debridement is important in crush injuries to reduce infection and optimize cosmetic and functional repair
  - Culture wound if signs of infection (erythema, necrosis or pus); obtain anaerobic cultures if wound foul smelling, necrotizing, or abscess; notify lab that sample is from bite wound
- Prophylactic antibiotics
  - Types of infections resulting from bites: cellulitis, lymphangitis, abscesses, tenosynovitis, osteomyelitis, septic arthritis, sepsis, endocarditis, meningitis
  - A 3-5 d course of antibiotics is recommended for all bite wounds to the hand and should be considered in other bites if any high-risk factors present (efficacy not proven)
  - Tetanus immunization if >10 yrs since last vaccine or incomplete primary series

Chest Pain/DVT/PE

ACUTE MYOCARDIAL INFARCTION (MI)

Management
- Immediate stabilization
  - Oxygen 4 L/min
  - IV access
  - Cardiac monitors
  - "STAT" ECG
  - Cardiac enzymes (CK, Troponins)
- ASA 160-325 mg chewed
- Nitroglycerin 0.3 mg SL q5min x 3 (IV for CHF, HTN, unresolved pain)
- Morphine 2-5 mg IV q5-30min if unresponsive to NTG
- Metoprolol 5 mg slow IV q5min x 3 if no contraindication (beware in inferior MI)
- Thrombolytics or primary percutaneous coronary intervention (PCI)
  - Agents include t-PA, r-PA, Streptokinase and TNK
  - Evaluate indications and contraindications prior to use
- Enoxaparin (Low Molecular Weight Heparin) 1 mg/kg SC bid (30 mg IV STAT post TNK infusion)
- Other – antiarrythmics, cardioversion, defibrillation, transthoracic pacing, angioplasty
- Cardiology consult

DEEP VEIN THROMBOSIS (DVT)

Wells' Score for DVT
- ≥2 DVT clinical pre-test probability likely, <2 DVT clinical pre-test probability unlikely

Clinical Parameter	Score	Clinical Parameter	Score
Active cancer (ongoing treatment, within 6 months, or palliative)	1	Calf swelling >3 cm compared to asymptomatic leg	1
Paralysis, paresis, or recent immobilization of the lower limbs	1	Pitting edema, greater in the symptomatic leg	1
Recently bedridden for >3 d or major surgery within 4 wks	1	Collateral superficial non-varicose veins	1
Localized tenderness along distribution of deep venous system	1	Alternative diagnosis likely	-2
Entire leg swelling	1		

PERC (Pulmonary Embolism Rule-Out Criteria) – assess prior to Well's criteria
- Age > 50 yrs
- HR >100 bpm
- O_2 sat on RA <94%
- Prior history DVT/PE
- Recent trauma or surgery
- Hemoptysis
- Exogenous estrogen
- Clinical signs suggesting DVT
- Score 1 for each question; a score 0/8 means patient has <1.6% chance having a PE and avoids further investigation

Wells' Score for PE
- <2 low probability, 2-6 intermediate probability, >6 high probability

Clinical Parameter	Score	Clinical Parameter	Score
Clinical finding suggestive of DVT	3	Previous DVT or PE	1.5
Alternative diagnosis unlikely	3	Malignancy (ongoing treatment, within 6 months, or palliative)	1
Recent bed rest for >3 d or major surgery within 4 wks	1.5	Hemoptysis	1
Heart rate >100	1.5		

PULMONARY EMBOLISM (PE)
Approach to Suspected PE

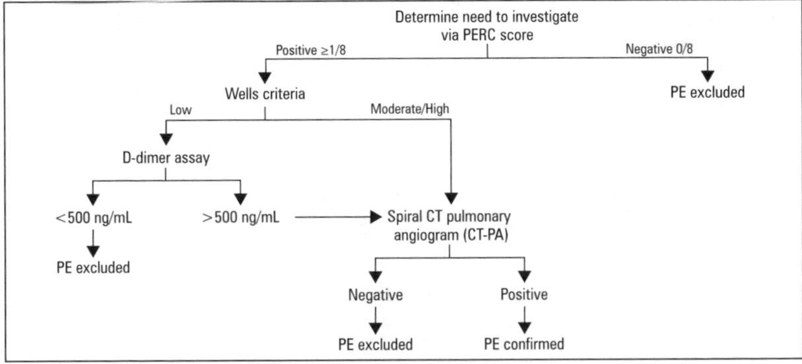

V/Q-Based Algorithm for Suspected PE

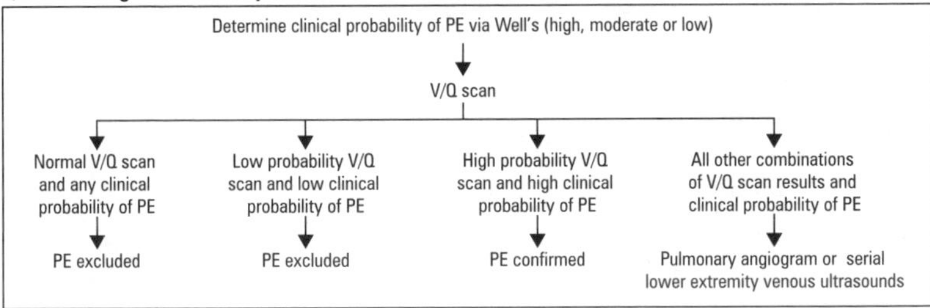

Headache

• See also Neurology

Etiology
- **The common**
  - Common migraine (no aura)/classic migraine (involves aura)
    - Gradual onset, unilateral/bilateral, throbbing
    - Nausea/vomiting, photo/phonophobia
    - Treatment: analgesics, neuroleptics, vasoactive meds
  - Tension/muscular headache
    - Never during sleep, gradual over 24 h
    - Posterior/occipital
    - Increased with stressors
    - Treatment: modify stressor, local measures, NSAIDs, tricyclic antidepressants

- **The deadly**
  - **Subarachnoid hemorrhage (SAH)** (see Neurosurgery)
    - Sudden onset, increased with exertion
    - "Worst" headache, nausea and vomiting, meningeal signs

  - ◆ Diagnosis: CT, LP (5-10% of patients with SAH have negative initial CT)
    – Sensitivity of CT decreases with time and is much less sensitive by 48-72 h
  - ◆ Management: urgent neurosurgery consult
- **Increased ICP**
  - ◆ Worst in morning, supine, or bending down
  - ◆ Physical exam: neurological deficits, cranial nerve palsies, papilledema
  - ◆ Diagnosis: CT scan
  - ◆ Management: consult neurosurgery
- **Meningitis** (see <u>Infectious Diseases</u>)
  - ◆ Fu-like presentation initially (fever, nausea/vomiting, malaise), meningeal signs, purpuric rash
  - ◆ Altered level of consciousness and confusion
  - ◆ Perform CT to rule out increased ICP then do LP for diagnosis
  - ◆ Treatment: early empiric antibiotics (depending on age group), steroid therapy
- **Temporal arteritis** (not immediately deadly but causes great morbidity) (see <u>Ophthalmology</u>)
  - ◆ Unilateral scalp tenderness, jaw claudication, visual disturbances
  - ◆ Labs: elevated ESR
  - ◆ Temporal artery biopsy is gold standard for diagnosis
  - ◆ Treatment: high-dose steroids immediately if TA suspected

Disposition
- Admit if underlying diagnosis is critical or emergent, if there are abnormal neurological findings, if patient is elderly or immunocompromised (don't manifest symptoms as well), or if pain is refractory to oral medications
- Most patients can be discharged with appropriate analgesia and follow-up with their family physician. Instruct patients to return for fever, vomiting, neurologic changes, or increasing pain

- **BEWARE**: every headache is serious until proven otherwise

Hypertensive Emergency/Urgency

- In hypertensive emergency (target organ damage present), urgent consult to varying services depending on type(s) of target organ damage:
  - Cardiology if ACS
  - Cardiac or vascular surgery if dissection
  - Neurology if acute stroke, possibly seizure d/o
  - Nephrology if renal failure
  - Otherwise general internal medicine
- In hypertensive urgency (no target organ damage), patient can usually be discharged home with follow-up
- Goal of treatment for hypertension in ER
  - In hypertensive emergency, the initial goal for BP reduction is to achieve a progressive, controlled reduction in BP to minimize the risk of hypoperfusion in cerebral, coronary, and renovascular beds. This can be done by reducing mean arterial blood pressure by 20-25% over a period of minutes to hours using IV agents
  - Ensure intensive monitoring of vitals and IV access
- **Exceptions**: in ischemic stroke do not use antihypertensive agents unless sBP >220 or dBP >120-140, in dissection or acute MI may lower BP more rapidly
- In hypertensive urgency, there is generally not good evidence to suggest that it is necessary to lower BP acutely in the ER
- If decision is made to administer antihypertensive drugs, use oral agents
- **Medications**
  - IV agents (choice in agent may depend on affected organ): nitroprusside 0.25-10 ug/kg/min, nitroglycerin 17-1000 ug/min, labetalol 20-80 mg bolus q10 min or 2-4 mg/min, hydralazine 5-20 mg q20-30 min, phentolamine 5-15 mg bolus prn
  - PO agents: captopril 25-50 mg, labetalol 200-400 mg, clonidine 0.1-0.2 mg loading dose then 0.1 mg qhr, hydralazine 10-25 mg
  - See *Common Medications* at end of chapter

Hospital/Inpatient
- Patients with organ damage usually require admission, rapid lowering of BP using IV medications and further medical workup
- Transition to oral medications as soon as possible

Pediatric Emergency

Modified GCS for Infants

Eye opening	Verbal Response	Motor Response
4 – Spontaneously	5 – Coos, babbles	6 – Normal, spontaneous movement
3 – To speech	4 – Irritable cry	5 – Withdraws to touch
2 – To pain	3 – Cries to pain	4 – Withdraws to pain
1 – No response	2 – Moans to pain	3 – Decorticate flexion
	1 – No response	2 – Decerebrate extension
		1 – No response

Modified GCS for Children <4 yrs

Eye opening	Verbal Response	Motor Response
4 – Spontaneously	5 – Oriented, social, speaks, interacts	6 – Normal, spontaneous movement
3 – To speech	4 – Confused speech, disoriented, consolable	5 – Localizes pain
2 – To pain	3 – Inappropriate words, not consolable/aware	4 – Withdraws to pain
1 – No response	2 – Incomprehensible, agitated, restless, not aware	3 – Decorticate flexion
	1 – No response	2 – Decerebrate extension
		1 – No response

- For pediatric respiratory emergencies, see *Shortness of Breath*

Pregnancy

Emergencies of Pregnancy

Trimester	Fetal	Maternal	
First **1-12 wks**	Pregnancy failure: Spontaneous abortion Fetal demise Gestational trophoblastic disease	Ectopic pregnancy Anemia Hyperemesis gravidarum UTI/pyelonephritis	
Second **13-28 wks**	Disorders of fetal growth: IUGR Oligo/polyhydramnios	Gestational diabetes mellitus Rh incompatibility UTI/pyelonephritis	
Third **29-41 wk**	Vasa previa	Preterm labour/PPROM Preeclampsia/eclampsia Placenta previa	Placental abruption Uterine rupture DVT

Seizure

STATUS EPILEPTICUS

Management of Status Epilepticus

Time (min)	Steps
0-5	Give oxygen; ensure adequate ventilation Monitor: vital signs, electrocardiography, oximetry Establish IV access; obtain blood samples for glucose level, CBC, electrolytes, toxins, and anticonvulsant levels
6-9	Give glucose (preceded by thiamine in adults)
10-20	Intravenously administer either 0.1 mg/kg of lorazepam at 2 mg/min or 0.2 mg/kg of diazepam at 5 mg/min Diazepam can be repeated if seizures do not stop after 5 min; if diazepam is used to stop the status, then phenytoin should be administered promptly to prevent the recurrence of status
21-60	If status persists, administer 15-20 mg/kg of phenytoin intravenously no faster than 50 mg/min in adults and 1 mg/kg/min in children
>60	If status does not stop after 20 mg/kg of phenytoin, give additional doses of 5 mg/kg to a maximal dose of 30 mg/kg. If status persists, then give 20 mg/kg of phenobarbital IV at 100 mg/min When phenobarbital is given after a benzodiazepine, ventilatory assistance is usually required. If status persists, then give general anaesthesia (e.g. pentobarbital). Vasopressors or fluid volume are usually necessary Electroencephalogram should be monitored. Neuromuscular blockade may be needed

Source: Cecil's Essentials of Medicine, 7th edition, Table 125-7. Used with permission.

Shortness of Breath

Stridorous Upper Airway Diseases: Diagnosis

Feature	Croup	Bacterial Tracheitis	Epiglottitis[1]
Age range (yrs)	0.5-4	5-10	2-8
Prodrome	Days	Hours to days	Minutes to hours
Temperature	Low grade	High	High
Radiography	Steeple sign	Exudates in trachea	Thumb sign
Etiology	Parainfluenza	*S. aureus*/GAS	*H. flu* type b
Barky Cough	Yes	Yes	No
Drooling	Yes	No	Yes
Appear Toxic	No	Yes	Yes
Intubation? ICU?	No	Yes	Yes
Antibiotics	No	Yes	Yes
NOTE:			No oral exam, consult ENT!

[1] Rare now with Hib vaccine in common use

Asthma Assessment and Management

Classifications	History and Physical Examination	Management
Respiratory Arrest Imminent	Exhausted, confused, diaphoretic, cyanotic Silent chest, ineffective respiratory effort Decreased HR O_2 sat <90% despite supplemental O_2	100% O_2, cardiac monitor, IV access Intubate β-agonist: MDI 4-8 puffs OR nebulizer 5 mg continually Anticholinergics: MDI 4-8 puffs q20min x 3 OR nebulizer 0.5 mg q20min x 3 IV steroids: methylprednisolone 125 mg, hydrocortisone 500 mg
Severe Asthma	Agitated, diaphoretic, laboured respirations Difficulty speaking in full sentences No relief from β-agonist O_2 sat <90%, FEV_1 <50%	Anticipate need for intubation Similar to above management β-agonist may be less frequent; q15-20min
Moderate Asthma	SOB at rest, cough, congestion, chest tightness Nocturnal symptoms Inadequate relief from β-agonist FEV_1 50-80%	O_2 to achieve O_2-sat >90% β-agonist: puffer of neb q1h Steroids: prednisone 40-60 mg PO Anticholinergics
Mild Asthma	Exertional SOB/cough with some nocturnal symptoms Good response to β-agonist FEV_1 >80%	β-agonist Monitor FEV_1 Consider steroids (nebulized or PO)

Acute Exacerbation of COPD (AECOPD)
- See Respirology pd 450

Stroke

Stroke Syndromes

Region of Stroke	Stroke Syndrome
Anterior Cerebral Artery	Primarily frontal lobe function affected Altered mental status, impaired judgement, contralateral lower extremity weakness and hypoesthesia, gait apraxia
Middle Cerebral Artery	Contralateral hemiparesis (arm and face weakness > leg weakness) and hypoesthesia, ipsilateral hemianopsia, gaze preference to side of lesion ± agnosia, receptive/expressive aphasia
Posterior Cerebral Artery	Affects vision and thought Homonymous hemianopsia, cortical blindness, visual agnosia, altered mental status, impaired memory
Vertebrobasilar Artery	Wide variety of CN, cerebellar and brainstem deficits: vertigo, nystagmus, diplopia, visual field deficits, dysphagia, dysarthria, facial hypoesthesia, syncope, ataxia Loss of pain and temperature sensation ipsilateral face and contralateral body

Acute Management
- ABCs: O_2, IV, cardiac monitor (>24 h), RSI if GCS ≤8, rapidly decreasing GCS, or inadequate airway protection reflexes
- Thrombolysis: immediate assessment for eligibility. Need acute onset <4.5 hrs from drug administration time AND compatible physical findings AND normal no-contrast CT head with no hemorrhage
- NPO, position (minimal elevation of head of bed if risk of aspiration)
- Within 24 h, aspirin therapy (initial dose 325 mg, thereafter 150 to 325 mg/d) be given to patients with ischemic stroke who are not receiving other forms of anticoagulation
- Hypertension: do not treat aggressively (in first 24 h) unless >220/120; hypotension: treat hypovolemia
- Fever: treat aggressively (Tylenol®) and search for a cause
- Anticoagulation: DVT prophylaxis if immobile; treat atrial fibrillation if present

Syncope

- Sudden, transient loss of consciousness and postural tone with spontaneous recovery
- Usually caused by generalized cerebral or reticular activating system hypoperfusion

Etiology
- Cardiogenic: arrhythmia, outflow obstruction (e.g. PE, tamponade, tension pneumo, pulmonary HTN), MI, valvular disease
- Non-cardiogenic: peripheral vascular (hypovolemia), vaso-vagal, cerebrovascular disorders, CNS, metabolic disturbances

History
- Signs and symptoms during presyncope, syncope and postsyncope
- Think anatomically in differential; pump (heart), blood (quality), vessels, brain
- Sudden loss of consciousness with no warning or prodrome means cardiac until proven otherwise

Physical Examination
- Postural BP and HR
- Cardiovascular, respiratory and neuro exam
- **Physical Findings in the Elderly Patient Who Falls (I HATE FALLING):**
    - **I**nflammation of joints (or joint deformity)
    - **H**ypotension (orthostatic blood pressure changes)
    - **A**uditory and visual abnormalities
    - **T**remor (Parkinson's disease or other causes of tremor)
    - **E**quilibrium (balance) problem
    - **F**oot problems
    - **A**rrhythmia, heart block or valvular disease
    - **L**eg-length discrepancy
    - **L**ack of conditioning (generalized weakness)
    - **I**llness
    - **N**utrition (poor; weight loss)
    - **G**ait disturbance

Investigations
- ECG (tachycardia, bradycardia, blocks, WPW, long QT interval), bedside glucose
- As indicated: CBC, electrolytes, BUN, creatinine, ABGs, Troponin, Mg^{2+}, Ca^{2+}, β-hCG
- Consider drug screen

Management
- ABCs, IV, O_2, monitor
- Examine for signs of trauma caused by syncopal episode
- Cardiogenic syncope: admit to medicine/cardiology
- Admit if >60 yrs old, cardiac RF's, recurrent syncope, or serious underlying illness
- Can safely discharge if:
    - No history of CHF
    - No history of shortness of breath
    - No ECG changes
    - SBP >90 at triage
    - Hct >30%

Toxicology

ABCs of Toxicology
- Basic axiom of care is symptomatic and supportive treatment
- Address underlying problem only once patient is stable
  - **A**   **A**irway (consider stabilizing the C-spine)
  - **B**   **B**reathing
  - **C**   **C**irculation
  - **D1**   **D**rugs
    - ACLS as necessary to resuscitate the patient
    - Universal antidotes – naloxone, glucose, thiamine, oxygen
  - **D2**   **D**raw bloods
  - **D3**   **D**econtamination (decrease absorption)
  - **E**   **E**xpose (look for specific toxidromes)/**E**xamine the patient
  - **F**   **F**ull vitals, ECG monitor, Foley, x-rays, etc.
  - **G**   **G**ive specific antidotes, treatments
- Go back and reassess
- Call Poison information
- Obtain corroborative history from family, bystanders

D1 – UNIVERSAL ANTIDOTES: treatments that will not harm patients and may be essential
Oxygen
- Do not deprive a hypoxic patient of oxygen no matter what the antecedent medical history (e.g. even COPD with CO_2 retention)
- If depression of hypoxic drive, intubate and ventilate
- Exception: paraquat or diquat (herbicides) inhalation or ingestion (oxygen radicals increase morbidity)

Glucose
- Give to any patient presenting with altered LOC
- Measure blood glucose prior to glucose administration if possible
- Adults: 0.5-1.0 g/kg (1-2 mL/kg) IV of D50W
- Children: 0.25 g/kg (2-4 mL/kg) IV of D25W

Thiamine (Vitamin B$_1$)
- 100 mg IV/IM to all patients with IV/PO glucose
- A necessary cofactor for glucose metabolism, but do not delay glucose if thiamine unavailable
- To prevent Wernicke-Korsakoff syndrome
- Must assume all undifferentiated comatose patients are at risk

Naloxone
- Antidote for opioids: administration is both diagnostic and therapeutic (1 min onset of action)
- Used for the undifferentiated comatose patient if opioids are suspected etiology
- Loading dose
  - Adults
    - 2 mg initial bolus IV/IM/SL/SC or via ETT (ETT dose = 2-2.5x IV dose)
    - If no response after 2-3 min, increase dose by 2 mg increments until a response or to max 10 mg
    - Known chronic user, suspicious history, or evidence of track marks, give 0.01 mg/kg
  - Child
    - 0.01 mg/kg initial bolus IV/IO/ETT
    - 0.1 mg/kg if no response and narcotic still suspected to max of 10 mg
- Maintenance dose
  - May be required because half-life of naloxone much shorter than many opioids
    - Hourly infusion rate at 2/3 of initial dose that produced patient arousal

D2 – DRAW BLOOD

Toxic Gaps

Metabolic Acidosis

Increased Anion Gap (AG): "MUDPILES CAT" (* = toxic)	**Increased Plasma Osmolar Gap (POG):**
Methanol*	**"MAE DIE"** (if "-ol", will likely ↑ POG)
Uremia	**M**ethanol
Diabetic ketoacidosis/Starvation ketoacidosis	**A**cetone
Phenformin*/Paraldehyde*	**E**thanol
Isoniazid, **I**ron, **I**buprofen	**D**iuretics (glycerol, mannitol, sorbitol)
Lactate (anything that causes seizures or shock)	**I**sopropanol
Ethylene glycol*	**E**thylene glycol
Salicylates*	
Cyanide, **C**arbon monoxide*	Note: normal osmolar gap does not rule out toxic alcohol; only an
Alcoholic ketoacidosis	elevated gap is helpful
Toluene, theophylline*	

Decreased AG	**Increased O_2 saturation gap**
Error	Carboxyhemoglobin
Electrolyte imbalance (increased $Na^+/K^+/Mg^{2+}$)	Methemoglobin
Hypoalbuminemia (50% fall in albumin	Sulfmethemoglobin
~5.5 mmol/L decrease in the AG)	
Li, Br elevation	
Paraproteins (multiple myeloma)	

Normal AG

High K^+: pyelonephritis, obstructive nephropathy, renal tubular acidosis (RTA), IV, TPN
Low K^+: small bowel losses, acetazolamide, RTA I, II

Use of the Clinical Laboratory in the Initial Diagnosis of Poisoning

Test	Finding	Selected Causes
ABG	Hypoventilation (↑ pCO_2)	CNS depressants (opioids, sedative-hypnotic agents, phenothiazines, EtOH)
	Hyperventilation (↓ pCO_2)	Salicylates, CO, other asphyxiants
Electrolytes	↑ AG metabolic acidosis	**"MUDPILES CAT"**: see "Metabolic Acidosis"
	Hyperkalemia	Digitalis glycosides, fluoride, potassium
	Hypokalemia	Theophylline, caffeine, β-adrenergic agents, soluble barium salts, diuretics, insulin
Glucose	Hypoglycemia	Oral hypoglycemia agents, insulin, EtOH, ASA
Osmolality and Osmolar Gap	Elevated osmolar gap	**"MAE DIE"**; see "Toxic Gaps"
ECG	Wide QRS complex	TCAs, quinidine, other class Ia and Ic antiarrhythmic agents
	Prolonged QT interval	Quinidine and related antiarrhythmics, terfenadine, astemizole
	Atrioventricular block	Ca^{2+} antagonists, digitalis glycosides, phenylpropanolamine
Abdominal X-Ray	Radiopaque pills or objects	**"CHIPES"**: **C**alcium, **C**hloral hydrate, **CCl**₄, **H**eavy metals, **I**ron, **P**otassium, **E**nteric coated **S**alicylates, and some foreign bodies
Serum Acetaminophen	Elevated level (>140 mg/L or 1000 μmol/L 4 h after ingestion)	May be only sign of acetaminophen poisoning

D3 – DECONTAMINATION AND ENHANCED ELIMINATION

Ocular Decontamination
- Saline irrigation to neutralize pH; alkali exposure requires ophthalmology consult

Dermal Decontamination (wear protective gear)
- Remove clothing, brush off toxic agents, irrigate all external surfaces

Gastrointestinal Decontamination
- Single dose activated charcoal (SDAC)
    - Absorption of drug/toxin to AC prevents availability
    - Contraindications: caustics, SBO, perforation
    - Dose: 10 g/kg drug ingested or 1 g/kg body weight
    - Odourless, tasteless, prepared as slurry with H_2O
- Whole bowel irrigation
    - 500 mL (child) to 2000 mL (adult) of balanced electrolyte solution/h by mouth until clear effluent per rectum (polyethylene glycol solution)
    - Indications
        - Awake, alert patient who can be nursed upright
        - Delayed release product
        - Drug/toxin not bound to charcoal
        - Drug packages (if any evidence of breakage → emergency surgery)
        - Recent toxin ingestion
    - Contraindications
        - Evidence of ileus, perforation, or obstruction
- Surgical removal in extreme cases
    - Indicated for drugs that are toxic, form concretions, or cannot be removed by conventional means
- No evidence for the use of cathartics (or ipecac)

EXTRA-CORPOREAL DRUG REMOVAL (ECDR)

Urine Alkalinization
- May be used for: ASA, methotrexate, phenobarb, chlorpropamide
- Weakly acidic substances can be trapped in alkali urine (pH >7.5) to increase elimination

Multidose Activated Charcoal (MDAC)
- May be used for: carbamazepine, *phenobarb*, quinine, theophylline
- For toxins which undergo enterohepatic recirculation
- Removes drug that has already been absorbed by drawing them back into GI tract
- Various regimens: 12.5 g (1/4 bottle) PO q1h or 25 g (1/2 bottle) PO q2h until non-toxic

Hemodialysis
- Indications/criteria for hemodialysis
    - Toxins that have high water solubility, low protein binding, low molecular weight, adequate concentration gradient, small volume of distribution (Vd) or rapid plasma equilibration
    - Removal of toxin will cause clinical improvement
    - Advantage is shown over other modes of therapy
    - Predicted that drug or metabolite will have toxic effects
    - Impairment of normal routes of elimination (cardiac, renal, or hepatic)
    - Clinical deterioration despite maximal medical support
- Useful for the following toxins:
    - Methanol
    - Ethylene glycol
    - Salicylates
    - Lithium
    - Phenobarbital
    - Chloral hydrate (g trichloroethanol)
- Others include theophylline, carbamazepine, valproate, methotrexate

E – EXAMINE THE PATIENT

TOXIDROMES: Specific Toxidromes

Toxidrome	Overdose Signs and Symptoms		Examples of Drugs
Anticholinergics	Hyperthermia Dilated pupils Dry skin Vasodilation Agitation/hallucinations Ileus Urinary retention Tachycardia	"Hot as a hare" "Blind as a bat" "Dry as a bone" "Red as a beet" "Mad as a hatter" "The bowel and bladder lose their tone and the heart goes on alone"	Antidepressants (e.g. TCAs) Cyclobenzaprine (Flexeril®) Carbamazepine Antihistamines (e.g. diphenhydramine) Antiparkinsonians Antipsychotics Antispasmotics Belladonna alkaloids (e.g. atropine)

Cholinergics	"DUMBELS"
	Diaphoresis, **D**iarrhea, **D**ecreased blood pressure
	Urination
	Miosis
	Bronchospasm, **B**ronchorrhea, **B**radycardia
	Emesis, **E**xcitation of skeletal muscle
	Lacrimation
	Salivation, **S**eizures
			Natural plants:
			  Mushrooms, trumpet flower
			Anticholinesterases:
			  Physostigmine
			  Insecticides (organophosphate)
			Nerve gases carbamates

Extrapyramidal	Dysphonia, dysphagia Rigidity and tremor Motor restlessness, crawling sensation (akathisia) Constant movements (dyskinesia) Dystonia (muscle spasms, laryngospasm, trismus, oculogyric crisis, torticollis)		Major tranquilizers Antipsychotics
Hemoglobin Derangements	Increased respiratory rate Decreased level of consciousness Seizures Cyanosis unresponsive to O_2 Lactic acidosis		Carbon monoxide poisoning (carboxyhemoglobin) Drug ingestion (methemoglobin, sulfmethemoglobin)
Opioids, Sedatives/Hypnotics, EtOH	Hypothermia Hypotension Respiratory depression Dilated or constricted pupils (pinpoint in opiate OD) CNS depression		EtOH Benzodiazepines Opiates (morphine, heroin, etc.) Barbiturates GHB
Sympathomimetics	Increased temperature CNS excitation (including seizures) Tachycardia, hypertension Nausea and vomiting Diaphoresis Dilated pupils		Caffeine Amphetamines Cocaine, LSD, PCP Ephedrine and other decongestants Thyroid hormone Sedatives, EtOH withdrawal
Serotonin Syndrome	Mental status changes, autonomic hyperactivity, neuromuscular abnormalities, hyperthermia, diarrhea, HTN		MAOI, TCA, SSRI, opiate analgesics Cough medicine, weight reduction medications

Note: ASA poisoning and hypoglycemia mimic sympathomimetic toxidrome

G – GIVE SPECIFIC ANTIDOTES AND TREATMENT
Protocol for Warfarin Overdose

INR	Management
<5.0	Cessation of warfarin administration, observation, serial INR/PT
5.1–9.0	If no risk factors for bleeding, hold warfarin x 1-2 d and reduce maintenance dose OR Vitamin K 1-2 mg PO if patient at increased risk of bleeding Consider Octoplex® if life-threatening bleed
9.1–20.0	Hold warfarin, vitamin K 2-4 mg PO, serial INR/PT, additional vitamin K if necessary Consider Octoplex® if life-threatening bleed
>20.0	Hold warfarin, vitamin K 10 mg IV over 10 min, increase vitamin K dosing (q4h) if needed Consider Octoplex® if life threatening bleed

Specific Antidotes and Treatments – call local poison information centre for specific doses and treatment recommendations

Toxin	Treatment	Considerations
Acetaminophen	Decontaminate (SDAC) N-acetylcysteine	Often clinically silent; evidence of liver/renal damage delayed >24 h Toxic dose >200 mg/kg (>7.5 g adult) Monitor drug level at 4 h post-ingestion; also liver enzymes, INR, PTT, BUN, Cr Hypoglycemia, metabolic acidosis, encephalopathy → poor prognosis
ASA	Decontaminate (SDAC) Alkalinize urine; want urine pH >7.5	Monitor serum pH and drug levels closely Monitor K^+ level; may require supplement for urine alkalinization Hemodialysis may be needed if intractable metabolic acidosis, very high levels, or end-organ damage (i.e. unable to diurese)
Anticholinergics	Decontaminate (SDAC) Supportive care	Special antidotes available. Consult PIC
Benzodiazepines	Decontaminate (SDAC) Supportive care	
β-blockers	Decontaminate (SDAC). Consider high dose insulin euglycemia therapy (HDIE)	Consult PIC
Calcium Channel Blockers	$CaCl_2$ 1-4 g of 10% solution IV if hypotensive Atropine or isoproterenol if severe Other: HDIE inotropes, intralipids	Order ECG, electrolytes (especially Ca^{2+}, Mg^{2+}, Na^+, K^+)
Cyanide	Cyanide antidote kit or hydroxocobalamin	
Digoxin	Decontaminate (SDAC) Digoxin-specific Ab fragments 10-20 vials IV if acute; 3-6 if chronic 1 vial (40 mg) neutralizes 0.5 mg of digoxin	Use for life-threatening arrhythmias unresponsive to conventional therapy, 6 h serum digoxin >12 nmol/L, initial K^+ >5 mM, ingestion >10 mg (adult)/>4 mg (child) Common arrhythmias include VFib, VTach, and conduction blocks
Acute Dystonic Rxn	Benztropine: 1-2 mg IM/IV then 2 mg PO x 3 d OR Diphenhydramine 1-2 mg/kg IV, then 25 mg PO qid x 3 d	Benztropine (Cogentin®) has euphoric effect and potential for abuse
Heparin	Protamine sulfate 25-50 mg IV	
Insulin/Oral Hypoglycemic	Glucose IV/PO/NG tube Glucagon: 1-2 mg IM (if no access to glucose)	Glyburide carries highest risk of hypoglycemia among oral agents Consider octreotide for oral hypoglycemics (50-100 µg SC q6h) in these cases; consult local PIC
Ethanol	Thiamine 100 mg IM/IV Manage airway and circulatory support	Hypoglycemia very common in children Mouthwash = 70% EtOH; perfumes and colognes = 40-60% EtOH Order serum EtOH level and glucose level; treat glucose level appropriately
Ethylene Glycol/Methanol	Ethanol (10%) 10 ml/kg over 30 min, then 1.5 ml/kg/h Or fomepizole (4-methylpyrazole) 15 mg/kg IV load over 30 min, then 10 mg/kg q12h	CBC, electrolytes, glucose, ethanol level Consider hemodialysis
TCAs	Decontaminate (SDAC) Aggressive supportive care $NaHCO_3$ bolus for wide QRS/seizures	Flumazenil antidote contraindicated in combined TCA/benzodiazepine overdose Also consider cardiac and hypotension support, gastric decontamination, seizure control Intralipid therapy (consult local PIC)
MDMA	Decontaminate (SDAC), supportive care	Monitor CK; treat rhabdomyolysis with high flow fluids Treat hyperthermia with aggressive external cooling
Cocaine	Decontaminate (SDAC) if oral Aggressive supportive care	β-blockers are contraindicated in acute cocaine toxicity

Common Medications

Most Commonly Used Agents for the Treatment of Hypertensive Crisis

Drug	Dosage*	Onset of Action	Duration of Action	Adverse Effects	Special Indications
VASODILATORS					
Sodium Nitroprusside 1st line	0.25 -10 µg/kg/min	Immediate	3-5 min	N/V, muscle twitching, sweating, cyanide intoxication, coronary	Most hypertensive emergencies (esp CHF, aortic steal syndrome dissection) Use in combination with β-blockers (i.e. esmolol) in aortic dissection Caution with high ICP and azotemia
Nicardipine (CCB)	2 mg IV bolus, then 4 mg/kg/h IV	15-30 min	40 min	Tachycardia, headache, (i.e. encephalopathy, RF, eclampsia, sympathetic crisis), flushing, local phlebitis	Most hypertensive emergencies Caution with acute CHF
Nitroglycerin	5-20 µg/min IV	1-2 min	3-5 min	Hypotension, bradycardia, headache, lightheadedness, dizziness	MI/Pulmonary edema
Hydralazine	5-10 mg IV/IM q20min Max 20 mg	5-20 min	2-6 h	Dizziness, drowsiness, headache, tachycardia, Na^+ retention	Eclampsia
Labetalol	20 mg IV bolus q10min or 0.5-2 mg/min	5-10 min	3-6 h	Vomiting, scalp tingling, burning in throat, dizziness, nausea, heart block, orthostatic hypotension	Most hypertensive emergencies (esp. eclampsia) Avoid in acute CHF, HB >1st degree
Esmolol	250-500 ug/kg/min for 1 min, then 50 ug/kg/min for 4 min; repeat	1-2 min	10-20 min	Hypotension, nausea, SVT, perioperative HTN bronchospasm	Aortic dissection, acute MI Avoid in acute CHF, HB >1st degree

Endocrinology

Common Presentations

Disorders of Calcium Homeostasis

- **Normal total serum Ca^{2+}**: 2.25-2.62 mmol/L (9.0-10.5 mg/dL)
- **Ionic/free Ca^{2+} levels**: 1.15-1.31 mmol/L (4.6-5.2 mg/dL)
- Corrected Ca^{2+} (mmol/L) = measured Ca^{2+} (mmol/L) + 0.02 (40 − albumin (mmol/L))

Parathyroid Hormone (PTH) Regulation

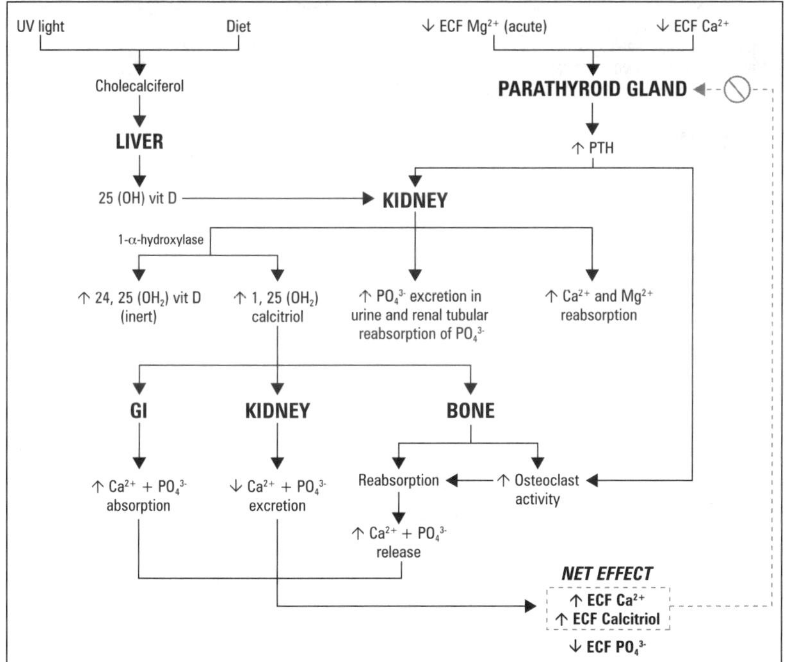

HYPERCALCEMIA
- Total corrected serum Ca^{2+} >2.62 mmol/L (10.5 mg/dL) OR ionized Ca^{2+} >1.35 mmol/L (5.4 mg/dL)

> **Differential Diagnosis: "GRIEF MD"**
> **G**ranulomas (sarcoid, TB)
> **R**enal failure (tertiary hyperparathyroidism)
> **I**mmobilization
> **E**ndocrine (primary hyperparathyroidism = #1 cause in healthy outpatients)
> **F**amilial hypocalciuric hypercalcemia (FHH)
> **M**alignancy (PTHrP-secreting tumour, eg. squamous cell lung ca, renal, breast, leukemia, lymphoma, myeloma, pheochromocytoma) = #1 cause in hospitalized patients
> **D**rugs – lithium, thiazides, antacids (milk-alkali syndrome)

Clinical Features
- "Bones, stones, moans, groans and psychiatric overtones" or asymptomatic
- CV: HTN, arrhythmias, short QT
- GI: anorexia, nausea, vomiting, constipation, abdo pain (PUD, pancreatitis)
- Renal: polyuria, polydipsia, nephrolithiasis, nephrogenic DI, renal failure
- MSK: bone pain, weakness
- Neuro: hypotonia, hyporeflexia
- Psych: anxiety, depression, confusion, psychosis

Investigations
- Ca^{2+}, PO_4^{3-}, albumin, ionized Ca^{2+}, PTH, PTHrP, 25- and 1,25-OH Vit. D, BUN, creatinine, urine Ca^{2+}

Management
- Based on Ca^{2+} level and severity of symptoms
  - Normal saline (4-6 L/d) — Hydration is most important therapy
  - Furosemide (IV) — Only when hypervolemic
  - Bisphosphonates — Takes 2-4 d for effect, but lasts wks
  - Calcitonin — Rapid but transient response, tachyphylaxis develops
  - Corticosteroids — Especially for hypervitaminosis D, malignancy, granulomatous diseases
  - Chelation therapy (EDTA) or dialysis if severe

HYPOCALCEMIA
- Total corrected serum Ca^{2+} <2.25 mmol/L (9.0 mg/dL)

Causes
- $1°$ hypoparathyroidism (usually iatrogenic), $2°$ hyperparathyroidism, pseudohypoparathyroidism, vitamin D deficiency, low Mg^{2+}, chronic renal failure, liver dysfunction, pregnancy

Clinical Features
- Tetany (most common), paresthesia (perioral, hands and feet), muscle cramping, weakness, stridor (laryngospasm), prolonged QT, lethargy, seizures, psychosis, increased ICP

Physical Examination
- Chvostek's sign (tap facial nerve and observe contraction of facial muscles)
- Trousseau's sign (prolonged inflation of BP cuff produces carpal spasm)
- Hyperreflexia, weakness

Investigations
- Ca^{2+}, Mg^{2+}, PO_4^{3-}, albumin, ionized Ca^{2+}, PTH, 25- and 1,25-OH Vit. D, BUN/creatinine, urine Ca^{2+}

Management
- Treat underlying condition; otherwise treat based on symptoms to increase Ca^{2+}
- If symptomatic: IV Ca gluconate, vitamin D; give Ca^{2+} slowly in order to promote endogenous PTH release
- If asymptomatic: oral Ca^{2+} and vitamin D

Disorders of Phosphate Homeostasis

HYPERPHOSPHATEMIA
- Serum PO_4^{3-} >1.45 mmol/L (4.1 mg/dL)

Etiology
- Increased PO_4^{3-} load
  - GI intake (rectal enema, GI bleeding)
  - IV PO_4^{3-} load (K-Phos®, blood transfusion)
- Shift of endogenous phosphate (tumour lysis syndrome, rhabdomyolysis, hemolysis, lactic and ketoacidosis)
- Reduced renal clearance
- ARF/CRF
- Hypoparathyroidism
- Acromegaly
- Tumour calcinosis (ability of kidney to specifically clear phosphate is defective)
- Pseudophosphatemia:
  - Hyperglobulinemia, hyperlipidemia, hyperbilirubinemia

Clinical Features
- Non-specific, include ectopic calcification, renal osteodystrophy

Treatment
- Low PO_4^{3-} diet, phosphate binders (e.g. $CaCO_3$), hemodialysis if acutely symptomatic

HYPOPHOSPHATEMIA
- Serum PO_4^{3-} <0.85 mmol/L (2.4 mg/dL)

Etiology
- Inadequate intake: starvation, malabsorption (diarrhea, steatorrhea), antacid use, alcoholism
- Renal losses: hyperparathyroidism, diuretics, X-linked or AD hypophosphatemic rickets, Fanconi syndrome
- Excessive skeletal mineralization: osteoblastic metastases, post parathyroidectomy (referred to as 'hungry bone syndrome')
- PO_4^{3-} shift into ICF: recovery from metabolic acidosis, respiratory alkalosis, starvation refeeding (stimulated by insulin)

Clinical Features
- Non-specific (CHF, coma, hypotension, weakness, defective clotting)

Treatment
- Treat underlying cause, supplement with oral PO_4^{3-} : 2-4 g/d divided bid-qid (start at 1000 mg/d to minimize diarrhea)

Disorders of Magnesium Homeostasis

HYPERMAGNESEMIA
- Serum Mg^{2+} >0.85 mmol/L (2.1 mg/dL)

Etiology
- ARF/ CRF
- Mg^{2+}-containing antacids or enemas
- IV administration of large doses of $MgSO_4$, e.g. for preeclampsia

Clinical Features
- Drowsiness, hyporeflexia, respiratory depression, heart block

Treatment
- Discontinue Mg^{2+}-containing products; calcium gluconate for $MgSO_4$ overdose

HYPOMAGNESEMIA
- Serum Mg^{2+} <0.70 mmol/L (1.7 mg/dL)

Etiology
- GI: starvation, malabsorption, vomiting, alcoholism, acute pancreatitis
- Excess renal loss: $2°$ hyperaldosteronism due to cirrhosis and CHF, hyperglycemia, hypokalemia, hypercalcemia, diuretics

Clinical Features
- Seizures, paresthesia, Chvostek and Trousseau signs, arrhythmia, ECG changes

Treatment
- Treat underlying cause
- Mg^{2+} IM/IV (note: cellular uptake of Mg^{2+} is slow therefore repletion requires sustained correction)
- Discontinue diuretics: in patients requiring diuretics, use a K^+-sparing diuretic to reduce the amount of magnesuria

Common Conditions

Osteoporosis

Definition
- A condition characterized by decreased bone mass and microarchitectrual deterioration of bone tissue with a consequent increase in bone fragility and susceptibility to bone fracture
- Bone mineral density (BMD) ≥2.5 standard deviations below the peak bone mass for young adults (i.e., T-score ≤−2.5)

Clinical Features
- Height loss >3 cm, weight <51 kg, kyphosis, tooth count <20, arm span-height difference >5 cm, wall-occiput distance >0 cm, rib-pelvis distance <2 finger breadth

Approach to Osteoporosis
1) Assess risk factors for osteoporosis on Hx and Px
2) Decide if patient requires BMD testing with dual-energy x-ray absorptiometry (DEXA)

3) Initial investigations:
  - For all patients with osteoporosis: Ca^{2+} corrected for albumin, CBC, creatine, ALP, and TSH
  - Also consider serum and urine protein electrophoresis, celiac workup and 24 h urinary Ca^{2+} excretion to r/o secondary causes
  - **25-OH-D level should only be measured after 3-4 months of adequate supplementation and should not be repeated if an optimal level ≥75 nmol/L is achieved**
4) Assess 10-yr fracture risk by combining BMD result and risk factors
  - 2 assessment tools: 1) WHO Fracture Risk Assessment Tool (FRAX); 2) Canadian Association of Radiologist and Osteoporosis Canada Risk Assessment Tool (CAROC)
5) For all patients being assessed for osteoporosis, encourage appropriate lifestyle changes

Low Risk **10-yr fracture risk <10%**	Unlikely to benefit from pharmacotherapy → reassess risk in 5 yrs
Medium Risk **10-yr fracture risk 10-20%**	Consider pharmacotherapy if risk factors present: vertebral fracture(s), previous wrist fracture in individuals older than age 65 or those with T-score ≤-2.5, rapid bone loss, aromatase inhibitor therapy, long-term glucocorticoid use, recurrent falls. If none of the above → reassess risk in 3 yrs; otherwise start pharmacotherapy
High Risk **10-yr fracture risk >20%; OR** **Prior fragility fracture of hip or spine; OR** **More than one fragility fracture**	Start pharmacotherapy (see *Common Medications*)

Treatment
- Diet: elemental Ca^{2+} 1000-1200 mg/d; Vit. D 800 IU/d
- Exercise: 3x30 min weight-bearing exercise per week
- Cessation of smoking, reduce caffeine intake, reduce EtOH intake, avoid osteoporosis-inducing medications

Thyroid Disorders

THYROTOXICOSIS

Causes of Hyperthyroidism

Disorder	TSH	T4/T3	Thyroid Antibodies	RAIU*
Graves' disease	Decreased	Increased	TSI	Increased
Toxic Nodular Goitre	Decreased	Increased	—	Increased
Toxic Nodule	Decreased	Increased	—	Increased
Thyroiditis				
Subacute Silent Postpartum	Decreased	Increased	Up to 50% of cases	Decreased
Extrathyroidal Sources of Thyroid Hormone				
Endogenous: (struma ovariae, ovarian teratoma, metastatic follicular ca) Exogenous (drugs)	Decreased	Increased	—	Decreased
Excessive Thyroid Stimulation				
Pituitary thyrotrophoma	Increased	Increased	—	Increased
Pituitary thyroid hormone receptor resistance	Increased	Increased	—	Increased
Increased hCG (e.g. pregnancy)	Decreased	Increased	—	Increased

*RAIU testing is contraindicated in pregnancy

Signs and Symptoms

Symptoms	Signs
General: heat intolerance, weight loss	Vitals: check for tachycardia, systolic hypertension, fever
Cardiac: palpitations, systolic hypertension, CHF, atrial fibrillation	Weight loss, agitation
GI: hyperdefecation	HEENT: fine hair, warm/moist skin, proptosis, lid lag, lid retraction, conjunctivitis
GU: menstrual irregularities	Thyroid: check for goiter, listen for bruit, Pemberton's sign (ask patient to raise both arms to the side and assess for carotid vascular compromise)
Derm: skin changes (fine hair, moist skin)	CV: atrial fibrillation (esp. elderly)
Neurologic: tremor, proximal muscle weakness	Neuro: proximal muscle weakness, tremor
	Derm: pretibial myxedema (thickening of dermis)

Risk Factors
- Family history, pregnancy (esp. post-partum period), excess iodine, amiodarone use, viral/bacterial infections, thyroxine overdose

Complications
- Thyroid storm (hyperthermia, tachycardia, arrhythmia, vascular collapse, hepatic failure, delirium, coma)
- CHF exacerbation

Investigations
- Thyroid function tests; (decreased TSH in 1° hyperthyroidism; increased TSH in 2° hyperthyroidism)
- TSI autoantibodies in Graves' disease

Management
- β-blockers (propanolol) for symptomatic control of tachycardia
- Graves' disease
    - Treat with propylthiouracil (PTU) or methimazole (MMI). Side effects include: fever, rash, arthralgias, hepatitis, agranulocytosis (rare). Avoid MMI in pregnancy (teratogenic)
    - Follow-up within 3-6 wks
    - Consider radioactive thyroid ablation or surgery if treatment resistant

HYPOTHYROIDISM

Causes of Hypothyroidism
- Primary hypothyroidism (90%):
    - Intrinsic thyroid defect
    - Autoimmune: Hashimoto's thyroiditis
    - Hypothyroid phase of subacute thyroiditis
    - Iatrogenic: thyroidectomy, drugs (goitrogens (iodine), PTU, MMI, lithium)
    - Iodine deficiency
    - Congenital (1/4000 births)
- Secondary hypothyroidism: pituitary hypothyroidism (insufficient TSH)
- Tertiary hypothyroidism: hypothalamic hypothyroidism (insufficient TRH)

Signs and Symptoms

Symptoms	Signs
General: fatigue, cold intolerance, hoarse voice, weight gain	Vitals: check for bradycardia, diastolic hypertension
Skin: dry and rough	HEENT: facial puffiness, periorbital edema, dry/rough skin, brittle hair, loss of lateral one-third of eyebrows
GI: constipation	Thyroid: check for goiter
GU: menorrhagia	CV: worsening CHF, pericardial effusion
Resp: decreased exercise capacity, muscle cramps	Neuro: slowing of mental processes, "hung reflexes" = delayed relaxation; carpal tunnel syndrome, sleep apnea (macroglossia)

Risk Factors
- Female, FHx of thyroid disease, family or personal hx of autoimmune disorders, smoking, radioactive iodine treatment, thyroid surgery, lithium or amiodarone use, infiltrative disease (e.g. amyloid), iodine deficiency, pituitary/hypothalamic disorders

Complications
- Myxedema coma (hypothermia, hyponatremia, hypoglycemia, hypotension, hypoventilation)

Investigations
- Thyroid function tests; (increased TSH in 1° hypothyroidism; decreased TSH in 2° hypothyroidism)
- Positive thyroid peroxidase and thyroglobulin antibodies (Hashimoto's thyroiditis)

Management
- L-thyroxine (0.05-0.2 mg/d), usually start at 1.5 times the weight in kg (microgram dosage)
- Elderly patients and those with CAD should be started at 0.025 mg/d and titrated up gradually
- Re-evaluate TSH in 3-6 wks and then follow-up with patient annually once reaching target levels

Disorders of Glucose Metabolism

DIABETES MELLITUS

Diagnostic Criteria

DM
- Presence of classic symptoms PLUS random glucose >11.1 mmol/L (200 mg/dL) OR
- On at least two occasions: fasting glucose ≥7.0 mmol/L (126 mg/dL) OR 2 h 75g OGTT ≥11.1 mmol/L (200 mg/dL)
- HbA1c ≥6.5% (American Diabetes Association Guidelines, 2011)

Impaired glucose tolerance (IGT): 2 h 75g OGTT 7.8-11.1 mmol/L (140-200 mg/dL)
Impaired fasting glucose (IFG): fasting glucose 6.1-6.9 mmol/L (110-125 mg/dL)

Etiologic Classification

I	Type 1 diabetes (immune-mediated β cell destruction, usually leading to absolute insulin deficiency)
II	Type 2 diabetes (ranges from predominantly insulin resistance with relative insulin deficiency to a predominantly insulin secretory defect with insulin resistance 2° to β cell dysfunction)
III.	Other causes of diabetes a. Genetic defects of β cell function (e.g. MODY – Maturity-Onset Diabetes of the Young) or insulin action b. Diseases of the exocrine pancreas • Pancreatitis, pancreatectomy, neoplasia, cystic fibrosis, hemochromatosis ("bronze diabetes") c. Endocrinopathies • Acromegaly, Cushing's syndrome, glucagonoma, pheochromocytoma, hyperthyroidism d. Drug-induced • Glucocorticoids, thyroid hormone, β-adrenergic agonists, thiazides, phenytoin, clozapine e. Infections • Congenital rubella, CMV, coxsackie f. Genetic syndromes associated with diabetes • Down's syndrome, Klinefelter's syndrome, Turner's syndrome
IV	Gestational Diabetes Mellitus

Comparisons of Type 1 and Type 2 DM

	Type 1 DM	Type 2 DM
Risk Factors	Personal Hx of other autoimmune diseases	Age ≥40 yrs Ethnicity (Black, Aboriginal, Hispanic, Asian-American, Pacific Islander) First-degree relative with DM Obesity, dyslipidemia, HTN Hx of IGT, IFG, PCOS, GDM
Natural History	β cell function / glucose / insulin / honeymoon period / time	insulin resistance / glucose / insulin / β cell defect / β cell decompensation / β cell failure
Clinical Features	Usually <30 yrs Normal to wasted body habitus	Usually >40 yrs but increasing incidence in pediatric population secondary to obesity Typically overweight with increased central obesity
Treatment	Carbohydrate counting Insulin	Weight loss, diet, lifestyle Oral anti-hyperglycemic agents (OHA) Insulin
Acute Complication	Diabetic ketoacidosis (DKA)	Hyperosmolar Hyperglycemic State (HHS, formerly known as HONK)

Chronic Complications

Microvascular	**Macrovascular**

Retinopathy
  Fundoscopy
  Annual ophthalmology assessment
Neuropathy
  Examine feet for sensory neuropathy (vibration sense, monofilament test)
  Autonomic neuropathy (postural hypotension, resting tachycardia, diarrhea/constipation)
Nephropathy
  Serum creatinine
  Albumin/creatinine ratio (microalbuminuria: male >2, female >2.8)
	Coronary artery disease
	Peripheral vascular disease
	Cerebral vascular disease/Ischemic stroke

Kinetics of Different Insulin Preparations

Insulin	Brand Names	Insulin Type	Onset	Peak	Duration of Action
Prandial (Bolus)					
Aspart	Novorapid®	Rapid	10-15 min	1-1.5 h	3-5 h
Lispro	Humalog®	Rapid	10-15 min	1-2 h	3.5-4.75 h
Glulisine	Apidra®	Rapid	10-15 min	1-1.5 h	3-5 h
Regular (R), Toronto	Humulin R®	Short	30 min	2-3 h	6.5 h
	Novolin Toronto®				
Basal					
NPH/(N)	Humulin N®	Intermediate	1-3 h	5-8 h	Up to 18 h
	Novolin NPH®	Intermediate	1-3 h	5-8 h	Up to 18 h
Detemir	Levemir®	Long	90 min	---	16-24 h
Glargine	Lantus®	Long	90 min	---	Up to 24 h

Insulin Regimens

1. Oral agent + basal insulin (DM2 only)	Start with 10 U basal insulin qhs Titrate up by 4 U q 4d until fasting glucose <10 Titrate up by 2 U q 4d until fasting glucose <7
2. Basal-bolus regimen + carbohydrate counting	Estimate total daily insulin requirement: 0.5 U/kg Give 40-50% as basal insulin qhs and divide the rest evenly as bolus insulin before each meal (breakfast, lunch, dinner)
3. Premixed insulin twice daily	Estimate total daily insulin requirement: 0.5 U/kg Give 2/3 of dose before breakfast and 1/3 dose before dinner

Titrating Insulin Doses

Insulin Regimen	Morning Blood Glucose	Lunch Blood Glucose	Dinner Blood Glucose	Bedtime Blood Glucose	Adjustments
MDI	Increased				Increase Evening I/L
Twice Daily	Increased			Increased	Increase Dinner Mixture
MDI		Increased			Increase Morning R/S
Twice Daily		Increased	Increased		Increase Morning Mixture
MDI			Increased		Increase Lunch R/S
MDI				Increased	Increase Evening R/S

** R=rapid acting, S=short-acting insulin, I= Intermediate Acting, L=Long-acting

VARIABLE INSULIN DOSING

Making a sliding scale for a patient on routine doses of insulin ± oral anti-hyperglycemics
1. Calculate Correction Factor (CF) = 100/Total Daily Dose (TDD) of Insulin (note: assume 30 U for a patient on oral anti-hyperglycemics). This number represents how many mmol/L that 1 unit of insulin decreases the blood sugar
2. BG <4: call MD and give 15 g carbohydrates
3. BG between 4 to 8: no additional/supplemental insulin (that is, pt will still receive usual meal bolus of insulin if eating)
4. BG between 8 to (8 + CF): give one additional unit
5. BG between (8 + CF) to (8 + 2CF): give two additional units
6. BG between (8 + 2CF) to (8 + 3CF): give three additional units
7. Review the extra units needed daily and add them to the TDD. Distribute the extra units based on usage (see *Table Titrating Insulin Doses*) and adjust the correction factor

SUMMARY OF MANAGEMENT GOALS IN DIABETES CARE

	Objective	Target
Self Monitoring of Blood Glucose	Develop self monitoring of blood glucose schedule Review records	Pre-prandial: 4-7 mmol/L 2-h post-prandial: 5-10 mmol/L (5-8 mmol/L if not achieving HbA1c target)
Blood Glucose Control	HbA1c q3months for most; q6 if lifestyle and glycemic targets are consistently achieved	HbA1c ≤7.0% for most patients
Blood Glucose Meter Accuracy	Annually check meter vs. lab measurement	Within 20%
Hypertension	Measure every visit	<130/80 mmHg
Waist Circumference/BMI	Indicators of body fat/size	Target WC: European Males <94 cm South Asian / Chinese / Japanese male <90 cm Females <80 cm Target BMI: 18.5-24.9
Nutrition	Encourage nutrition as a part of treatment and self management (can reduce HbA1c by 1.5-2%)	Cholesterol <200 mg/d Protein 15-20% of total calories Carbohydrates 45-60% of total calories Saturated fats <7% of total calories with minimal trans fat
Physical Activity	Encourage aerobic exercise ECG stress test can be considered before activity in previously sedentary individuals at high risk of CAD	Aerobic >150 min/wk Resistance: 3 sessions/wk
Smoking	Encourage cessation	Encourage cessation
Retinopathy	**Type 1 DM:** screen annually after 5 yrs from dx **Type 2 DM:** screen at dx, then every 1-2 yrs if no retinopathy present Screening done by eye care professional	Early detection and treatment
Chronic Kidney Disease	Screening: 1) random albumin to creatinine (ACR) AND 2) eGFR (from serum creatinine) **Type 1 DM:** screen annually after 5 yrs from dx **Type 2 DM:** screen at dx, then every 1-2 yrs if no CKD present If CKD present, do ACR and eGFR q6months	ACR (mg/mmol) **Normal:** Males <2.0, females <2.8 **Microalbuminuria:** Males 2-20, females 2.8-28 **Macroalbuminuria:** Males >20, females >28 **CKD:** eGFR <60 ml/min
Neuropathy/Foot Exam	Screening: Neuropathy with 10 gm monofilament or 128 Hz tuning fork Foot exam: structural abnormalities, neuropathy, arterial disease, ulcers, infection **Type 1 DM:** screen annually after 5 yrs from dx **Type 2 DM:** screen at dx, then every 1-2 yrs if no neuropathy present	Early detection and treatment

SUMMARY OF MANAGEMENT GOALS IN DIABETES CARE (continued)

	Objective	Target
CAD Assessment	ECG at baseline then q2yrs if age 40, duration of diabetes >15 yrs, symptoms, hypertension, proteinuria, bruits, reduced pulses High risk: based on age >45 if male, >50 if female, micro or macrovascular disease, cardiac risk factors, extremely elevated LDL (>5 mmol/L) or systolic BP (>180)	Vascular protection Optimize BP, glycemic control, lifestyle (weight, exercise, smoking) If high risk: ACE/ARB, antiplatelet therapy, lipid lowering drugs If known CVD: antiplatelet therapy
Dyslipidemia	Measure fasting lipid levels (TC, HDL, LDL, TG) at dx, then q 1-3 yrs or more often based on treatment initiation	LDL <2.0 or ≥50% reduction in LDL-C, if high risk

DIABETIC KETOACIDOSIS (DKA)

Precipitants (6 I's)	Infection, Ischemia/Infarction, Iatrogenic (glucocorticoids), Intoxication, Insulin missed, Intra-abdominal process (e.g. pancreatitis, cholecystitis)
Clinical Features	Polyuria, polydipsia, polyphagia with marked fatigue, nausea, vomiting ECF volume contraction (orthostatic changes) LOC may be decreased with acidosis and/or high serum osmolality (osm >330 mmol/L) Abdominal pain Fruity smelling breath (acetone) Kussmaul's respiration
Serum	Increased BG (11-55 mmol/L, 198-990 mg/dL), decreased Na^+ (2° to shift with hyperglycemia (for every increase in BG by 10 mmol/L (180 mg/dL) there is a decrease in Na^+ by 3 mmol/L) Normal or increased K^+, decreased HCO_3^-, increased BUN, increased Cr, increased anion gap, ketonemia, decreased PO_4^{3-} Increased osmolality
ABG	Metabolic acidosis with increased AG plus possible 2° respiratory alkalosis If severe vomiting/ECF volume contraction, there may be a metabolic alkalosis
Urine	+ve for glucose and ketones
Treatment	Immediate resuscitation and emergency measures if patient is stuporous or comatose Monitor degree of ketoacidosis with AG, not BG or serum ketone level ECF volume reexpansion: 　1L/h NS in first 2 h 　After 1st 2 L, usually switch to 0.45% NS at 300-400 ml/h (as long as serum osmolality is not falling too rapidly (<3 mosm/kg water) 　Once BG reaches 13.9 mmol/L (250 mg/dL) switch to D5W to maintain BG in the range of 13.9-16.6 mmol/L (250-300 mg/dL) Insulin therapy: 　If serum K^+ < 3.3 mmol/L, hold insulin and give 40 mmol/L/h K^+ replacement 　Critical to resolve acidosis, not hyperglycemia 　Use intravenous insulin infusion (mixed using regular insulin) 　Initially load 0.1 U/kg body weight IV insulin bolus 　Maintenance 0.1 U/kg/h IV insulin infusion 　Check serum glucose hourly 　Maintain IV insulin infusion until the acidosis is resolved and the patient is able to eat and drink K^+ replacement: 　With Insulin therapy, hypokalemia may develop 　When K^+ 3.5- 5.5 mmol/L add KCL 20-40 mmol/L IV fluid to keep K^+ in the range of 3.5-5 mmol/L HCO_3^-: 　If pH <7.0 or if hypotension, arrhythmia, or coma is present with a pH of <7.1 give HCO_3^- in 0.45% NS 　Do not give if pH >7.1 (risk of metabolic alkalosis!) 　Can give in case of life-threatening hyperkalemia ± mannitol (for cerebral edema)

HYPERGLYCEMIC HYPEROSMOLAR STATE (HHS, formerly HONK)

Precipitants	Sepsis, stroke, MI, CHF, renal failure, trauma, burns, recent surgery, drugs (glucocorticoids, diuretics)
Clinical Features	Onset is insidious; preceded by weakness, polyuria, polydipsia History of decreased fluid intake History of ingesting large amounts of glucose containing fluids Dehydration (orthostatic changes) Decreased LOC, lethargy, confusion, comatose Kussmaul's respiration is absent unless the underlying precipitant has also caused a metabolic acidosis
Serum	Increased BG (typically 44.4-133.2 mmol/L, 800-2400 mg/dL) In mild dehydration, may have hyponatremia (shift of water from ICF $2°$ to hyperglycemia for every increase in BG by 10 mmol/L (180 mg/dL) there is a decrease in Na^+ by 3 mmol/L If dehydration progresses, may get hypernatremia Ketosis usually absent or mild if starvation occurs Increased osmolality
ABG	Metabolic acidosis absent unless underlying precipitant leads to acidosis (e.g. lactic acidosis in MI)
Urine	-ve for ketones unless there is starvation ketosis Glycosuria
Treatment	*Same resuscitation and emergency measures as DKA: Rehydration K^+ replacement Search for precipitating event Insulin therapy

*HCO_3^- is not indicated in HHS

HYPOGLYCEMIA

Characterized by Whipple's Triad
1. BG <2.5 mmol/L (45 mg/dL) in males or BG <2.2 mmol/L (40 mg/dL) in females
2. Adrenergic and neuroglycopenic symptoms
3. Resolution of symptoms with ingestion of carbohydrate

Differential Diagnosis

Hyperinsulinemia	Exogenous – insulin, insulin secretagogues Endogenous – insulinoma, islet hyperplasia
Ectopic	IGF-2 – sarcoma, mesenchymal tumours
Low BG	Major organ failure Endocrine organ failure – decreased glucagon, decreased cortisol (Addison's), decreased catecholamines (pheochromocytoma resection), decreased GH (hypopituitarism) Glycogen storage disease Starvation
Drugs	EtOH, ASA, pentamidine, quinine, haloperidol, Septra, unripened akee fruit

Investigations
1. 48-72 h fast to rule out insulinoma
   - Obtain baseline BG, insulin and C-peptide
   - Monitor BG regularly and monitor for neuroglycopenia q1-2h once BG <3.3
   - When BG <2.2 and symptomatic, determine BG, insulin, C-peptide, β-hydroxybutyrate, urine sulfonylurea, cortisol, GH
2. Localization (endoscopic ultrasound, selective arterial calcium injection, laparoscopic ultrasound)

Laboratory Findings in Different Causes of Hypoglycemia

Dx	BG	Insulin	C-peptide	β-hydroxybutyrate	Urine sulfonylurea
Exogenous insulin	Decreased	Increased	Decreased	Decreased	—
Insulinoma	Decreased	Increased	Increased	Decreased	—
Sulfonylurea	Decreased	Increased	Increased	Decreased	+
Low glucose states	Decreased	Decreased	Decreased	Increased	—
Ectopic IGF-2	Decreased	Decreased	Decreased	Decreased	—

Management
1. Medical (e.g. diazoxide, octreotide, chemoembolization for large metastases)
   - Patient awake and taking fluids, eat/drink 15 g carbohydrate if BG <4 mmol/l (20 g if BG <2 mmol/l)
2. Surgery (e.g. partial pancreatectomy)

Dyslipidemia

Etiology

Primary Disorders	Secondary Disorders
Primary hypercholesterolemia • Familial hypercholesterolemia • Polygenic hypercholesterolemia **Primary hypertriglyceridemia** • Familial hypertriglyceridemia • Familial lipoprotein lipase deficiency **Combined hyperlipidemia** • Familial dysbetalipoproteinemia • Familial combined hyperlipidemia	**Secondary hypercholesterolemia** • Diet, anorexia nervosa, hypothyroidism, cholestatic liver disease, nephrotic syndrome, monoclonal gammopathy, drugs (e.g. cyclosporin, anabolic steroids, carbamazepine) **Secondary hypertriglyceridemia** • Obesity/metabolic syndrome, alcohol, DM, drugs (e.g. corticosteroids, estrogen, HCTZ, β-blockers, atypical antipsychotics, anti-retroviral drugs), chronic liver failure, hepatitis, glycogen storage disease, hypothyroidism, hypopituitarism, acromegaly, Cushing's disease

Risk Factors
- Family history, poor diet, sedentary lifestyle, obesity, smoking, alcoholism (high triglycerides), OCP

Physical Examination
- Tendon xanthomas: lipid deposits on elbows, dorsum of hand, Achilles tendon; seen mostly in Familial hypercholesterolemia
- Xanthelasma: yellow fatty streak on eyelids; seen in most cases of elevated cholesterol
- Arcus corneae: grayish-white ring on surface of eye at corneal margin, common in elderly, suspect hypercholesterolemia if young

Complications
- Atherosclerosis: CAD, CVD, PVD in elevated cholesterol
- Pancreatitis with elevated triglycerides

Management
- Conservative: diet, smoking cessation, reduced alcohol consumption, exercise, weight loss
- Medical: please see *Common Medications* at end of chapter; standard treatment usually statin
  - For Statin Follow-Up:
    - Lipids and LFTs: LFTs once at beginning of treatment, lipids once/yr after stabilized, both ordered if patient complains of jaundice, RUQ pain, dark urine
    - CK at baseline and if patient complains of myalgia
    - d/c statin if CK >10x upper limit of normal

Lipid Targets

Level of Risk	Target LDL	Alternate Target
High	<2.0 mmol/L or ≥50% reduction in LDL-C	apoB <0.80 g/L
Moderate	<2.0 mmol/L or ≥50% reduction in LDL-C	apoB <0.80 g/L
Low	≥50% reduction in LDL-C	

As per established Canadian guidelines – *Can J Cardiol* 2009. 25(10): 567-79.

Disorders of the Pituitary Gland

Pathological Conditions Associated with Pituitary Gland Hormones

Hormone	Investigations	Treatment

Growth hormone (GH)
• GH excess
  • Gigantism
  • Acromegaly
	Glucose suppression test (OGTT)
	Insulin-like growth factor-1 (IGF-1)
		Surgery, octreotide, growth hormone receptor antagonist, bromocriptine (dopamine agonist), radiation

Prolactin (PRL) • Hyperprolactinemia (due to pregnancy/breastfeeding, prolactinoma, pituitary stalk lesions, 1° hypothyroidism, renal failure, liver failure medication side-effects)	Serum PRL, β-HCG, TSH, liver enzyme tests, creatinine	Long-acting dopamine agonist e.g. bromocriptine, cabergoline Possibly no treatment If medication side-effect, consider discontinuing medication
Luteinizing hormone (LH) and Follicle Stimulating hormone (FSH) • Hypogonadotropism	Serum LH, FSH, in males: testosterone, in females: estradiol and administration of medroxyprogesterone to look for vaginal bleeding	Pergonal® (combined FSH/LH hormone therapy), hCG, GnRH analogue for fertility Symptomatic treatment with estrogen/testosterone
Adrenocorticotropic hormone (ACTH)	See *Disorders of Adrenal Cortex*	
Thyroid Stimulating hormone (TSH)	See *Thyroid Disorders*	
Antidiuretic hormone (ADH) • ADH deficiency: diabetes insipidus (DI)	Plasma and urine Na^+ concentration, plasma and urine osmolality, water restriction test, plasma ADH level if water restriction test equivocal	DDAVP/vasopressin for total DI DDAVP, chlorpropamide, clofibrate, carbamazepine for partial DI Solute restriction and thiazide diuretics for nephrogenic DI

Disorders of the Adrenal Cortex

HORMONES

Markers of Adrenocortical Function

Serum or salivary cortisol	Diurnal variation: elevated at midnight means hyperfunction Response of serum cortisol to stimulation or suppression also informative
24 hour urinary free cortisol	Correlates well with secretory rates Good screening test for adrenal hyperfunction
Serum ACTH	High in primary adrenal insufficiency Low in secondary adrenal insufficiency High in ACTH-dependent Cushing's Low in adrenal Cushing's
Serum DHEA-S	Primary adrenal androgen

Mineralocorticoids (Aldosterone)
- Na^+ (and Cl^-) retention and K^+ (and H^+) excretion, ECF volume expansion
- Regulated by the renin-angiotensin-aldosterone system
- Negative feedback to juxtaglomerular apparatus (JGA) by long loop (aldosterone via volume expansion) and short loop (angiotensin II via peripheral vasoconstriction)

Physiological Effects of Glucocorticoids

Stimulatory Effects	Inhibitory Effects
Stimulate hepatic glucose production (gluconeogenesis)	Inhibit bone formation; stimulate bone resorption
Increase insulin resistance in peripheral tissues	Inhibit fibroblasts, causing collagen and connective tissue loss
Increase protein catabolism	Suppress inflammation; impair cell-mediated immunity
Stimulate leukocytosis and lymphopenia	

Sex Steroids (Androgens)
- Regulated by ACTH; primarily responsible for adrenarche (growth of axillary and pubic hair)
- Principal adrenal androgens are dihydroepiandrosterone (DHEA), androstenedione and 11-hydroxyandrostenedione

Cushing's Syndrome (Hypercortisolism)

Definition
- Results from chronic glucocorticoid excess (endogenous or exogenous sources)

Etiology
- ACTH-dependent (85%) – bilateral adrenal hyperplasia and hypersecretion due to:
  - ACTH-secreting pituitary adenoma (Cushing's disease responsible for 80% of ACTH-dependent)
  - Ectopic ACTH-secreting tumour (e.g. small cell lung carcinoma, bronchial, carcinoid, pancreatic, adrenal or thyroid tumours)
- ACTH-independent (15%)
  - Long-term use of exogenous glucocorticoids (10 mg/d for >3 wks duration)
  - Primary adrenocortical tumours: adenoma and carcinoma (uncommon)
  - Bilateral adrenal nodular hyperplasia
  - Major depression and alcoholism

Hypercortisolism: Algorithm for Diagnosis

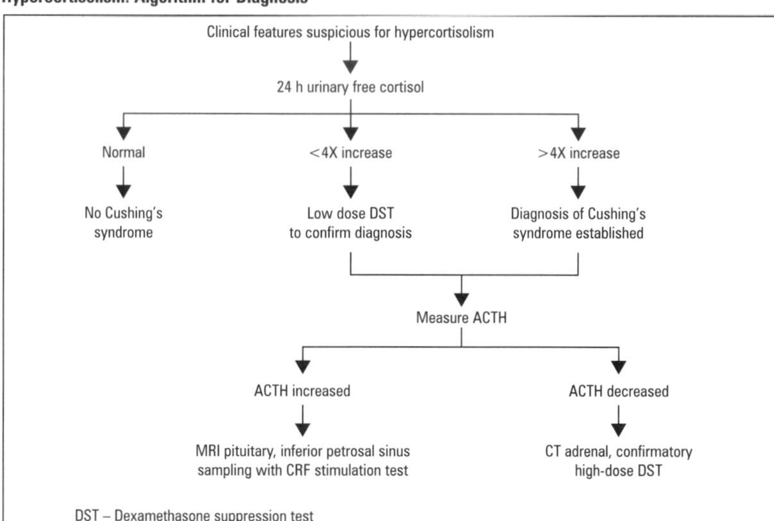

Clinical Features of Cushing's Syndrome
- Head and Neck: red cheeks, cataracts, acne, moon facies
- Back/Abdomen: central obesity, purple striae, dorsal and supraclavicular fat pads
- MSK: osteoporosis, avascular necrosis, arthralgia
- Skin: easy bruising, poor wound healing, hyperhydrosis, telangiectasia
- GU: impotence, amenorrhea, infertility
- Psych: depression, psychosis

INVESTIGATIONS

Dexamethasone (DXM) Suppression Test (DST)
- Gold standard to determine presence and etiology of hypercortisolism
- Principle: DXM suppresses pituitary ACTH, so plasma cortisol should be lowered by negative feedback if HPA axis were normal

Plasma ACTH Assay
- Supplements DST for differentiation of the various etiologies of Cushing's

Treatment
- Pituitary
  - Transsphenoidal resection, with glucocorticoid supplementation peri- and post-operatively
  - Irradiation: only 50% effective, with significant risk of hypopituitarism
- Adrenal
  - Adenoma: unilateral adrenalectomy (curative)
  - Carcinoma: palliative (frequent metastases, poor prognosis); adjunctive chemotherapy often not useful
- Ectopic ACTH tumour – usually bronchogenic cancer (paraneoplastic syndrome)
  - Chemotherapy/radiation for primary tumour
  - Agents blocking adrenal steroid synthesis: metyrapone or ketoconazole
  - Poor prognosis

Adrenal Insufficiency

Etiology of Primary Adrenocortical Insufficiency

Etiology	Notes
Autoimmune (70-90%) (most common in developed world) (60-75% of pts have antibodies against adrenal enzymes and 3 zones of the cortex)	Isolated adrenal insufficiency Polyglandular autoimmune syndrome type I and II
Infection	TB (7-20%) (most common in developing world) Fungal: histoplasmosis, paracoccidioidomycosis HIV, syphilis, African trypanosomiasis
Metastatic cancer	Lung, breast, stomach, colon, lymphoma
Adrenal hemorrhage or infection	Coagulopathy in adults or Waterhouse-Friderichsen syndrome in children (meningococcal or Pseudomonas septicemia)
Drugs	Ketoconazole, rifampin, phenytoin, barbituates, megestrol acetate, heparin, coumadin
Others	Adrenoleukodystrophy Congenital adrenal hypoplasia Familial glucocorticoid deficiency or resistance

Etiology of Secondary Adrenocortical Insufficiency
• Inadequate pituitary ACTH secretion due to: withdrawal of exogenous steroids and any cause of hypopituitarism

Clinical Features of Adrenocortical Insufficiency

	1° Adrenal Insufficiency (Addison's or Acute)	2° Adrenal Insufficiency (normal aldosterone)
Clinical Features	Weight loss Weakness Dehydration Hypotension Vitiligo Hyperpigmentation (buccal mucosa, flexor/palmar creases) N/V + Hx of wt loss + anorexia Acute abdomen Unexplained hypoglycemia Unexplained fever Other autoimmune endocrine deficiencies (e.g. hypothyroidism, gonadal failure)	Many of the signs and symptoms seen in primary adrenal insufficiency are also present here EXCEPT: NO hyperpigmentation NO salt craving GI: less common
Labs	Hyponatremia Hyperkalemia Hypercalcemia Azotemia Eosinophilia Anemia Lymphocytosis Hypoglycemia	NO hyperkalemia Hyponatremia often present Low cortisol, low ACTH Hypoglycemia is more common

Investigations
• Measure ACTH and cortisol at baseline
• Administer cosyntropin IV or IM at time 0; measure cortisol at time 0, 30, and 60 min
• Appropriate response after cosyntropin IV: plasma cortisol >500 nmol/L (>18 µg/dL)

Treatment
• Acute condition – can be life-threatening
  ▪ IV NS in large volumes (2-3 L)
  ▪ May need to add D5W if hypoglycemic from adrenal insufficiency
  ▪ Hydrocortisone 50-100 mg IV q6-8h for 24h, then gradual tapering
  ▪ Identify and correct precipitating factors
• Maintenance
  ▪ Hydrocortisone 15-20 mg PO daily, divided into 2-3 doses, highest dose in the AM
  ▪ Florinef® (fludrocortisone, synthetic mineralocorticoid) 0.05-0.2 mg PO daily if mineralocorticoid deficient
  ▪ Increase dose of steroids 2-3 fold for a few days during illness or surgery
  ▪ Medical alert bracelet for patient

Adrenal Medulla

MEN Syndromes

Type	Tissues Involved	Clinical Manifestations
MEN I **(Wermer's syndrome)** Chromosome 11 (PYGM gene)	Pituitary	Ant. pituitary adenomas, often non-secreting but may secrete GH and PRL
	Parathyroid	Primary hyperparathyroidism from hyperplasia
	Entero-pancreatic endocrine	Pancreatic islet cell tumours Gastrinoma (peptic ulcers) Insulinomas (hypoglycemia) VIPomas (secretory diarrhea)
MEN II **3 distinct syndromes** Chromosome 10 (RET proto-oncogene) autosomal dominant		
IIa **(Sipple's syndrome)**	Thyroid	Medullary thyroid cancer (MTC) (>90%)
	Adrenal medulla	Pheochromocytoma (40-50%)
	Parathyroid	1° parathyroid hyperplasia (10-20%)
	Skin	Cutaneous lichen amyloidosis
IIa Variant **(Familial medullary thyroid ca.)**	Thyroid	Medullary thyroid ca without other clinical manifestations of MEN IIa or IIb
IIb	Thyroid	Medullary thyroid ca: most common component, more aggressive and earlier onset than MEN IIa
	Adrenal medulla	Pheochromocytoma
	Neurons	Mucosal neuroma, intestinal ganglioneuromas
	MSK	Marfanoid habitus (no aortic abnormalities) Parathyroid hyperplasia – NOT a feature Chronic constipation Megacolon

Common Medications

Common Medications for Metabolic Bone Disorders

Drug Class	Mechanism of Action	Generic Drug Name	Canada Name	Dosing	Indications	Contraindications	Side Effects
Bisphosphonates	Inhibit osteoclast-mediated bone resorption	alendronate	Fosamax®	5-10 mg OD 70 mg once weekly 40 mg OD for 6 months	• Prevention of postmenopausal osteoporosis • Treatment of osteoporosis • Glucocorticoid-induced osteoporosis • Paget's disease	• Esophageal stricture or achalasia (oral) • Unable to stand or sit upright for >30 min (oral) • Hypersensitivity • Hypocalcemia • Renal insufficiency	• GI • MSK pain • Headache • Osteonecrosis of the jaw
		risedronate	Actonel®	5 mg OD 35 mg once weekly 150 mg once monthly 30 mg OD for 2 months	• Treatment and prevention of postmenopausal osteoporosis • Treatment and prevention of glucocorticoid-induced osteoporosis • Paget's disease		
		etidronate	Didronel®	5-10 mg /kg OD x 6 months	• Osteoporosis • Symptomatic Paget's disease • Prevention and treatment of heterotopic ossification after total hip replacement or spinal cord injury		
		ibandronate	Boniva®	2.5 mg OD or 150 mg once monthly	• Treatment and prevention of postmenopausal osteoporosis (US only)		
		pamidronate	Aredia®	IV	• Hypercalcemia of malignancy • Paget's disease • Osteolytic bone metastases of breast cancer • Osteolytic lesions of multiple myeloma		
		zoledronate	Zometa® Aclasta®	5 mg IV once yearly IV	• Treatment of osteoporosis • Hypercalcemia of malignancy • Treatment and prevention of skeletal complications related to cancer		
Selective Estrogen Receptor Modulators	• Decreases resorption of bone through binding to estrogen receptors	raloxifene	Evista®	60 mg OD	• Treatment and prevention of postmenopausal osteoporosis (2nd line)	• Lactation • Pregnancy • Active or past history of DVT, PE or retinal vein thrombosis	• Hot flashes • Leg cramps • Increased risk of fatal stroke, venous thromboembolism

Common Medications for Metabolic Bone Disorders (continued)

Drug Class	Mechanism of Action	Generic Drug Name	Canada Name	Dosing	Indications	Contraindications	Side Effects
Calcitonin	• Inhibits osteoclast-mediated bone resorption	salcatonin	Miacalcin®	One spray (200 IU) per day, alternating nostrils	• Treatment of postmenopausal osteoporosis, greater than 5 yrs postmenopause	• Clinical allergy to calcitonin-salmon	• Rhinitis • Epistaxis • Sinusitis • Nasal dryness
PTH	• Stimulates new bone formation by preferential stimulation of osteoblastic activity over osteoclastic activity	teriparatide	Forteo®	20 µg SC OD X 18-24 months	• Treatment of postmenopausal women with osteoporosis who are at high risk for fracture • Treatment of men with primary or hypogonadal osteoporosis who are at high risk for fracture	• Paget's disease • Prior external beam or implant radiation therapy involving the skeleton • Bone metastases • Metabolic bone diseases other than osteoporosis	• Orthostatic hypotension • Hypercalcemia • Dizziness • Leg cramps
Calcium	• Inhibits PTH secretion			1200 mg/d (including diet) Divided in 3 doses	• Osteopenia • Osteoporosis • Prevention of metabolic bone disease	• Caution with renal stones	• Vomiting • Constipation • Dry mouth
Vitamin D	• Regulation of calcium and phosphate homeostasis	cholecalciferol (vitamin D3)		800 IU/d	• Osteopenia • Osteoporosis • Prevention of metabolic bone disease	• Caution in patients on digoxin (risk of hypercalcemia may precipitate arrhythmia)	• Hypercalcemia • Headache • Nausea, vomiting • Constipation
		ergocalciferol (vitamin D2)	Osteoforte® Deltalin®	50000 IU	• Osteoporosis in patients with liver dysfunction, refractory rickets, hypoparathyroidism	• Hypercalcemia • Malabsorption syndrome • Decreased renal function	
		calcitriol $(1,25(OH)_2\text{-}D)$	Rocaltrol®	Start 0.25 µg/d Titrate up by 0.25 µg/d at 4-8 wk intervals to 0.5-1 µg/d	• Hypocalcemia and osteodystrophy in patients with chronic renal failure on dialysis	• Hypercalcemia • Vitamin D toxicity	
			Calcijex®	Start 0.25 µg/d Titrate up by 0.25 µg/d at 2-4 wk intervals to 0.5-2 µg/d	• Hypoparathyroidism		

Common Medications for Thyroid Disorders

Drug Class	Mechanism of Action	Generic Drug Name	Canada Name	US Name (if different)	Dosing	Indications	Contraindications	Side Effects
Antithyroid Agent	• Decreases thyroid hormone production by inhibiting iodine and peroxidase from interacting with thyroglobulin to form T_4 and T_3 • Also interferes with conversion of T_4 to T_3	propylthiouracil (PTU)	Propyl-Thyracil® Tapazole®		Start 100 mg PO tid, then adjust accordingly Thyroid storm: start 200-300 PO qid, then adjust accordingly	• Hyperthyroidism	• Hypersensitivity • Relative: renal failure, liver disease	• Nausea, vomiting • Rash • Drug-induced hepatitis • Agranulocytosis
		methimazole (MMI)			Start 5-20 mg PO OD, then adjust accordingly		• Pregnancy, lactation	• Hepatitis
Thyroxine	• Synthetic form of thyroxine (T_4)	levothyroxine l-thyroxine	Synthroid® Levothroid® Unithroid®	Levoxyl®	0.05-2.0 mg/d, in elderly patients start at 0.025 mg/d	• Hypothyroidism	• Recent MI, thyrotoxicosis	• Symptoms of hyperthyroidism • Tachycardia • Angina • Weight loss • Hyperthermia • Diarrhea • Insomnia • Tremors • Muscle weakness

Medical Management of Diabetes Mellitus

Drug Class	Mechanism of Action	Generic Drug Name	Canada Name	US Name (if different)	Dosing	Indications	Contraindications	Side Effects	Comments
Biguanide	• Sensitizes peripheral tissues to insulin → increases glucose uptake • Decreases hepatic glucose production	metformin	Glucophage® Glumetza®		500 mg OD titrated to 1000 mg bid maximum	• Useful in obese Type 2 DM • Improves both fasting and postprandial hyperglycemia • Also ↓ TG	ABSOLUTE: • Moderate to severe liver dysfunction • Moderate renal dysfunction • Cardiac dysfunction	• GI upset (abdo discomfort, bloating, diarrhea) • Lactic acidosis • Anorexia	↓ HbA1c 1.0-1.5%
Insulin secretagogue	• Stimulates insulin release from β cells by causing K^+ channel closure → depolarization → Ca^{2+} mediated insulin release • Use in nonobese Type 2 DM	sulfonylureas: glyburide gliclazide glimepiride	Diabeta® Euglucon® Diamicron® Diamicron® MR Amaryl®	Micronase® Glynase PreTab®	2.5-5.0 mg/d titrated to >5 mg bid Max: 20 mg/d 40-160 mg bid 30-120 mg OD 1-8 mg OD		ABSOLUTE: • Moderate to severe liver dysfunction RELATIVE: • Adjust dose in patients with severe kidney dysfunction (and avoid glyburide in these patients) • Avoid glyburide in the elderly INTERACTIONS: Do not combine with a non-sulfonylurea or preprandial insulin	• Hypoglycemia • Weight gain	↓ HbA1c 1.0-1.5%
		non-sulfonylureas: repaglinide nateglinide	GlucoNorm® Starlix®		0.5-4 mg tid 60-120 mg tid	Short $t_{1/2}$ of 1 hour causes brief but rapid ↑ in insulin, therefore effective for post prandial control	ABSOLUTE: • Severe liver dysfunction • Severe renal dysfunction INTERACTIONS: Do not combine with a non-sulfonylurea or preprandial insulin	• Hypoglycemia • Weight gain	↓ HbA1c 1.0-1.5% for repaglinide and 0.5-1.0% for nateglinide

Medical Management of Diabetes Mellitus (continued)

Drug Class	Mechanism of Action	Generic Drug Name	Canada Name	US Name (if different)	Dosing	Indications	Contraindications	Side Effects	Comments
Insulin sensitizers (thiazolidinedione)	• Sensitizes peripheral tissues to insulin → increases glucose uptake • Decreases FFA release from adipose • Binds to nuclear receptor	rosiglitazone pioglitazone	Avandia® Actos®		2-8 mg OD 15-45 mg OD		ABSOLUTE: • Severe liver dysfunction • NYHA > class II CHF INTERACTIONS: • Do not combine with insulin	• Peripheral edema • Pulmonary edema • CHF • Anemia • Weight gain • Fractures	↓ HbA1c 1.0-1.5%
α-glucosidase inhibitor	• ↓ carbohydrate GI absorption by inhibiting brush border α-glucosidase	acarbose	Glucobay®		25 mg OD titrated to 100 mg tid	• ↓ postprandial hyperglycemia	ABSOLUTE: • Inflammatory bowel disease • Severe liver dysfunction	• Flatulence • Abdominal cramps • Diarrhea	↓ HbA1c 0.5-1.0%
Dipeptidyl peptidase-IV (DPP-IV) inhibitor	• Inhibits degradation of endogenous antihyperglycemic incretin hormones • Incretin hormones stimulate insulin secretion, inhibit glucagon release, and delay gastric emtyping	sitagliptan	Januvia®		100 mg OD		ABSOLUTE: • Type 1 DM • DKA RELATIVE: • Adjust dose in patients with kidney dysfunction	Nasopharyngitis • URTI • Headache	↓ HbA1c 0.5-1.0%

Common Medications for Dyslipidemia

Drug Class	Mechanism of Action	Generic Drug Name	Canada Name	US Name (if different)	Dosing	Indications	Contraindications	Side Effects
HMG CoA reductase inhibitor (Statins)	• Inhibit cholesterol biosynthesis, ↓ LDL synthesis, ↑ LDL clearance, modest ↑ HDL, limited ↓ VLDL	atorvastatin fluvastatin lovastatin pravastatin rosuvastatin simvastatin	Lipitor® Lescol® Mevacor® Pravachol® Crestor® Zocor®		10-80 mg/d 20-80 mg/d 20-80 mg/d 10-40 mg/d 5-40 mg/d 10-80 mg/d	• 1st line monotherapy for dyslipidemia • Used for ↑ LDL, ↑ TG • 1st prevention of LAD CAD; post MI	• Active liver disease • Persistent ↑ in AST, ALT	• GI symptoms • Rash, pruritus • ↑ liver enzymes • Myositis (↑ risk if combined with fibrates) • Rhabdomyolysis (dose >80 mg)
Fibrates	• Upregulate lipoprotein lipase + Apo A1, ↓ VLDL, ↓ TG, modest ↓ LDL, modest ↑ HDL	bezafibrate fenofibrate gemfibrozil	Bezalip® Lipidil® Lopid®		400 mg/d 48-200 mg/d 600-1200 mg/d	• Used for ↑ TG, hyperchylomicronemia	• Hepatic disease • Renal disease	• GI upset • ↑ risk of gallstone formation • ↑ risk of rhabdomyolysis when combined with statins
Niacin	• Inhibits secretion of hepatic VLDL via lipoprotein lipase (LPL) pathway → decreased VLDL and LDL; decreased clearance of HDL	nicotinic acid	Niaspan® generic niacin	Niacor®	0.5-2 g/d 1-3 g/d	• Used for ↑ LDL, ↑ VLDL	• Hypersensitivity • Hepatic dysfunction • Active PUD • Overt DM • Hyperuricemia	• Generalized flushing • Abnormal liver enzymes • Pruritus • IGT • Severe hypertension
Bile acid sequestrants	• Resins that bind bile acids in intestinal lumen and prevent absorption thereby ↓ LDL	cholestryamine colestipol	Questran® Prevalite® Colestid®		2-24 g/d 5-30 g/d	• Used for ↑ LDL • Use as adjunct with statins or fibrates	• Complete biliary obstruction • Pregnancy, lactation • TG > 300 mg/dL • GI motility disorder	• Constipation • Nausea • Flatulence • Bloating
Cholesterol absorption inhibitors	• Inhibits cholesterol absorption at the small intestine brush border	ezetimibe	Ezetrol®	Zetia®	10 mg/d	• Used for ↑ LDL, Apo B	• Hypersensitivity • Hepatic dysfunction • Don't combine with fibrates or bile acid resins	• Fatigue • Pharyngitis • Sinusitis • Abdominal pain • Diarrhea • Arthralgia

Family Medicine

Essential History and Physical Exam

PERIODIC HEALTH EXAM

	General Population	Special Population

DISCUSSION	• Dental hygiene (community fluoridation, brushing, flossing) (A)
	• Noise control and hearing protection (A)
	• Smokers: counsel on smoking cessation, provide
	  • Nicotine replacement therapy (A)
	  • Referral to smoking cessation program (B)
	  • Dietary advice on leafy green vegetables and fruits (B)
	• Seat belt use (B)
	• Injury prevention (bicycle helmets, smoke detectors) (B)
	• Moderate physical activity (B)
	• Avoid sun exposure and wear protective clothing (B)
	• Problem drinking screening and counselling (B)
	• Counselling to protect against STIs (B)
	• Nutritional counselling and dietary advice on fat and cholesterol (B)
	• Dietary advice on calcium and vitamin D requirements
	(see http://www.canadiantaskforce.ca for up to date guidelines)
		Pediatrics:
		Home visits for high risk families (A)
		Inquiry into developmental milestones (B)
		
		Adolescents:
		Counsel on sexual activity and contraceptive methods (B)
		Counsel to prevent smoking initiation (B)
		
		Adults >50:
		Assess for RF for osteoporosis and fracture (A)
		
		Perimenopausal women:
		Counsel on osteoporosis
		Counsel on risks/benefits of hormone replacement therapy (B)
		
		Adults >65:
		Follow-up on caregiver concern of cognitive impairment (A)
		Multidisciplinary post-fall assessment (A)

PHYSICAL	• Clinical breast exam (women age 50-69) (A) • Blood pressure measurement (B) • BMI measurement in obese adults (B)	**Pediatrics:** Repeated examinations of hips, eyes and hearing (especially in first year of life) (A) Serial heights, weights and head circumference (B) Visual acuity testing after age 2 (B) **Adults >65:** Visual acuity (Snellen sight chart) (B) Hearing impairment (inquiry, whispered voice test, audioscope) (B) **First degree relative with melanoma:** Full body skin exam (B)

PERIODIC HEALTH EXAM (continued)

	General Population	Special Population

TESTS	• Multiphase screening with the Hemoccult test (adults age >50 q1-2yrs) (A)
	• Sigmoidoscopy (adults >50) (frequency not established) (B)
	• Bone mineral density: age 50 if at risk (1 major or 2 minor criteria), otherwise age 65
	• Fasting lipid profile (C):
	  • Women age >50 or post-menopausal; earlier if at risk
	  • Men age >40; earlier if at risk (optimal frequency unknown, at least q5yrs)
	• Fasting blood glucose: age >40 q3yrs (or sooner and more frequently if risk factors present)
	• Syphilis screen if at risk (D)
	• **Men:** PSA testing screening guidelines not established (I)
	• **Women:** Mammography (women age 50-69) q1-2yrs (A)
	Pap smear annually (women age 18-69 if ever sexually active, start after sexual debut); q3yrs after 3 normal results (more frequently if concerns) Stop at age 70 once have 4 normals in 10 yrs prior Rubella titres in women of childbearing age, vaccinate if non-immune (A)
		Pediatrics:
		Routine hemoglobin for high risk infants (B)
		Blood lead screening of high risk infants (B)
		
		Diabetics:
		Urine dipstick (A)
		Fundoscopy (B)
		
		TB high risk groups: Mantoux skin testing (A)
		
		STI high risk groups:
		Voluntary HIV antibody screening (A)
		Gonorrhea screening (A)
		Chlamydia screening in women (B)
		FAP: Sigmoidoscopy and genetic testing (B)
		
		HNPCC: Colonoscopy (B)
		
		Syphilis risk group: VDRL test (A)

THERAPY	• Folic acid supplementation to women of child-bearing age (A) • Varicella vaccine for children age 1-12 and susceptible adolescents/adults (A) • Rubella vaccine for all non-pregnant women of child-bearing age (B) • Pharmacologic treatment of hypertension with dBP >90 mmHg (adults age 21-64, elderly specific subgroups) (A) • Tetanus vaccine: routine booster q10yrs if had 1° series (A) • Pertussis vaccine: routine booster of acellular vaccine once during adulthood (can be given as dTap) (A)	**Pediatrics:** Routine immunizations (A) Hepatitis B immunization (A) **Influenza high risk groups:** Outreach strategies for vaccination (A) annual immunization (B), now recommended for all **TB high risk groups:** INH prophylaxis for household contacts/skin test converters (B) INH prophylaxis for high risk sub-groups (B) **Immunocompromised/age ≥65/COPD:** Pneumococcal vaccine (A)

Reference: Canadian Task Force on Preventative Health Care, 2005. http://www.ctfphc.org

Classification of Recommendations (from the Canadian Taskforce on Preventative Health Care)

A	–	**good** evidence to recommend the clinical preventative action
B	–	**fair** evidence to recommend the clinical preventative action
C	–	existing evidence is **conflicting** and does not allow to make a recommendation for or against use of the clinical preventative action; however, other factors may influence decision-making
D	–	**fair** evidence to recommend against the clinical preventative action
E	–	**good** evidence to recommend against the clinical preventative action
I	–	**insufficient** evidence (in quantity or quality) to make a recommendation; however, other factors may influence decision-making

Common Presentations

Abdominal Pain

- Most common diagnosis = "non-specific abdominal pain" (no identifiable cause, self-limited)

Differential Diagnosis
- GI disorders – PUD, pancreatitis, IBD, appendicitis, gastroenteritis, IBS, diverticular disease, biliary tract disease
- Urinary tract disorders – UTI, renal calculi
- Gynecological disorders – PID, ectopic pregnancy, endometriosis
- Cardiovascular – CAD, AAA, ischemic bowel
- Other – toxic ingestion, foreign body, psychogenic

Investigations
- Bloodwork – CBC, electrolytes, BUN, Cr, amylase, lipase, AST, ALT, ALP, bilirubin, glucose, INR/PTT, tox screen, β-hCG
- Imaging – abdominal x-ray (gas pattern, free air), ultrasound (gallbladder disease, gynecological problems), CT scan (AAA, appendicitis)
- Other – urinalysis, fecal occult blood, endoscopy, *H. pylori* testing (breath test, serology, biopsy)

Chest Pain

Differential Diagnosis

Cardiac	Pulmonary	GI	MSK/Neuro	Psychologic
Angina*	Pneumonia	GERD	Costochondritis	Anxiety
MI*	Pneumothorax*	PUD	Intercostal strain	Panic
Pericarditis*	PE*	Perforated viscus*	Arthritis	Depression
Myocarditis	Pulmonary HTN	Esophageal spasm	Rib fractures	
Aortic dissection*	Lung CA	Cholecystitis	Herpes zoster	
Endocarditis		Hepatitis		

*Emergent

Clinical Features
- High-risk symptoms and signs of chest pain include:
  - Severe pain, pain for >20 min, new onset pain at rest, severe SOB
  - Loss of consciousness, hypotension, tachycardia, bradycardia
  - Cyanosis

Investigations
- ECG, CXR, and others if indicated (cardiac enzymes, D-dimers, LFTs, etc.)

Management of Common Causes of Chest Pain
- Angina/ischemic heart disease:
  - Acute: nitroglycerin (NTG) (wait 5 min between sprays) – if no effect after 3 sprays call ambulance or go to Emergency Department
- Post-MI:
  - MONA (Morphine, Oxygen, NTG, ASA)
  - Reperfusion therapy with tPA or streptokinase if within 6 h (Note: can only use SK once in lifetime)
  - Start β-blocker (e.g. metoprolol starting dose 12.5 mg PO OD, increase gradually to 50 mg PO bid)

Treatment Algorithm for Stable Ischemic Heart Disease

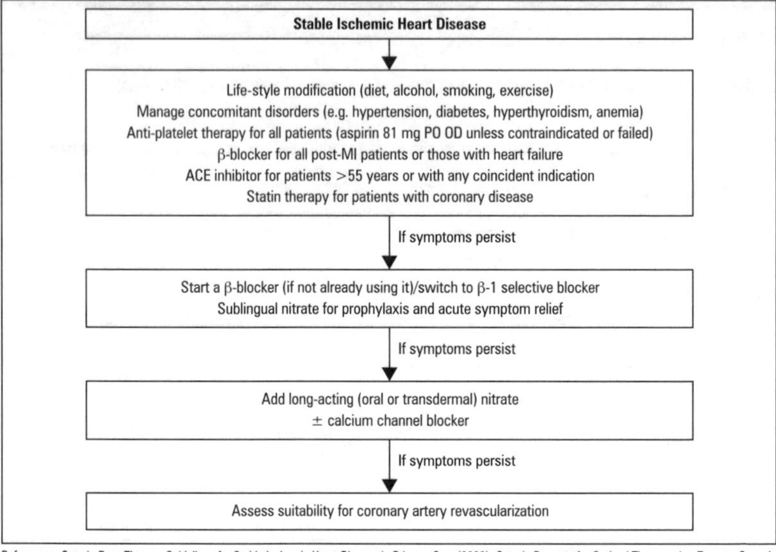

References: Ontario Drug Therapy Guidelines for Stable Ischemic Heart Disease in Primary Care (2000). *Ontario Program for Optimal Therapeutics*. Toronto: Queen's Printer of Ontario, pp. 10.
Guidelines on the management of stable angina pectoris. *Recommendations of the Task Force of the European Society of Cardiolology*; 2006. 63 p.

Common Cold (Acute Rhinitis)

Definition
• Viral upper respiratory tract infection (URTI) with inflammation

Epidemiology
• Organisms
  ▪ Mainly rhinoviruses (30-35% of all colds)
  ▪ Others: coronavirus, adenovirus, RSV, influenza, parainfluenza, echovirus, coxsackie virus
• Incubation: 1-5 d
• Transmission: person-person contact via secretions on skin/objects and by aerosol droplets

Risk Factors
• Psychological stress, excessive fatigue, allergic nasopharyngeal disorders, smoking, sick contacts

Etiology
• **PRIMA** – **P**aramyxoviruses, **R**hinoviruses, **I**nfluenza viruses, **M**yxoviruses, **A**denoviruses

Differential Diagnosis
• Allergic rhinitis, pharyngitis, influenza, laryngitis, croup, sinusitis, bacterial infections

Clinical Features
- Symptoms
  - Local – nasal congestion, clear to mucopurulent secretions, sneezing, sore throat, conjunctivitis, cough
  - General – malaise, headache, myalgias, mild fever
- Signs
  - Boggy and erythematous nasal/oropharyngeal mucosa, enlarged lymph nodes
  - Normal chest exam
- Complications
  - Secondary bacterial infection: otitis media, sinusitis, bronchitis, pneumonia
  - Asthma/COPD exacerbation

Management
- Patient education
  - Symptoms peak at day 1-3 and usually subside within 1 wk
  - Cough may persist for days to weeks after other symptoms disappear
  - No antibiotics indicated because of viral etiology
  - Secondary bacterial infection can present within 3-10 d after onset of cold symptoms
- Prevention
  - Frequent hand washing, avoidance of hand to mucous membrane contact, use of surface disinfectant
- Symptomatic relief
  - Rest, hydration, gargling warm salt water, steam
  - Analgesics and antipyretics: acetaminophen, ASA (not in children because risk of Reye's syndrome)
  - Cough suppression: dextromethorphan or codeine if necessary
  - Zinc gluconate lozenge use is controversial
  - Decongestants, antihistamines
- Patients with reactive airway disease will require increased use of bronchodilators and inhaled steroids

Influenza vs. Colds: A Guide to Symptoms

Questions...	Flu	Cold
Onset of illness	Sudden	Slow
Fever	High fever	None
Exhaustion level	Severe	Mild
Cough	Dry severe or hacking	±
Throat	Normal	Sore
Nose	Dry and clear	Runny
Head	Achy	Headache-free
Appetite	Decreased	Normal
Muscles	Achy	Normal
Chills	Yes	No

Contraception

Contraindications to Combined Oral Contraceptives
- Absolute: known/suspected pregnancy, undiagnosed abnormal vaginal bleeding, prior thromboembolic events, thromboembolic disorder (protein C/S, antithrombin III deficiency, Factor V Leiden mutation), active thrombophlebitis, cerebrovascular or coronary artery disease, estrogen dependent tumours (breast, uterus), impaired liver function associated with acute liver disease, familial hypertriglyceridemia, smoker age >35 yrs, migraines with focal neurological symptoms, uncontrolled HTN
- Relative: migraines – nonfocal with aura <1 h, DM complicated by vascular disease, SLE, controlled HTN, hyperlipidemia, sickle cell anemia, gallbladder disease

Contraception Table

	Advantages	Disadvantages
Combined OCP	Effectiveness: 99.9% with perfect use, 97-99% with typical use, cycle control, ↓ dysmenorrhea, ↓ menstrual flow, ↓ ovarian cancer, ↓ endometrial cancer, ↓ risk of fibroids, ↓ acne, ↓ hirsutism	Irregular bleeding, systemic hormonal side effects (breast tenderness, nausea, mood changes, H/A, bloating), no STI protection, slightly increased risk of venous thromboembolism (VTE), MI, and stroke, decreased quantity of breast milk postpartum
Progestin Only Pill (e.g. Micronor®)	At least 95% effective with perfect use, ↓ menstrual flow, ↓ cramping, no ↑ risk of VTE, MI or stroke, suitable for postpartum	Irregular bleeding, no STI protection, contraceptive reliability requires taking pill at the same time each day (within 3 h), no pill free interval
Transdermal Patch (e.g. Evra®)	Same as OCP, easy to use, changed weekly, 99% effective with correct use	Same as OCP, skin irritation
NuvaRing® (inserted by patient)	Same as OCP, easy to use (in for 3 wks, out for 1), less systemic hormonal side effects, 99% effective with correct use	Same as OCP, vaginitis, some women may be uncomfortable with self-insertion
DMPA IM progesterone injection q12 wks (e.g. DepoProvera®)	99.7% effective against pregnancy, infrequent dosing, ↓ menstrual flow or amenorrhea, ↓ risk of endometrial cancer	Irregular bleeding, delayed return of fertility, no STI protection, systemic hormonal side effects (most common is headache), wt gain, ↓ bone mineral density (check after 5 yrs)
Male Condom	97% effective against pregnancy and STIs when used properly When used properly WITH spermicide they are close to 99.9% effective, no Rx required	Latex allergy, irritation, only effective before the expiry date, must be applied properly, can only be used once
Diaphragm	92-96% effective with perfect use, non-hormonal, female-controlled method of contraception, decreased risk of cervical cancer	Must be left in for 6h after intercourse, must be used with spermicide, incomplete STI protection, latex allergy, must be fitted by health care worker, increased risk of UTI, risk of toxic shock syndrome
Sponge	One-size-fits-all barrier method, does not require fitting by MD, available in pharmacies, 90% effective without a condom, 98% effective with a condom	Relatively expensive, only ~60% effective in parous women, incomplete STI protection, risk of toxic shock syndrome
Intrauterine Device (IUD)	99% effective against pregnancy, effective for 5 yrs, no daily regimen required, can be easily removed, ideal in post-partum women	No STI protection, increased relative risk of PID in first month, must be inserted by MD, risk of post-insertion vaso-vagal response, risk of uterine rupture is 0.6-1.6 per 1000, 2-10% expulsion rate
Levonorgestrel IUD (e.g. Mirena®)	↓ menstrual flow, ↓ systemic hormonal side effects than OCP	Hormonal side effects (see *combined OCP*), expensive (~$400)
Copper IUD (e.g. Nova T®)	↓ risk of endometrial cancer, less expensive (~$170)	Irregular bleeding or ↑ menstrual flow, 6-20% women discontinue use in first 5 yrs because of pain or ↑ bleeding
Fertility Awareness/ Natural Family Planning (e.g. symptothermal method)	Effectiveness: 95-98% with perfect use, 75-88% with typical use, increased awareness of gynecological health, reasonable for couples for whom an unplanned pregnancy would be acceptable	High probability of failure if not used consistently and correctly, no STI protection
Lactational amenorrhea	Very effective in breastfeeding women if menses not returned, fully or nearly fully breastfeeding baby and baby is under 6 months old	Not effective if infant receives any food supplementary to breastfeeding, must breastfeed regularly, even through the night (at least q6h)

Emergency Contraception (EC)
- Hormonal EC (Yuzpe or Plan B, usually 2 doses taken 12 h apart) or post-coital IUD insertion
- Hormonal EC is effective if taken within 72 h of unprotected intercourse (reduces chance of pregnancy by 75-85%); does not affect an established pregnancy
- Post-coital IUDs inserted within 5 d of unprotected intercourse are significantly more effective than hormonal EC (reduces chance of pregnancy by ~99%)
- Pregnancy test should be performed if no menstrual bleeding within 21 d of either treatment
- Advance provision of hormonal emergency contraception increases the use of emergency contraception without decreasing the use of regular contraception
- Pharmacists across Canada can dispense Plan B without a doctor's prescription

Fatigue

Differential Diagnosis of Fatigue: PS VINDICATE

P	Psychogenic	**Depression, sleep disorder, life stresses**, anxiety disorder, chronic fatigue syndrome, fibromyalgia
S	Sedentary	Unhealthy/sedentary lifestyle
V	Vascular	Stroke
I	**Infectious**	Viral (e.g. mononucleosis, hepatitis), bacterial (e.g. TB), fungal, parasitic, HIV
N	**Neoplastic**	Any malignancy
	Nutrition	**Anemia** (Fe deficiency, B_{12} deficiency)
	Neurogenic	Myasthenia gravis, multiple sclerosis, Parkinson's Disease
D	**Drugs**	β-blockers, antihistamines, anticholinergics, benzodiazepines, antiepileptics
I	Idiopathic	
C	Chronic illnesses	CHF, lung diseases (e.g. COPD, sarcoidosis), renal failure, chronic liver disease
A	**Autoimmune**	SLE, RA, mixed connective tissue disease, polymyalgia rheumatica
T	Toxin	**Substance abuse** (e.g. alcohol), heavy metal
E	Endocrine	**Hypothyroidism, diabetes**, Cushing's syndrome, adrenal insufficiency, pregnancy

Common causes are in bold

Fatigue Red Flags
- Fever, wt loss, night sweats, neurological deficits, ill-appearing

Investigations
- Psychosocial causes are common, so usually minimal investigation is warranted
- Physical causes of fatigue usually have associated symptoms/signs that can be elicited from a focused history and physical examination
- Investigations should be guided by findings on history and physical and may include the following:
  - CBC + differential, electrolytes, BUN, Cr, ESR, glucose, TSH, ferritin, B_{12}
  - Total protein, albumin, AST, ALT, ALP, bilirubin, calcium, phosphate, ANA, hCG
  - Urinalysis, CXR, ECG
  - Additional tests: serologies (lyme disease, hepatitis B and C screen, HIV, ANA) and PPD skin tests

Treatment
- Treat the cause
- If etiology is not identified (1/3 of patients)
  - Physician support, REASSURANCE and follow-up, especially with fatigue of psychogenic etiology
  - Counselling: sleep hygeine
  - Supportive counselling, behavioural, or group therapy
  - Encourage patient to stay physically active to maximize function
  - Review all medications, OTC, and herbal remedies, watching for drug-drug interactions and side effects
  - Prognosis: after 1 yr, 40% are no longer fatigued

Headache

Primary Headaches

	Migraine	Tension-type	Cluster	Caffeine withdrawal
Epidemiology	12% of adults F>M 20% with aura 80% without aura	38% of adults, can be episodic or chronic	<0.1% of adults, M>>F	~50% of people drinking >2.5 cups/d
Duration	5-72 h	May occur as isolated incident or daily, duration is variable	<3 h at same time of day	Begins 12-24 h after last caffeine intake, can last ~1wk
Pain	Classically unilateral and pulsatile, but 40% are bilateral, moderate-severe intensity, nausea/vomiting, photo/phonophobia	Mild to moderate pain, bilateral, fronto-occipital or generalized pain, band-like pain, ± contracted neck/ scalp muscles, associated with little disability	Sudden, unilateral, severe, usually centered around eye, frequently awakens patient	Severe, throbbing, associated with drowsiness, anxiety, muscle stiffness, nausea, waves of hot or cold sensations
Triggers	Numerous (e.g. food, sleep disturbance, stress, hormonal, fatigue, weather, high altitude) Aggravated by physical activity	Stressful events, NOT aggravated by physical activity	Often alcohol	Discontinuing caffeine
Treatment of Acute Headache	1st line- acetaminophen, ASA, ± caffeine 2nd line- NSAIDs 3rd line- 5HT agonists ± antiemetic	Rest and relaxation NSAIDs	Sumatriptan Dihydroergotamine High-flow O_2 Intranasal lidocaine	Caffeine Acetaminophen or ASA ± caffeine
Prophylactic Therapy	1st line – β-blockers 2nd line – TCAs 3rd line – anticonvulsants	Rest and relaxation, physical activity, biofeedback	Lithium carbonate, prednisone, methysergide	Cut down on caffeine

Secondary Headaches
- Caused by underlying organic disease
- Account for <10% of all headaches, may be life-threatening
- Etiology
  - Space-occupying lesion
  - Systemic infection (meningitis, encephalitis)
  - Stroke
  - Subarachnoid hemorrhage
  - Systemic disorders (thyroid disease, hypertension, pheochromocytoma, etc.)
  - Temporal arteritis
  - Traumatic head injuries
  - TMJ or C-spine pathology
  - Serious ophthalmological and otolaryngological causes of headache

Treatment
- Based on underlying disorder
- Analgesics may provide symptomatic relief

- **Red Flags**: sudden onset of severe headache, worst headache ever, new headache after age 50, headache present on awakening, impaired mental status, fever, neck stiffness, seizures, focal neurologic deficits, jaw claudication, scalp tenderness

Investigations
- Indicated only when red flags are present, may include:
  - CBC for suspected systemic or intracranial infection
  - ESR for suspected temporal arteritis
  - Neuro-imaging (CT or MRI) to rule out intracranial pathology
  - CSF analysis for suspected hemorrhage, infection

Low Back Pain

Differential Diagnosis
- Mechanical back pain (95% of low back pain): ligamentous/muscle strain, facet joint degeneration, disc injury, spondylosis, spondylolisthesis, compression fracture, spinal stenosis, pregnancy)
- Surgical emergencies: cauda equina syndrome, AAA
- Medical conditions: neoplasm (1° vs. mets vs. multiple myeloma), infection (TB, osteomyelitis), metabolic (Paget's disease, osteomalacia, osteoporosis), rheumatologic (ankylosing spondylitis, polymyalgia rheumatica), referred pain (ectopic pregnancy, perforated ulcer, pancreatitis, pyelonephritis, herpes zoster)

History and Diagnosis
- Pain characteristics, history of trauma
- Remember to ask about
  - **RED FLAGS**: neurologic symptoms (numbness/tingling), urinary retention, fecal incontinence, constitutional symptoms, IV drug use, age >50, neuromotor deficits, chronic disease, Hx cancer

Definitions
- Acute: <6 wks
- Subacute: 6-12 wks
- Chronic: >12 wks

Pain Pattern

BACK DOMINNANT

Pattern I	Pattern II
Worse with flexion	Worse with extension
Constant/intermittent	Always intermittent
Disc pathology	Facet joint pathology

LEG DOMINANT

Pattern III	Pattern IV
Constant pain (currently or previously)	Intermittent pain (short duration)
Pain changes with back movement/position	Worse with activity, improves with rest
Root compression, sciatica	Spinal stenosis, neurogenic claudication

Associated Symptoms
- Depend on the etiology (see above under DDx)
- Make sure to do a thorough review of systems to elicit any associated symptoms that may help point to a specific etiology

Predisposing/Precipitants
- Trauma/strain is often a precipitating factor in mechanical back pain

Complications/PMHx/FmHx
- Ask about family history of malignancy, rheumatologic disease, metabolic disease, etc.

Physical Exam
- Inspection: curvature, posture, gait
- Palpation: paraspinal, bony tenderness, point of maximal tenderness
- ROM: flexion, extension, lateral flexion, rotation
- Neuro exam: focus on L4, L5, S1 to determine level of spinal involvement (power, sensation, reflexes)
- Peripheral pulses
- Special tests: (1) straight leg raise (+ve if sciatica pain at <70°, aggravated by ankle dorsiflexion); (2) crossed straight leg raise (+ve if raising uninvolved leg elicits pain in leg with sciatica, more specific than straight leg raise); (3) femoral stretch test (pt. prone, examiner extends hip)
- Examine other systems if suspect non-mechanical causes of back pain (hip, peripheral vascular, abdominal)

Management

ER
- Urgent surgical consult if: suspected cauda equina syndrome, worsening neurologic deficit, intractable pain not responding to conservative therapy, suspected AAA

Hospital/Inpatient
- Patients not normally admitted unless suspected cauda equina syndrome

Outpatient

Imaging
- Plain films are generally not recommended in initial evaluation
- Indications for lumbar spine x-ray: no improvement after 1 month, fever >38°, significant trauma, progressive neuromotor deficit, suspicion of ankylosing spondylitis, history of cancer (to r/o mets), and alcohol/drug abuse (increased risk of osteomyelitis, trauma, fracture). If there are worsening neurologic deficits or if infection/tumour suspected consider CT or MRI

Bloodwork
- If suspect non-mechanical cause, consider: CBC/ESR (cancer/infection), urinalysis (infection), bone scan (tumour, infection, occult fracture)

Treatment
- Reassurance/education if no underlying serious condition (70% improve in 2 wks, 90% improve by 6 wks)
- Comfort measures: stay active (within limits of pain), limit bed rest (up to 2 d), activity modification (temporarily avoid activities that stress the spine), heat/cold therapies, low-stress aerobic exercise (start during first 2 wks)
- Pharmacological:
    1. Acetaminophen (Tylenol®), 325 mg 1-2 tabs PO q4-6h (dose not to exceed 4 g/24h)
    2. NSAIDs (many available) Ibuprofen (Advil®) 200 mg 1-2 tabs, PO q4-6h (no specific NSAID has been shown to be superior over others)
    3. Muscle relaxants (many available) methocarbamol (Robaxin®) 1.5 g PO qid for the first 48-72 h after acute muscle spasm and then reduce to 1 g PO qid
    4. AVOID narcotics
- Physical methods:
    - Short course of massage therapy has been shown to be effective. Spinal manipulation has not shown to be superior to other treatments (no proven efficacy of TENS, spinal traction, biofeedback, acupuncture or injections)
    - Follow-up with family physician in 2-4 wks
    - Consider further investigations (x-ray, bloodwork) if no improvement after 1 month of conservative therapy

Common Conditions

Asthma/COPD

	COPD	Asthma
Age of Onset	Usually in 6th decade	Any age (but 50% of cases diagnosed in children <10 yrs)
Role of Smoking	Directly related	Known trigger
Reversibility of Airflow obstruction	Airflow obstruction is chronic and persistent	Airflow obstruction is episodic and usually reversible with therapy
Evolution	Slow, cumulative disabling pattern	Episodic, less than 50% will out grow
History of Allergy	Infrequent	Over 50% patients
Precipitators	Environmental irritants (air pollution), cigarette smoking, antiprotease deficiency, viral infection, occupational exposure	Environmental irritants (dust, pollen), furry animals, cold air, exercise, URTIs, cigarette smoke, use of β-blockers/ASA (firefighters, dusty jobs)
Symptoms/Signs	Chronic cough, sputum and/or dyspnea	Wheeze (hallmark symptom), dyspnea, chest tightness, cough which is worse in cold, at night, and in early am prolonged expiration
Diffusion Capacity	Decreased (more so in pure emphysema)	Normal (for pure asthma)
Hypoxemia	Chronic in advanced stages	Not usually present Episodic with severe attacks
Spirometry	May have improvement with bronchodilators but not universally seen	Marked improvement with bronchodilators or steroids
Chest X-Ray	Often normal Increased bronchial markings (chronic bronchitis) and chronic hyperinflation	Often normal or episodic hyperinflation Hyperinflation during asthma attack (emphysema) often co-exist
Management	1° Line: Ipratropium bromide (Atrovent®) Others: salbutamol (Ventolin®), fluticasone (Flovent®),tiotropium bromide (Spiriva®), oral prednisone, oxygen, salmeterol (Serevent®) at bedtime Get flu shot and Pneumovax®	Combination of reliever medications (SABAs) taken prn and controller medications (see below) taken regularily to achieve control of asthma symptoms Controller Medications

Asthma Management:
Step 1: Low-dose ICS
Step 2: Medium/high-dose ICS or low-dose ICS plus either LABA, LT modifier, or long-acting theophylline
Step 3: Medium/high-dose ICS plus either LABA, LT modifier, or long-acting theophylline
Step 4: As above plus immunotherapy ± oral glucocorticosteroids

SABA = short-acting β-agonist   LABA = Long-acting β-agonist   ICS = inhaled glucocorticosteroids   LT modifier = leukotriene modifier

Asthma Control Targets
- Daytime symptoms <3x per wk
- No limitation of activities
- No nocturnal symptoms
- Use of reliver medication <3x per wk
- Normal lung function (PEF, FEV_1)
- No exacerbations

Bronchitis (acute)

Definition
- Acute infection of the tracheobronchial tree causing inflammation with resultant bronchial edema and mucus formation

Etiology
- 80% viral: rhinovirus, coronavirus, adenovirus, influenza, parainfluenza, RSV
- 20% bacterial: *M. pneumoniae, C. pneumoniae, S. pneumoniae*
- How to tell if viral or bacterial
    - Bacterial infections tend to give a higher fever, excessive amounts of purulent sputum production, and may be associated with concomitant COPD
    - NB: purulent sputum is not necessarily bacterial

Differential Diagnosis
- URTI, asthma, acute exacerbation of chronic bronchitis, sinusitis, pneumonia, bronchiolitis, pertussis, environmental/occupational exposures, post-nasal drip, others: reflux esophagitis, CHF, bronchogenic CA, aspiration syndromes, CF, foreign body

Investigations
- Acute bronchitis is typically a clinical diagnosis
- Sputum culture/Gram stain is not very informative
- CXR if suspect pneumonia (cough >3 wks, abnormal vital signs, localized chest findings) or CHF
- Pulmonary function tests with methacholine challenge if suspect asthma

Management
- Primary prevention
    - Frequent hand washing, smoking cessation, avoid irritant exposure
- Symptomatic relief: rest, fluids (3-4 L/d when febrile), humidity, analgesics and antitussives as required
- Bronchodilators, i.e. albuterol, may offer improvement of symptoms
- Current literature does not support routine antibiotic treatment for the management of acute bronchitis because it is most likely to be caused by a viral infection
    - Antibiotics may be useful if elderly, comorbidities, pneumonia is suspected, or if the patient is toxic (refer to <u>Antibiotic Quick Reference</u> chapter)
    - Antibiotics in children show no benefit

Diabetes

Epidemiology
- Major health concern, affecting up to 10% of Canadians
- Type 1 Diabetes (DM1): 10-15% of DM, peak incidence age 10-15
- Type 2 Diabetes (DM2): 85-90% of DM, peak incidence age 50-55, up to 60 000 new cases in Canada per yr
- Gestational diabetes mellitus (GDM): 2-4% of all pregnancies
- Incidence of DM2 is rising dramatically because of a number of different factors: aging population, rising rates of obesity, and sedentary lifestyles
- Leading cause of new-onset blindness and renal dysfunction
- Canadian adults with diabetes are twice as likely to die prematurely, compared to persons without diabetes

Risk Factors
- Type 1
  - Personal history of autoimmune disease, family history
- Type 2
  - First degree relative with DM
  - Age >40 yrs
  - Obesity (especially abdominal), hypertension, hyperlipidemia, coronary artery disease, vascular disease
  - Prior GDM, macrosomic baby (>4 kg)
  - PCOS
  - History of IGT or IFG
  - Presence of complications associated with diabetes
- Both
  - Member of a high risk population (e.g. Aboriginal, Hispanic, Asian or African descent)

Diagnosis
- Persistent hyperglycemia is the hallmark of all forms of diabetes

Diagnosis of Insulin Associated Disorders

Condition	Diagnostic Criteria
Diabetes mellitus	One of the following on 2 occasions: 1. Random BG ≥11.1 mmol/L (200 mg/dL) with symptoms of DM (fatigue, polyuria, polydipsia, unexplained weight loss) OR 2. Fasting BG ≥7.0 mmol/L (126 mg/dL) OR 3. BG 2 h post 75 g OGTT ≥11.1 mmol/L (200 mg/dL) OR 4. HbA1c ≥6.5%
Impaired fasting glucose (IFG)	Fasting BG = 6.1-6.9 mmol/L (110-124 mg/dL)
Impaired glucose tolerance (IGT)	BG 2 h post 75 g OGTT = 7.8-11.0 mmol/L (141-198 mg/dL)

Screening
- Type 2 diabetes
  - Mass screening for Type 2 DM is not recommended
  - Test FBG in everyone >40 yrs q3 yrs
  - More frequent or earlier testing (or both) if presence of >1 risk factor (as previously listed)
- GDM
  - All pregnant women between 24-28 wks gestation
  - Non-fasting 1 h 50 g OGCT ≥10.3 mmol/L (186 mg/dL) is diagnostic
  - If between 7.8-10.2 mmol/L (141-184 mg/dL) do confirmatory fasting 2 h 75 g OGTT
  - If develop GDM, 50% chance of developing Type 2 DM in next 20 yrs

Goals of Therapy
- General
  - To avoid the acute complications (e.g. ketoacidosis, hyperglycemia, infection)
  - To prevent long-term complications
    - Microvascular: nephropathy, retinopathy, neuropathy
    - Macrovascular: CAD, CVD, PVD
  - To minimize negative sequelae associated with therapies (e.g. hypoglycemia, weight gain)
- Specific
  - Fasting or preprandial glucose
    - Ideal: 4-6 mmol/L (72-108 mg/dL)
    - Recommended: 4-7 mmol/L (72-126 mg/dL)
    - Suboptimal (action may be required): 7.1-10.0 mmol/L (128-180 mg/dL)
    - Inadequate (action required): >10.0 mmol/L (180 mg/dL)

- 2 h postprandial glucose
  - Ideal: 5-8 mmol/L (90-144 mg/dL)
  - Recommended: 5-10 mmol/L (90-180 mg/dL)
- HbA1c
  - Ideal: ≤0.06
  - Recommended: ≤0.07
  - Suboptimal: 0.07-0.084
  - Inadequate: >0.084
- Blood pressure
  - Adults: <130/80 (DM and HTN guidelines)
- Lipids
  - LDL cholesterol <2.0 mmol/L (<77 mg/dL)
  - Total cholesterol/HDL ratio <4.0
  - Triglyceride <1.5 mmol/L (132 mg/dL)

Nonpharmacologic Management

- Education
  - Refer to Diabetes Education Program
- Diet
  - All people with DM should see a registered dietician
  - Strive to attain healthy body weight
  - Decrease combined saturated fats and trans fatty acids to <10% of calories
  - Avoid simple sugars, encourage complex carbohydrates, choose low-glycemic index foods
- Physical activity and exercise
  - Encourage 30-45 min of moderate exercise 3-5 d/wk
  - Promotes cardiovascular fitness, increases insulin sensitivity, lowers BP and improves lipid profile
  - If insulin treated, may require alterations of diet, insulin regimen, injection sites and self-monitoring

Pharmacologic Management – see Endocrinology

Dyslipidemia

Assessment

- Measure fasting serum TC, LDL-C, HDL-C, and TG
- Often measured in adults over age 20 at least once every 5 yrs
- Screen for secondary causes: hypothyroid, chronic kidney disease, DM, nephritic syndrome, liver disease
- Assess for presence of CAD risk factors
- Risk category
  - Estimated using the model for 10-yr CAD risk developed from the Framingham data
  - Gives recommended values for LDL-C and TC:HDL-C ratio (no longer gives target TG levels, keep TG as low as possible)
- Hyperlipidemia signs
  1. Atheromata – plaques in blood vessel walls
  2. Xanthoma – plaques or nodules composed of lipid-laden histiocytes in the skin (especially the eyelids)
  3. Tendinous xanthoma – lipid deposits in tendon (especially Achilles)
  4. Corneal arcus (arcus senilis) lipid deposit in cornea

Model for Calculating the 10-year Risk of CAD in a Patient Without Diabetes Mellitus or Clinically Evident Cardiovascular Disease*, Using Framingham Data

STEP 1: DETERMINE RISK POINTS

	Risk Points				Risk Points	
Risk Factor	Men	Women		Risk Factor	Men	Women
Age, year						
30-34	-1	-9		55-50	4	7
35-39	0	-4		60-64	5	8
40-44	1	0		65-69	6	8
45-49	2	3		70-74	7	8
50-54	3	6				
Total cholesterol level, mmol/L						
<4.14	-3	-2		6.22-7.24	2	2
4.15-5.17	0	0		≥7.25	3	3
5.18-6.21	1	1				
HDL-C level, mmol						
<0.90	2	5		1.30-1.55	0	0
0.91-1.16	1	2		≥1.56	-2	-3
1.17-1.29	0	1				
Systolic blood pressure, mmHg						
<120	0	-3		140-159	2	2
120-129	0	0		≥160	3	3
130-139	1	1				
Smoker						
No	0	0		Yes	2	2

STEP 2: CALCULATE RISK**

Total Risk	10-year Risk, %			Total Risk	10-year Risk, %	
Points	Men	Women		Points	Men	Women
1	3	2		10	25	10
2	4	3		11	31	11
3	5	3		12	37	13
4	7	4		13	45	15
5	8	4		14	≥53	18
6	10	5		15		20
7	13	6		16		24
8	16	7		17		>27
9	20	8				

*For example, a 55-year-old man who has a total cholesterol level of 5.43 mmol/L, an HDL-C level of 1.23 mmol/L, a systolic blood pressure of 148 mmHg and who smokes would have a total risk score of 9. His 10-year risk for CAD would be 20%, the risk for the average person of his age in the study population is 16%.

**Risk of CAD outcomes including angina pectoris, unstable angina, nonfatal myocardial infarction and coronary death over subsequent 10 years for a Framingham Study participant with that specific risk score.

Reference: Recommendations for the management of dyslipidemia and the prevention of cardiovascular disease: Summary of the 2003 update. Reprinted from *CMAJ* 28 October 2003; 169(1):921-924 by permission of the publisher. © 2003 Canadian Medical Association.

CLINICAL DEFINITION OF METABOLIC SYNDROME

1) Central obesity
   Men – waist circumference ≥94 cm
   Women – waist circumference ≥80 cm

2) Plus any TWO of the following four factors:

Risk Factor	Defining Level
TG level	>1.7 mmol/L (150 mg/dL)
HDL-C level	
Men	<1.0 mmol/L (40 mg/dL)
Women	<1.3 mmol/L (50 mg/dL)
Blood Pressure	>130/85 mmHg
Fasting glucose level	≥5.6 mmol/L (100 mg/dL)

Management

- Use level of risk to guide intensity of treatment
- Lifestyle modification
  - Dietary modification: <7% of calories from saturated fat, increase soluble fibre
  - Increased physical activity, smoking cessation
  - Patient should employ consistent lifestyle modifications for at least 3 months before considering drug therapy
- Pharmacologic therapy (lipid-lowering agents)
  - Statins
    - HMG-CoA reductase inhibitor
    - Currently recommended as 1st line mono-therapy following unsuccessful lifestyle modifications (most commonly used)
    - Risk of myopathy and hepatotoxicity with intensive therapy, is rare but must consider risk-benefit ratio in individual patients
  - Other agents: bile acid sequestrants, nicotinic acid, fibrates, psyllium, cholesterol absorption inhibitors (e.g. ezetimibe)
  - After initiating drug therapy, lipids should be measured after 6 wks, and at 3 months, if adequate response monitor lipids q 4-6 months
  - When prescribing statins, monitor ALT, AST, CK at baseline then q6wks for signs of transaminitis or myositis; tolerate rise in CK or creatinine ≤25%
- Isolated hypertriglyceridemia
  - Normal HDL-C and TC, elevated TG
  - Mild >2.0 mmol/L (>200 mg/dL) : marked >4.5 mmol/L (>400 mg/dL)
  - Principal therapy is lifestyle modifications: weight loss, exercise, avoidance of smoking and alcohol, effective blood glucose control in diabetics
  - Omega-3 fatty acid intake
  - Drug therapy: nicotinic acid or fibrates
- Emerging risk factors (from Framingham group)
  - Lipoprotein (a)
  - Metabolic syndrome
  - Genetic risk
  - Hormone replacement therapy
  - Infectious agents

Target Lipid Values for Primary Prevention of CAD in mmol/L (mg/dL)

Risk Category	LDL-C (mmol/L)		Total-C:HDL-C ratio
High (10-yr risk of CAD ≥20%, or history of DM or any atherosclerotic disease)	<2.0 (<100)	and	<4
Moderate (10-yr risk 11-19%)	<3.5 (<130)	and	<5
Low (10-yr risk ≤10%)	<5.0 (<130 with ≥2 risk factors) (<160 with ≤1 risk factors)	and	<6

Reference: McPherson, Ruth et al. (2006). Canadian Cardiovascular Society position statement – Recommendations for the diagnosis and treatment of dyslipidemia and prevention of cardiovascular disease. Can J Cardiol 6;22(11):913-927.

Hypertension

Differential Diagnosis
1. Essential (primary) hypertension: >90%, undetermined cause, positive family history, onset 30-55
2. Secondary hypertension: 10%, several causes

Causes of Secondary Hypertension

Renal	Renovascular HTN, renal parenchymal disease, glomerulonephritis, pyelonephritis, polycystic kidney, renal artery stenosis
Endocrine	$1°$ hyperaldosteronism Pheochromocytoma Cushing's syndrome Hyperthyroidism/hyperparathyroidism Hypercalcemia of any cause
Vascular	Coarctation of the aorta Renal artery stenosis
Drug-induced	Estrogens Steroids NSAIDs MAOIs Lithium Decongestants Cocaine Amphetamines Alcohol
Other	Obstructive aleep apnea (common cause of $2°$ HTN) Eclampsia White coat (labile)

History
- Symptoms of hypertension (especially mild HTN) are usually NOT PRESENT (HTN = "the silent killer")
- Patients may have occipital headache upon awakening or organ specific complaints if advanced
- Complete functional inquiry with focus on cardiac/vascular, neurologic, and renal systems (SOB, angina, seizures, mental status changes, oliguria)
- Ask about visual disturbances and retinopathy
- Rule out emergencies (e.g. chest pain for MI, back pain for dissection, morning headache)
- Detailed assessment of prescription, OTC medications and recreational drug use
- Assess duration and severity of previously diagnosed hypertension if applicable, treatments and compliance

Risk Factors/Predisposing/Precipitants
- Family history of HTN, CVD, DM, obesity (especially abdominal), sedentary lifestyle, alcohol consumption, smoking, stress, male gender, age >40, dyslipidemia, excessive salt intake/fatty diet, African ancestry

Complications/PMHx/FmHx
- Ask about history of: CAD (angina/MI), LVH, CHF, TIA/CVD, PVD (i.e. claudication), renal disease, DM, other medical conditions
- Ask about family history of the same above conditions, for CVD inquire about age of onset in family members as age <55 in males and <65 in females most significant

Physical Exam
- Vital signs including ER/clinic BP monitoring, ensure cuff is appropriate size, do bilateral readings and include upper and lower extremities if pulses markedly reduced
- Cardiovascular exam: murmurs, signs of LVH, volume status with JVP, orthostatic vitals, etc.
- Neuro exam: focal neurological signs and mental status
- Peripheral vascular exam: carotid, femoral and brachial pulses, bruits
- Abdominal exam: masses or bruits
- Fundoscopic exam: papilledema, exudates, hemorrhages
- Note: physical exam will aid in assessing degree of organ damage and clues to possible secondary HTN

Diagnosis
- Requires >2 measurements separated by >2 mins over >2 office visits; should verify in contralateral arm
- If patient presents with urgency or emergency (see definition section for details) – diagnosis of hypertension is made immediately
- When not a hypertensive crisis, diagnosis of hypertension usually takes place over several visits – specific algorithm for approach to diagnosis of hypertension available from the Canadian Hypertension Society; can use home blood pressure monitoring and ambulatory BP monitors in addition to manual cuff

Definition
- Hypertension: any BP >140/90 mmHg, can be divided into stage I HTN – sBP 140-159 or dBP 90-99 and stage II HTN – sBP >160 or dBP >100
- Isolated hypertension: sBP >140 and dBP <90, usually begins in 5th decade
- Hypertensive crisis: urgency or emergency
  a) Urgency: BP >210 or dBP >120 with minimal or no target-organ damage
  b) Emergency: high BP + acute target-organ damage (neurologic, cardiac, renal), not defined by an absolute BP value, rather by clinical status of patient
- Two subtypes of emergencies: 1. accelerated hypertension – significant increase in BP over previous hypertensive levels associated with evidence of vascular damage on fundoscopy but without papilledema and 2. malignant hypertension – sufficient elevation in hypertension to cause papilledema and other manifestations of vascular damage (retinal hemorrhages, bulging discs, mental status changes, increasing creatinine)

Management

Outpatient
- Close outpatient follow-up is required for patients with hypertensive emergencies to prevent further episodes
- Patients discharged from ER with urgencies should be evaluated and treated promptly as outpatients by their family physicians or a hypertension specialist
- Initial investigations for HTN (non-hypertensive crisis): CBC, Na^+, K^+, creatinine, urinalysis, blood glucose, lipids (HDL, LDL, total chol, TG), ECG
- Suspect secondary cause if: onset of HTN <30 or >55, HTN is refractory to >3 drugs, patient presents with accelerated/malignant HTN or the clinical situation is suspicious for a renal/endocrine abnormality
  - If DM/renal disease → urinary protein excretion, renal ultrasound, captopril scan
  - If endocrine cause → plasma aldosterone and plasma renin
  - If pheochromocytoma suspected → 24 h urine metanephrines

Treatment
- Target BP <140/90, <130/80 if DM or renal disease
- Lifestyle modification in all patients, in fact may be sole treatment in stage 1 HTN (140-159/90-99):
  - Smoking cessation
  - Alcohol restriction to low drinking guidelines
  - Weight loss if BMI >25
  - Exercise
  - Diet (low sodium, saturated fat and cholesterol)
- Pharmacological treatment when lifestyle modification alone is not successful:
  - First-line monotherapy with one of: thiazide diuretic, β-blocker, ACEI, or calcium channel blocker
  - ACEI should not be used as 1st line agent for those of African American descent
  - If ACEI not tolerated prescribe angiotensin receptor blocker
  - When only partial response with monotherapy, use combination therapy, useful combination: (thiazide or dihydropyridine CCB) + (ACEI or β-blocker)
    - Not recommended as 1st line agents for patients >60 yrs old due to lack of benefit (A)
  - Choice of particular drug(s) to start with will depend on the patient's age, other medical conditions and past medical history, whether HTN is isolated systolic or not, BP level
  - At follow-up visits, discuss adherence/healthy lifestyle
  - Visits q1 month until meet target, q3-6 months after
- Referral for refractory HTN, 2° causes, renal failure, etc.

Osteoporosis

Epidemiology
- Age-related disease characterized by decreased bone mass and increased susceptibility to fractures
- Affects 1 in 6 Canadian women over the age of 50

Risk Factors for Osteoporosis

Major Risk Factors	Minor Risk Factors
Age >65 yrs	Rheumatoid arthritis
Vertebral compression fracture	Past history of clinical hyperthyroidism
Fragility fracture after age 40	Chronic anticonvulsant therapy
Family history of osteoporotic fracture	Low dietary calcium intake
(especially maternal hip fracture)	Smoker
Systemic glucocorticoid therapy of >3 months duration	Excessive alcohol intake
Malabsorption syndrome	Excessive caffeine intake
Primary hyperparathyroidism	Weight <57 kg
Propensity to fall	Weight loss >10% of weight at age 25
Osteopenia apparent on x-ray film	Chronic heparin therapy
Hypogonadism	
Early menopause (before age 45)	

Diagnosis
- Defined in terms of a bone mineral density (BMD) < -2.5 SD
- Osteopenia defined by BMD T-score between -1 SD and -2.5 SD
- Mass BMD screening is not recommended
- Measure BMD in:
    - All patients >65 yrs of age
    - All patients with one major or two minor risk factors for osteoporosis
- Measure BMD using dual energy x-ray absorptiometry (DEXA)
- Suspect osteoporosis in women with back pain, a decrease in height or thoracic kyphosis

Management
- Institute a fall prevention program for those at risk, optimize eyesight
- Lifestyle
    - Weight bearing exercise, smoking cessation, decrease EtOH intake
- Diet
    - For women without documented osteoporosis, calcium and vitamin D supplementation alone prevents osteoporotic fractures
    - Calcium (1200 mg/d) and vitamin D (800 IU/d) intake in diet or supplements
- Pharmacological
    - For women with osteoporosis, alendronate, risedronate or raloxifene prevent osteoporotic fractures (grade A to B recommendation)
    - For women with severe osteoporosis (osteoporosis plus at least 1 fragility fracture), alendronate, risedronate, parathyroid hormone (limited duration), raloxifene, etidronate and oral palmidronate therapy. If none of these drugs is tolerated, hormone replacement therapy (HRT) or calcitonin can be considered. Severe esophagitis is the major side effect of bisphosphonate use
- HRT, calcitonin
    - There is fair evidence that combined estrogen–progestin therapy decreases the incidence of total, hip and nonvertebral fractures; however, for most women the risks may outweight the benefits

Pharyngitis

Definition
- Acute pharyngitis is an inflammation of the oropharynx
- May be caused by a wide range of infectious organisms, most of which produce a self-limited infection with no significant sequelae

Differential Diagnosis
- Viral pharyngitis, bacterial pharyngitis, infectious mononucleosis, laryngotracheobronchitis, tonsillitis, epiglottitis, parapharyngeal abscess

Etiology
- Viral
    - Adenovirus, rhinovirus, influenza virus, RSV, EBV, coxsackie virus, herpes simplex virus
- Bacterial
    - Group A, β-hemolytic *Streptococcus* (GABHS)
    - Other bacterial causes:
        - Group C and G, β-hemolytic *Streptococcus, Neisseria gonorrhoeae, Chlamydia pneumoniae, Haemophilus influenzae, Mycoplasma pneumoniae, Corynebacterium diphtheriae*

Epidemiology
- Viral
    - Most common cause, occurs year round
- Bacterial
    - Group A β-hemolytic *Streptococcus*
    - Most common bacterial cause
    - 5-15% of adult cases and up to 50% of all pediatric cases of acute pharyngitis
    - Most prevalent between 5-17 yrs old
    - Occurs most often in winter months

Clinical Features
- Viral
    - Pharyngitis, conjunctivitis, rhinorrhea, hoarseness, cough
    - Nonspecific flu-like symptoms such as fever, malaise, and myalgia
    - Often mimics bacterial infection
    - **Coxsackie virus** (hand, foot and mouth disease)
        - Primarily late summer, early fall
        - Sudden onset of fever, pharyngitis, headache, abdominal pain and vomiting
        - Appearance of small vesicles that rupture and ulcerate on soft palate, tonsils, pharynx
        - Ulcers are pale gray, several mm in diameter, have surrounding erythema, may appear on hands and feet
    - **Herpes simplex virus**
        - Like coxsackie virus but ulcers are fewer and larger
    - **EBV** (infectious mononucleosis)
        - Pharyngitis, tonsillar exudate, fever, lymphadenopathy, fatigue, rash
- Bacterial
    - Symptoms: sore throat, absence of cough, fever, malaise, headache, abdominal pain
    - Signs: fever, tonsillar or pharyngeal erythema/exudate, swollen/tender anterior cervical nodes
    - Complications
        - Rheumatic fever, glomerulonephritis, suppurative complications (abscess, sinusitis, otitis media, pneumonia, cervical adenitis), meningitis, impetigo

- Seven danger signs in patients with "sore throat"
  1. Persistence of symptoms longer than 1 wk without improvement
  2. Respiratory difficulty, particularly stridor
  3. Difficulty in handling secretions
  4. Difficulty in swallowing
  5. Severe pain in the absence of erythema
  6. A palpable mass
  7. Blood in the pharynx or ear

Investigations

- Suspected GABHS
  - See Table for approach to diagnosis and management of GABHS
  - Gold standard for diagnosis is throat culture
  - Rapid test for streptococcal antigen: high specificity (95%), low sensitivity (50-90%)
  - If rapid test positive, treat patient
  - If rapid test negative, take culture and call patient if positive to start antibiotics
- Suspected EBV (infectious mono)
  - Peripheral blood smear, heterophile anitobody test (i.e. the latex agglutination assay, or "monospot" test)

Management

- GABHS
  - Treat if patient presents with a sore throat score >4 or once culture confirms diagnosis
  - No increased incidence of rheumatic fever with 48-hour delay in treatment
  - Incidence of glomerulonephritis is not decreased with antibiotic treatment
  - 7-10 d antibiotic course
    - Adults: penicillin V 600 mg PO tid
    - Children: amoxicillin 40 mg/kg/d PO divided q8h
    - Erythromycin if penicillin allergic
    - Routine follow-up and/or post-treatment throat cultures are not required for most patients
    - Follow-up throat culture recommended only for: patients with history of rheumatic fever, patients whose family member has history of acute rheumatic fever, suspected strep carrier
- Viral pharyngitis
  - Antibiotics NOT indicated
  - Symptomatic therapy: acetaminophen/NSAIDs for fever and muscle aches, decongestants
- Infectious mono (EBV)
  - Antibiotics NOT indicated; administering ampicillin produces rash
  - Self-limiting course; rest during acute phase is beneficial
  - If acute airway obstruction give corticosteroids, consult ENT
  - Supportive care, i.e. acetaminophen or NSAIDS for fever, sore throat, malaise
  - Avoid heavy physical activity and contact sports for at least one month or until splenomegaly resolves because of risk of splenic rupture

Sore Throat Score: Approach to Diagnosis and Management of GABHS

	POINTS	SCORE
Cough absent?	1	0
History of fever >38°?	1	1
Tonsillar exudate?	1	2
Swollen, tender anterior nodes?	1	3
Age 3-14 yrs?	1	4
Age 15-44 yrs?	0	
Age >45 yrs?	−1	

In communities with moderate levels of strep infection (10-20% of sore throats):

Score	0	1	2	3	4
Chance patient has strep	2-3%	3-7%	8-16%	19-34%	41-61%
Suggested action		NO culture or antibiotic		Culture all, treat only if culture is positive	Culture all, treat with antibiotics on clinical grounds[1]

[1]Clinical grounds include a high fever or other indicators that the patient is clinically unwell and is presenting early in the course of the illness.
Limitations: *This score is not applicable to patients less than 3 yrs of age.. *If an outbreak or epidemic of illness caused by GAS is occuring in any community, the score is invalid and should not be used. Adapted from: Centor RM et al (1981). *Med Decis Making.* 1: 239-46. McIssac WI, White D, Tannenbaum D, Low DE (1998). *CMAJ.* 158(1):75-83.

Gastroenterology

Essential History, Physical Exam and Investigations

History and Physical Exam
- See *Common Presentations* and <u>General Surgery</u>

Essential Investigations

LIVER FUNCTION TESTS
- Prothrombin time (PT) (most sensitive): marker of hepatic protein synthesis, must exclude vitamin K deficiency
- Bilirubin: product of liver heme metabolism, must exclude extrahepatic causes of hyperbilirubinemia
- Albumin: decreased by hepatic dysfunction, must exclude malnutrition, renal and GI losses

LIVER ENZYMES
- AST and ALT are released due to inflammation (hepatitis) or ischemia
- AST or ALT >1000: viral hepatitis, drugs, passed common bile duct stones, hepatic ischemia, autoimmune hepatitis
- AST:ALT >2:1 and AST <300: alcoholic hepatitis, cirrhosis, nonhepatic sources (e.g. hemolysis, myopathy)

PATTERNS OF LIVER TESTS
- Hepatocellular pattern: transaminases (ALT/AST) relatively more increased than ALP (alkaline phoshatase)
  - Viral hepatitis: HAV, HBV, HCV, HDV, HEV, CMV, EBV, HSV, VZV
  - Drugs and toxins: acetaminophen, alcohol, drugs (e.g. isoniazid, phenytoin, carbamazepine, antidepressants (especially TCAs))
  - Non-alcoholic fatty liver disease (NAFLD) (including steatohepatitis). Risk factors include obesity, DM type 2, hyperlipidemia; ALT>AST unless cirrhosis has developed
  - Vascular: veno-occlusive disease, CHF, Budd-Chiari syndrome
  - Hereditary: Wilson's disease, hemochromatosis, α-1 anti-trypsin deficiency
- Cholestatic pattern: ALP relatively more increased than transaminases
  - With duct dilatation (biliary obstruction): choledocholithiasis, carcinoma at the head of the pancreas, cholangiocarcinoma, sclerosing cholangitis
  - Without duct dilatation (intrahepatic cholestasis): sepsis, primary biliary cirrhosis, medications (e.g. EPO)

VISUALIZING THE GI TRACT

Esophagus, Stomach, Duodenum
- In most circumstances endoscopy is best (esophagogastroduodenoscopy) – most sensitive visualization of mucosa
- Allows for therapeutic intervention (band varices, cauterize/clip/inject bleeding ulcers)
- Consider barium swallow first if dysphagia, decreased level of consciousness (increases risk of aspiration), inability to cooperate (increases risk of pharyngeal trauma during intubation), extrinsic compression of bowel suspected
- Endotracheal intubation first if massive upper GI bleed, acidosis, or unable to protect airway

Small Bowel
- Most difficult to visualize
- CT enterography (use enteroclysis if suspect obstruction) is more accurate than small bowel swallow with follow-through, but both have low sensitivity
- Wireless endoscopy capsule (26 x 11 mm capsule is swallowed, transmits images to a computer; contraindicated if bowel obstruction because capsule can become impacted)
- Is more accurate than radiology, but not covered by OHIP
- MRI enteroclysis increasingly available
- "Double balloon" endoscopy (endoscope with balloons proximally and distally to propel endoscope: into jejunum from mouth, into ileum from anus) may be most sensitive but currently available only in selected centres; technically demanding

Colon and Terminal Ileum
- Usually colonoscopy, with biopsy if required. Contraindicated in acute diverticulitis and severe colitis (increased risk of perforation)
- CT colonography ("virtual colonoscopy") more accurate in diagnosing diverticulosis, extrinsic pressure on colon (e.g. ovarian cancer compressing sigmoid colon), and fistulae

Pancreatic/Biliary Duct
- MRCP (magnetic resonance cholangiopancreatography = MRI of pancreas/bile duct) almost as sensitive as ERCP (endoscopic retrograde cholangiopancreatography) to determine if bile duct obstruction present, but less accurate in determining cause of obstruction (tumour, stone, stricture)
- Use ERCP if therapeutic intervention likely to be required, such as endoscopic draining if strong suspicion of stone or ampullary tumour
- MRCP reported to have lower sensitivity in sclerosing cholangitis than ERCP

Common Presentations

- Note: see <u>General Surgery</u> for DDx of acute abdominal pain

Dysphagia

Definition
- Difficulty in swallowing, the sensation of food sticking with swallowing

Differential Diagnosis
- **"DISPHAGIA"** – **D**iffuse esophageal spasm, **I**ntrinsic lesion, **S**cleroderma, **P**haryngeal disorders, **H**eart (especially left atrial enlargement), **A**chalasia, **G**oiter, **I**nfection, **A**merican trypanosomiasis

History
- Difficulty with solids, liquids, or both; intermittent or progressive heartburn, change in eating habits/diet, weight loss, chest pain

Investigations
- Barium swallow – motility and mechanical
- Oesophagogastroduodenoscopy (OGD) – mechanical
- Manometry – motility

Approach to Dysphagia

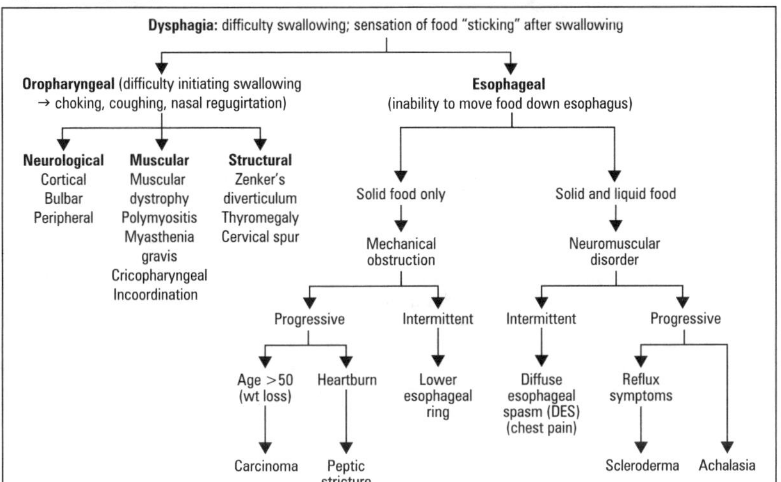

GASTROENTEROLOGY

Dyspepsia/Indigestion

Definition
• Intermittent epigastric discomfort, characteristically develops after eating

Etiology – If upper GI endoscopy and other investigations are normal:
• NERD (non-esophagitis reflux disease)
• Gastroparesis (non-obstructive gastric stasis, common in diabetes)
• Medication side-effect
• Celiac disease, submucosal infiltration of stomach e.g. by cancer/lymphoma or pancreatic disease missed on abdominal imaging

Nausea and Vomiting

History
• Sx: abdominal pain, diarrhea, bloody stools, headache, fever, weight loss
• Risk factors (based on differential below)

Differential Diagnosis of Nausea/Vomiting

With Abdominal Pain Relieved by Vomiting	With Abdominal Pain Not Relieved by Vomiting	Without Abdominal Pain/Non-GI Associated with CNS Sx	Without Abdominal Pain/ Non-GI Not Relieved by Vomiting
Gastric outlet obstruction	Gallbladder disease	Cerebral tumour	Drugs
Small bowel obstruction	Pancreatitis	Migraine	Uremia
	Myocardial infarction	Vestibular	Pregnancy
	Hepatitis	Cerebellar hemorrhage	Metabolic (e.g. hypercalcemia)
			Gastroparesis (e.g. diabetes)
			Ketoacidosis

Diarrhea

Definition
- Passage of frequent, unformed stools >200 g stool/24 h
- Acute: duration <14 d
- Chronic: duration >14 d

Classification
- Secretory: large volume, normal stool osmotic gap, fasting improves but does not resolve diarrhea
    - Bacterial toxins (cholera toxin, clostridial endotoxin), non-invasive gastroenteritis, bile salt absorption, neuroendocrine tumours (carcinoid syndrome, pancreatic cholera syndrome, Zollinger-Ellison syndrome, thyroid cancer), villous adenoma, laxative abuse, Addison's disease, congenital electrolyte absorption defects
- Osmotic: watery stool with no blood or pus, resolves with fasting, increased stool osmotic gap, water drawn into bowel lumen by osmotically active particles in lumen
    - Medications (e.g. Mg-containing laxatives), poorly absorbed carbohydrates (lactase deficiency=lactose intolerance, most common; sorbitol, lactulose, mannitol), diarrhea of pancreatic insufficiency, celiac sprue and other causes of malabsorption (partially explained by osmotic mechanism)
- Inflammatory: small, infrequent stools with blood or pus, damaged mucosal lining, decreased ability to absorb lost fluids
    - IBD = Crohn's disease or ulcerative colitis, ischemic colitis, radiation-induced enteritis, invasive gastroenteritis
- Steatorrheal: decreased stool volume with fasting, increased fecal fat, increased stool osmotic gap
    - Intraluminal maldigestion (pancreatic insufficiency, bacterial overgrowth, liver disease), mucosal malabsorption (celiac sprue, Whipple's disease, infection), postmucosal obstruction (primary or seconday lymphatic obstruction)
- Altered motility: variable volume related to malabsorption
    - Thyrotoxicosis, irritable bowel syndrome, neurological disease (DM-associated enteropathy)

Investigations
- Stool
    - WBC: positive if >3 PMNs in 4 high-power fields
    - C+S, O+P: in acute diarrhea, highest yield is from WBC's present in stool
    - Routinely only cultured for *Campylobacter, Salmonella, Shigella, E. coli* O157:H7
    - Fecal fat
    - Stool osmotic gap: OSM_{stool} (usually 290) – [2 x (Na_{stool} + K_{stool})]
    - *C. difficile* toxin: especially if recent antibiotic use, hospitalization, nursing home resident or chemotherapy
- Sigmoidoscopy if inflammatory diarrhea suspected

Management of Acute Diarrhea
- Fluid and electrolyte replacement – encouraging intake of salt and sugar more important than encouraging intake of water
- Antimotility agents: diphenoxylate, loperamide (contraindicated if mucosal inflammation)
- Diet: only rarely changes underlying disease (celiac disease is exception), but avoiding fresh fruits/cereals/ vegetables (fibre), encouraging bananas, rice, apple sauces, toast (BRAT diet) decreases stool volume
- Antibiotics: refer to <u>Infectious Diseases</u> for agents: uncommonly indicated (before stool analysis results available) as risks for prolonged excretion of enteric pathogen, side effects including *C. difficile* colitis, development of resistant strains
- Indications for antibiotics:
    - Clear indications: *Shigella, V. cholera, C. difficile*, Traveler's diarrhea, enterotoxigenic *E. coli* (ETEC), *Giardia, Entamoeba histolytica, Cyclospora*
    - Indicated in certain situations: *Salmonella* (if *S. typhi* or immunodeficiency, hemolytic anemia, extremes of age, prosthetic valves or grafts), *Campylobacter, Yersinia*, non-enterotoxigenic *E. coli*

Jaundice

Definition
- Yellow pigmentation of the skin, sclerae and mucus membranes due to increased serum bilirubin

Clinical Features
- Dark urine or pale stools suggests an increase in direct bilirubin
- Pruritus suggests a chronic problem
- Abdominal pain is suggestive of biliary tract obstruction (e.g. stone or pancreatic tumour)

Differential Diagnosis
- Predominantly unconjugated (indirect) hyperbilirubinemia
  - Overproduction: hemolysis (spherocytosis, autoimmune hemolytic anemia), ineffective erythropoiesis (megaloblastic anemia)
  - Decreased hepatic uptake: Gilbert's syndrome, drugs (e.g. rifampin, radiocontrast)
  - Decreased conjugation: hepatocellular disease, drug inhibition (e.g. chloramphenicol), Crigler-Najjar syndromes I and II, neonatal jaundice, Gilbert's syndrome
- Predominantly conjugated (direct) hyperbilirubinemia
  - Impaired hepatic secretion: hepatocellular disease (most common), drug-induced cholestasis (e.g. OCP, chlorpromazine), primary biliary cirrhosis, sepsis, post-operative
  - Extrahepatic biliary obstruction: intraductal obstruction (gallstones, biliary stricture, infection, cholangiocarcinoma, sclerosing cholangitis), extraductal obstruction (pancreatic cancer, lymphoma, pancreatitis)

Investigations
- Bilirubin direct (conjugated) and total, liver enzymes (AST, ALT, GGT, ALP), hepatitis serology
- Imaging of bile ducts: ultrasound, ERCP, MRCP, PTC
- Liver biopsy

Approach to Jaundice

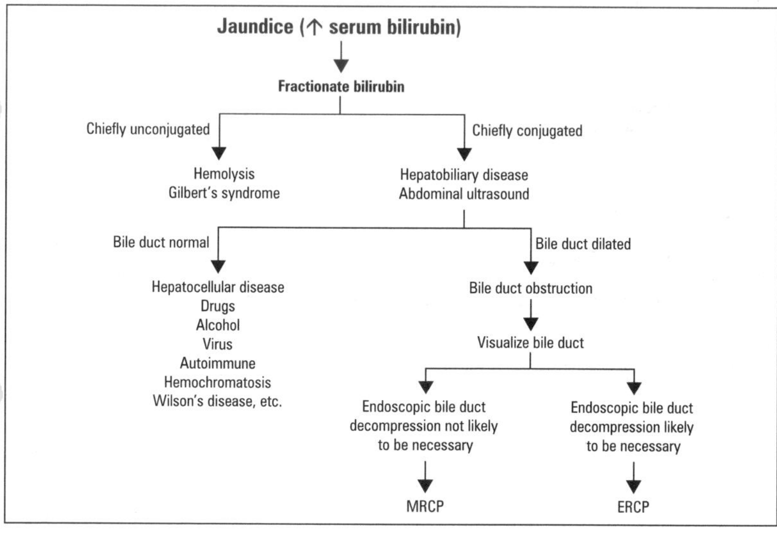

Upper GI Bleed (UGIB)

Definition
• Bleeding proximal to the ligament of Treitz

Differential Diagnosis
• Above the gastro-esophageal junction: epistaxis, esophageal varices, esophagitis, esophageal cancer, Mallory-Weiss tear
• Stomach: gastric ulcer, gastritis (e.g. alcohol, post-surgery), gastric cancer
• Duodenum: ulcer in bulb, aortoenteric fistula (if previous aortic graft)
• Coagulopathy: drugs, renal disease, liver disease
• Vascular malformations: Dieulafoy's lesion, AVM

Differential Diagnosis of Upper GI Bleeding

Common	Uncommon	Rare
Ulcers (*H. pylori*, ASA, NSAIDs)	Tumours	Aorto-enteric fistulas
Esophageal varices	Arteriovenous malformation	Hemobilia
Mallory-Weiss tears	Dieulafoy's lesion	
Erosive esophagitis	Gastric antral vascular ectasia	
Erosive gastritis	Portal hypertensive gastropathy	

History
• OPQ (BRB vs. coffee grounds) RSTUVW
• BM – black tarry (UGI bleed) vs. BRBPR (massive upper UGI bleed or lower GI bleed of any severity)
• N/V/D, abdominal pain
• Acid reflux, heartburn (PUD, GERD)
• B symptoms – appetite, weight loss/gain, fever, night sweats, chills
• Recent episode of retching/forceful vomiting
• Aortic aneurysm repair, GI surgery or procedures
• Family or personal history of coagulation disorder
• Personal history of previous GI bleed
• History of alcohol abuse

Predisposing Factors
• Use of NSAIDs, ASA, warfarin or heparin
• *H. pylori* infection
• End-stage liver disease (cirrhosis)
• Age >70 yrs
• Excessive alcohol consumption

Factors Associated with Mortality
• High rate of bleeding (as indicated by hemodynamic instability, hemoglobin concentration, transfusion requirement), liver disease, co-existing illness, age >60, bleeding developed in hospital

Physical Exam
• Vitals including postural changes, abdominal exam including systemic manifestations of liver disease, cardiac exam, JVP, DRE for fecal occult blood (if not frank)

Investigations
• CBC, PT/INR, aPTT, Electrolytes, BUN, CR, LFTs, ± NG tube aspirate

Management
- Esophageal Variceal Bleed or Unstable Patient:
  - NPO
  - Maintain hemodynamic stability: IV fluids, cross and type, blood transfusion
  - If coagulopathy: vit K, FFP, stop antithrombotic drugs (warfarin, heparin, aspirin)
  - PPI (IV) if peptic ulcer suspected
  - Octreotide if varices suspected
  - Foley to monitor fluid status
  - Surgery if perforated duodenal ulcer
- Consult GI: endoscopy provides definitive diagnosis and management via coagulation /epinephrine injection of bleeding ulcer, banding of varices
- Active bleeding/visible vessel/varices at endoscopy, indicate poor prognosis, consider ICU
- Consider erythromycin 250 mg IV prior to endoscopy to dissolve clots
  - If variceal bleed, loading dose of octreotide 50 µg IV followed by infusion of 50 µg/h; balloon tamponade or TIPS if varical bleeding cannot be controlled
  - If peptic ulcer bleed with active bleeding, visible vessel, clot – IV PPI
- Consider General Surgery consult if: prolonged bleeding, high blood loss, high rate of bleeding, failure of medical management

Lower GI Bleed

Definition
- Bleeding distal to the ligament of Treitz

Clinical Features
- Hematochezia, often associated with anemia/fatigue, anorexia, abdominal pain, syncope, changes in bowel habits, occult blood in stool; rarely melena

Differential Diagnosis
- Massive bleeding: diverticulosis, angiodysplasia, occasionally massive upper GI bleed, aortoenteric fistula (history of AAA repair)
- Non-massive bleeding: hemorrhoids, colitis infectious, IBD, anorectal lesions
- Occult bleeding: neoplasms, colon cancer
- Other: systemic diseases including vascular malformations (e.g. Osler-Weber-Rendu syndrome), vasculitides (e.g. Henoch-Schonlein purpura, polyarteritis nodosa); blood dyscrasias (e.g. thrombocytopenia), coagulation disorders (e.g. DIC) predispose to bleeding but usually an underlying cause is found

Differential Diagnosis of Lower GI Bleeding

Common	Uncommon	Rare
Diverticulosis	Upper GI bleed (brisk)	Intussusception
Ischemia	Post-polypectomy	Vasculitides
Angiodysplasia (elderly)	Radiation colitis	Stercoral ulcer
Infectious	IBD	Coagulopathies
Anorectal (hemorrhoids, fissure, ulcer)		

History
- Characterization of hematochezia or melena, onset, amount, duration
- Bowel habits, especially recent change
- Abdominal pain, nausea, vomiting
- Rectal urgency or tenesmus
- B symptoms: fever, night sweats, chills, weight loss, decreased appetite
- Travel and sick contacts
- Previous medical or surgical history (particularly AAA repair), treatment with radiation

- Family history of colon cancer, IBD, coagulopathy, liver disease
- Personal history of GI bleed, hemorrhoids, GI investigations (e.g. colonoscopy, FOBT, etc.)
- Medications including anticoagulants

Approach to Lower GI Bleed

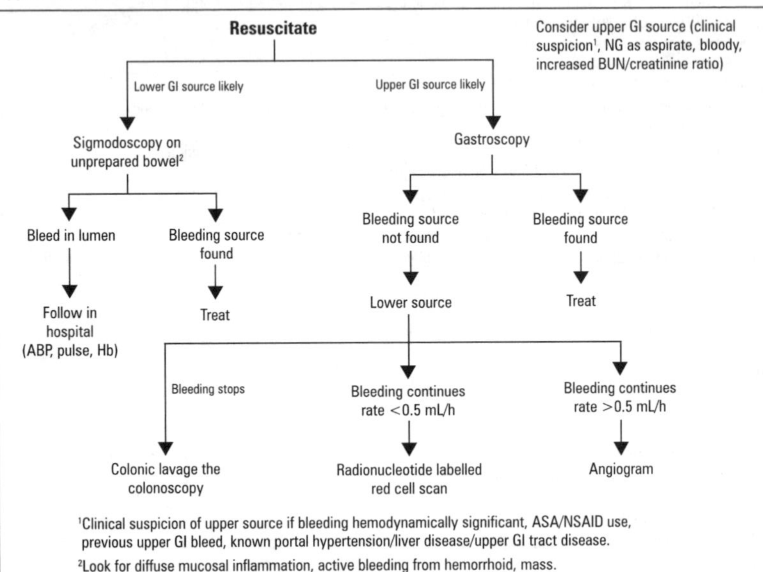

Investigations
- CBC, PT/INR, aPTT, electrolytes, BUN, CR, LFTs, NG tube, colonoscopy/sigmoidoscopy: ID site and coag/clip
- If can't ID bleeding site or if profuse bleeding: radionucleotide-labelled red cell scan, CT angiography – can localize and embolize

Management
- NPO
- Maintain hemodynamic stability: IV fluids, cross and type, blood transfusion
- If coagulopathy: vit K, FFP, stop warfarin

Common Conditions

Gastroesophageal Reflux Disease (GERD)

Definition
- Reflux of stomach and duodenal contents severe enough to produce symptoms and complications

Presentation
- Heartburn, bitter regurgitation, cough, halitosis

Etiology
- Inappropriate relaxation of lower esophageal sphincter (LES) is most common/important mechanism
- Less common/important are: low basal LES tone, increased intra-abdominal pressure (e.g. pregnancy), delayed esophageal clearance, delayed gastric emptying, acid hypersecretion (uncommon), sliding hiatus hernia

Management
- If no established esophagitis, (e.g. if the diagnosis is NERD), then over-the-counter antacids PRN are acceptable
- PPIs (e.g. omeprazole) most potent, H2 antagonists (e.g. ranitidine) less potent, prokinetic agents (e.g. metoclopramide) are not well established in the management of GERD
- Among the lifestyle modifications advocated in the past, only weight loss if overweight and elevating the head of bed as evidence-based
- If responds to PPI but cannot afford or tolerate life-long therapy, anti-reflux surgery (e.g. Nissen fundoplication) may be considered

Complications
- Reflux esophagitis: esophageal inflammation from prolonged acid regurgitation, may cause ulceration and bleeding
- Stricture, less often bleeding
- Barrett's esophagus (squamous to columnar metaplasia): increased risk of esophageal adenocarcinoma

Inflammatory Bowel Disease (IBD)

Important Features of Crohn's Disease and Ulcerative Colitis

	Crohn's Disease	Ulcerative Colitis
Location	Any part of GI tract ("gum to bum") • Small bowel + colon: 50% • Small bowel only: 30% • Colon only: 20%	Isolated to large bowel Always involves rectum, may progress proximally
Rectal Bleeding	Uncommon	Very common (90%)
Diarrhea	Less prevalent	Frequent small stools
Abdominal Pain	Post-prandial/colicky	Pre-defecatory urgency
Fever	Relatively common	Uncommon
Palpable Mass	Frequent (25%), RLQ	Rare (if present, cecum full of stool)
Recurrent After Surgery	Common	None post-colectomy
Endoscopic Features	Discrete aphthous ulcers, patchy lesions, pseudopolyps if chronic	Continuous diffuse inflammation, erythema, friability, loss of normal vascular pattern, pseudopolyps if chronic
Histologic Features	Transmural distribution with skip lesions Focal inflammation ± noncaseating granulomas, deep fissuring and aphthous ulcerations, strictures Glands intact	Mucosal distribution, continuous disease (no skip lesions) Granulomas absent Gland destruction, crypt abscess
Radiologic Features	Cobblestone mucosa Frequent strictures and fistulae XR: Bowel wall thickening, "string sign"	Features mucosa; lack of haustra Strictures rare, suggests complicating cancer
Complications	Strictures, fistulae, perianal disease, abscesses	Toxic megacolon
Colon Cancer Risk	Increased if more than 30% of colon involved	Increased

Management
- Traditional "step-up approach":
  - Recent studies suggest that if 5-ASA drugs/antibiotics are not helpful, proceeding next to immunomodulators may be preferable to a course of corticosteroids, especially if there are factors suggesting aggressive disease (young age, perianal disease, corticosteroids used in past)

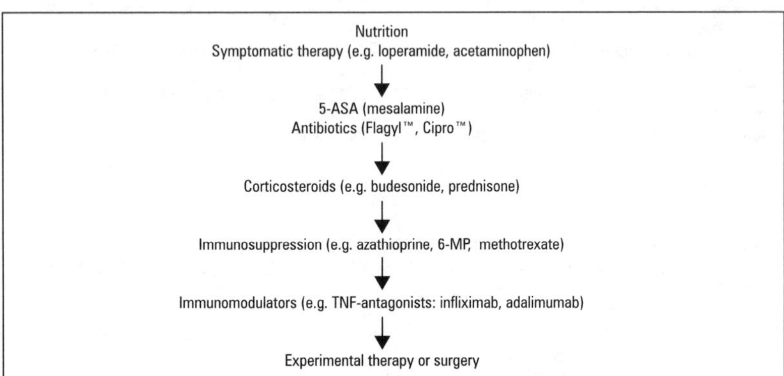

Irritable Bowel Syndrome (IBS)

IBS Rome III Criteria
- ≥12 wks in the past 12 months of abdominal discomfort or pain that has 2 out of 3 features:
  - Relieved with defecation
  - Associated with a change in frequency of stool
  - Associated with a change in consistency of stool
- The following are supportive, but not essential to the diagnosis:
  - Abnormal stool frequency (>3/d or <3/wk)
  - Abnormal stool form (lumpy/hard/loose/watery) >1/4 of defecations
  - Abnormal stool passage (straining, urgency, feeling of incomplete evacuation) >1/4 of defecations
  - Passage of mucus >1/4 of defecations
  - Abdominal gas, bloating

Diagnosis of IBS less likely in presence of "Alarm" Features
- Weight loss, fever, nocturnal defecation, anemia, blood or pus in stool, abnormal gross findings on flexible sigmoidoscopy

Acute Pancreatitis

Differential Diagnosis
- Biliary colic/acute cholecystitis/cholangitis, mesenteric infarction, nephrolithiasis,
- Before diagnosis, consider MI, perforated peptic ulcer, perforated/ischemic bowel, dissection, ruptured aneurysm, small bowel obstruction, ischemic colitis

Etiology
- Gallstones, alcohol, medications (protease inhibitiors, Septra, dexamethasone, valproic acid, etc.), trauma (e.g. post-ERCP), metabolic (hypertriglyceridemia, TG >11), hypercalcemia, renal failure, tumours (pancreas, ampula), SLE, infections (mumps, Coxsackie virus B, hepatitis A/B), vascular disease

History (S/Sx)
- **Common chief complaints**: epigastric pain, constant, radiating to the back, improving with leaning forward; nausea and vomiting, fever
- Pain history (OPQRSTUVW)
- N/V, alcohol consumption, jaundice, ileus
- B symptoms: fever, weight loss, chills, loss of appetite
- Previous hx of gallstones, recent medications use

Physical Exam
- Vitals (including postural changes and temp), cardiac exam (including JVP), abdo exam (look for guarding, distention, dec. bowel sounds), signs of retroperitoneal hemorrhage (Cullen's and Grey Turner's)

Investigations
- CBC, electrolytes, creatinine, urea, blood glucose, liver enzymes (ALT >3x ULN suggestive of gallstone pancreatitis), amylase (>3x ULN very suggestive of pancreatitis), lipase (more specific than amylase), Ca^{2+}, triglyceride level
- Abdominal CT (to diagnose, exclude other abdo processes, stage, and identify local complications)

Management
- ABCs, IV fluids (depending on the volume status of patient), NPO (consider NG tube for vomiting), analgesics to control pain, antibiotics (controversial except on documented infection)
- Analgesia, antiemetics, consider prophylactic antibiotics for severe necrotizing pancreatitis, stop NSAIDS and anticoagulation if possible
- Specific Rx not available; mainstay of therapy is supportive, treatment of complications

Complications
- Local: necrosis, infection (abscess), pancreatic pseudocyst (after wks)
- Systemic: multiorgan failure, non-cardiac pulmonary edema, renal failure

Prognosis
- Better prognosis if high proportion of pancreas taking up contrast dye on CT scan (areas of pancreas not taking up dye are necrotic)
- Ranson's Criteria, APACHE II score to determine severity of pancreatitis
- Ranson's Criteria for alcoholic pancreatitis (>2 for difficult course, >3 high mortality)
  - At admission: glucose >11 mM, age >55, LDH >350 IU/L, AST >250 IU/L, WBC >16x10^6/L
  - In first 48 h: Ca^{2+} <2 mM, hematocrit decreased >10%, arterial PO_2 <60 mmHg, base deficit >4 mM, BUN increase >1.8 mM, fluid sequestration >6 L

Approach to Liver Disease

Common Etiologies of Hepatitis
- Viral, alcohol, drugs, immune-mediated, toxins

VIRAL HEPATITIS

Time Course of Acute Hepatitis B (Resolving Spontaneously)

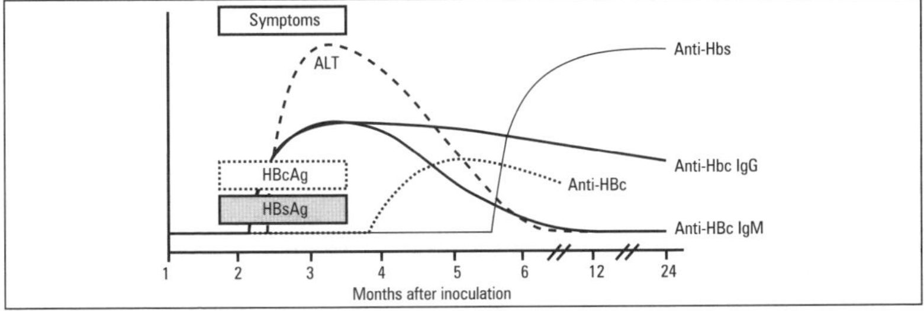

Viral Hepatitis

	Hepatitis A	Hepatitis B	Hepatitis C	Hepatitis D	Hepatitis E
Transmission	Fecal-oral Contaminated food, H_2O, shellfish	Percutaneous Sexual Perinatal	Percutaneous Sexual (rare)	Percutaneous Sexual Requires concomitant Hep B infxn	Fecal-oral Travel to tropical areas
Incubation	2-6 wks	2-6 months	1-3 months	–	5-60 d
Natural History	Always acute No chronicity	Acute: 70% asympt., 30% jaundice, fulminant hep. rare Chronic: divided into replicative vs. nonreplicative phases	Acute: 75% asympt., 25% jaundice Chronic: ~30% will develop cirrhosis; HCC (3%)HBsAg rapidly progressive liver disease in ~5%	Rare in Canada complicates Hep B (superinfection) Consider if: (1) HBSAg positive flares (2) HBsAg positive anti-HBe significant liver disease	Rare in Canada, acute illness mortality in pregnancy
Serology	Acute: anti-HAV IgM Past exposure: anti-HAV IgG	HBsAg + : (infxn; carrier) Anti-HBs – : (immunity) Anti-HBc – : (exposure) HBeAg + : (viral replic) Anti-HBe – : (seroconversion)	HCV RNA + in 2 wks implies active infection Anti-HCV does not imply recovery!	Anti-HDV	Anti-HEV IgM
Treatment	Supportive	Acute: supportive Chronic: IFN lamivudine adefovir tenofovir entecavir	PEG-IFN + ribavarin	? IFN ?	Supportive
Vaccine	Yes	Yes	No	Immunize against Hep B	No

Hepatocellular Carcinoma Risk
- Chronic hepatitis B increased in all cases. Chronic hepatitis C increased only if cirrhotic
- Liver Transplant can be considered for all cases if deterioration despite Rx

Investigations for Hepatitis
- HBsAg, anti-HBs (to check for immunity; anti-HBc least useful); anti-HCV, ANA, anti-Sm, protein electrophoresis (high gamma globulin in autoimmune hepatitis), ferritin, cerulopasmin
- If anti-HCV positive, measure serum HCV-RNA (and genotype); if HBsAg positive, measure serum HBV-DNA
- Serum glucose, lipids tend to be elevated in fatty liver
- AFP for hepatocellular carcinoma
- Abdominal ultrasound
- Liver biopsy in selected cases

Liver Cirrhosis

Definition
- Diffuse, irreversible fibrosis plus hepatocellular nodular regeneration

Etiology
- Alcohol (85%), viral (HBV, HBV+HDV, HCV; not HAV or HEV), autoimmune, genetic (e.g. Wilson's disease, hemochromatosis, glycogen storage diseases), Gaucher's disease, α-1-antitrypsin deficiency, drugs (e.g. methotrexate), primary or secondary biliary cirrhosis, chronic hepatic congestion (e.g. chronic right heart failure, constrictive pericarditis, hepatic vein thrombosis [Budd-Chiari]), idiopathic

Child-Pugh Classification of Liver Cirrhosis (for prognosis)

	1	2	3
Serum bilirubin (μmol/L)	<34	34-51	>51
Serum albumin (g/L)	>35	28-35	<28
Presence of ascites	Absent	Controllable	Refractory
Encephalopathy	Absent	Minimal	Severe
INR	<1.7	1.7-2.3	>2.3

Score: 5-6 (Child's A), 7-9 (Child's B), 10-15 (Child's C)

*Note: Child's classification is rarely used for shunting, but is still useful to quantitate the severity of cirrhosis

Complications and Management
- Minimize alcohol intake
- Identify and treat precipitating cause of the complications (e.g. sedatives, GI bleed, diuretics for hepatic encephalopathy, increased sodium intake, hepatoma)
- Portal hypertension:
  - With ascites: sodium restriction, diuretics, therapeutic paracentesis
  - With varices: endoscopic banding, β-blockers/nitrates decrease risk of bleeding
  - With encephalopathy: lactulose, minimize dietary protein, consider non-absorbable antibiotics (e.g. neomycin)
- Transjugular Intrahepatic Portosystemic Shunt (TIPS) – decreases portal venous pressure; can benefit varices and ascites, may worsen encephalopathy
- Hepatopulmonary syndrome: intrapulmonary vasodilation leading to hypoxia from V/Q mismatch
- Improves with supplemental oxygen, no medical therapy available
- Hepatorenal syndrome – due to peripheral vasoconstriction because the body perceives hypovolemia when fluid is sequestered in ascites

Clinical Features of Liver Disease

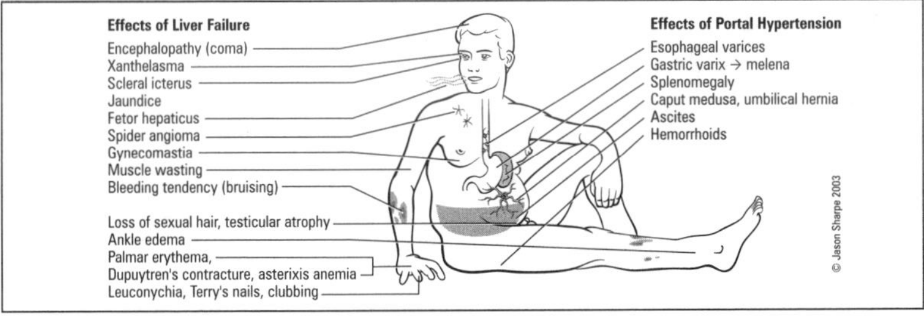

Common Medications

Class	Generic Drug Name	Trade Name	Dosing	Mechanism of Action	Indications	Contraindications	Side Effects
Proton Pump Inhibitors (H^+- K^+ ATPase inhibitors)	omeprazole	Losec®/Prilosec®	20 mg OD	Inhibits gastric enzymes H^+/ K^+ ATPase (proton pump)	Duodenal ulcer, gastric ulcer, NSAID-associated gastric and duodenal ulcers, reflux esophagitis symptomatic GERD, dyspepsia, Zollinger-Ellison Syndrome, eradication of *H. pylori* (combined with antibiotics)	Hypersensitivity to drug	Dizziness, headache, flatulence, abdo pain, nausea, rash, increased risk of osteoporotic fracture (secondary to impaired calcium absorption)
	lansoprazole	Prevacid®	Oral therapy: 15-30 mg OD (before breakfast) IV therapy: 30 mg OD	Same as above	Same as above	Same as above	Same as above
	pantoprazole	Pantoloc® Protonix®	40 mg OD for UGIB: 80 mg bolus then 8 mg/h infusion	Same as above	Same as above and UGIB	Same as above	Same as above
	rabeprazole	Pariet®/Aciphex®	40 mg OD	Same as above	Same as above	Same as above	Same as above
	esomeprazole	Nexium®	20-40 mg OD	Same as above	Same as above	Same as above	Same as above
Histamine H_2-receptor Antagonists	ranitidine	Zantac®	300 mg OD or 150 mg bid IV therapy: 50 mg q8h (buttachyphylaxis a problem)	Inhibits gastric histamine H_2-receptors	Duodenal ulcer, gastric ulcer, NSAID-associated gastric and duodenal ulcers, ulcer prophylaxis, reflux esophagitis, symptomatic GERD, Zollinger-Ellison syndrome	Hypersensitivity to drug	Confusion, dizziness, headache, arrhythmias, constipation, nausea, agranulocytosis, pancytopenia, depression
	famotidine	Pepcid®	Oral therapy: duodenal/gastric ulcers: 40 mg qhs GERD: 20 mg bid IV therapy: 20 mg bid	Same as above	Same as above	Same as above	Same as above

Class	Generic Drug Name	Canada Name	Dosing Schedule	Mechanism of Action	Indications	Contraindications	Side Effects
Antidiarrheal Agents	loperamide	Imodium®	Acute diarrhea: 4 mg initially, followed by 2 mg after each unformed stool	Acts as antidiarrheal via cholinergic, oncholinergic, opiate and nonopiate receptor-medicated mechanisms; decreases activity of myenteric plexus	Adjunctive therapy for acute non-specific diarrhea, chronic diarrhea associated with IBD, and for reducing the volume of discharge for ileostomies, colostomies and other intestinal resections	Children <2 yrs, known hypersensitivity to drug, acute dysentery characterized by blood in stools and fever, acute ulcerative colitis or pseudomembranous colitis associated with broad-spectrum antibiotics	Abdo pain or discomfort, drowsiness or dizziness, tiredness, dry mouth, nausea and vomiting, hypersensitivity reaction
	diphenoxylate/ atropine	Lomotil®	5 mg tid to qid	Inhibits GI propulsion via direct action on smooth muscle, resulting in a decrease in peristaltic action and in transit time	Adjunctive therapy for diarrhea, as above	Hypersensitivity to diphenoxylate oratropine, jaundice, pseudomembranous enterocolitis, diarrhea caused by enterotoxin producing bacteria	Dizziness, drowsiness, insomnia, headache, nausea, vomiting, cramps, allergic reaction
IBD Agents	mesalamine	Pentasa® Salofalk® Asacol® Mesasal®	CD: 1g tid/qid Active UC: 1g qid Maintenance UC: 1.6 g divided doses daily also as suppositories and enemas	5-ASA: Blocks arachidonic acid metabolism to prostaglandins and leukotrienes	IBD	Hypersensitivity to mesalamine salicylates	Abdo pain, constipation, arthralgia, headache
	sulfasalazine	Salazopyrin®	3-4 g/d in div doses	Compound composed of 5-ASA bound to sulfapyridine, hydrolysis by intestinal bacteria releases 5-ASA, the active component	Colonic disease	Hypersensitivity to sulfasalazine, sulfa drugs, salicylates; intestinal or urinary obstruction, porphyria	Rash, loss of appepitite, nausea, vomiting, headache, oligospermia (reversible)
	prednisone		20-40 mg OD for acute exacerbation	Anti-inflammatory	Mod-severe CD and UC		Complications of steroid therapy
Immuno-Suppressive Agents	6-mercaptopurine (6-MP)	Purinethol®	CD: 1.5 mg/kg/d	Immunosuppressive	IBD: active inflammation and to maintain remission	Hypersensitivity to mercaptopurine, prior resistance to mercaptopurine or thioguanine, history of treatment with alkylating agents, hypersensitivity to azathioprine, pregnancy	Pancreatitis, bone marrow suppression, increased risk of cancer
	azathioprine	Azasan® Imuran®	IBD: 2-3 mg/kg/d	Same as above	Same as above	Same as above	Same as above
Immuno-modulators	infliximab	Remicade®	5-10 mg/kg IV over 2 h	Antibody to tumour necrosis factor	Medically refractory CD	Heart failure, moderate to severe, doses greater than 5 mg/kg	Reported cases of reactivated TB, PCP, lymphoma, other infections

Class	Drug Name	Brand Name	Dosing Schedule	Indications	Contraindications	Side Effects	Mechanism of Action
Laxatives							
	bran	All-Bran®	1 cup/d	Constipation		Bloating, flatus	Bulk-forming laxative
	psyllium	Metamucil® Prodium Plain®	1 tsp PO tid	Constipation, hypercholesterolemia	N/V, fever, abdo pain, obstruction	Bloating, flatus	Bulk-forming laxative
	docusate	Colace® Docusoft®	100 mg PO bid	Constipation	Abdo pain, N/V, fever Not to be used with mineral oil	Mild cramps	Emollient, stool softener
	lactulose	Chronulac® Cephulac® Kristalose®	15-30 cc PO daily/bid	Constipation, hepatic encephalopathy, bowel evacuation following barium exam	Patients on low galactose diets Abdo pain, N/V, fever	Flatus, cramps, nausea, diarrhea	Hyperosmolar agent, lowers pH of colon to decrease blood ammonia levels
	senna	Senokot®/Ex-lax® Glysennid®	1-2 tabs PO daily or 10-15 cc syrup PO daily	Constipation	Abdo pain, N/V, fever	Cramps, griping, dependence	Stimulant laxative
	bisacodyl	Dulcolax®	5-15 mg PO (10 mg PR)	Constipation	Ileus, obstruction, abdo pain, N/V, fever, severe dehydration	Cramps, diarrhea	Stimulant laxative
Osmotic diuretics	mannitol (Osmitrol®) glycerol urea	Renal tubules (proximal and collecting duct)	Non-reabsorbable solutes increase osmotic pressure of glomerular filtrate – inhibits reabsorption of water and ↑ urinary excretion of toxic materials	To ↓ intracranial or intraoccular pressure Mobilization of excess fluid in renal failure or edematous states	mannitol: ↓ ICP: 0.25-2 g/kg IV over 30-60 min	Transient volume expansion Electrolyte abnormalities ($\downarrow/\uparrow$ Na$^+$, $\downarrow/\uparrow$ K$^+$)	

General Surgery

Essential History, Physical Exam and Investigations

History

Symptoms	Risk Factors and Other Key Questions
Pain – OPQRST	Appetite, energy, weight
Vomiting, hematemesis	Medications (esp. NSAIDs)
Changes in bowel habits – diarrhea, constipation, passing flatus, distention/bloating	Alcohol history, smoking history
Bleeding – melena, hematochezia	Travel history, recent illness, sick contacts
GU – frequency, urgency, hematuria, dysuria	Past medical history, previous GIB, hepatitis, malignancy
Gyne – LMP, sexual and contraceptive history	Investigations: FOBT, colonoscopy, endoscopy
Chest/Resp symptoms	Family history: colon, ovarian, breast cancer, IBD
	Food intolerance, relation of symptoms to meals, last meal
	Ancestry
	Last BM

Physical Exam

Vitals

Inspection
Abdomen (distension, scars, hernias)
Ascites
Skin, hands, nails
JVP, edema
Stigmata of liver disease

Percussion (percuss region of pain last)
Quadrants (normal: tympanic; pathology: dull)
Liver (normal: 9-11 cm)
Spleen (Castell's sign: percussion in 10th IC space, dullness on inspiration suggests enlargement)
Ascites (flank dullness, shifting dullness, fluid wave)

Auscultation (performed BEFORE palpation)
Bowel sounds (1 quadrant is sufficient)
Bruits (aortic, renal artery, liver)
Rubs (splenic, hepatic)

Palpation
Light: tenderness, involuntary/voluntary guarding
Deep: masses
Liver, spleen, kidney

Special Tests (acute abdomen)
Cough, shake tenderness (if present, no need to do rebound)
Rebound tenderness
McBurney's sign, Rovsing's sign, psoas, obturator tests (for appendicitis)
Cullen's sign (acute hemorrhagic pancreatitis, ectopic pregnancy)
Grey-Turner's sign (acute hemorrhagic pancreatitis, ruptured AAA, bowel strangulation)
Murphy's sign (cholecystitis)
Courvoisier's sign (pancreatic cancer)
Check for hernias
DRE
Pelvic exam in all females

Investigations

- Tailor to differential diagnosis

Bloodwork
- CBC
- Electrolytes with Ca^{2+}, Mg^{2+}, PO_4^{3-} (extended electrolytes)
- Creatinine, BUN
- Liver function tests: albumin, PT/INR, aPTT, bilirubin (direct and indirect)
- Liver enzymes: AST, ALT, ALP, GGT
- Amylase or lipase (lipase is more specific)
- β-HCG
- Hep A, B, C serology
- Troponins
- As per patient assessment: acetaminophen level, toxicology screen
- In diffuse abdominal pain: blood glucose and ketones (if diabetic r/o DKA); norepinephrine derivatives in urine r/o pheochromocytoma; lead levels r/o lead toxicity; endocrine profile r/o Addisonian crisis

Imaging/Visualization
- 3 views abdominal x-ray (lateral, supine, erect)/CXR to r/o free air
- Abdominal ultrasound with focus on liver/GB/pancreas (if upper abdomen) or appendix/cecum/ureters ± gyne organs (if lower abdomen)
- CT scan thorax/abdo/pelvis ± triple contrast
- Triphasic liver protocol abdo/pelvic
- ± OGD
- ± Flex sig/C-scope

Other
- Urinalysis
- ECG
- Diagnostic/therapeutic paracentesis if ascites
- If suspect ruptured AAA, do not investigate: stat OR

Common Presentations

Differential Diagnosis Abdominal Pain

RUQ Pain	Epigastric Pain	LUQ Pain
Hepatobiliary	**Cardiac**	**Pancreatic**
Biliary Colic	Aortic Dissection/Ruptured AAA	Pancreatitis (acute vs. chronic)
Cholecystitis	MI (ischemia)	Pancreatic Pseudocyst
Cholangitis	Pericarditis	Pancreatic Tumours (note Courvosier's
Choledocholithiasis (stone, tumour)		Sign = painless jaundice and palpable gall
Hepatitis (infection, toxic,	**Gastrointestinal**	bladder)
Budd-Chiari, etc.)	Gastritis	
Hepatic Abcess	Peptic Ulcer Disease	**Gastrointestinal**
Hepatic Mass	GERD/Esophagitis	see Epigastric causes
	Pancreatitis	Splenic flexure pathology (i.e. CRC,
Gastrointestinal	Appendicitis	ischemia)
Gastric/duodenal pathology	Mallory-Weiss Tear	Splenic Rupture
Pancreas (pancreatitis)		Splenic Infarct/Abscess
Appendicitis in pregnancy >20 wks	**Other**: Pneumonia	Splenic Aneurysm (ruptured)
Hepatic flexure pathology (CRC, subcostal		
incisional hernia)		**Cardiopulmonary**
		see RUQ and Epigastric causes
Genitourinary		MI (ischemia)
Nephrolithiasis/Renal Colic		
Pyelonephritis		**Genitourinary**
Renal: mass, trauma, ischemia		see RUQ causes
Cardiopulmonary		
RLL Pneumonia or Empyema		
CHF (causing hepatic congestion		
and R pleural effusion)		
MI (ischemia)		
Pericarditis		
Pleuritis		
Miscellaneous		
Herpes Zoster		
Trauma		
Costochondritis		

RLQ Pain	Suprapubic Pain	LLQ Pain
Gastrointestinal Appendicitis Appendiceal Phlegmon (post perforated appendicitis) Perforated duodenal ulcer Crohns Disease Tuberculosis of the ileocecal junction Inflamed/Hemorrhagic cecal tumour Intussuception Mesenteric Lymphadenitis Cecal Diverticulitis Cecal Volvulus Hernia: Amyand's, Femoral, Inguinal Obstruction (and resulting cecal distension) Pancreatitis **Gynecological** see Suprapubic **Genitourinary** see Suprapubic **Extraperitoneal** Abdominal wall hematoma/abscess Psoas Abscess	**Gastrointestinal** Any etiology of the lower quadrants Acute appendicitis IBD **Gynecological** Ectopic Pregnancy Mittelschmirtz (Ruptured Graffian Follicle) PID Ovarian Torsion Hemorrhagic Fibroid Endometriosis Threatened/Incomplete Abortion Tubo-Ovarian Abcess Hydrosalpinx/Salpingitis Gynecological Tumours **Genitourinary** Cystitis (infectious, hemorrhagic) Hydroureter/Urinary Colic Epididymitis Testicular Torsion Acute Urinary Retention **Vascular** IVC thrombus	**Gastrointestinal** Diverticulitis Diverticulosis Colon/Sigmoid/Rectal Ca Fecal Impaction Proctitis (Ulcerative Colitis, infectious; i.e gonococcus or chlamydia) Sigmoid Volvulus **See gynecological, urological, vascular, and extraperitoneal as per RLQ and suprapubic**

Diffuse Abdominal Pain	
Peritonitis Hemo/pneumo/fecoperitoneum Perforated viscus (duodenal ulcer, sigmoid diverticulitis, Meckels, appendicitis, anastamotic leak, trauma) Spontaneous bacterial peritonitis Post laparoscopic insufflation **Pancreatitis** Often better on leaning forward and more of a 'retroperitoneal pain' **Gastrointestinal** Mesenteric Ischemia ('pain out of proportion to physical findings') Inflammatory Bowel Disease (Crohns, Ulcerative Colitis, IBD NOS) Irritable Bowel Syndrome Gastroenteritis Medications (e.g. stimulant laxatives, chemotherapy) Pan-colitis (pseudomembranous, ischemic, infectious) Visceral Hypersensitivity Syndrome Constipation Bowel obstruction Early appendicitis, perforated appendicitis Ogilvie's syndrome	**Cardiovascular/Hematological** Aortic Dissection/ Ruptured AAA Sickle Cell Crisis Porphyria **Genitourinary/Gynecological** Perforated Ectopic Pregnancy PID Acute Urinary Retention **Endocrine** Carcinoid Syndrome Diabetic Keto-Acidosis Addisonian Crisis Uremia Hypercalcemia **Psychological** Munchausen Syndrome Depression **Other** Lead poisoning Tertiary syphillis

Principles of Management of Surgical Patient

ABC (airway, breathing, circulation)
If GCS <8 or unstable patient
Monitor and stabilize vitals
IV N/S @ 100 cc/h (or as per 4-2-1 rule for maintenance)
(2L RL wide open over 1h if unstable)
Titrate O_2 sat by NP >92% (or if COPD 88-92%)

Provisionals
NG tube to lo gomco suction if persistent vomiting
NPO until assessed and cleared by G/S for possible OR
Foley catheter to straight drainage (monitor urine output)
Two large bore anticubital IVs if require aggressive fluid resuscitation
Antibiotics as appropriate (cholecystitis, cholangitis, abscess)
VTE Prophylaxis in all surgery patients: Fragmin 5000 U SQ BID

Condition Specific (see *Common Conditions*)

Surgical Site Infection Prevention in elective patients
1. Warn patients pre-op and intra-op
2. Ancef®/Flagyl® 1hr pre-op
3. No hair removal
4. Chlorhexdine to prep

GI Bleeding

- See Gastroenterology

Post-Op Complications

Post-Operative Fever

POD 0-2	Atelectasis Aspiration Pneumonia Early wound infection (Clostridium, GAS)
POD 3 (Infection becomes more likely)	Wound infection (POD 3-6) UTI Line site (e.g. IV) infection – IV's should be changed q72h
POD 5+	Intra-abdo abscess (POD 5-10) DVT/PE (can occur ANY time post-op, but most commonly POD 7-10) Drug fever (POD 6-10) Leakage of bowel anastomosis (tachycardia, hypotension, oliguria, abdominal pain) **Management**: treat underlying cause, antipyrexia (e.g. acetaminophen)

Wound Complications

Wound Infection	Early, POD 0-2: Clostridum, GAS Typically POD 3-6: *S. aureus, E. coli, Enterococcus, Streptococcus* spp, *Clostridium* spp Clinical features: pain, erythema, induration, frank pus or purosanguinous discharge, warmth Treatment: re-open incision, culture wound, pack, heal by secondary intention, Abx if cellulitis or immunodeficiency
Wound Dehiscense	Definition: failure/disruption of fascial layer Treatment: surgical closure, evisceration is surgical emergency

Urinary and Renal Complications

Urinary Retention	Occurs with GA or spinal anesthesia. Beware in pt with BPH Treatment: Foley or I/O catheterization PRN
Oliguria/Anuria	Definition: <0.5 cc/kg/h (in general: <30 cc/h) Pre-renal vs. renal vs. post-renal. Pre-renal ± ischemic ATN is most common Treatment: according to underlying cause

Common Conditions

Appendicitis

Definition
- Appendix distension and ischemia following luminal obstruction

Etiology
- Children or young adult: hyperplasia of lymphoid follicles, initiated by infection
- Adult: fibrosis/stricture, fecolith, obstructing neoplasm, idiopathic
- Other causes: parasites, foreign body
- Classically: luminal obstruction allows bacterial overgrowth. Subsequent inflammation/swelling/distention increases pressure
- Localized ischemia predisposes to perforation and localized abscess or peritonitis

Clinical Features
- Most reliable feature is progression of signs and symptoms; classic pattern: pain initially periumbilical, constant, dull, poorly localized (visceral) → well localized pain over McBurney's point (peritoneal)
- Low grade fever (38°C), rises if perforation
- Abdominal pain THEN anorexia, nausea, vomiting

Signs

Location of Appendix	Description
Inferior appendix	McBurney's sign (tenderness 1/3 from ASIS to umbilicus) Rovsing's sign (palpation pressure to left abdomen causes McBurney's point tenderness)
Retrocecal appendix	Psoas sign (pain on flexion of hip against resistance or passive hyperextension of hip)
Pelvic appendix	Obturator sign (flexion then external or internal rotation about right hip causes pain)

Management
- ABCs, lines – IV NS bolus for resusc, then maintenance+losses
- Investigations: CBC, electrolytes, Cr, G&S, INR, PTT, β-HCG, urinalysis
- Imaging: Abdo/pelvic US to help r/o gyne pathology, CT optimal, CXR pre-op where indicated
- Admit acute appendicitis for emergent surgery
- Admit subacute (>5 d) for antibiotics ± percutaneous drainage of abscess. NPO, AAT, VSR, cefazolin+metronidazole for 24 h if not perforated
- If perforated, 2nd or 3rd generation cephalosporin + fluoroquinolone + metronidazole
- Opioid analgesia perioperatively (morphine 2-10 mg IV/SC q2h PRN)
- Post-op: admit to floor, Sips-DAT, AAT, VSR, SLIV WDW, Fragmin 5000 U SC OD
- D/C home following uncomplicated lap-appy POD1 with T3s and Colace. F/U with FP MD within two wks
- F/U with general surgeon in 4-6 wks

Complications
- Perforation (especially if >24 h duration), abscess, phlegmon

Perforated Bowel

Definition
- Rupture wall of intestines

Etiology
- Traumatic (e.g. colonoscopy), post-op anastomosis failure, or secondary to other intra-abdominal pathology: PUD, BO with ischemic segments, cecal volvulus, perforated appendicitis or diverticulitis

Management
- ABCs, lines – two large bore IVs, aggressive crystalloid resuscitation
- Investigations: CBC, electrolytes, Cr, INR, PTT, lactate, cross+match for 4U RBC
- Imaging: CXR/CT
- Emergency – emergent OR to resect diseased bowel ± primary anastomosis
- Admit to General Surgery step down unit NPO, AAT, VSR
- Broad spectrum antibiotics (i.e. cefazolin 1 g q8h + metronidazole 500 mg IV q8h), opioid analgesia perioperatively (morphine 2-10 mg IV/SC q2h prn)
- Fragmin 5000 IU SC OD
- Foley with I/Os, IV NS @ maintenance usually 75-125 cc/h
- D/C home when stable and tolerating PO, pain well managed
- F/U within two wks with FP
- F/U with general surgeon within 6 wks

Bowel Obstruction

History
- Abdominal pain, abdominal distension, nausea, vomiting, constipation/obstipation

Physical Exam
- Signs of dehydration: tachycardia, hypotension, decreased urine output, decreased skin turgor, sunken eyes
- Auscultation: rushing/tinkling/high pitched bowel sounds initially, absent BS if advanced
- Tympanic percussion
- Palpation: tenderness/guarding, abdominal distension, ± peritoneal signs
- Rectal exam: mass, hematochezia, fecal impaction

Investigations
- CBC, Electrolytes, BUN, Cr., Amylase, LDH
- Upright CXR, AXR
- ± contrast – contrast contraindicated if suspect perforation/peritonitis, CT abdomen

CLASSIFICATION

Mechanical vs. Functional
- Mechanical
  - Small bowel (adhesions > hernias > cancer)
    - Extramural (adhesions, hernia, volvulus, neoplasm), intramural (Crohn's, radiation stricture, adeno CA), intraluminal (intussusception, gallstones)
  - Large bowel (cancer > diverticulitis > volvulus)
    - Extramural (volvulus), intraluminal (colon CA, diverticulitis, IBD or radiation stricture)
- Functional
  - Ileus, neurogenic

Partial vs. Complete
- Partial: may allow gas, fluid, stool to pass
- Complete: no passage of any substances

Closed vs. Open Loop in LBO
- Closed Loop: loop of bowel obstructed at both ends (afferent and efferent limbs) – no flow of contents in either direction (usually requires OR)
- Open Loop: incompetent ileocecal valve – allows reflux into ileum

Bowel Obstruction vs. Paralytic Ileus

	SBO	LBO	Paralytic ileus
Nausea, Vomiting	Early, may be bilious	Late, may be feculent	Present
Abdominal Pain	Colicky	Colicky	Minimal or absent
Abdominal Distention	+ (prox) < + + (distal)	+ +	+
Constipation/Obstipation	+	+	+
Other	± visible peristalsis	± visible peristalsis	
Bowel Sounds	Normal, increased Absent if secondary ileus	Normal, increased (borborygmi) absent if secondary ileus	Decreased, absent
AXR Findings	Air-fluid levels "Ladder" pattern (plicae circularis) Proximal distention (>3 cm) + no colonic gas	Air-fluid levels "Picture frame" appearance Proximal distention + distal decompression No small bowel air if competent ileocecal valve	Air throughout small bowel and colon

Management
- Manage ABC's
- Keep patient NPO!
- Lines – IV NS, NG Tube (only if decompression is needed), Foley to monitor u/o
- Monitor and maintain hemodynamic stability, Cross and Type
- Investigations – CBC + diff, electrolytes, BUN, Cr, PTT, INR, G&S, lactate, LDH, β-HCG, urinalysis
- Imaging – CXR (free air), AXR (3 views), CT (for level of obstruction, cause)
- IV Antibiotics: to cover anaerobes and GN (only if suspected perforation)
- Dimenhydrinate 25-50 IM/IV q4-6h
- Morphine 2.5-5 mg IM/IV q4-6h prn
- Surgical correction of complete obstruction, may observe for 24-48h if secondary to adhesion if no fever or white count
- Sigmoid volvulus: sigmoidoscopy decompression (if not ischemic) + sigmoid resection (rarely)
- D/C home when tolerating PO intake and passing flatus or stool
- F/U with FP in 2 wks
- F/U with general surgeon in 4-6 wks (if OR during admission)

Cholecystitis

History
- Fever, RUQ pain >24 h, abdominal tenderness, nausea, vomiting, anorexia, r. infrascapular pain (referred)

Cholangitis: Charcot's Triad (Fever, RUQ pain, jaundice) and/or Reynold's Pentad (Charcot's Triad + shock, confusion) requires urgent CBD decompression via ERCP, PTC or surgery

Physical Exam
- +ve Murphy's sign, palpable mass, jaundice, tenderness, focal peritoneal signs, fever, tachycardia

Investigations
- CBC (leukocytosis), PT/INR, aPTT, LFTs, liver enzymes, ALP, bili, electrolytes, BUN, Cr, amylase, β-HCG, urinalysis
- Abdominal U/S: GB wall thickening (>3 mm), distended GB, pericholecystic fluid, + U/S Murphy's

Classification
- Acute, chronic, calculous, acalculous

Management
- ABCs: fluid resuscitation, oxygen, monitored setting (BP, O_2 sat)
- Analgesia
- Antibiotics (amp and gent/cipro and metronidazole)
- Early laparoscopic cholecystectomy (w/in 3 d of onset) vs. medical management

Intestinal Ischemia

Etiology
- Acute: occlusive (thrombotic, embolic, compression), non-occlusive (mesenteric vasoconstriction secondary to systemic hypoperfusion), trauma/dissection
- Chronic: atherosclerotic disease (CVD risk factors)

Clinical Features
- Acute: severe pain, vomiting, bloody diarrhea, bloating, minimal peritoneal signs early on (therefore difficult Dx)
- Chronic: postprandial pain (fear of food), weight loss

> **Pain** "out of keeping with physical findings" is the hallmark of early intestinal ischemia if thromboembolic event to SMA (RARE)
>
> Acute abdomen + metabolic acidosis is bowel ischemia until proven otherwise

Investigations
- Leukocytosis, lactic acidosis (late), hypercoag. work-up (if suspecting venous thrombosis)
- Observe progress: amylase, LDH, CK, ALP
- AXR: portal venous gas, intestinal pneumatosis, free air if perforation
- Contrast CT: thickened bowel wall, luminal dilation, SMA or SMV thrombus, mesenteric/portal venous gas, pneumatosis
- CT angiography: gold standard

Treatment
- Fluid resusc., NPO, ABx prophylaxis, exploratory laparotomy, angiogram, embolectomy/thrombectomy, bypass/graft, mesenteric endarterectomy, anticoagulation, segmental resection of necrotic intestine

Diverticular Disease

- Diverticulum – abnormal sac or pouch protruding from the wall of a hollow organ
- Right sided (true) diverticuli – contain all layers (congenital)
- Left sided (false) diverticuli – contains only mucosal and submucosal layers (acquired)
- Diverticulosis – presence of multiple false diverticuli, increased incidence in 5th-8th decade
- Diverticulitis – inflammation of diverticuli

DIVERTICULOSIS

Risk Factors
- Low fibre diet, genetics

Clinical Presentation
- Uncomplicated: asymptomatic
- Episodic LLQ abdominal pain (poorly localized), bloating, flatulence, constipation, diarrhea
- NO fever/leukocytosis
- Complications: diverticulitis (15-20%), PAINLESS rectal bleeding (2/3 of lower GIB)

Treatment
- Asymptomatic: high fibre, education
- Diverticular bleed: as per lower GI bleed, resect involved area if hemorrhage does not stop

DIVERTICULITIS

Clinical Features
- LLQ pain/tenderness, present for several days before admission, alternating constipation and diarrhea, urinary sx, palpable mass (if phlegmon), N/V, low-grade fever, mild leukocytosis
- Occult or gross blood in stool LESS common, generally no blood
- Generalized tenderness suggests macroperforation and peritonitis
- Complications: abscess (palpable O/E), fistula, obstruction, macroperforation, peritonitis
  - Note: recurrent attacks RARELY lead to peritonitis

Investigations
- AXR, upright CXR, CT scan (optimal), Hypaque enema
- Barium enema (NOT during acute attack – risk of chemical peritonitis)
- Sigmoidoscopy/colonoscopy (NOT during acute attack, use to r/o other lesions)

Treatment
- Admit, NPO, fluid resusc, IV cipro or metranidazole (B. fragilis)
- Indications for surgery: unstable, complications (generalized peritonitis, free air, abscess, fistula, obstruction, inability to r/o colon cancer on endoscopy, or failure of medical management
- Consider surgery after 1 attack if: a) immunosuppressed, b) abscess needing percutaneous drainage, consider after 2+ attacks for others

Hernias

INGUINAL HERNIA

History
- Mass of variable size, tenderness worse at end of day, relieved with supine position or reduction, abdominal fullness, vomiting, constipation

Physical Exam
- Inguinal mass increases with coughing/straining

Investigations
- U/S ± CT

Classification

	Direct Inguinal	Indirect Inguinal	Femoral
Epidemiology	1% of all men	Males > females	Affects mostly elderly females
Etiology	Acquired weakness of transversalis fascia "Wear and tear" Increased intra-abdominal pressure	Congenital persistence of processus vaginalis in 20% of adults	Pregnancy – weakness of pelvic floor musculature Increased intra-abdominal pressure
Anatomy	Through Hesselbach's triangle **Medial** to inferior epigastric Usually does not descend into scrotal sac	Originates in deep inguinal ring **Lateral** to inferior epigastric artery Often descends into scrotal sac (or labia majora)	Into femoral canal, below inguinal ligament but may override it Medial to femoral vein within femoral canal
Treatment	Surgical repair	Surgical repair	Surgical repair
Prognosis	3-4% risk of recurrence	<1% risk of recurrence	

HIATUS HERNIA

History
• Heartburn – 1-3 h post-prandial, chest pain, regurgitation, relief w/ sitting, standing, water, antacids, dysphagia

Physical Exam
• No specific findings, respiratory + precordial exam to help rule out other causes

Investigations
• CXR, barium swallow, 24h esophageal pH monitoring, esophageal manometry, gastroscopy with biopsy

Classification
• Type I – sliding
• Type II – paraesophageal
• Type III – mixed
• Type IV – herniation of other abdominal organs into thorax

Management
• Lifestyle modification, medical (antacids, H2 antagonists, PPI's), surgical (antireflux procedures – usually laparoscopic)
• Risk of GERD and esophageal adenocarcinoma

Colorectal Cancer (CRC)

Clinical Presentation of CRC

	Right Colon	Left Colon	Rectum
Frequency	25%	35%	30%
Pathology	Exophytic lesions with occult bleeding	Annular, invasive lesions	Ulcerating
Symptoms	Weight loss, weakness, rarely obstruction	Constipation ± overflow (alternating bowel patterns), abdominal pain, decreased stool caliber, rectal bleeding	Obstruction, tenesmus, rectal bleeding
Signs	Fe-deficiency anemia, RLQ mass (10%)	BRBPR, LBO	Palpable mass on rectal exam (DRE), BRBPR

TNM Classification System for Staging of Colorectal Carcinoma

Primary Tumour (T)		Regional Lymph Nodes (N)		Distant Metastasis (M)	
T0	No primary tumour found	N0	No regional node involvement	M0	No distant metastasis
Tis	Carcinoma in situ	N1	Metastasis in 1-3 pericolic nodes	M1	Distant metastasis
T1	Invasion into submucosa	N2	Metastasis in 4 or more pericolic nodes		
T2	Invasion into muscularis propria	N3	Metastasis in any nodes along the course of named vascular trunks		
T3	Invasion through muscularis and serosa				
T4	Invasion into adjacent structures/organs/ serosa				

Breast Cancer

History	Physical Exam	Investigations
Spectrum of presentation: incidental finding on routine mammography to shortness of breath with diffuse lung mets **Constitutional symptoms**: fevers, night sweats, weight loss Breast 'lump' detected by patient or family MD Hx of nipple discharge or breast changes (i.e. Paget's disease, Peau D'Orange, asymmetry) **Risk Factors**: female gender, age, prior history of breast CA, prior breast biopsy, 1st degree relative with breast Ca (especially if relative was premenopausal), nulliparity, first pregnancy >30 yrs, menarche <12 yrs., menopause >55 yrs, HRT >5 yrs, radiation exposure, FHx of CRC, BRCA status **Decreased risk** with lactation, early menopause, early childbirth	**HEENT**: Lymphadenopathy suggestive of mets **Resp**: Absent air entry at bases suggestive of pleural effusions (met) **Breast Exam**: **Inspection**: Inspect breasts with patient supine, sitting, and leaning forward characterize lesion Examine for asymmetry, skin puckering, color changes, nipple discharge **Palpation**: Palpate both breasts checking for masses Superior border: clavicle; medial border: sternum; inferior border: costal margin; lateral border: mid axillary line. Palpate for lymphadenopathy in axilla and along sternum **General Resp**, CVS, Abdo exam. Neuro exam if suspect metastatic disease	**General Investigations**: CBC, electrolytes with bone minerals, BUN, Cr, INR **Investigation of Palpable Lesions**: Mammography to the breasts If mass suspected to be malignant: FNA or core biopsy If malignant pathology: MRI head, CXR, bone scan **Investigation of Non Palpable Lesions**: Detected by routine mammography. If lesion is suspicious for malignancy investigations as per palpable lesion Mets: Bone, brain, lung are most common sites **Tumour Markers and Specific Investigations**: Estrogen receptors, Progesterone receptor, HER2/NEU

TNM Classification System for Staging Breast Cancer

Primary Tumour (T)	Regional Lymph Nodes (N)	Distant Metastasis (M)
TX Primary cannot be assessed	NX Regional N cannot be assessed	MX Distant mets cannot be assessed
T0 No primary tumour found	N0 No regional node involvement	M0 No distant metastasis
Tis Carcinoma in situ	N1 Mets to movable ipsilateral axillary N	M1 Distant metastasis (includes ipsilateral supraclavicular nodes)
T1 Tumour <2 cm	N2 Mets to ipsilateral axillary N fixed to one another or other structures	
T2 Tumour >2 cm but <5 cm	N3 Mets to ipsilateral internal mammary N	
T3 Tumour >5 cm		
T4 Tumour any size with direct extension to chest wall or skin; includes inflammatory Ca		

Management

Breast Cancer Treatment by Stage

Stage	Primary Treatment Options	Adjuvant Systemic Therapy
0 (in situ)	Breast-conserving surgery (BCS) + radiotherapy BCS alone if margins >1 cm and low nuclear grade Mastectomy* ± sentinel lymph node biopsy (SLNB)	None
I	BCS + SLNB + radiotherapy Mastectomy* + SLNB	May not be needed; discuss risks/benefits of chemotherapy and tamoxifen
II	BCS + SLNB + radiotherapy Mastectomy* + axillary node dissection/SLNB	Chemotherapy for premenopausal women or postmenopausal and estrogen receptor (ER) negative, follow by tamoxifen if ER positive
III	Likely mastectomy + axillary node dissection (if SLNB positive) + radiotherapy	Neoadjuvant therapy may be considered i.e. preoperative chemotherapy and/or hormone therapy. Adjuvant radiation
Inflammatory	Likely mastectomy + axillary node dissection + radiotherapy	Neoadjuvant therapy
IV	Surgery as appropriate for local control	Primary treatment is systemic therapy i.e. chemotherapy and/or hormone therapy

* If no reason to select mastectomy, the choice between BCS + radiotherapy and mastectomy can be made according to patient's preference since choice of local treatment does not significantly affect survival if local control is achieved

- "Probably Benign" lesions (well defined solitary masses <5 cm) and patient low risk for breast cancer: counselling and F/U mammogram in 6 mos
- Surgical (see Table): Breast conserving surgery (BCS)
  - Lumpectomy with wide local excision, SLNB
  - Must be combined with radiation for survival equivalent to mastectomy
  - For patients with advanced breast cancer (T >5 cm) or inflammatory breast disease, patients get neoadjuvant chemotherapy followed by surgery

Pre-Op/Post-Op Orders

Admit to Ward X under Dr. Y
Diagnosis
Diet: NPO, sips to DAT when passing gas
Activities: AAT (activity as tolerated)
Vitals: VSR (vital signs routine)
IV: NS @ 100cc/h + 20Meq/L KCl
Investigations: CBC, electrolytes, creatinine, BUN
Drains: Foley to urometer, JP to straight drainage, NG to low gomco
Drugs (6As): Analgesia (with concurrent laxatives), Antiembolics (DVT prophylaxis), Antiemetics, Anxiolytics, Antibiotics, Antecedents (pt's own medication)

Geriatric Medicine

Essential History

- **Geriatric Giants**: Memory, Falls, Incontinence, Polypharmacy
- **5 I's of Geriatrics**: Immobility, Intellect, Incontinence, Iatrogenesis, Impaired homeostasis

Functional Assessment: ADLs and IADLs

ADLs: ABCDE-TT	IADLs: SHAFT-TT
Ambulating	**S**hopping
Bathing	**H**ousework
Continence	**A**ccounting/Managing finances
Dressing	**F**ood preparation
Eating	**T**ransportation
Transferring	**T**elephone
Toileting	**T**aking medications

Sensory Issues
- Vision
  - Do you wear corrective lenses?
  - How would you describe the quality of your vision?
- Hearing
  - Can you hear me clearly?
  - Have you experienced any difficulty with your hearing?
- Balance
  - Have you ever fallen or lost your balance?
  - Did this cause any injuries?

Social Data
- Living arrangements, marital status, family/social support structures
- Caregiver status, caregiver burnout, elder abuse screening
- Financial status, drug benefit plan
- Substance use, occupational history, cultural background, interests
- Advance directives: power of attorney, living will, etc.

Mood and Anxiety (see Psychiatry)
- Depression
  - How is your mood?
  - Have you been feeling sad, down or depressed? For how long?
  - Have you lost interest in or get less pleasure from things you used to enjoy?
- Anxiety
  - Are you frequently worried or anxious about a number of things in your daily life?
  - Do you find it difficult to control your worrying?

Geriatric Giants

Memory

Mini-Mental Status Exam (MMSE)

Domain	Score	Task
Orientation	/5	Time: Year, Season, Month, Day, Date
	/5	Place: Country, Province, City, Building, Floor
Registration	/3	Immediate Recall: 3 unrelated items
Attention and Concentration	/5	Spell 'WORLD' backwards or do Serial 7s
Recall	/3	Delayed recall of previous 3 items
Language	/2	Naming: Pen, Watch
	/1	Repetition: 'No ifs, ands, or buts'
	/3	3-Step Command: "take this paper in your left hand, fold it in half and place it on the floor with your right hand"
	/1	Read and obey: 'CLOSE YOUR EYES'
	/1	Writing: Write a full sentence
Drawing	/1	Copy: Intersecting Pentagons (10 angles, 2 bisecting)
TOTAL	/30	Cognitive impairment if <24/30

+ Clock drawing (test executive functioning): ask patient to draw clock face with hands pointing to "10 past 11"
Note: MMSE score affected by education level, language, etc.

Delirium, Dementia and Depression

	Delirium	Dementia	Depression
Onset	Acute (hours-days)	Gradual/step-wise decline	Subacute
Duration	Days-weeks	Months-years	Variable
Natural History	Fluctuating, reversible, high morbidity/mortality in very old	Progressive, usually irreversible	Recurrent, usually reversible
Level of Consciousness	Fluctuating (over 24 h)	Normal	Normal
Attention	Decreased (wandering, easy distraction)	Not initially affected	Difficulty concentrating
Orientation	Impaired (usually to time and place), fluctuates	Intact initially	Intact
Behaviour	Severe agitation/retardation	Disinhibition, impairment in ADL/IADL, personality change, loss of social graces	Importuning, self-harm/suicide
Psychomotor	Fluctuates between extremes	Normal	Slowing
Sleep Wake Cycle	Reversed sleep/wake cycle	Fragmented sleep at night	Early morning awakening
Mood and Affect	Anxious, irritable, fluctuating	Labile, but not usually anxious	Depressed, stable
Cognition	Fluctuating, preceded by mood changes	Decreased executive functioning, paucity of thought	Not affected
Memory Loss	Marked recent	Recent, eventually remote	Recent

Delirium, Dementia and Depression (continued)

	Delirium	Dementia	Depression
Language	Dysnomia, dysgraphia, speech rambling, irrelevant, incoherent, subject changes	Agnosia, aphasia, decreased comprehension, repetition, speech (echolalia, palilalia)	Not affected
Delusions	Nightmarish and poorly formed	Compensatory	Nihilistic, somatic
Hallucinations	Visual common	Variable	Less common, auditory predominates
Quality of Hallucinations	Frightening/bizarre	Vacuous/bland	Self-deprecatory (if any)
Medical Status	Acute illness, drug toxicity	Variable	Rule out systemic illness, meds
Non-pharmacological Management	Environment quiet and well-lit, optimize hearing and vision, room near nursing station for close observation, orientation cues, family member presence for reassurance and re-orientation, physical restraints if necessary	Orientation cues (clock, calendar), education and support for patient and family, consider LTC facility	Individual therapy (psychodynamic, interpersonal, CBT), family therapy, group therapy, vocational/rehabilitation/ social skills training, etc.
Pharmacological Management	Stop all non-essential medications, haloperidol, low dose risperidone	Anti-cholinesterase inhibitors low dose neuroleptics, anti depressants, NMDA agonists (memantine) reassess pharmacological therapy every 3 months	Antidepressants, lithium, antipsychotics, anxiolytics, ECT, light therapy

DEMENTIA

Dementia DDx: VITAMIN D VEST

- **V**itamin deficiency (B_{12}, thiamine), **I**ntracranial tumour, **T**rauma (head injury), **A**noxia, **M**etabolic (diabetes), **I**nfection (postencephalitis, HIV), **N**ormal pressure hydrocephalus, **D**egenerative (Alzheimer's, Huntington's, CJD), **V**ascular (multi-infarct dementia), **E**ndocrine (hypothyroid), **S**pace-occupying lesion (chronic subdural hematoma), **T**oxic (alcohol)

Common Causes of Dementia

	Etiology	Key Clinical Features	Investigations
Primary Degenerative	Alzheimer's disease	Memory impairment Aphasia, apraxia, agnosia	CT or MRI, SPECT
	Lewy body disease	Hallucinations Parkinsonism Fluctuating cognition	CT or MRI, SPECT
	Frontotemporal dementia (e.g. Pick's disease)	Disinhibition, perseveration Decreased social awareness Progressive non-fluent aphasia Memory relatively spared	MRI, SPECT
	Huntington's disease	Chorea	Molecular testing
Vascular	Multi-infarct dementia	Abrupt onset Stepwise deterioration Dysexecutive syndrome	MRI, SPECT
	CNS vasculitis	Systemic S&S of vasculitis	ANA; ANCA; RF MRI Angiography

Delirium – see <u>Neurology</u>

Etiology of Delirium – I WATCH DEATH
- **I**nfectious, **W**ithdrawal from drugs, **A**cute metabolic disorder, **T**rauma, **C**NS pathology, **H**ypoxia, **D**eficiencies in vitamins, **E**ndocrinopathies, **A**cute vascular insults, **T**oxins, **H**eavy metals

Depression – see <u>Psychiatry</u>

Falls

History
- **Risk Factors**: previous falls (especially within the last year), sensory impairment (hearing/vision), gait/balance impairment, cognitive impairment; impairment in IADLS; polypharmacy, orthostatic hypotension
- **Pre-fall**: prodrome – lightheadedness, palpitations, diaphoresis, flushing, chest pain, shortness of breath, nausea, weakness, objects
- **Fall**: loss of consciousness, head injury, tongue biting, incontinence
- **Post-fall**: confusion, injury, bleeding

Investigations
- CBC, electrolytes, BUN, creatinine, glucose, Ca^{2+}, TSH, B_{12}, urinalysis, cardiac enzymes, ECG, CT head

Approach to Falls in the Elderly

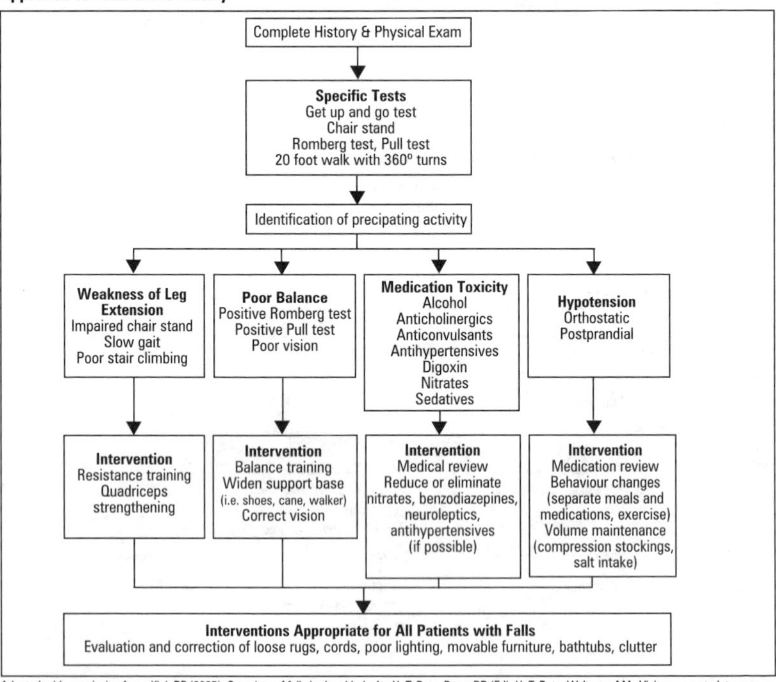

Adapted with permission from: Kiel, DP (2005). Overview of falls in the elderly. In: *UpToDate*, Rose, BD (Ed), UpToDate, Waltman, MA. Visit www.uptodate.com for more information

Failure to Thrive (Frailty)

- Declining independence and functional capacity in older adults – NOT an inevitable consequence of aging

Evaluation of the Geriatric Patient who is Failing in the Community

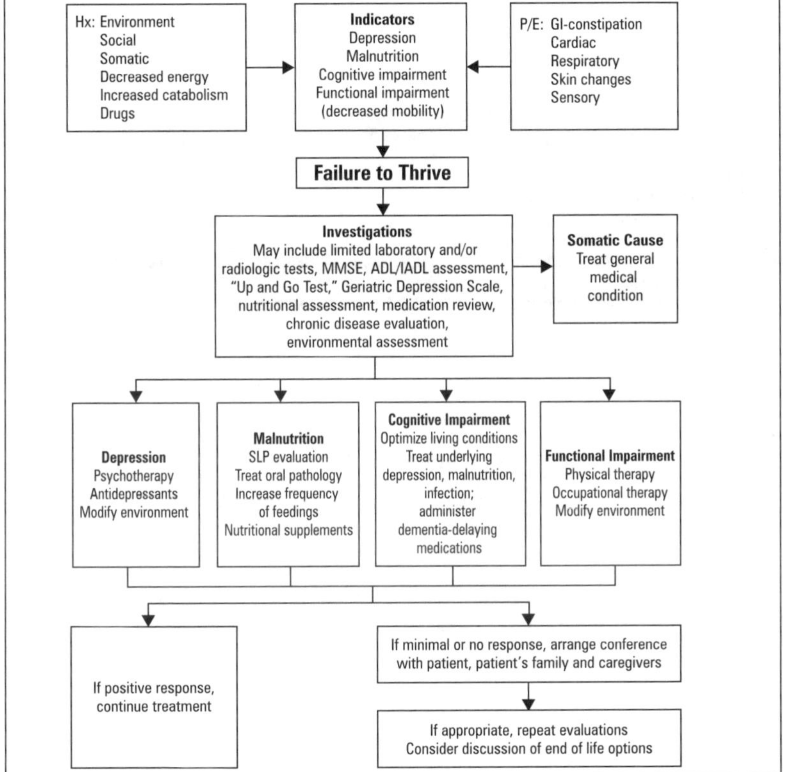

Sarkisian CA, Lachs MS. "Failure to Thrive" in older adults. *Ann Intern Med* 1996; 124:1072-1078

Incontinence

Fecal Incontinence
- Etiology: pelvic floor intact (neurological, overflow, diarrhea) vs. pelvic floor affected (trauma, surgery, sphincter damage)
- Risk factors: prior vaginal delivery, anorectal surgery, pelvic radiation, diabetes, neurological disease, diarrheal conditions
- Investigations: stool studies, endorectal U/S, colonoscopy/anoscopy, anorectal/functional testing
- Management: disimpaction, diet/bulk-forming agent, anti-diarrheal, regular defecation program (in dementia), biofeedback therapy (retraining of pelvic floor muscles)

URINARY INCONTINENCE

Transient causes of incontinence = DIAPERS
Delirium
Infection
Atrophic vaginitis/urethritis
Pharmaceuticals
Excessive urine output
Restricted mobility
Stool impaction

Elder Abuse

Red Flags
- Delay in seeking medical attention
- Disparity in histories
- Implausible or vague explanations
- Frequent emergency room visits for exacerbations of chronic disease despite plan for medical care and adequate resources
- Presentation of functionally impaired patient without designated caregiver
- Lab findings inconsistent with history

Palliative Care

Suggested Topics for Discussion
- Goals of care
- Advance directives, power of attorney, public guardian and trustee
- Treatment options and likelihood of success
- Common medical interventions: mechanical ventilation, antibiotics, feeding tubes
- Resuscitation options

Polypharmacy

Principles for prescribing in the elderly = CARE
Caution, **C**ompliance
Age-adjusted dose
Review regimen regularly
Educate

Beers Criteria
- 48 medications to avoid in adults 65 yrs and older due to safety concerns
- Examples – long-acting benzodiazepines, strong anticholinergics, high dose sedatives

Gynecology

Essential History and Physical Exam

History

Obstetrical History
- GTPAL (see Obstetrics)
- Year, location, mode of delivery, duration of labour, sex of child, gestational age, weight, complications
- History of infertility including work-up and treatment
- Ectopic pregnancy, including treatment

Menstrual History
- LNMP = last normal menstrual period
- Age of thelarche, age of menarche
- Age of menopause, menopausal symptoms (hot flashes, mood, vaginal dryness, etc.), postmenopausal bleeding, HRT
- Cycle characteristics (length, duration, regularity, flow)
- Associated features (dysmenorrhea, PMS, intermenstrual bleeding)

Sexual History
- Age of coitarche
- Number and sex of partners
- Oral, anal, vaginal
- Dyspareunia, post-coital bleeding
- History of sexual assault or abuse
- Current relationship, partner's health, satisfaction

Contraceptive History
- Present and past contraception modalities, compliance, complications, failure, side-effects

Gynecological Infections
- STIs, PID
- Vaginitis, vulvitis
- Lesions
- Include treatments, complications

Gynecological Procedures
- Pap test
  - Date of most recent Pap test and results
  - History of abnormal Pap – include treatment and follow-up
- Gynecological surgery
- Colposcopy

Medications
- **Past Medical/Surgical History**: include mammograms, breast disease, cancer, abdominal surgery including laparoscopic
- **Family History**: include endometriosis, infertility, breast disease, cancer (breast, uterine, ovary, crevix)
- **Review of Systems**: include breast, gastrointestinal (constipation, dyschezia), urinary (incontinence, LUTS), pelvis (feeling of pressure, prolapse), MSK (osteoporosis)

Physical Exam

- Important: need for proper consent, especially as this pertains to cross-cultural communication and cultural-sensitivity
- Pelvic Exam
  - Inspection of external genitalia
  - Speculum
    - Inspect cervix and vaginal walls (colour, shape, discharge, polyps, lesions, ulcerations, inflammation, odour)
    - Pap smear
      - Endocervical: insert brush into os with all bristles inside, rotate 360°, remove, smear against slide, and spray with fixative or remove brush and place in labeled bottle solution
  - Vaginal/cervical swabs: insert cotton swab into os for cervical cultures and hold for 10-20 sec. Do GC swab before chlamydia
- Bimanual exam
  - Cervix, uterus, adnexa and ovaries
  - Palpate for position, size, contour, mobility, shape, cervical motion tenderness, prolapse
- Rectal exam
  - Inspect for bleeding, polyps, ulcerations
  - Bimanual for sphincter tone and tenderness

Common Presentations

Pelvic Pain

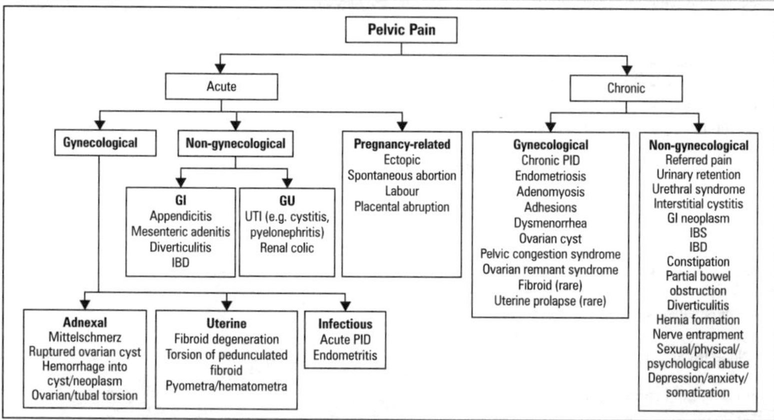

Amenorrhea

Definition

- Primary: No menses by age 14 in the absence of secondary sexual characteristics or no menses by age 16 with secondary sexual characteristics
- Secondary: Absence of menses for >6 months or 3 cycles after documented menarche

Differential Diagnosis

- Amenorrhea is pregnancy until proven otherwise
- Hypothalamic dysfunction (low or normal FSH, LH): anorexia, extreme exercise/stress/systemic illness, tumour, GnRH deficiency (e.g. Kallman's syndrome)

- Pituitary dysfunction: tumour, primary hypopituitarism, Sheehan syndrome
- Ovarian dysfunction: menopause, radiation/chemotherapy, gonadal dysgenesis (e.g. Turner's), PCOS, tumour
- Uterine/outflow tract defects: Mayer-Rokitansky-Kuster-Hauser syndrome, imperforate hymen, cervical stenosis, intrauterine adhesions (e.g. Asherman's syndrome)
- Endocrine: hyperprolactinemia, hyper/hypothyroidism, hyperandrogenism (PCOS, tumour, etc.), Cushing's syndrome
- Other – androgen insensitivity syndrome, drugs (metoclopramide, neuroleptics, danazol)

History/Physical Exam
- Signs of pregnancy (rule out pregnancy), lifestyle, Tanner Staging, hirsutism/virilization, galactorrhea/visual changes/headache, thyroid, external genitalia and vagina, bimanual exam, family history of delayed puberty (rare)

Investigations
- Hormonal blood work: β-hCG, FSH, LH, DHEAS, androstenedione, testosterone (free and total), estradiol, TSH, prolactin
- U/S (transabdominal and/or transvaginal) for anatomy, PCOS, etc.
- Progesterone challenge to assess estrogen status
- CT or MRI if tumour suspected
- Karyotype (e.g. premature ovarian failure, primary amenorrhea)

Diagnostic Approach to Amenorrhea

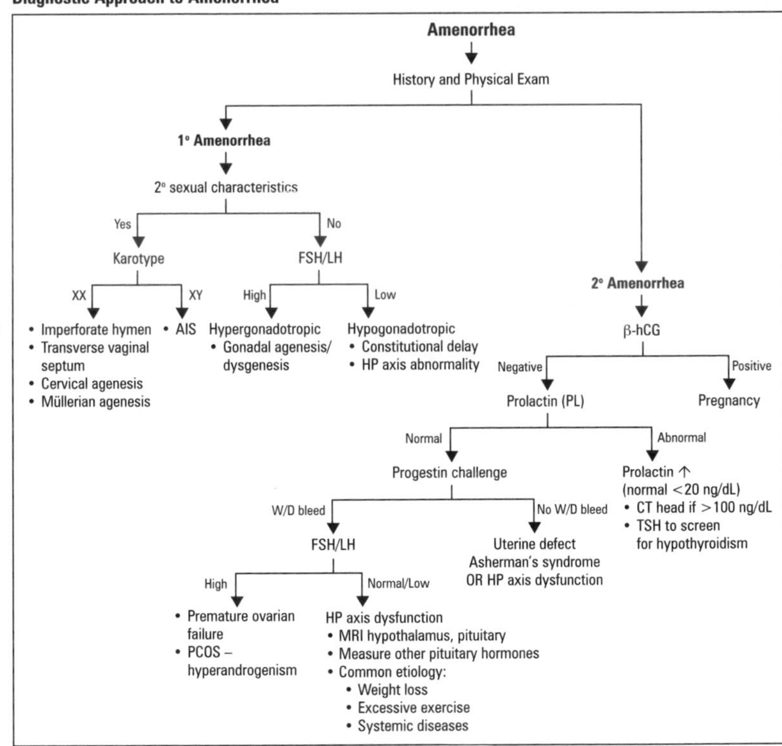

Treatment
- Hypothalamic dysfunction: stop any medication, reduce stress/exercise, adequate nutrition; may require GnRH pump if pregnancy desired, otherwise OCP to induce menstruation (withdrawal bleed)
- Hyperprolactinemia: bromocriptine if fertility desired, OCP if not; rarely, surgery for macroadenoma
- Premature ovarian failure (high FSH, LH): look for associated autoimmune disorder (thyroid, adrenal), HRT/OCP for symptomatic relief, removal of gonadal tissue if Y chromosome present

Abnormal Uterine Bleeding (AUB)

Etiology/Differential Diagnosis
- Pregnancy related (bleeding following a missed period): implantation bleed, abortion (missed, threatened, inevitable, incomplete, complete), molar pregnancy, ectopic pregnancy, etc.
- Exogenous hormones: breakthrough bleeding (OCP, patch, HRT, etc.)
- IUD
- Benign growths: cervical/endometrial polyp, fibroids, ectropion, adenomyosis
- Malignant tumours: cervical, vaginal, vulvar, ovarian (granulosa-theca cell), uterine postmenopausal bleeding is endometrial cancer until proven otherwise
- Trauma, sexual abuse, foreign body
- Infection: endometritis, cervicitis, STI
- Non-gynecologic: blood dyscrasias, hepatic disease, renal failure, endocrine (thyroid, DM, CAH, Cushing's, prolactinoma, PCOS), drugs (anticoagulants, spironolactone, danazol, etc.)
- Adolescent: exogenous hormone (e.g. OCP), clotting disorder (e.g. VWD), trauma
- Reproductive/premenopausal: exogenous hormone (e.g. OCP, patch, etc.), uterine fibroids, cervical/endometrial polyp, thyroid dysfunction, trauma, pregnancy-related
- Postmenopausal: endometrial cancer, endometrial lesion/polyp, exogenous hormone (e.g. HRT), atrophic vaginitis (most common), other tumour (vulvar, vaginal cervical), trauma
- Dysfunctional uterine bleeding (DUB): diagnosis of exclusion

History
- Psychological history (mood changes, stressors), menopausal symptoms, hirsutism, diabetes, weight loss, fever, thyroid symptoms

Labs
- Blood work (CBC, serum ferritin, β-hCG, TSH; depending on presentation: coagulation profiles, prolactin, FSH, LH, serum androgens, day 21 progesterone to confirm ovulation)
- Pap test ± vaginal/cervical swabs
- Endometrial sampling in women >40 yrs, postmenopausal, or high risk of endometrial cancer

Imaging
- Pelvic/transvaginal ultrasound (detect polyps, myomata; measure endometrial thickness in postmenopausal women)
- Sonohysterogram (sensitive for intrauterine pathology, e.g. polyps, submucosal fibroids)
- Hysteroscopy

Treatment
- Treat underlying disorder
- If anatomical lesion and systemic disease have been ruled out, consider dysfunctional uterine bleeding (DUB)
- Rhogam® if Rh-negative and cause of AUB is either ectopic pregnancy or miscarriage

- Medical
  - Mild DUB
    - NSAID, anti-fibrinolytic, combined OCP, progestins (Provera®) on 1st 10-14 d each month, Mirena® IUD, danazol
    - Anovulatory patients wishing to get pregnant: clomiphene citrate
  - Acute/severe DUB: replace fluid losses, consider admission, treatments include:
    - A) Estrogen (Premarin®) 25 mg IV q4h x 24 h with Gravol® 50 mg IV/PO q4h, or
    - B) Ovral®, or any OCP with minimum 50 μg estradiol. 1 tab PO q4h x 24h with Gravol® 50 mg IV/PO q4h (taper Ovral to 1 tab tid x 2 d, then bid x 2 d, then OD)
    - After A) or B), OCP for several months (anovulatory patients wishing to get pregnant: clomiphene citrate)
- Surgical
  - D&C for diagnosis (rarely done)
  - Endometrial ablation after pretreatment with danazol or GnRH agonists to improve efficacy and safety (if finished childbearing)
  - Hysterectomy

Vaginal Discharge

Differential Diagnosis
- Physiologic (pH <4.5): normal midcycle discharge, increased estrogen states (e.g. pregnancy)
- Local: allergic/irritative vaginitis, atrophic vaginitis, poor hygiene, foreign body
- Infectious
  - Bacterial vaginosis: thin, white/grey, 'fishy' odour with KOH whiff test, pH >4.5
  - *Candidiasis*: white, thick, adherent, cottage-cheese like, pH <4.5, pruritic
  - *Trichomonas*: yellow/green, frothy, pH >4.5
  - *N. gonorrhoeae, C. trachomatis*: mucopurulent cervicitis
- Neoplastic: invasive cervical cancer, fallopian tube cancer (watery), vaginal squamous cell cancer, endometrial
- Systemic: Crohn's, collagen disease, dermatologic (e.g. lichen sclerosis)
- Other: enterovaginal fistula

History/Physical Exam/Investigations
- Duration/timing of symptoms
- Colour/amount/consistency of discharge
- Odour
- Irritative symptoms
- Dysuria, dyspareunia,
- Topical product use, sexual activity
- Current medications
- Associated skin changes: erythema, vesicles, ulcers
- Bimanual exam: cervical motion tenderness, adnexal masses/tenderness/mobility
- pH test of secretions, wet mount slide with normal saline and 10% KOH, KOH whiff test
- Cervical swabs and cultures, nucleic acid amplification for gonorrhea

Treatment
- Local: enhance hygiene, change products (e.g. detergents, soaps), local estrogen (e.g. Premarin® cream) for atrophic vaginitis
- Candidiasis: clotrimazole, butoconazole, etc. suppositories/creams for 1, 3, or 7 d or fluconazole 150 mg PO once
- Bacterial vaginosis: metronidazole 500 mg PO bid x 7 d (no treatment if non-pregnant or asymptomatic)
- *Trichomonas*: metronidazole 2 g PO once (treat partner)
- *N. gonorrhoeae*: ceftriaxone 125 mg IM once or cefixime 400 mg PO once (treat partners, co-treat for *C. trachomatis*)
- *C. trachomatis*: azithromycin 1 g PO once or doxycycline 100 mg PO bid x 7 d (treat partners; co-treat for *N. gonorrhoeae*)

Infectious Vulvovaginitis

	Candidiasis (Moniliasis)	Bacterial Vaginosis (BV)	Trichomoniasis
Organisms	*Candida albicans* (90%) *Candida glabrata* (<5%) *Candida tropicalis* (<5%)	*Gardnerella vaginalis* *Mycoplasma hominis* anaerobes: *Prevotella,* *Mobiluncus, Bacteroides*	Trichomonas vaginalis (flagellated protozoan)
Pathophysiology or Transmission	Predisposing factors include: Immunosuppressed host (diabetes, AIDS, etc.) Recent antibiotic use Increased estrogen levels, e.g. pregnancy, OCP	Replacement of vaginal *Lactobacillus* with organisms above	Sexually transmitted
Discharge	Whitish, "cottage cheese", minimal	Grey, thin, diffuse	Yellow-green, malodorous, diffuse, frothy
Other Signs/ Symptoms	20% asymptomatic Intense pruritus Swollen, inflamed genitals Vulvar burning, dysuria, dyspareunia	Absence of vulvar/vaginal irritation	50-75% asymptomatic 25% symptomatic Fishy odour, especially after coitus Petechiae on vagina and cervix Occasionally irritated tender vulva Dysuria, frequency
pH	≤4.5	>4.5	≥4.5
Saline Wetmount	KOH wetmount reveals hyphae and spores	1. >20% clue cells = squamous 2. Paucity of WBC 3. Paucity of Lactobacillli 4. Positive whiff test = fishy odour with addition of KOH to slide due to formation of amines	1. Motile flagellated organisms, epithelial cells dotted with coccobacilli (Gardnerella) 2. Many WBCs 3. Inflammatory cells (PMNs)
Treatment	Recommended if uncomplicated: Fluconazole 150 mg PO in single dose Clotrimazole, butoconazole, terconazole suppositories and/or creams for 1, 3, or 7-d treatments Treatment in pregnancy is usually topical treatment	No treatment if non-pregnant and asymptomatic unless scheduled for gyne procedure Oral: Metronidazole 500 mg PO bid x 7 d Topical: Clindamycin 2% 5 g intravaginally at bed time x 7 d May use during pregnancy	Treat if asymptomatic! 2 g PO single dose metronidazole, miconazole, for pelvic surgery or procedure (recom.) or 500 mg bid x 7d (alternative) Symptomatic pregnant women should be treated with 2 g metronidazole once or metronidazole gel 0.75% OD x 5 d
Other	For repeat infections prophylaxis, vaginal suppositories, luteal phase fluconazole Routine treatment of partner(s) not recommended	Associated with recurrent and preterm endometritis in pregnancy Need to warn patients on metronidazole: do not consume alcohol (disulfiram-like action) Routine treatment of partner(s) not recommended	Warnings accompanying metronidazole use Treat partner(s)

Genital Lesions

Differential Diagnosis
- Infectious
  - Painful: herpes/HSV (may be multiple vesicles), chancroid (may be multiple papules/pustules), Bartholin's abscess
  - Painless: syphilis (chancre), condylomata acuminata/genital warts/HPV (hyperkeratotic, verrucous or flat, macular lesions)
- Malignant: vulvar cancer (red/white ulcerative or exophytic lesions)
- Other: trauma, foreign body

Treatment
- Genital warts – podofilox 0.5% solution or gel bid x 3 d in a row and repeat x 4 wks (patient-applied), provider may use cryotherapy q1-2wk or TCA q1-2wks, Imiquimod (Aldara® 5% cream 3x/wk qhs x 16 wks)
- Herpes: acyclovir 400 mg PO tid x 7-10 d for first episode; 5 d for recurrent episodes; consider daily bid therapy if 6-8 attacks per yr
- Syphilis: benzathine penicillin G 2.4 million units IM single dose (treat partners)
- Bartholin's abscess: antibiotics, incision and drainage or marsupialization
- Vulvar cancer: excision (additional treatment depends on stage)

Common Conditions

Pelvic Inflammatory Disease (PID)

Definition
- Inflammation of the uterus, fallopian tubes and adjacent pelvic structures (not associated with pregnancy)

Pathogenesis
- Ascending infection from the cervix and vagina to the upper portions of the genital tract
- Causative organisms: *C. trachomatis*, *N. gonorrhoeae* (often co-exist) > endogenous flora (e.g. *E. coli, Staph, Strep, Enterococcus, Bacteroides, Peptostreptococcus, H. flu, G. vaginalis*) > *Actinomyces israelii*
- Others (e.g. TB, Gram negs, *U. urealyticum*)
- NB: Must treat with polymicrobial coverage

Differential Diagnosis
- Ruptured ovarian cyst, ovarian torsion, ectopic pregnancy (β-hCG to rule out), endometriosis, acute appendicitis, urinary tract infection

History
- Common symptoms; ask about risk factors (see below)
- Lower abdominal pain, usually bilateral (most common symptom): OPQRSTUVW
- Abnormal vaginal discharge, fever, nausea/vomiting, abnormal uterine bleeding, dysuria, dyspareunia
- Take full gynecologic, obstetric and sexual history, and contraceptive use

Physical Exam
- General appearance (sick/septic), vitals, abdominal exam (tenderness, peritoneal signs, palpable mass), speculum exam (odour, discharge), bimanual exam (adnexal tenderness, cervical motion tenderness)

Risk Factors (*C. trachomatis* and *N. gonorrhoeae*)
- Sexually active, <25 yrs of age, history of previous STI, new partner in last 3 months, multiple partners, no barrier contraception, contact with infected person, vaginal douching, IUD (within 10 d of insertion), invasive gynecological procedures (e.g. endometrial biopsy), cigarette smoking

Complications
- Abscess, peritonitis
- Adhesion formation leading to chronic pelvic pain, tubal obstruction, infertility, ectopic pregnancy
- Disseminated infection (bacteremia, septic arthritis, endocarditis)

Criteria for Diagnosis
- Must have:
    - Abdominal tenderness
    - Cervical motion tenderness
    - Adnexal tenderness (may be unilateral)
- Confirmatory findings (minimum one):
    - Fever >38°C
    - Leukocytosis
    - Mucopurulent cervical discharge
    - Cul-de-sac fluid, abscess or inflammatory mass on ultrasound
    - Positive culture for *C. trachomatis, N. gonorrhoeae, E.coli* or other vaginal flora
    - Elevated ESR or CRP (not commonly used)
    - High risk partner

Investigations
- Blood work: CBC, blood cultures if suspect bacteremia, β-hCG
- Speculum exam: swabs (gram stain), cervical cultures
- Endometrial biopsy will give definitive diagnosis but is rarely done
- Pelvic U/S: fluid in cul-de-sac, pelvic or tubo-ovarian abscess, hydrosalpinx
- Laparoscopy is not considered a diagnostic "gold-standard" because it is invasive and costly

MANAGEMENT

Hospital (Inpatient)
- Indications for hospitalization: severe/atypical infection, unable to tolerate oral therapy, abscess, immunocompromised, pregnant, adolescent/first episode
- Medical treatment (CDC recommendations):
    - 1. Cefoxitin 2 g IV q6h or cefotetan 2 g IV q12h + doxycycline 100 mg IV PO q12h OR
    - 2. Clindamycin 900 mg IV q8h + gentamicin 2 mg/kg IV/IM loading dose + gentamicin 1.5 mg/kg q8h maintenance dose
    - Continue IV Abx for at least 48 h after symptoms have improved then doxycycline 100 mg PO bid to complete 14 d
    - If abscess: percutaneous drainage under U/S guidance or laparascopic drainage. If failure, salpingectomy or TAH-BSO

Discharge (Outpatient)
- Indications for outpatient therapy: mild-moderate infection, compliant with oral meds and will follow-up within 48-72 h
- Medical treatment:
    - 1. Cefoxitin 2 g IM + probenecid 1 g PO + doxycycline 100 mg PO bid to complete 14 d OR ceftriaxone 250 mg IM + doxycycline 100 mg PO bid to complete 14 d OR
    - 2. Ofloxacin 400 mg PO bid X 14d + metronidazole 500 mg bid X 14d
- Follow-up: report to Public Health, treat partners, consider rescreening for *C. trachomatis* and *N. gonorrhoeae* 4-6 wks after treatment

Sexually Transmitted Infections (STIs)

HUMAN PAPILLOMAVIRUS (HPV)

Etiology and Epidemiology
- Most common viral STI in Canada
- >200 subtypes of which >30 are genital subtypes
- Types 16, 18, 31, 33, 35, 45, 36 (and others) are associated with increased incidence of cervical and vulvar intraepithelial hyperplasia and carcinoma
- HPV types 6 and 11 are classically associated with anogenital warts/condylomata acuminata
- HPV types 16 and 18 are the most oncogenic (classically associated with cervical HSIL)

Clinical Features
- Latent infection
    - No visible lesions
    - Detected by DNA hybridization tests
    - Asymptomatic
- Subclinical infection
    - Visible lesion found during colposcopy, or found on Pap test
- Clinical infection
    - Visible wart-like lesion without magnification
    - Hyperkeratotic, verrucous or flat, macular lesions
    - Vulvar edema

Investigations
- Cytology
- Biopsy of lesions at colposcopy
- Detection of HPV DNA subtype using nucleic acid probes not routinely done but can be done in presence of abnormal Pap test to guide treatment

Treatment
- Patient administered
    - Podofilox 0.5% solution or gel bid x 3 d in a row (4 d off) then repeat x 4 wks
    - Imiquimod (Aldara®) 5% cream 3x/wk qhs x 16wks
- Provider administered
    - Cryotherapy with liquid nitrogen – repeat q1-2wks
    - Podophyllin resin in tincture of benzoin – weekly
    - Trichloroacetic acid (TCA) or bichloroacetic acid weekly (80-90%) (safe in pregnancy)
    - Surgical removal/laser
    - Intralesional interferon
- Cannot be prevented by using condoms

Prevention
- HPV types 6, 11, 16, 18: preventable with Gardasil® (Quadrivalent HPV recombinant vaccine)
- HPV types 16 and 18: preventable with Cervarix® (Bivalent HPV recombinant vaccine)

HERPES SIMPLEX VIRUS OF VULVA (HSV)

Etiology
* 90% are HSV-2, 10% are HSV-1

Clinical Features
* May be asymptomatic
* Initial symptoms
    * Present 2-21 d following contact
* Prodromal symptoms: tingling, burning, pruritus
* Multiple, painful, shallow ulcerations with small vesicles (absent in many infected persons)
    * Lesions are infectious
    * Appear 7-10 d after initial infection
* Inguinal lymphadenopathy, malaise and fever often with first infection
* Dysuria and urinary retention if urethral mucosa affected
* Recurrent infections: less severe, less frequent and shorter in duration

Investigations
* Viral culture preferred in patients with ulcer present: decreased sensitivity as lesions heal
* Cytologic smear
    * Multinucleated giant cells
    * Acidophilic intranuclear inclusion bodies
* Type specific serologic tests for antibodies to HSV-1 and HSV-2 (not available routinely in Canada)
* HSV DNA PCR

Treatment
* First episode
    * Acyclovir 400 mg PO tid x 7-10d (also famciclovir 250 mg PO tid x 7-10d, valacyclovir 1 g PO bid x 7-10d)
* Recurrent episode
    * Acyclovir 400 mg PO tid x 3-5d, or famciclovir 125 mg PO bid x 3-5d or valacyclovir 500 mg PO bid x 3d
* Daily suppressive therapy
    * Consider if 6-8 attacks per yr
    * Acyclovir 400 mg PO bid, or famciclovir 250 mg bid, or valacyclovir 500 mg-1 g PO qid
* Severe disease
    * Consider IV therapy acyclovir 5-10 mg/kg IV q8h x 5-7d
* Treat pregnant women with a history at 36 wks gestation onwards with Acyclovir 400 mg PO TID
* Education regarding transmission
* Avoid contact from onset of prodrome until lesions have cleared
* Use barrier contraception

CHLAMYDIA

Etiology
* *Chlamydia trachomatis*

Clinical Features
* Asymptomatic (80% of women)
* Muco-purulent endocervical discharge
* Urethral syndrome: dysuria, frequency, pyuria, no bacteria
* Pelvic pain
* Post-coital bleeding or intermenstrual bleeding, particularly if on OCP and prior history of good cyclic control

Risk Factors
* Previous STI, sexually active <2.5 yrs, multiple partners, contact with untreated person, new partner in last 3 months, not using condoms, street involvement (IVDU, homelessness)

Investigations
- Cervical culture or nucleic acid amplification test
- Obligate intracellular parasite; tissue culture is the definitive standard

Treatment
- Doxycycline 100 mg PO bid for 7d or azithromycin 1 g PO in a single dose (may use in pregnancy)
- Treat partners
- Reportable disease
- Test of cure for chlamydia required in pregnancy (cure rates lower in pregnant patients), retest in 3-4 wks post-initiation of therapy

Screening
- High risk groups, pregnancy

Complications
- Acute salpingitis, PID
- Fitz-Hugh-Curtis syndrome (liver capsule inflammation)
- Conjunctivitis, urethritis, reactive arthritis (male predominance, HLA-B27)
- Infertility: tubal obstruction from low grade salpingitis
- Ectopic pregnancy
- Chronic pelvic pain
- Perinatal infection: conjunctivitis, pneumonia

GONORRHEA

Etiology
- *Neisseria gonorrhoeae*
- Symptoms and risk factors same as *Chlamydia*

Investigations
- Gram stain shows Gram-negative intracellular diplococci + cervical, rectal and throat culture

Treatment
- Single dose of ceftriaxone 125 mg IM or cefixime 400 mg PO or ciprofloxacin 500 mg PO
- Plus doxycycline or azithromycin to treat chlamydia, because of high rate of co-infection
- If pregnant: cephalosporin regimen (as above) or 2 g spectinomycin IM (avoid quinolones)
- Treat partners, reportable disease
- Screening as with chlamydia

Endometriosis

Symptoms
- May be asymptomatic
- Cyclic symptoms due to swelling and bleeding of ectopic endometrium, often precede menses and continue throughout and after flow
    - Secondary dysmenorrhea
    - Deep dyspareunia
    - Sacral pain with menses
    - Pain may eventually become constant but remains worse perimenstrually
- Premenstrual and postmenstrual spotting
- Infertility
    - 30-40% of patients with endometriosis will be infertile
    - 15-30% of those who are infertile will have endometriosis
- Bowel and bladder symptoms
    - Frequency, dysuria, hematuria
    - Diarrhea, constipation, hematochezia, dyschezia
- Tender nodularity of uterine ligaments and cul-de-sac felt on rectovaginal exam
- Fixed retroversion of uterus
- Firm, fixed adnexal mass (endometrioma)

Investigations
- Definitive diagnosis requires
  - Direct visualization of lesions typical of endometriosis at laparoscopy
  - Biopsy and histologic exam of specimens (2 or more of: endometrial epithelium, glands, stroma, hemosiderin-laden macrophages)
- Laparoscopy
  - Mulberry spots: dark blue or brownish-black implants on the uterosacral ligaments, cul-de-sac or anywhere in the pelvis
  - Endometrioma: "chocolate" cysts in the ovaries
  - "Powder-burn" lesions on the peritoneal surface
  - Pearly white lesions and clear blebs
  - Peritoneal "pockets"
- CA-125
  - May be useful for confirming endometriosis but nonspecific

Treatment
- Depends on the certainty of the diagnosis, severity of symptoms, extent of disease, desire for future fertility and threat to GI/GU systems
- **Medical**
  - NSAIDs (e.g. naproxen, Anaprox®)
  - Pseudopregnancy: cyclic/continuous estrogen-progestin (OCP), medroxyprogesterone (Depo-Provera®)
  - Pseudomenopause: 2nd line: only short-term (<6 months) due to osteoporotic potential with prolonged use
    - Danazol (Danocrine®) = weak androgen
      - Side effects: weight gain, fluid retention, acne, hirsutism, voice change
    - Leuprolide (Lupron®) = GnRH agonist (suppresses pituitary)
      - Side effects: hot flashes, vaginal dryness, reduced libido
      - Can use >12 months with add-back progestin and estrogen
- **Surgical**
  - Laparoscopy using laser, electrocautery ± laparotomy
    - Ablation/resection of implants, lysis of adhesions, ovarian cystectomy of endometriomas
    - Best time to become pregnant is immediately after surgery
  - Total pelvic clean-out if post childbearing
  - ± follow-up with medical treatment for pain control NOT preservation of fertility

Leiomyomata (fibroids)

Investigations
- Bimanual exam: uterus asymmetrically enlarged, mobile
- CBC: anemia
- Ultrasound: assess location of fibroids
- Sonohysterogram: can differentiate endometrial polyps from submucosal fibroids
- Endometrial biopsy to rule out uterine cancer if abnormal uterine bleeding: especially if age >40 yrs
- Occasionally MRI is used for pre-op planning for myomectomy

Treatment
- Only if symptomatic, rapidly enlarging, menorrhagia, or menometrorrhagia
- Treat anemia if present
- Conservative approach (watch and wait) if
  - Symptoms absent or minimal
  - Fibroids <6-8 cm or stable in size
  - Not submucosal (i.e. submucosal fibroids are more likely to be symptomatic)

- Medical approach
    - Antiprostaglandins (ibuprofen)
    - Tranexamic acid (Cyklokapron®)
    - OCP/Depo-Provera®
    - GnRH agonist: leuprolide (Lupron®) or androgen derivative, danazol (Danocrine®); short-term use only (6 months); often used pre-myomectomy to facilitate surgery (reduces fibroid size)
    - Selective progesterone receptor modulators: currently in clinical trials; prototype is RU486 which reduces fibroid volume by 50% after 3 months without the side effects of GnRH agonists
- Interventional radiology approach
    - Uterine artery embolization occludes both uterine arteries and shrinks fibroids by 50% at 6 months. Improves menorrhagia in 90% of patients within 1-2 months (not an option in women considering childbearing)
- Surgical approach
    - Myomectomy (hysteroscopic, transabdominal or laparoscopic approach) preserves childbearing capabilities
    - Hysterectomy: abdominal, vaginal, or laparoscopic depending on fibroid size
    - Endometrial resection of fibroid and endometrial ablation if submucosal in location
    - Note: avoid operating on fibroids during pregnancy (due to increased vascularity); expectant management only

Endometrial Carcinoma

Investigations
- Office endometrial biopsy, D&C ± hysteroscopy

Treatment
- Based on tumour grade and depth of myometrial invasion
- Surgical: hysterectomy/BSO and pelvic washings ± pelvic and periaortic node dissection – laparoscopic preferred
    - General trend (controversial)
        - Grade 1: BSO and washings
        - Grades 2, 3 and high risk histologies: hysterectomy/BSO/nodes ± omentectomy
- Adjuvant radiotherapy: for selected patients based on depth of myometrial invasion, tumour grade, and/or lymph node involvement
- Hormonal therapy: progestins for distant or recurrent disease
- Adjuvant chemotherapy: if disease progresses

Cervical Cancer

Decision Making Chart for Pap Smear (not applicable to adolescents)

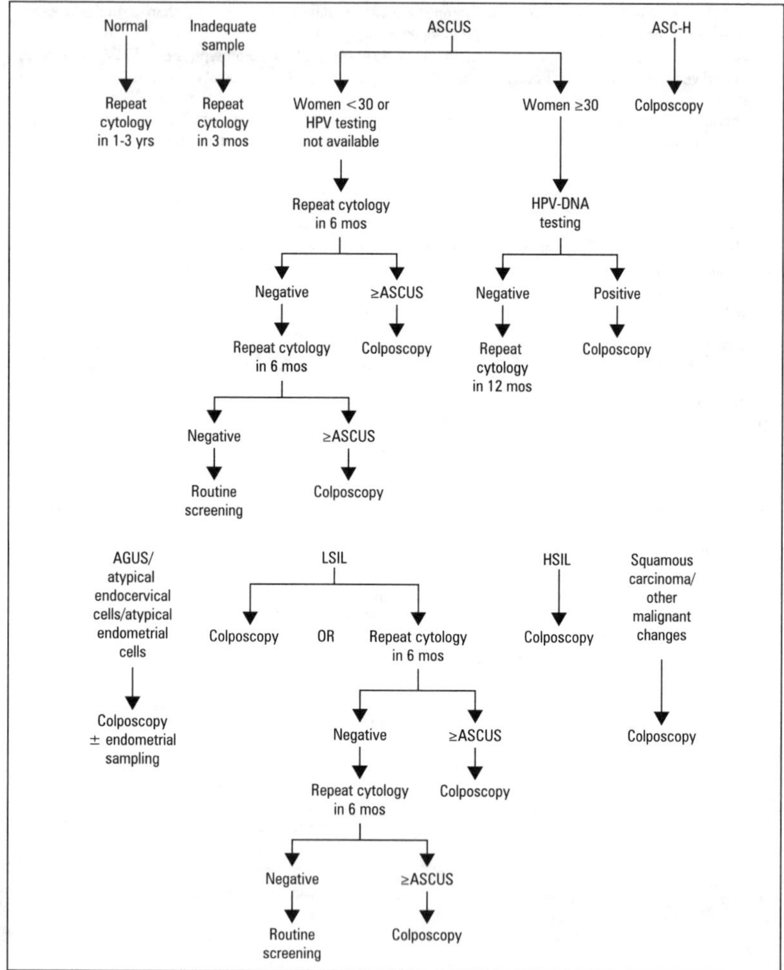

Adapted from *Ontario Cervical Screening Practice Guidelines*. June 2005.

Treatment of Abnormal Pap Test and Cervical Cancer

	Treatment
CIN I (LSIL)	Observe with regular cytology (every 6 months) Many lesions will regress or disappear (60%) Colposcopy if positive on 2 consecutive tests Lesions which progress should have area excised by either LEEP, laser, cryotherapy or cone biopsy (with LEEP, tissues obtained for histological evaluation)
CIN II, III (HSIL)	Colposcopy referral LEEP, laser, cryotherapy, cone excision Hysterectomy: if no desire for future childbearing and only after ruling iconfirmingn cancer with LEEP or cone biopsy
Stage 1A + B	Fertility desired: cone vs. radical trachelectomy No fertility desired: radical hysterectomy ± nodes If lesion >4 cm: chemotherapy/radiotherapy
Stages 2,3,4	Chemotherapy/radiotherapy

Ovarian Tumours

Ultrasound Characteristics of Benign vs. Malignant Ovarian Tumours

Benign	Malignant
<8-10 cm in diameter	>10 cm in diameter
Unilateral	Bilateral
Cystic	Solid elements (internal papillary structures/mural nodules)
Uniloculated	Multiloculated
Thin septations	Thick septations
No ascites	Ascites

Investigation of Suspicious Ovarian Mass
- Bimanual examination: solid, irregular, fixed pelvic mass is suggestive of ovarian cancer
- Bloodwork: CA-125 for baseline, CBC, liver function tests, electrolytes, creatinine
- Radiology: chest x-ray, abdo/pelvic U/S ± transvaginal U/S; CT or U/S to assess urinary tract
- Rule out primary if metastatic:
  - Occult blood: if positive, endoscopy ± barium enema
  - If gastric symptoms, gastroscopy ± upper GI series
  - If abnormal vaginal bleeding, Pap test and endometrial biopsy to rule out concurrent endometrial or cervical cancer
  - Mammogram
- Use Risk of Malignancy Index (RMI = U x M x CA-125) to guide next step (if RMI >200, refer to Gynecologic Oncology)

Risk of Malignancy Index (RMI) RMI = U x M x CA-125 **ULTRASOUND FINDINGS** (1 pt for each) • Multilocular cyst • Evidence of solid areas • Evidence of metastases • Presence of ascites • Bilateral lesions U = 1 (for U/S scores of 0 or 1) U = 4 (for U/S scores of 2-5)	**MENOPAUSAL STATUS** • Postmenopausal: M = 4 • Pre-menopausal: M = 1 **ABSOLUTE VALUE OF CA-125 SERUM LEVEL** Jacobs et al. *BJOG*, 1990.

Menopause

Definitions
- Physiological: average age 51 yrs (follicular atresia)
- Premature ovarian failure: before age 40 (autoimmune disorder, infection, Turner's syndrome)
- Iatrogenic (surgical/radiation/chemotherapy)

Clinical Features
- Associated with estrogen deficiency
  - Vasomotor instability (tends to dissipate with time)
    - Hot flashes, night sweats, sleep disturbances, formication, nausea, palpitations
  - Urogenital atrophy involving vagina, urethra, bladder
    - Dyspareunia, pruritus, vaginal dryness, bleeding, urinary frequency, urgency, incontinence
  - Skeletal
    - Osteoporosis, joint and muscle pain, back pain
  - Skin and soft tissue
    - Decreased breast size, skin thinning/loss of elasticity
  - Psychological
    - Mood disturbance, irritability, fatigue, decreased libido, memory loss

Investigations
- Increased levels of FSH (>35 IU/L) on day 3 of cycle (if still cycling) and LH (FSH>LH), decreased levels of estradiol (later). FSH level not diagnostic, due to cyclic fluctuation. Use absence of menses x 1 yr to diagnose

Treatment
- Goal is for individual symptom management
  - Vasomotor instability
    - HRT (first line), clonidine, SSRIs, venlafaxine, gabapentin, propanolol
  - Vaginal atrophy
    - Local estrogen: cream (Premarin®)/vaginal suppository (VagiFem®)/ring form (Estring®)
    - Lubricants (Replens®)
  - osteoporosis
    - 1000-1200 mg calcium daily, 400-800 IU vitamin D, weight-bearing exercise, quit smoking
    - Bisphosphonates (e.g. alendronate)
    - Selective estrogen receptor modifiers (SERMs): raloxifene (Evista®): mimics estrogen effects on bone, avoids estrogen-like action on breast and uterine cancer; does not help hot flashes
    - HRT: second-line treatment (unless for vasomotor instability as well)
  - Decreased libido
    - Vaginal lubrication, sexual counseling, rarely androgen replacement (testosterone cream, Andriol® PO)
  - Cardiovascular disease
    - Management of cardiovascular risk factors
  - Alternative choices (not evidence-based)
    - Black cohosh, phytoestrogens, St. John's wort, gingko biloba, valerian, evening primrose oil, ginseng, Dong Quai
  - Well-being
    - Physical exercise, relaxation, yoga

Hormone Replacement Therapy (HRT)

Examples of HRT Regimens

HRT Regimen	Estrogen Dose	Progestin Dose	Notes
Unopposed Estrogen	CEE 0.625 mg PO OD	N/A	1. If no intact uterus
Standard-dose	CEE 0.625 mg PO OD	MPA 2.5 mg PO OD, or micronized progesterone 100 mg PO OD	1. Withdrawal bleeding occurs in a spotty, unpredictable manner 2. Usually abates after 6-8 months due to endometrial atrophy 3. Once patient has become amenorrheic on HRT, significant subsequent bleeding episodes require evaluation (endometrial biopsy)
Standard-dose Cyclic	CEE 0.625 mg PO OD	MPA 5-10 mg PO days 1-14 only, or micronized progesterone 200mg PO days 1-14 only	1. Bleeding occurs monthly after day 14 of progestin (can continue for years) 2. PMS-like symptoms (breast tenderness, fluid retention, headache, nausea) are more prominent with cyclic HRT
Pulsatile	CEE 0.625 mg PO OD	MPA low-dose	1. 3 days on, 3 days off
Transdermal	Estroderm® – Estradiol 0.05 mg/d or 0.1 mg/d Estalis® – Estradiol 140 µg/d or 250 µg/d	Estroderm® – MPA 2.5 mg PO OD Estalis® – NEA 50 µg/d MPA 2.5 mg PO OD MPA 5-10 mg days 1-14	1. Use patch twice weekly 2. Can use combined patched (Estroderm® MPA) and (Estalis® NEA)

CEE = conjugated equine estrogen (e.g. Premarin®)
MPA = medroxyprogesterone acetate (e.g. Provera®)
Micronized progesterone (e.g. Prometrium®)
NEA = norethindrone acetate
Consider lower dose regimens, PREMPRO® 0.45/1.5 (Premarin 0.45 mg and Provera 1.5 mg) recently released in the United States

Contraception

Classification of Contraceptive Methods

Type	Effectiveness (perfect use, typical use)
Physiological	
Withdrawal/coitus interruptus	77%
Rhythm method/calendar/mucus/symptothermal	98%, 76%
Lactational amenorrhea	98% (first 6 months postpartum)
Chance – no method used	10%
Abstinence of all sexual activity	100%
Barrier Methods	
Male condom alone	98%, 85%
Spermicide alone	82%, 71%
Sponge – Parous	80%, 68%
– Nulliparous	91%, 84%
Diaphragm with spermicide	94%, 84%
Female condom	95%, 79%
Cervical cap – Parous	74%, 68%
– Nulliparous	91%, 84%

Classification of Contraceptive Methods (continued)

Type	Effectiveness (perfect use, typical use)
Hormonal	
OCP	99.7%, 92%
Nuva Ring®	99.7%, 92%
Transdermal (Ortho Evra®)	99.7%, 92%
Depo-Provera®	99.7%, 97%
Progestin-only pill (Micronor®)	90-99%
Mirena® IUD	99.9%
Copper IUD	99.3%
Surgical	
Tubal ligation	99.65%
Vasectomy	99.9%
Emergency Postcoital Contraception (EPC)	
Yuzpe® method	98% (within 24 h), decreases by 30% at 72 h
"Plan B" levonorgestrel only	98% (within 24 h), decreases by 70% at 72 h
Postcoital IUD	99.9%

Effectiveness: percentage of women reporting no pregnancy after 1 yr of use.

Barrier Methods

Examples of Barrier Contraceptive Methods

	Advantages	Disadvantages
Male Condom	98% effective against pregnancy and STIs with perfect use No prescription required	Latex allergy Irritation Must be applied properly One-time use
Diaphragm	94% effective with spermicide Female-controlled	Must be in place for 6h after intercourse Must be used with spermicide Incomplete STI protection Latex allergy Must be fitted by health care provider Increased risk of UTI Risk of toxic shock syndrome
Sponge	80-91% effective Does not require fitting by MD Available in pharmacies	Relatively expensive Only 80% effective in parous women Incomplete STI protection Risk of toxic shock syndrome

Hormonal Methods

Starting Hormonal Contraceptives
- Thorough history and physical examination including blood pressure and breast exam
- Follow-up visit 6 wks after hormonal contraceptives prescribed

Combined Estrogen and Progestin Contraceptive Methods

Mechanism of Action	Advantages	Side Effects	Contraindications
• Ovulatory suppression through inhibition of LH and FSH • Decidualization of endometrium • Thickening of cervical mucus resulting in decreased sperm penetration	• Highly effective • Reversible • Cycle regulation • Decreased dysmenorrhea and menorrhagia (less anemia) • Decreased benign breast disease and ovarian cyst development • Decreased risk of ovarian and endometrial cancer • Increased cervical mucus which may lower risk of STIs • Decreased PMS symptoms • Improved acne • Osteoporosis protection (possibly)	**Estrogen-related** • Nausea • Breast changes (tenderness, enlargement) • Fluid retention/bloating/edema • Weight gain (rare) • Migraine, headaches • Thromboembolic events • Liver adenoma (rare) • Breakthrough bleeding (low estradiol levels) **Progestin-related** • Amenorrhea/breakthrough bleeding • Headaches • Breast tenderness • Increased appetite • Decreased libido • Mood changes • Hypertension • Acne/oily skin* • Hirsutism* * Androgenic side effects may be minimized by prescribing formulation containing desogestrel, norgestimate, drospirenone or cyproterone acetate	**Absolute** • Known/suspected pregnancy • Undiagnosed abnormal vaginal bleeding • Prior thromboembolic events, thromboembolic disorders (Factor V Leiden mutation; protein C, S or antithrombin III deficiency), active thrombophlebitis • Cerebrovascular or coronary artery disease • Estrogen-dependent tumours (breast, uterus) • Impaired liver function associated with acute liver disease • Congenital hypertriglyceridemia • Smoker age >35 yrs • Migraines with focal neurological symptoms (excluding aura) • Uncontrolled hypertension **Relative** • Migraines – non-focal with aura <1 hour • Diabetes mellitus complicated by vascular disease • SLE • Controlled hypertension • Hyperlipidemia • Sickle cell anemia • Gallbladder disease **Drug Interactions/Risks** • Rifampin, phenobarbital, phenytoin and primidone can decrease efficacy, requiring use of back-up method • No evidence of fetal abnormalities if conceived on OCP • No evidence that OCP is harmful to nursing infant but may decrease milk production, not recommended until at least 6 wks postpartum

Reference: World Health Organization Guidelines for Oral Contraceptive Pill (OCP) Use

Missed Combined OCPs

Miss 1 pill	Miss 2 pills in a row during first 2 wks of the cycle	Miss 2 pills in a row during third wk of the cycle OR miss 3 in a row at any time
Take 1 pill as soon as patient remembers, and the next pill at the usual time OR 2 pills at the next dose	Take 2 pills the day patient remembers, and 2 pills the next day Then 1 pill per day until pack is finished Back-up method of birth control required during next 7 d	Throw out pack and start a new pack immediately Back-up method of birth control required during the next 7 d

Other Hormonal Methods

	Active Compounds	Route	Efficacy	Disadvantages	Advantages
Transdermal ('Ortho Evra®)	Continuous release of 6 mg norelgestromin and 0.60 mg ethinyl estradiol into bloodstream	• Patch applied to lower abdomen, back, upper arm, buttocks, NOT breast • Worn for 3 consecutive wks (changed every wk) with 1 wk break to allow for menstruation	• As effective as OCP in preventing pregnancy (>99% with perfect use)	• May be less effective in women >90 kg • May not be covered by drug plans	
Contraceptive Ring (Nuva Ring®)	Continuous release of etonogestrel 120 µg/d and estradiol 15 µg/d	• Thin flexible plastic ring inserted into vagina for 3 wks then removed for 1 wk to allow for menstruation	• As effective as OCP in preventing pregnancy (98%)	• Avoids first pass effect • Side effects: vaginal infection/ irritation, vaginal discharge	• May have better cycle control, i.e. decreased breakthrough bleeding

PROGESTIN-ONLY METHOD

Progestin Only Contraceptive Methods

Contraceptive	Mechanism of Action	Side Effects	Contraindications	Missed Doses
Suitable for postpartum women (does not affect breast milk supply) Women with contraindications to combined OCP (e.g. thromboembolic or myocardial disease) Women intolerant of estrogenic side effects of combined OCPs	Progestin prevents LH surge Thickening of cervical mucus Decrease tubal motility Endometrial decidualization Ovulation suppression – oral progestins (not IM) do not consistently suppress compared to combined OCPs	Irregular menstrual bleeding Weight gain Headache Breast tenderness Mood changes Functional ovarian cysts Acne/oily skin Hirsutism	**Absolute** None	IF MISSED PILL > 3 h: Use back-up contraceptive method for at least 48 h. Continue to take remainder of pills as prescribed IF MISSED DMPA (Depo-Provera®) >14 wks, do β–hCG, then give shot. No evidence of fetal abnormalities if conceived on DMPA

Selected Examples of Progestin-Only Methods

	Active Compounds	Timing of dose	Efficacy	Effect on menses	Disadvantages
Progestin-Only Pill ("minipill") Micronor®	0.35 mg norethindrone	Taken daily at same time of day to ensure reliable effect; no pill free interval	Higher failure rate (1.1-13% with typical use, 0.51% with perfect use) than other hormonal methods Highly effective if also post-partum breastfeeding	Ovulation inhibited in 60% of women; most have regular cycles (but may cause oligo/amenorrhea)	Higher failure rate than other hormonal methods Efficacy depends on reliable dosing
Depo-Provera®	Injectable depot medroxyprogesterone acetate Dose 150 mg IM q12-14wks	Initiate within 5 d of beginning of normal menses, immediately postpartum in breastfeeding and non-breastfeeding women	Highly effective 99%; failure rate 0.3%	Irregular spotting progresses to complete amenorrhea in 70% of women (after 1-2 yrs of use)	Decreased bone density (may be reversible) Restoration of fertility may take up to 1-2 yrs

Intrauterine Device (IUD)

IUD Contraceptive Methods

Mechanism of Action	Side Effects	Contraindications
Copper-containing IUD (Nova-T®): mild foreign body reaction in endometrium toxic to sperm and alters sperm motility **Progesterone-releasing IUD (Mirena®):** decidualization of endometrium and thickening of cervical mucus; minimal effect on ovulation Highly effective (95-99%); failure rate 0-1.2% Contraceptive effects last 5 yrs Reversible, private, convenient May be used in women with contraindications to OCPs or wanting long-term contraception	**Copper IUD:** increased blood loss and duration of menses, dysmenorrhea **Progesterone IUD:** bloating, headache **Both Copper and Progesterone IUD:** Breakthrough bleeding Expulsion (5% in the first yr, greatest in first month and in nulliparous women) Uterine wall perforation (1/1000) on insertion If pregnancy occurs with an IUD, increased risk of ectopic Increased risk of PID (within first 10 d of insertion only)	**Absolute** Known or suspected pregnancy Undiagnosed genital tract bleeding Acute or chronic PID Lifestyle risk for STIs* Known allergy to copper (copper IUD only) Wilson's disease (copper IUD only) **Relative** Valvular heart disease Past history of PID or ectopic pregnancy Presence of prosthesis Abnormalities of uterine cavity Severe dysmenorrhea or menorrhagia (copper IUD only) Cervical stenosis Immunnosuppressed individuals (e.g. HIV) Intracavitary fibroids

*Cervical swabs for gonorrhea and chlamydia should be done prior to IUD insertion

Emergency Postcoital Contraception (EPC)

Emergency Contraceptive Methods

	Mechanism of Action	Side Effects	Contraindications
HORMONAL **Yuzpe Method** Used within 72 h of unprotected intercourse; limited evidence of benefit up to 5 d Any OCP can be used as EPC: 100 µg ethinyl estradiol PO q12h x 2 doses E.g. Ovral® 2 tablets then repeat in 12 h (ethinyl estradiol 100 µg/levonorgestrel 500 µg) 2% overall risk of pregnancy Efficacy decreased with time (e.g. less effective at 72 h than 24 h)	Unknown; suggestions include: Suppresses ovulation or causes deficient luteal phase Alters endometrium to prevent implantation Affects sperm/ova transport	Nausea (due to estrogen; treat with Gravol®) Irregular spotting	Pre-existing pregnancy (although not teratogenic) Caution in women with contraindications to OCP (although NO absolute contraindications)
"Plan B" Consists of levonorgestrel 750 µg q12h for 2 doses (can also take 2 doses together); taken within 72 h of intercourse Greater efficacy (75-95% if used within 24 h) and better side effect profile than Yuzpe method but efficacy decreases with time. Efficacy decreases less than Yuzpe, so should be 1st choice If >24 h No estrogen thus very few contraindications/side effects (less nausea)			
NON-HORMONAL **Postcoital IUD (Copper)** Insert up to 7 d postcoitus Prevents implantation 1% failure rate Can use for short duration in higher risk individuals Mirena® IUD cannot be used as EPC	See *IUD Contraceptive Methods* above	See *IUD Contraceptive Methods* above	See *IUD Contraceptive Methods* above

Follow-up
- 3-4 wks post treatment to confirm efficacy (confirmed by spontaneous menses or pregnancy test)
- Contraception counseling

Common Medications

Drug Name (Brand Name)	Action	Dosing Schedule	Indications	Side Effects (S/E), Contraindications (C/I), Drug Interactions (D/I)
bromocriptine (Parlodel®)	Dopaminomimetic Agonist at D_2Rx Antagonist at D_1Rx Acts directly on anterior pituitary cells to inhibit synthesis and release of prolactin	**Initial**: 1.25-2.5 mg PO qhs with food **Then**: 2.5 mg PO bid with meals	Galactorrhea + amenorrhea 2° to hyperprolactinemia Prolactin-dependent menstrual disorders and infertility Prolactin-secreting adenomas (microadenomas, prior to surgery of macroadenomas)	**S/E**: nausea, vomiting, headache, postural hypotension, somnolence **C/I**: uncontrolled hypertension, pregnancy-induced hypertension, CAD **D/I**: domperidone, macrolides, octreotide
clomiphene citrate (Clomid®)	Increases output of pituitary gonadotropins which induces ovulation	50 mg PO daily x 5 d Try 100 mg PO daily if ineffective for 3 courses	Patients with persistent ovulatory dysfunction (e.g. amenorrhea, PCOS) who desire pregnancy	**S/E**: Common – hot flashes, abdominal discomfort, exaggerated cyclic ovarian enlargement, accentuation of Mittelschmerz Rare – ovarian hyperstimulation syndrome, multiple pregnancy, visual blurring, birth defects **C/I**: pregnancy, liver disease, hormone-dependent tumours, ovarian cyst, undiagnosed vaginal bleeding
clotrimazole (Canesten®)	Antifungal; disrupts fungal cell membrane	**Tablet**: 100 mg/d intravaginally x 7d or 500 mg PO x 1 dose **Cream** (1 or 2%): 1 applicator intravaginally qhs x 3-7d **Topical**: apply bid x 7d	Vulvovaginal candidiasis	**S/E**: vulvar/vaginal burning
danazol (Cyclomen® – CAN) (Danocrine® – US)	Synthetic steroid that inhibits pituitary gonadotropin output and ovarian steroid synthesis Has mild androgenic properties	200-800 mg PO in 2-3 divided doses Used for 3-6 months Biannual hepatic U/S required if >6 months use	Endometriosis 1° menorrhagia/DUB	**S/E**: weight gain, acne, mild hirsutism, hepatic dysfunction **C/I**: pregnancy, undiagnosed vaginal bleeding, breastfeeding, severely impaired renal/hepatic/cardiac function, porphyria, genital neoplasia **D/I**: warfarin, carbamazepine, cyclosporine, tacrolimus, anti-hypertensives
doxycycline	Tetracycline derivative; inhibits protein synthesis	100 mg PO bid x ≥7d	Chlamydia, gonococcal infection, syphillis	**S/E**: GI upset, hepatotoxicity **C/I**: pregnancy, severe hepatic dysfunction **D/I**: warfarin, digoxin
fluconazole (Diflucan®)	Antifungal; disrupts fungal cell membrane	150 mg PO x 1 dose	Vulvovaginal candidiasis unresponsive to clotrimazole	**S/E**: headache, rash, nausea, vomiting, abdominal pain, diarrhea **D/I**: terfenadine, cisapride, astemizole, hydrochlorothiazide, phenytoin, warfarin, rifampin
leuprolide (Lupron®)	Synthetic GnRH analog Induces reversible hypoestrogenic state	3.75 mg IM q1month or 11.25 mg IM q3months Usually ≤6 months, check bone density if >6 months	Endometriosis Leiomyomata DUB Precocious puberty	**S/E**: hot flashes, sweats, headache, vaginitis, reduction in bone density **C/I**: pregnancy, undiagnosed vaginal bleeding, breastfeeding
menotropin (Pergonal®)	Human Gonadotropin with FSH and LH effects; induces ovulation and stimulates ovarian follicle development	75-150 U of FSH and LH IM qd x 7-12d, then 10 000 U hCG one day after last dose	Infertility	**S/E**: bloating, irritation at injection site, abdominal/pelvic pain, headache, nausea and vomiting **C/I**: primary ovarian failure, intracranial lesion (e.g. pituitary tumour), uncontrolled thyroid/adrenal dysfunction, ovarian cyst (not PCOS), pregnancy
oxybutinin (Ditropan®)	Anticholinergic – relaxes bladder smooth muscle, inhibits involuntary detrusor contraction		Overactive bladder (urge incontinence)	**S/E**: dry mouth/eyes, constipation, palpitations, urinary retention **C/I**: glaucoma, GI ileus, severe colitis, obstructive uropathy, use with caution if impaired hepatic/renal function

Drug Name (Brand Name)	Action	Dosing Schedule	Indications	Side Effects (S/E), Contraindications (C/I), Drug Interactions (D/I)
tolterodine (Detrol®)	Anticholinergic		Overactive bladder (urge incontinence)	**S/E**: anaphylaxis, psychosis, tachycardia, dry mouth/eyes, headache, constipation, urinary retention, chest pain **C/I**: glaucoma, gastric/urinary retention, use with caution if impaired hepatic/renal function
tranexamic acid (Cyklokapron®)	Anti-fibrinolytic, reversibly inhibits plasminogen activation		Menorrhagia Rare cases of thrombosis	**S/E**: nausea, vomiting, diarrhea, dizziness **C/I**: thromboembolic disease, acquired disturbances of colour vision, subarachnoid hemorrhage, age <15 yrs
urofollitropin (Metrodin®)	FSH		Ovulation induction in PCOS	**S/E**: ovarian enlargement or cysts, edema and pain at injection site, arterial thromboembolism, fever, abdominal pain **C/I**: primary ovarian failure, intracranial lesion (e.g. pituitary tumour), uncontrolled thyroid/adrenal dysfunction, ovarian cyst (not PCOS), pregnancy

Hematology

Approach to Common Bloodwork

COMPLETE BLOOD COUNT
- Red blood cells (RBC): count of actual RBCs per volume of blood
  - If low: see *Approach to Anemia*
  - If high: spurious erythrocytosis, reticulocytosis, polycythemia vera (PV), secondary polycythemia (e.g. hypoxia, CO poisoning, renal cell carcinoma, renal artery stenosis)
- Hemoglobin (Hb): concentration of oxygen-carrying protein in blood
  - If low: see *Approach to Anemia*
  - If high: see *Differential for Increased RBC*
- Hematocrit (Hct): % of blood volume occupied by packed RBCs
  - If low: see *Approach to Anemia*
  - If high: profound diuresis, hemoconcentration (burn injury, trauma, shock) or see *Differential for Increased RBC*
- Mean corpuscular volume (MCV): measurement of RBC size
- Red cell distribution width (RDW): measurement of variability of RBC size
  - If high: combined nutritional deficiency (Fe, folate, B_{12}), reticulocytosis, immune hemolytic anemia, liver disease
- White blood cells (WBC): count of actual WBCs per volume of blood; differential includes neutrophils, lymphocytes, eosinophils, basophils and monocytes; flags presence of abnormal cells including blasts, reactive lymphocytes, lymphoma cells, mononuclear granulocytes
- Platelets (PLT): count of actual platelets per volume of blood
  - If low: see *Approach to Thrombocytopenia*
  - If high: reactive thrombocytosis, myeloproliferative neoplasm

BLOOD FILM INTERPRETATION

Red Blood Cells
- Size
  - Microcytic (MCV <80), normocytic (80< MCV <100) or macrocytic (MCV >100)
  - Normocytic RBC: approximately the size of the nucleus of a lymphocyte
  - Anisocytosis: RBCs of variable sizes
- Colour
  - Hypochromic: central pallor more than 1/3 of the RBC diameter as seen in iron deficiency and sideroblastosis
  - Hyperchromic: increase in blue cells as in megaloblastic anemia, spherocytosis and increased marrow production
- Shape
  - Normal: biconcave disc or discocyte
  - Poikilocytosis: abnormal degree in variation of RBC shape
  - Spherocyte: spherical RBC with loss of central pallor due to hereditary spherocytosis or immune hemolytic anemia
  - Elliptocyte (ovalcyte): elongated RBC due to hereditary elliptocytosis, megaloblastic anemia or iron deficiency
  - Schistocyte (helmet cell): fragmented cell from traumatic disruption of its membrane due to microangiopathic hemolytic anemias (e.g. TTP, DIC, vasculitis or glomerulonephritis) or prosthetic heart valves
  - Codocyte (target cell): cell with "bull's eye" appearance due to liver disease, Hb S and C, thalassemia, Fe deficiency

- Dacrocyte (teardrop cell): cell with a single pointed end due to myelofibrosis, extramedullary hematopoeisis
    - Acanthocyte (spur cell): RBC with multiple, irregularly-distributed cytoplasmic projections due to severe liver disease, starvation/anorexia, post-splenectomy
    - Echinocyte (burr cell): RBC with multiple indentations (shrivelled) due to uremia or artifact
- Distribution
    - Rouleaux formation: RBC aggregates resembling a stack of coins due to artifact, multiple myeloma, macroglobinemia, tissues disorders, inflammatory conditions, pregnancy
- Inclusions
    - Nucleated: immature RBCs, extramedullary hematopoiesis, hypoxia or hemolysis
    - Heinz bodies: denatured and precipitated Hb due to G6PD deficiency
    - Howell-Jolly bodies: small nuclear remnant due to asplenism, hemolytic anemia, megaloblastic anemia
    - Basophilic stippling: deep blue granulations of variable size and number (RNA aggregations) due to lead intoxication, thalassemia, hemolysis, megaloblastic anemia or hereditary cause

White Blood Cells
- Lymphocytes: usually comprise 30-40% of white cells
    - Reed-Sternberg (RS) cell: giant, multinucleated B-lymphocyte of Hodgkin's lymphoma **not circulating – seen in lymph nodes
    - Smudge cells: lymphocytes damaged during preparation of blood smear indicating cell fragility; seen in chronic lymphocytic leukemia (CLL) and other lymphoproliferative disorders
    - Granulocytes: consist of neutrophils, monocytes, eosinophils
    - Neutrophils: usually only mature and band (immediate precursor) neutrophils with 3-4 lobed nuclei in peripheral blood
    - Hypersegmented neutrophils (>5 lobes): megaloblastic, iron deficiency anemia, myelodysplasia (MDS)
    - Pelger-Huet (< 2 lobes): "pinced nez" appearance seen in Pelget-Huet abnormality or MDS

TESTS OF HEMOSTASIS

Prothrombin Time (PT), International Normalized Ratio (INR)
- Measures extrinsic pathway (factor VII) and common pathway; INR validated only for use to monitor warfarin therapy
- If high: Factor VII deficiency, warfarin use, vitamin K deficiency, DIC, liver disease

Partial Thromboplastin Time (PTT)
- Measures intrinsic pathway (factors VIII, IX, XI, XII) and common pathway; used to monitor heparin therapy and intrinsic pathway factors
- If high: Factor VIII and IX deficiencies (e.g. hemophilias A and B), DIC, liver disease, von Willebrand's disease, nephrotic syndrome, heparin use, lupus anti-coagulant, factor inhibitor

Common Presentations

Anemia

Approach to Anemia

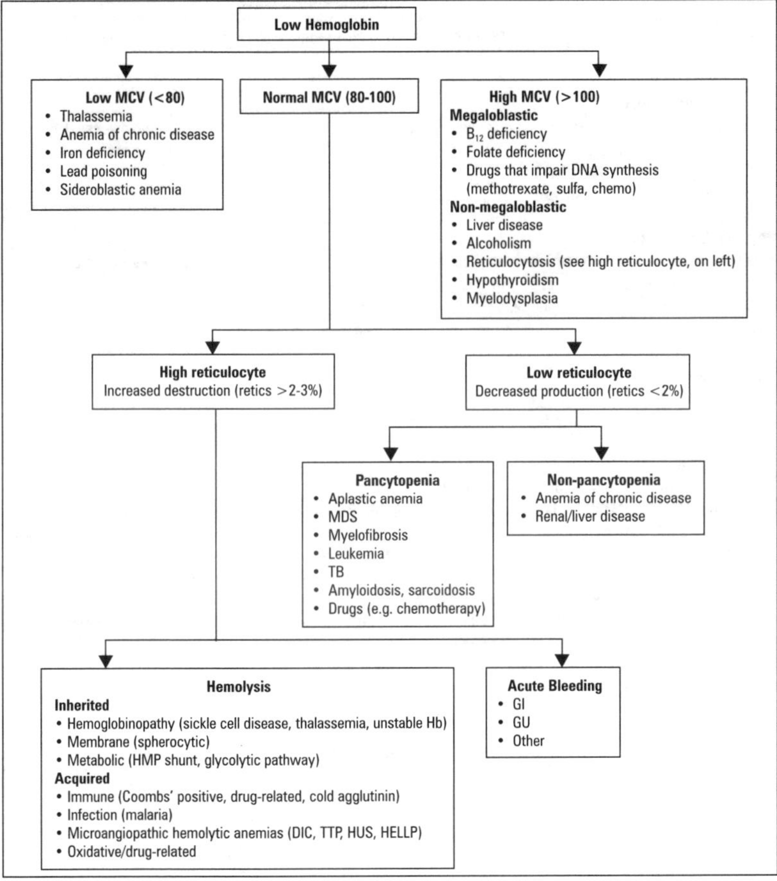

Definition

• Hb <135 g/L in males or <120 g/L in females

History

• Ethnicity, recent blood loss (e.g. blood donation, surgery, trauma, menstrual history), recent blood transfusion, signs of hemolysis (e.g. jaundice, dark urine), rule out GI bleed (e.g. melena, BRBPR), personal or family history of anemia and treatments, chronic diseases, medications, diet, alcohol consumption

Associated Symptoms
- Fatigue, weakness, exercise intolerance, syncope, dyspnea, headache, palpitations, postural dizziness, tinnitus, feeling cold, confusion, difficulty with concentration

Predisposing Factors
- Mediterranean/Asian (thalassemia) or African (sickle cell) descent, active bleeding or recent blood loss, medications (chemotherapy, methotrexate, anti-retrovirals), excessive alcohol consumption, lead exposure
- Diet: Low in leafy, green vegetables (folate deficiency), vegan (vitamin B_{12} deficiency), "tea and toast" (Fe deficiency)

Past Medical History
- Chronic disease: malignancy, infections, inflammatory conditions, rheumatic disease, renal disease, liver disease, endocrine disorders
- Malabsorption: IBD, celiac disease
- Occult blood loss: PUD, ASA use, GI malignancy

Physical Examination
- HEENT: pallor of mucous membranes and conjunctiva, icterus (hemolysis), glossitis (nutrient deficiencies), thyroid abnormalities, orbital bruits (Hb <50)
- CVS: tachycardia, postural hypotension, systolic flow murmur, wide pulse pressure
- GI: hepatosplenomegaly (thalassemia, neoplasm, chronic hemolysis, hereditary spherocytosis), digital rectal exam (for occult blood)
- Derm: pallor in skin creases, jaundice (hemolysis), telangiectasia (hemolysis), koilonychias (Fe deficiency), petechiae and purpura (bleeding disorder)
- Neuro: decreased vibration and proprioception, numbness, parasthesias, ataxia (all severe B_{12} deficiency)

Investigations
- CBC, MCV, reticulocytes, blood film, PT/INR, PTT, consider TSH
- If microcytic anemia (MCV <80): ferritin – if ferritin in "grey zone" or high index of suspicion then consider serum Fe, TIBC, transferrin saturation, soluble transferrin receptor, bone marrow stain for iron (gold standard), Hb electrophoresis for thalassemia, GI endoscopy for occult bleeding/malignancy
- If macrocytic anemia (MCV >100): RBC folate, serum B_{12}, Ab to intrinsic factor (note: must rule out B_{12} deficiency before initiating folate replacement)
- If normocytic anemia (80< MCV <100): LDH, bilirubin, haptoglobin, Coombs' test, Hb electrophoresis and genetic analysis for thalassemia or sickle cell (see *Hemolysis Studies*)

Approach to Microcytic Anemia

	Lab Tests				Blood Film
	Ferritin	Serum Iron	TIBC	RDW	
Iron-Deficiency Anemia	↓↓	↓	↑	↑ (>15)	• Hypochromic, microcytic
Anemia of Chronic Disease	N/↑	↓	↓	N	• Normocytic/microcytic
Sideroblastic Anemia	N/↑	↑	N	↑	• Dual population • Basophilic stippling
Thalassemia	N/↑	N/↑	N	N/↑	• Hypochromic, microcytic • Basophilic stippling • Poikilocytosis

Medications for Anemia

Drug	Common Formulary	Mechanism of Action	Dosing Schedule	Indications	Contraindications	Side Effects
iron	Iron gluconate Iron sulphate Iron fumarate Palafer® Femiron®	Synthesis of hemoglobin	2-3 mg/kg/d of elemental iron in 3 divided doses PO	Iron deficiency anemia treatment and prevention Pregnancy	Iron overload	In children: acute iron toxicity Constipation
B$_{12}$	cyanocobalamin hydroxycobalamin Bedoz® Cobex®	Synthesis of folic acid and DNA	Up to 1000 µg/d PO	B$_{12}$ deficiency	Hypersensitivity	Diarrhea
folic acid	Folic acid Novo Folacid® Folvite®	Synthesis of purines and thymidylate, thus DNA	up to 5 mg/d PO	Folic acid deficiency Pregnancy	Uncorrected pernicious anemia	Rash
erythropoietin	epoetin Epogen® Eprex® dabrepoetin Aranesp®	Stimulation of RBC synthesis	50-1000 U/kg SC/IV, 3 times weekly	Renal failure Marrow failure Autologous blood donation	Uncontrolled hypertension Myelodysplastic syndrome	Hypertension

Thrombocytopenia

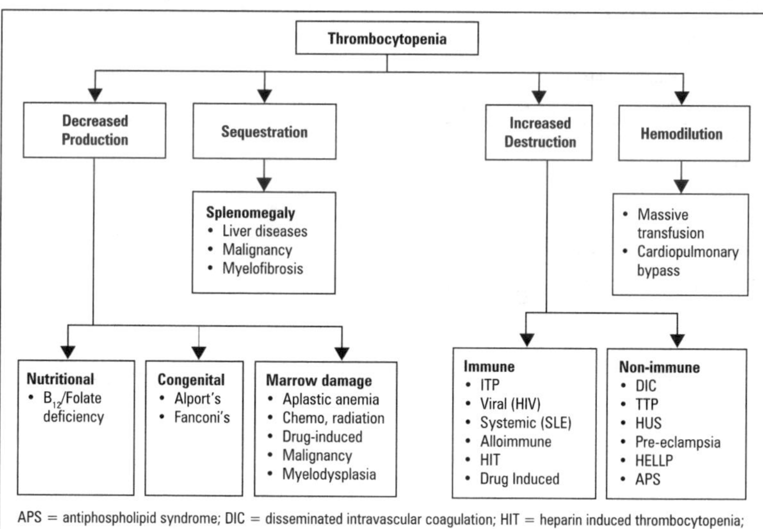

APS = antiphospholipid syndrome; DIC = disseminated intravascular coagulation; HIT = heparin induced thrombocytopenia; HUS = hemolytic uremic syndrome; ITP = idiopathic thrombocytopenic purpura; TTP = thrombotic thrombocytopenic purpura

Splenomegaly

Differential Diagnosis of Splenomegaly

Increased Demand for Splenic Function			Congestive	Infiltrative
Hematological	**Infectious**	**Inflammatory**	**Cirrhosis**	**Non-malignant**
Spherocytosis	CMV	Felty syndrome	Splenic vein thrombosis	Benign metaplasia
Hemoglobinopathies	Bacterial endocarditis	Still's disease	Portal vein obstruction	Amyloidosis, sarcoidosis
Hemolysis	TB	SLE	Portal HTN (including	Lysosomal storage diseases
Sequestration crisis	HIV/AIDS	Sarcoidosis	right heart failure)	(Gaucher's, Niemann-Pick)
Nutritional anemias	EBV			Glycogen storage diseases
Elliptocytosis	Malaria			
	Histoplasmosis			**Malignant**
	Leishmaniasis			Leukemia (CML)
				Lymphoproliferative disease
				Hodgkin lymphoma
				Myeloproliferative disorders
				Metastatic tumour

Lymphadenopathy

History
- Enlarged lymph nodes, swelling of extremities, family/personal history of malignancy, chronic inflammatory diseases, recent infection, TB history, sexual history (STIs), occupational history (infection, carcinogens)
- Constitutional symptoms
- Previous surgeries, medications
- Joint pain, swelling, rashes (connective tissue disease)

Differentiating Inflammatory vs. Neoplastic Lymph Nodes

Feature	Inflammatory Nodes	Neoplastic
Consistency	Rubbery	Firm/hard
Mobility	Mobile	Matted/Immobile
Tenderness	Tender	Non-tender
Size	<2 cm	>2 cm

* Note: these classifications are not absolute; lymphoma and CLL nodes can feel rubbery and are frequently mobile, non-tender

Differential Diagnosis of Generalized Lymphadenopathy

Reactive	Inflammatory	Neoplastic
Bacterial (TB, Lyme, Cat-scratch disease)	Autoimmune (RA, SLE)	Lymphoma
Viral (EBV, CMV, HIV)	Drug hypersensitivity	Lymphocytic leukemias
Parasitic (toxoplasmosis)	Sarcoidosis	Metastatic cancer
Fungal (histoplasmosis)	Amyloidosis	Histiocytosis X
	Serum sickness	

Common Conditions

Disorders of Primary Hemostasis

IMMUNE THROMBOCYTOPENIC PURPURA (ITP)

Etiology
- Anti-platelet antibodies → increased splenic destruction and clearence

Clinical Features
- Mucosal and skin bleeding, epistaxis, menorrhagia, no splenomegaly

Investigations
- Diagnosis of exclusion; normal PT and PTT, numerous of megakaryocytes in BM (note: BM biopsy is a critical test to rule out other causes of thrombocytopenia like myelodysplasia in people >60 yrs old)

Management
- Conservative with steroids or IVIG; splenectomy if refractory
- Platelet transfusion does NOT assist therapy
- Major concern is cerebral hemorrhage at platelet counts $<5 \times 10^9$/L

HEPARIN INDUCED THROMBOCYTOPENIA (HIT)

Diagnosis
- 50% reduction in platelets while on heparin within 5-15 d of initiation (if previously exposed to heparin, HIT can develop in hours)

Etiology
- Non-immune (heparin-associated thrombocytopenia) versus immune-mediated (heparin-induced thrombocytopenia)

Clinical Features
- Arterial thrombosis (MI, stroke, limb and mesenteric arteries, adrenal gland involvement), venous thrombosis (DVT, PE), heparin-induced skin necrosis, acute platelet activation syndromes (fever/chills, flushing, etc.), transient global amnesia
- Bleeding is uncommon

Investigations
- ELISA for HIT-Ig (most sensitive) or serotonin release assay

Management
- Discontinue heparin and use alternative agent for anti-coagulation (argatroban, danaparoid)

HEMOLYTIC UREMIC SYNDROME (HUS)

Etiology
- Shiga toxin (*E. coli* serotype 0157:H7)

Clinical Features
- Severe thrombocytopenia (primarly in children):
  1. Purpura, epistaxis, GI bleed, hematuria, hemoptysis
  2. Mircroangiopathic haemolytic anemia (MAHA)
  3. Renal failure (abnormal urinalysis, oliguria, ARF)

Investigations
- As per TTP, stool C&S

Management
- Plasmapheresis ± steroids or plasma infusion if not available, platelets contraindicated

THROMBOTIC THROMBOCYTOPENIC PURPURA (TTP)

Epidemiology
- Predominantly adults

Etiology
- Deficiency of metalloproteinase that breaks down vWF multimers; may be congenital (genetic absence of ADAMTS-13) or acquired (drugs), malignancy, transplant, HIV-associated, idiopathic

Clinical Features
- Pentad of 1) thrombocytopenia, 2) microangiopathic hemolytic anemia (MAHA), 3) fever, 4) renal failure, 5) neurological symptoms (H/A, confusion, focal defects, seizures) – full pentad is rare in a single patient
- If #1 and #2 are present with suggestive history, one can consider management with plasmapharesis presumptively because of the high cure rate vs. high mortality for those not treated with plasma exchange

Investigations
- CBC, blood film (schistocytes and decreased platelets), normal PT/PTT, normal fibrinogen, Cr, urea; unconjugated bilirubin (↑), LDH (↑), haptoglobin (↓), negative Coombs' test, ADAMTS13 assay

Management
- Plasmapheresis ± steroids or plasma infusion if not available, platelets contraindicated
- 90% mortality if untreated

Disorders of Secondary Hemostasis

Classification of Secondary Hemostasis Disorders

Hereditary	Acquired
Factor VIII: Hemophilia A, vWD	Liver disease
Factor IX: Hemophilia B (Christmas Disease)	DIC
Factor XI	Vitamin K deficiency
Other factor deficiencies are rare	Acquired inhibitors

Screening Test Abnormalities in Coagulopathies

Increased INR Only	Increased PTT Only	Increased Both
Factor VII deficiency	Hemophilia A and B	Prothrombin deficiency
Vitamin K deficiency	vWD	Fibrinogen deficiency
Warfarin	Heparin	Factor V and X deficiency
Liver disease	Antiphospholipid Ab	Severe liver disease
Factor VII inhibitors	Factor inhibitors	Factor V and X, prothrombin, and fibrinogen inhibitors
DIC	F XI/XII deficiency	Excessive anticoagulation

DISSEMINATED INTRAVASCULAR COAGULATION (DIC)

Definition
- An acquired syndrome characterized by the intravascular activation of coagulation with loss of localization arising from different causes
- Can originate from and cause damage to the microvasculature, can produce organ dysfunction
- Hemorrhage or thrombotic events may occur

Etiology
- Trauma, shock, infection, malignancy, obstetric complications

Clinical Features
- Spectrum of both bleeding (intracranial bleeding, ecchymosis, hematuria, epistaxis, massive bleeding) and thrombosis (multifocal brain infarcts, superficial gangrene, oliguria, ARDS, acute GI ulceration, MAHA)

Investigations
- ↓ platelets, MAHA, ↑ INR, ↑ aPTT, ↓ fibrinogen, ↑ FDPs, ↑ D-dimers, short euglobin lysis time, extent of fibrin deposition (urine output, urea, RBC fragmentation)

Management
- Treat underlying disorder, replacement of hemostatic elements with platelet transfusion, FP, cryoprecipitate

Anticoagulant Therapy

VENOUS THROMBOEMBOLISM PROPHYLAXIS
- Consider for those with a moderate to high risk of thrombosis without contraindications
- Non-pharmacological measures include: early ambulation, elastic compression stockings (TEDs), intermittent pneumatic compression (IPC)
- UFH 5000 IU SC bid for moderate risk
- UFH 5000 IU SC tid or enoxaparin 40 mg SC OD for high risk

RISK OF VTE IN HOSPITALIZED PATIENTS
- Low risk surgical patients: <40 yrs, no risk factors for VTE, general anesthetic (GA) <30 min, minor elective, abdominal or thoracic surgery.
- Moderate risk surgical patients: >40 yrs, >1 risk factor for VTE, GA >30 min
- High risk surgical patients: >40 yrs, surgery for malignancy or lower extremity orthopedic surgery lasting >30 min, inhibitors deficiency or other risk factor
- High risk medical patients: heart failure, severe respiratory disease, ischemic stroke and lower limb paralysis, confined to bed and have >1 additional risk factor (e.g. active cancer, previous VTE, sepsis, acute neurological disease, IBD)

CONTRAINDICIATIONS

Absolute Contraindications
- Active bleeding, severe bleeding diathesis or platelet count $<20 \times 10^9/L$ ($<20,000/mm^3$), intracranial bleeding, neurosurgery or ocular surgery within 10 d

Relative Contraindications
- Mild-moderate bleeding diathesis or thrombocytopenia, brain metastases, recent major trauma, major abdominal surgery within the past 2 d, GI or GU bleeding within 14 d, endocarditis, severe hypertension (sBP >200 or DBP >120), recent stroke

COMPARISON OF HEPARIN AND WARFARIN

	Heparin	Warfarin
Structure	Large anionic polymer, acidic	Small lipid soluble molecule
Route Administration	Parenteral (IV, SC)	Oral (PO)
Site of Action	Blood (via Antithrombin)	Liver
Onset	Rapid (seconds)	Slow (limited by half-life of clotting factors)
Mechanism	Accelerates activity of Antithrombin	Vitamin K antagonist, inhibits production of II, VII, IX, X, Protein C and S
Duration of Action	Acute (hours)	Chronic (days)
Acute Overdose	Protamine sulphate	IV Vitamin K + FFP
Monitoring	aPTT (intrinsic pathway)	PT/INR (extrinsic pathway)
Pregnancy	Safe (does not cross placenta)	Not used (can cross placenta), teratogenic

ADVERSE REACTIONS OF HEPARIN
- Hemorrhage: depends on dose, age, concomitant use of antiplatelet agents or thrombolytics
- Heparin-induced thrombocytopenia: associated with venous or arterial thrombosis
- Osteoporosis: with long term use

Hematologic Malignancies

Overview of Hematologic Malignancies

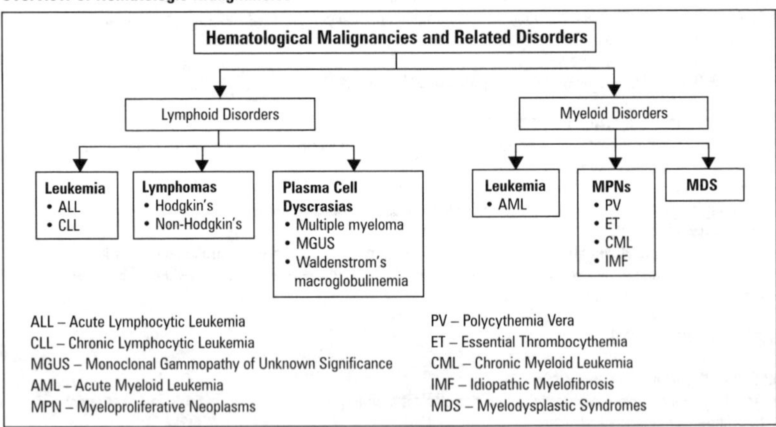

ACUTE MYELOID LEUKEMIA

Definition
- Rapidly progressive malignancy characterized by failure of myeloid cells to differentiate beyond blast stage
- Subtypes are characterized by genetic abnormality or lineage affected.

Risk Factors
- MDS, benzene, radiation, previous chemotherapy (alkylating agents)

Clinical Features
- Pancytopenia, fatigue, infection, easy bruising and bleeding, bony tenderness (infiltration of the bone marrow)

Investigations
- CBC + differential, electrolytes, uric acid, LDH, peripheral blood smear (Auer rods), bone marrow aspirate (Blasts >20%, cytogenetics and immunophenotyping), markers of renal and liver function
- Tumour lysis syndrome: hyperuricemia, hyperkalemia, hyperphosphatemia, hypocalcemia

Treatment
- All AML treated similarly except promyelocytic variant (APL) which is treated with all trans retinoic acid (ATRA)
- Induction therapy: several regimens (e.g. cytarabine + anthracycline)
- Consolidation: treatment varies depending on prognosis, in general consists of high dose chemotherapy followed by either autologous or allogeneic hematopoietic cell transplant

MYELODYSPLASTIC SYNDROMES (MDS)

Definition
- Heterogeneous group of malignant stem cell disorders characterized by dysplastic and ineffective blood cell production, resulting in peripheral cytopenias
- Diagnosis: anemia ± thrombocytopenia ± neutropenia
- Dependent on subclassification, risk of transformation to AML ranges from 5-15% in pts with RA or RARS to 40-50% for those with RAEB
- Most patients die of progressive bone marrow failure rather than transformation to leukemia

Risk Factors
- Elderly, post-chemo, benzene or radiation exposure

Clinical Features
- Insidious onset of fatigue, weakness, pallor, infections, bruising, epistaxis
- RARELY weight loss, fever, HSM

Investigations
- CBC, peripheral blood film: macrocytic anemia (macro-ovalocytes), decreased reticulocytes
- WBC: decreased granulocytes, abnormal morphology (e.g. bilobed or unsegmented nuclei called "Pelger Huet cells")
- Platelets: thrombocytopenia, size/cytoplasm abnormalities (hypogranular)
- BM aspirate and biopsy with cytogenetic analysis required for definitive diagnosis
- BM (normocellular/hyper/hypocellular, ± micromegakaryocytes, fibrosis (10%)
- Cytogenetics – partial/total loss of chromosomes 5, 7, Y, or trisomy 8

Treatment (depends on risk of progression to acute leukemia)
- Low risk (<5% blasts in marrow): supportive, weekly Epo SC, hematopoietic growth factors (G-CSF, GM-CSF)
- High risk (>5% blasts in marrow): supportive, chemotherapy, allo stem cell transplantation

MYELOPROLIFERATIVE NEOPLASMS

Definition and Features
- Clonal myeloid stem cell abnormalities leading to qualitative and quantitative changes in erythroid, myeloid and platelet cells
- Includes polycythemia vera (PV), chronic myeloid leukemia (CML), idiopathic myelofibrosis (IMF) and essential thrombocythemia (ET)
- Mostly middle-aged and older patients (peak 60-80 yrs)
- May develop marrow fibrosis with time
- All disorders may progress to AML

Chronic Myeloproliferative Disorders

	PV	CML	IMF	ET
Hct	↑↑	↓/N	↓	N
WBC	↑	↑↑	↑/↓	N
Plt	↑	↑/↓	↑/↓	↑↑↑
Marrow fibrosis	±	±	+++	±
Splenomegaly	+	+++	+++	+
Hepatomegaly	+	+	++	−
Genetic Assoc.	JAK2 mut. (95%)	Bcr-Abl mut. (90+%)	JAK2 mut. (~50%)	JAK2 mut. (~50%)

PV = polycythemia vera   CML = chronic myeloid leukemia   IMF = idiopathic myelofibrosis   ET = essential thrombocythemia

ACUTE LYMPHOCYTIC LEUKEMIA

Definition
- Bone marrow malignancy in which early lymphoid cells proliferate and replace normal hematopoietic cells of the marrow. Two main subtypes: B-cell and T-cell

Epidemiology
- Most common cancer in childhood, peak incidence between 2-5 yrs old, associated with some genetic syndromes (Trisomy 21, NF1)
- Can also occur in adults

Clinical Features
- Generalized fatigue and infections from pancytopenia. Features of organ infiltration include tender bones, lymphadenopathy, hepatosplenomegaly, and meningeal signs (CNS involvement)

Investigations
- Similar to AML, except morphology on peripheral smear is distinctly different
- Bone marrow aspirate for immunophenotyping and cytogenetics (BCR-ABL +ve in 25% of adult ALL)
- CXR to assess for mediastinal mass and LP to look for CNS involvement

Treatment
- Induction: to induce complete remission using chemotherapeutic agents both systemically and intrathecally
- Consolidation/intensification: high dose chemotherapy to eliminate resistant cells
- Maintenance (2-3 yrs) to prevent relapse
- CNS radiation or methotrexate prophylaxis
- Allogeneic hematopoietic cell transplant in select cases (especially for patients who have relapsed)

LYMPHOMA

Definition
- Malignant T- or B-lymphocytes accumulate in lymph nodes and lymphoid tissues
- Two main divisions: Hodgkin Lymphoma (HL) and Non-Hodgkin Lymphoma (NHL, many histological subtypes)
- Hodgkin Lymphoma is characterized by Reed-Sternberg cells (multinucleated giant cells)

Risk Factors
- NHL: immunodeficiency, autoimmune diseases, infections (EBV)

Clinical Features
- Asymptomatic lymphadenopathy
- Splenomegaly ± hepatomegaly
- B symptoms (unexplained fever >38°C, unexplained weight loss, night sweats)
- HL features: pruritis, cervical, mediastinal & retroperitoneal nodes
- NHL: extranodal involvement – GI tract, testes, bone, kidney, CNS

Investigations
- CBC + diff, peripheral smear, uric acid, LDH, liver enzymes
- CXR, CT chest, pelvis, abdomen for staging
- LN excisional biopsy and BM biopsy to assess involvement

Treatment
- HL: Chemotherapy (adriamycin, bleomycin, vinblastine, dacarbazine) + radiation
- NHL: varies with histological subtype, indolent types: watchful waiting, radiation for local disease, chemo for advanced disease
- Aggressive NHL: chemotherapy CHOP + rituximab if B-cell

MULTIPLE MYELOMA

Etiology
- Malignant proliferation of plasma cells producing a monoclonal Ig; either M protein (heavy + light chain, 80%) or light chain only (20%). 1-2% are non secretory

Clinical Features
- **CRAB** (hyper**C**alcemia, **R**enal insufficiency, **A**nemia, **B**ony disease – related to myeloma) or evidence of lymphoma

Investigations
- SPEP, 24 hour UPEP, immunofixation, free light chains, CBC (normocytic anemia, thrombocytopenia, leukopenia), electrolytes and renal function (Cr may be incr.), calcium (incr.), ESR (incr.), bone marrow biopsy (often focal abnormality, greater than 10% plasma cells, abnormal morphology, clonal plasma cells), skeletal series (lytic lesions, areas at risk of pathologic fracture). $\beta2$ microglobulin and albumin for staging

Management
- Chemotherapy (on a backbone of steroids), bisphosphonates (osteoporosis, lytic bone lesions, severe hypercalcemia), radiation, stem cell transplant
- Treat complications: hydration for hypercalcemia and renal failure, bisphosphonates (e.g. pamidronate) for severe hypercalcemia, prophylactic antibiotics (if on high dose steroids), prophylactic anticoagulation (dependent on therapy as high risk of DVT/PE), erythropoietin for anemia

MONOCLONAL GAMMOPATHY OF UNKONWN SIGNIFICANCE (MGUS)

Definition
- Presence of M protein in serum in absence of any clinical or laboratory evidence of myeloma or lymphoproliferative disorder (MGUS is a plasma cell dyscrasia)
- May undergo malignant transformation (1% per year or higher if IgM MGUS, cumulative risk)

Diagnosis
- Presence of serum M-protein at a concentration <30 g/L, <10% plasma cells in BM, absence of **CRAB** (hyper**C**alcemia, **R**enal insufficiency, **A**nemia, **B**ony disease – related to myeloma) or evidence of lymphoma

WALDENSTROM'S MACROGLOBULINEMIA

Definition
- Proliferation of lymphoplasmacytoid cells → secrete large quantities of monoclonal IgM

Clinical Features
- Sx: weakness, fatigue, bleeding (oronasal), weight loss, recurrent infections, dyspnea, CHF, neuro sx
- Signs: pallor, HSM, lymphadenopathy, retinal lesions
- Complication: hyperviscosity syndrome

Investigations and Diagnosis
- Normocytic anemia, rouleaux, high ESR, serum viscosity
- BM: plasmacytoid lymphocytes
- Cold hemagglutinin disease (possible) – Reynaud's phenomenon, hemolytic anemia precipitated by cold weather

Blood Products and Common Medications

Blood Products and Transfusion

PACKED RED BLOOD CELLS (pRBCs)
- **Indications**
  - Keep Hb >70 g/L in acute blood loss, critical care and perioperatively; higher target in those with ischemic heart disease, impaired pulmonary function, increased oxygen consumption and uncontrolled, unpredictable bleeding although unlikely benefit with Hb >100 g/L; in chronic anemia, goal is to keep the Hb concentration above the lowest level that produces symptoms
- **Reactions**
  - Early: most common to least common are allergic, febrile non-hemolytic, TACO, TRALI, ABO-incompatability, bacterial sepsis
  - Late: infection (HBV, HCV, HIV, HTLV, West Nile virus), delayed hemolytic transfusion reaction, iron overload, transfusion-associated graft versus host disease (GVHD)

PLATELETS
- **Indications**
  - Platelets <10 x 10^9 or ITP and bleeding; platelets <50 x 10^9 and bleeding from minor procedures or upcoming major surgery; platelets <100 x 10^9 and neurosurgery or head trauma; any platelet count with platelet dysfunction and marked bleeding
- **Possible Reactions**: bacterial sepsis (1:10,000) and same for RBC transfusion

FROZEN PLASMA (FP)
- **Indications**
  - Emergent warfarin reversal, active bleeding or major surgery with PT/PTT >1.5x normal

PROTHROMBIN COMPLEX CONCENTRATES (PCC Octaplex)
- Plasma derivative (from pooled human plasma) containing coagulation factors II, VII, IX, and X as well as Protein C and S. Also contains heparin as a non-medicinal ingredient
- Indicated for the **Urgent** reversal of warfarin (Coumadin®) therapy with INR greater than 1.5. Examples would include intracranial bleeds, emergency surgery and life-threatening bleeding
- Note: PCC- Octaplex is a **warfarin/vit K deficiency antidote** and will not work with other coagulation disorders (bleeding after trauma, liver disease)

CRYOPRECIPITATE (Fibrinogen, vWF and Factor VIII)
- Indications: microvascular bleeding in patients with a fibrinogen concentration <0.8-1.0 g/L (usually trauma or severe obstetrical bleeding or DIC)

Antiplatelet Therapy

ASPIRIN (ASA)
- Irreversibly acetylates COX enzyme, inhibiting TXA2 synthesis, thus inhibiting platelet aggregation
- ASA is currently indicated for:
  - Stroke and MI prophylaxis
  - To reduce the incidence of recurrent MI
  - To decrease mortality in post-MI patients
- Dosage: single loading dose of 200-300 mg, followed by daily dose of 75-100 mg PO OD

AGGRENOX®
- Combination of ASA and dipyridamole
- Dipyridamole increase intracellular cAMP levels which inhibits TXA2 synthesis, leading to decreased platelet aggregation
- Aggrenox® is more effective than aspirin in secondary prevention of stroke
- Dosage: ASA/dipyridamole (25/200 ER), 1 cap PO bid

CLOPIDOGREL (Plavix®)
- ADP activates GP IIb/IIIa, allowing platelets to bind to fibrinogen and aggregate
- Clopidogrel and ticlopidine (Ticlid®) inhibit ADP binding to platelets, thus inhibiting aggregation
- Useful for prevention of cardiovascular events in high-risk patients
- Clopidogrel may cause TTP
- Ticlodipine (Ticlid®) is associated with a risk of agranulocytosis and is rarely used
- Dosage: 75 mg PO OD; for ACS, start 300 mg PO x 1 dose then 75 mg PO OD

GLYCOPROTEIN IIb/IIIa INHIBITORS
- Reopro® (abciximab), Integrelin® (eptifibatide), Aggrastat® (tirofiban)
- Blocking GP IIb/IIIa receptor inhibits fibrinogen and vWF binding, leading to decreased platelet aggregation
- Used most commonly in patients undergoing cardiac catheterization

Infectious Diseases

Common Conditions

Meningitis

Etiology	Neonates: *E. coli*, GBS, *L. monocytogenes* Infants/Children/Adults: *H. influenzae*, *S. pneumoniae*, *N. meningitidis* Elderly/Immunocompromised: *S. pneumoniae*, *N. meningitides*, *L. monocytogenes*, HIV – *C. neoformans*
Risk Factors	Preceding URTI, otitis media or sinusitis, head trauma, neurosurgery, immunocompromised states, crowded living conditions, alcoholism, IV drug use
History	Neck stiffness, headache, fevers/chills, lethargy, malaise, nausea/vomiting confusion, decreased LOC, focal neurological deficits, seizures, petechial rash
Physical Exam	"Toxic" appearance, full neuro exam, nuchal rigidity Kernig's (resisted knee extension with hip flexion) Brudzinski's (neck flexion causes knee/hip flexion) Jolt accentuation of headache (most sensitive sign)
Investigations	CBC, blood cultures, electrolytes, BUN/Cr Lumbar puncture for C&S/chemistry/viral PCR/cell count Consider CT, x-rays for primary site of infection
Management	Neonates: ampicillin + aminoglycoside All others: vancomycin 1 g IV q12h + ceftriaxone 2 g IV q12h ± ampicillin if risk factors for *Listeria* Dexamethasone: 10 mg IV q6h x 4 d started before or with Abx for suspected bacterial meningitis

Note: encephalitis presents similarly and should always be considered on the DDx

Pneumonia

Etiology	See Table next page
Risk Factors	Community-Acquired Pneumonia (CAP): Comorbidity (especially neoplastic disease, neurologic disease, and alcoholism) Age >65 Use scoring systems such as Port Score or CURB 65 to assess risk Hospital-Acquired/Nosocomial: Aspiration, COPD or other chronic severe illnesses, thoracic and upper abdominal surgery, treatment in an ICU, mechanical ventilation Aspiration pneumonia: Decreased level of consciousness, GERD, dysphagia secondary to stroke/multiple sclerosis/myasthenia gravis/dementia, vomiting, ETT, upper gastrointestinal endoscopy
History	Symptoms: cough, sputum production, pleuritic chest pain, chills, rigors, tachypnea, dyspnea *Fever without a concomitant rise in pulse rate may be seen in legionellosis, mycoplasma infections and other non-bacterial pneumonias – not sensitive or specific *Elderly often present atypically; altered LOC is sometimes the only sign

Physical Exam	Vitals: Hypoxia, fever, tachycardia
	Inspection – look for signs of respiratory distress such as accessory muscle use, pursed lip breathing
	Percussion – dullness to percussion over area of consolidation
	Palpation – increased tactile fremitus over area of consolidation
	Auscultation – bronchial breath sounds, rales, ronchi, crackles, whisper pectoriloquy, egophony
Investigations	Bloodwork: CBC, BUN, Cr, electrolytes, random blood glucose
	ABGs
	Sputum C&S and Gram stain, blood C&S, ± pleural fluid C&S, ± serology/viral detection, ± nasopharyngeal swab for patients requiring hospitalization (Note: no organism found in >50% of cases)
	Urine for Legionella antigen if suspected
	CXR: shows distribution (lobular consolidation or interstitial pattern), extent of infiltrate ± cavitation
	Bronchoscopy ± washings for severely ill patients unresponsive to treatment and for the immunocompromised
Management	For CAP, determine whether in-patient or out-patient treatment is required using PORT score and clinical judgment
	Begin empiric therapy – see Table + *Common Medications* section
	Use directed therapy against the specific organism if one is identified from sputum, blood cultures, etc.
Complications	Empyema

IDSA/ATS Community Acquired Pneumonia Treatment Guidelines 2007

Setting	Circumstances	Treatment	Example
Outpatient	Previously well No antibiotic use in last 3 mos	macrolide OR doxycycline	clarithromycin 500 mg PO bid OR doxycycline 100 mg PO bid
	Comorbidities (listed above) Antibiotic use in last 3 mos (use different class)	Respiratory fluoroquinolone OR β-lactam + macrolide	Respiratory fluoroquinolone OR amoxicillin 1000 mg PO tid + clarithromycin 500 mg PO bid
Inpatient	Ward	Respiratory fluoroquinolone OR β-lactam + macrolide	Respiratory fluoroquinolone OR amoxicillin 1000 mg PO tid + clarithromycin 500 mg PO bid
	ICU	β-lactam PLUS azithromycin PLUS a respiratory fluoroquinolone	ceftriaxone 1g IV q24h + (azithromycin 500 mg IV q24h x 5 d) Step-down to oral therapy when tolerated

β-lactam – ceftriaxone,
Macrolide – azithromycin, clarithromycin
Respiratory fluoroquinolone – moxifloxacin, levofloxacin at the 750 mg dose ONLY
http://www.thoracic.org/sections/publications/statements/pages/mtpi/idsaats-cap.html

Common Organisms in Pneumonia

Community Acquired		Nosocomial	HIV-associated	Alcoholic
Healthy Adults	**Elderly/Comorbidity*/** **Nursing Home**			
S. pneumoniae	*S. pneumoniae*	Enteric Gram-neg rods	Pneumocystis jiroveci	*Klebsiella*
Mycoplasma	*H. influenzae*	*Pseudomonas*	(PCP/PJP)	Gram-neg bacilli
Chlamydophila	Gram-neg bacilli	*S. aureus*	Gram-neg bacilli	*S. aureus*
(Chlamydia)	*S. aureus*			Anaerobes (aspiration)
H. influenzae	*Legionella*			
Viral				

* Comorbidity includes COPD, CHF, diabetes, renal failure, recent hospitalization

Infective Endocarditis

Definition:	Infection of cardiac endothelium			

Etiology	**Native Valve**	**IVDU**	**Prosthetic Valve** **(surgery <1 yr)**	**Prosthetic Valve** **(surgery >1 yr)**
	Strep[1]	**S. aureus**	**S. epidermidis**	**Streptococcus**
	S. aureus	**Strep**	**S. aureus**	**S. aureus**
	Enterococcus	Enterococcus	**Enterococcus**	**S. epidermidis**
	GNB	GNB	GNB	**Enterococcus**
	Other	Candida	Other	Other
		Other		

Organisms in bold are the most common isolates.

1. Strep = *Streptococcus* includes mainly *Viridans* group

Risk Factors	1) valve problem: prosthetic cardiac valve, previous IE, congenital heart disease, cardiac transplant with valve disease, valvular dysfunction, cardiomyopathy, 2) source of bacteremia: IV drug use, indwelling venous catheter, poor dentition, mucosal injury
Physical Exam	Vital signs: ABCs, fever, chills, weight loss, night sweats Cardiac: dyspnea, chest pain, clubbing, regurg murmur, signs of CHF Abdo: splenomegaly Embolic and immune: petechiae, splinter hemorrhages, Janeway lesions, Roth`s spots, Osler`s nodes, arthritis, glomerulonephritis
Investigations	Blood work: anemia, ESR/CRP Urinalysis: proteinuria, hematuria, red-cell casts Blood cultures: 3 sets, different sites, >1hr apart before antibiotics echo: vegetations, regurgitation, abscess ECG: increased PR interval may indicate perivalvular abscess

Diagnosis

Modified Duke Criteria (see Table below)
- Definite diagnosis if: 2 major OR 1 major + 3 minor OR 5 minor
- Possible diagnosis if: 1 major + 1 minor OR 3 minor

Major Criteria

Positive blood cultures for IE
- Typical microorganisms for IE from 2 separate blood cultures (Streptococcus viridans, HACEK group, Streptococcus bovis, Staphylococcus aureus, community-acquired enterococci) OR
- Persistently positive blood culture, defined as recovery of a microorganism consistent with IE from blood drawn >12 h apart or all of 3 or a majority of 4 or more separate blood cultures, with first and last drawn >1 h apart
- Single positive blood culture or Coxiella burnetii or antiphase I IgG antibody titer >1:800

Evidence of endocardial involvement
- Positive echocardiogram for IE (oscillating intracardiac mass on valve or supporting structures, or in the path of regurgitant jets, or on implanted material in the absence of an alternative anatomic explanation OR abscess OR new partial dehiscence of prosthetic valve)
- New valvular regurgitation (insufficient if increase or change in preexisting murmur)

Minor Criteria

Predisposing condition (abnormal heart valve, IVDU)

Fever (38.0°C/100.4°F)

Vascular phenomena: major arterial emboli, septic pulmonary infarcts, mycotic aneurysms, ICH, conjunctival hemorrhages, Janeway lesions

Immunologic phenomena: glomerulonephritis, rheumatoid factor, Osler's nodes, Roth's spots

Positive blood culture but not meeting major criteria OR serologic evidence of active infection with organism consistent with IE

Echocardiographic minor criteria eliminated

Management	1) Medical: Start empiric antibiotics immediately after cultures are drawn. First line – cloxacillin 2 g IV q4h & gentamicin 1 g/mg IV q8h; if native valve and non-IVDU add ampicillin 2 g IV q4h; if prosthetic valve add rifampin 600 mg po daily. 2) Surgical: Relative indications – refractory CHF, valve ring abscess, fungal etiology, valve perforation, unstable prosthesis, >1 major emboli, antimicrobial failure, mycotic aneurism, staphylococci on prosthetic valve
Prognosis	Mortality approaches 30%

Acute Infectious Diarrhea

Etiology	Invasive bacterial – *Campylobacter jejuni, enteroinvasive E. coli* (EIEC), *Salmonella typhi, S. paratyphi, S. typhimurium, S. enteritidis, Shigella dysenteriae, Yersinia enterocolitica, Y. pseudotuberculosis* Non-invasive/Toxin-mediated bacterial – *Bacillus cereus*, enterohemorrhagic *E. coli* (EHEC), enterotoxigenic *E.coli* (ETEC), *Clostridium difficile, C. perfringens, Staphylococcus aureus, Vibrio cholerae* Parasites – *Cryptosporidium, Entamoeba histolytica, Giardia lamblia* Viruses – Norovirus, Rotavirus
Risk Factors	Fecal-oral spread (poor hand hygiene); sick household contacts, healthcare or daycare exposure Contaminated food/water (poultry – *Campylobacter and Salmonella*, beef – *E. coli*, seafood – *Vibrio*, rice dishes – *Bacillus cereus*) Recent antibiotic use (*C. difficile*) Travel (Asia, Africa, Central and South America, cruise ships anywhere) Immunosuppression
History	Frequent unformed stools, abdominal pain, cramping, hematochezia, tenesmus, nausea and vomiting, fever, headache, myalgia, rash (rose spots in *S. typhi*), food Hx, travel Hx, recent antibiotic use, sick contacts
Physical Exam	Volume status is most important! Vitals – do postural vitals and look for signs of hypovolemia such as tachycardia and hypotension, fever CVS – JVP (may be low if hypovolemic) Abdo – DRE Derm – rashes (esp. Rose spots seen in *Salmonella typhi* infection)
Investigations	Usually none required – typically self-limiting in healthy individuals with community-acquisition in Canada Stool for Ova and Parasites if >10 d symptoms Stool culture for *Salmonella, Shigella, Campylobacter, Yersinia, E. coli* Stool for *C. difficile* toxins
Management	Symptomatic treatment Loperamide (Immodium®) ONLY if no fever or dysentery Fluid and electrolyte replacement Antibiotics may cause *C. difficile* infection and usually not required in healthy individuals with community acquisition Antibiotics clearly indicated: *Salmonella typhi* (ceftriaxone or azithromycin), *Shigella* (ciprofloxacin), *V. cholera* (tetracycline or ciprofloxacin), *C. difficile* (metronidazole or PO vancomycin), *Cryptosporidium* (Nitazoxanide), *Entamoeba histolytica* (metronidazole + iodoquinol), immunocompromised patients Antibiotics indicated in some situations (severe symptoms): Non-typhoidal *Salmonella* (Ciprofloxacin), *Campylobacter* (Macrolide), *Yersinia* (flouroquinolone), *Giardia* (Metronidazole), ETEC (Quinolone or Azithromycin) Antibiotics NOT indicated: EIEC, *Bacillus cereus*, EHEC/STEC, *Clostridium perfringens, Staphylococcus* aureus, Entamoeba dispar, viral

Chronic Hepatitis B

Epidemiology	Develops in ≤5% of healthy adults with acute HBV hepatitis and 90% of those infected at birth
Clinical Features	Many asymptomatic If symptomatic, generally only mild and intermittent fatigue; correlates poorly with disease severity Signs and symptoms of liver disease: advanced histological disease

Types of Chronic Infection	Inactive (formerly termed chronic persistent hepatitis or carrier):
	    Virus reactivation can occur at any time, especially if immunosuppressed (e.g. corticosteroids, lymphoma)
	    Reactivation clinically resembles acute hepatitis B
	"Core or precore mutant": active virus replication with elevated HBV DNA but HBeAg negative because of promoter gene mutation
	Poor prognosis, difficult to treat

Hepatitis B Serology

	HBsAg	Anti-HBs	HBeAg	Anti-HBe	Anti-HBc	HBV DNA	ALT, AST
Acute HBV	+	–	+	–	IgM	High	Elevated
Chronic Active HBV (high infectivity)	+	–	+	–	IgG	High	Elevated
Chronic Inactive HBV (low infectivity)	+	–	–	+	IgG	Low	Normal
Recovery	–	+	–	+/-	IgG	Low	Normal
Immunization	–	+	–	–	–	None	Normal
Perinatal	+	-	+	-	IgM	High	Normal

*HBeAg and high viral load are indicators of high infectivity

Treatment
- No treatment is indicated if in immune-tolerant, inactive carrier/low replicative, or latent HBV infection phases
- Treatment of chronic replicative hepatitis with IFN-α, pegylated or standard
  - Pegylated: 24 wk course of 180 µg SC 1x per wk
  - Standard: 5 million units SC OD or 10 million units SC 3x/wk
  - Increases annual rate of cessation of viral replication from 7% to 40%; loss of HBsAg less common
  - Relapse after successful therapy is rare (1 to 2%)
- Lamivudine (Heptovir®): resolves hepatic inflammation and leads to HBeAg negative/anti-HBe positive ("seroconversion") in >90% of patients
  - 100 mg PO OD
  - Relapse common when drug is stopped; drug resistance can develop after 1-2 yrs of use
- Other antivirals used in hepatitis B treatment include adefovir dipivoxil, entecavir and tenofovir (nucleoside analogues used to decrease viral load)
- End-stage treatment is transplant, although reinfection occurs in 80-100%
- Recurrence reduced with use of HBIg
- Increased incidence of hepatocellular carcinoma (HCC), especially if HBeAg positive, cirrhosis, male

Chronic Hepatitis C

Epidemiology	Most common chronic liver disease; antibody prevalence in the USA is 1.6% 60-80% of acute HCV infections go on to become chronic; of those 20-30% go on to cirrhosis, and of those 25% per yr develop HCC Key findings include abnormal AST, history of IVDU, and history of blood transfusion <1992 Time course: 　Clinical chronic hepatitis at 10 yrs 　Cirrhosis at 20-30 yrs 　HCC at 30 yrs 　Time course accelerated if co-infected with HIV
Clinical Features	Usually asymptomatic May have non-specific symptoms: fatigue, nausea, anorexia, myalgia, arthralgia, weakness, weight loss, abdominal pain, pruritis, dark urine, cognitive impairment
Investigations	Anti-HCV: positive in chronic and resolved acute infections HCV RNA: positive in chronic, negative in resolved acute infection
Treatment	Ondansetron 4 mg PO bid for fatigue Pegylated IFN + ribavirin for 48 wks; dosing dependent on patient weight and HCV genotype 　30-50% are non-responders 　If no early response in patient without liver decompensation, stop therapy early because sustained remission is unlikely 　Multiple side effects including depression and fever/chills/malaise from IFN use, hemolytic anemias commonly from ribavirin HAV and HBV vaccination suggested if HCV patient is not immune

Urinary Tract Infection

• See Urology

Etiology	Common organisms: *Klebsiella, E. coli, Enterococcus, Proteus, Pseudomonas, S. saprophyticus*
Risk Factors	Stasis and obstruction: residual urine in poorly flushing system, foreign body: introduce pathogen or acts as nidus of infection, history of instrumentation (Foley), decreased resistance to organisms (diabetes, immunosuppression), other factors (trauma, anatomic variance, female, previous UTI, sexual activity)
Management	Aymptomatic bacteruria: treat only in pregnant women and those undergoing GU instrumentation Treatment options include: TMP/SMX 1 DS tab PO bid x 3 d (7-10 d for males) Ciprofloxacin 500 mg PO bid x 3 d Nitrofurantoin 100 mg PO qid x 7 d

Acute Pyelonephritis

• See Urology, pg 482

Osteomyelitis

Etiology	Hematogenous spread (indwelling lines, IVDU, sickle cell) (20%)
	   Most common organism is *Staphylococcus aureus*
	   Consider *Salmonella* sp. in patients with sickle cell disease, *Pseudomonas* in diabetics
	   25% Gram negatives: *E. coli, Pseudomonas aeruginosa* in vertebrae, *Serratia* in IVDU (usually vertebral)
	   TB in endemic areas (Pott's disease)
	   10% progress to chronic osteomyelitis
	Contiguous spread (i.e. from open fracture or soft tissue infection) (50%)
	   30-50% polymicrobial: *S. aureus, S. epidermidis*, Gram negatives, anaerobes
	   Gram negatives in ICU patients, multiple procedures
	   Anaerobes in human bite, associated with dental infection, intra-abdominal abscess, decubitus ulcer
	Associated with vascular insufficiency (30%)
	Diabetes mellitus or severe peripheral vascular disease
	Usually in the feet associated with infected neuropathic ulcers

Risk Factors	Poor circulation – diabetes, sickle cell disease, decubitus ulcer, sternotomy with use of LITA for cardiothoracic surgery (complication in 1-5%), orthopedic surgery or trauma, indwelling lines
History	Localized extremity pain (pinpoint tenderness) Fever (<50%) Associated cellulits or wound/ulcer infection

Physical Exam	Probe-to-bone in a diabetic foot ulcer is highly predictive of underlying osteomyelitis
	Warmth, swelling, erythema, tenderness over the area of infection
	Purulent drainage from an open wound
	± Fever
Investigations	Bone biopsy – send for C&S, blood culture (positive in 50%), CBC (leukocytosis), ESR, CRP (non-specific)
	Swabs of associated skin ulcers do not reflect organisms in bone (*Clin Infect Dis* 2006;42:57-62)
	Imaging: X-ray (will be normal for first 2 wks), bone scan (increased blood flow, pooling, and reactive new bone formation) (good sensitivity, poor specificity), CT, MRI is the most sensitive and specific
Management	Surgical debridement of infected bone and intraosseous abscess (aka Brodie's abscess)
	Foot ulcer associated: extensive debridement ± amputation + antibiotics
	Directed IV therapy at organism(s) found in bone culture
	Treat for at least 6 wks
	If acutely ill, start empiric treatment against likely organisms

Septic Arthritis

DDx	Reactive arthritis
	Reiter's syndrome (urethritis, conjunctivitis, arthritis, uveitis, rash) – after infection with *C. trachomatis, Campylobacter jejuni, Yersinia enterocolitica, Shigella sp., Salmonella sp.*
	Post-streptococcal – may also have rheumatic fever
Etiology	Bacterial infection of a joint by hematogenous (adults) or contiguous (children) spread, direct
	N. gonorrhoeae: accounts for 75% of septic arthritis in young sexually active adults
	S. aureus: affects all ages, rapidly destructive, accounts for 50% of non-gonococcal cases of septic arthritis in adults (and 80% of those in rheumatoid arthritis)
	Gram negatives: affects neonates, elderly, IVDU, immunocompromised. *E. coli* and *Pseudomonas* most common
	S. pneumoniae: affects children
	Kingella kingae: affects children <2 y.o. since HIB immunization
	Salmonella spp.: characteristic of HIV, sickle cell
	Coagulase-negative *Staphylococcal*: recent joint surgery
	If culture negative: *Borrelia sp.* (Lyme disease) or *Tropheryma whippeli* (Whipple's disease)
Risk Factors	Extra-articular infection with hematogenous seeding, IVDU, chronic illness (e.g. RA, DM, malignancy), prior joint damage (e.g. OA, RA, joint surgery, prosthetic joints), unprotected sexual activity, skin infection
History	Sudden onset monoarthritis. Migratory polyarthritis and tenosynovitis possible in gonococcal infection
	Severe pain with passive range of motion
	Knee > hip > ankle > wrist > shoulder > elbow (most to least common)
	Redness and swelling of affected joint
	Fever, chills
	Rash in gonococcal: 2-10 necrotic pustules on palms or soles
Physical Exam	Vital signs – fever
	Examine affected joint looking for erythema, warmth, effusion

Investigations	Also endocervical, urethral, rectal and oropharyngeal swabs if gonorrhea suspected
	Blood culture Culture and sensitivity: joint aspirate, blood, urine positive in ~50%
	Arthrocentesis
	Send synovial fluid for: CBC + diff, Gram stain, culture, examine for crystals
	Infectious = opaque, increased WBC count (inflammatory), PMNs >85%, culture positive, low glucose (see <u>Rheumatology</u>)
	Growth of gonococci from synovial fluid is successful in <50% of cases ± imaging
	X-ray may be negative early on
	Bone scan, CT and MRI are all non-specific
Management	Admit to hospital
	Start IV antibiotics empirically, delay may result in joint destruction: Acute monoarticular: vancomycin 1 g IV q24h ± cefazolin 1 g IV q8h
	Add ciprofloxacin or gentamicin if risk for Gram neg. (i.e. diabetes)
	If suspecting gonococcal: ceftriaxone 1 g IM/IV q24h
	Post intra-articular injection: no empiric antibiotics, wait for Gram stain, C&S
	Prosthetic joint: no empiric antibiotics, wait for gram stain, C&S, Ortho consult – possible replacement of prosthesis, debridement
	Gram stain guides subsequent treatment
	Duration of antibiotic therapy depends on causative organism
	No need for intra-articular antibiotics
	Intra-articular corticosteroids are contraindicated in septic arthritis
	Surgical incision and drainage if:
	Persistent positive joint cultures on repeat arthrocentesis
	Hip joint involvement
	Failure to improve after 2-4 d of treatment
	Prosthetic joint
	Repeated joint aspiration to relieve symptoms if fluid reaccumulates
	Physiotherapy
Complications	10-30% mortality due to sepsis
	Up to 50% morbidity (decreased joint function/motility)

Tuberculosis (TB)

Etiology	*Mycobacterium tuberculosis*
Risk Factors	For exposure: travel to endemic countries, aboriginal, crowded living conditions, low SES/homeless
	For progression to active disease: immunocompromised, seroconversion in the past 2 yrs, concurrent local disease process (e.g. lung), recent immigration
Signs and Symptoms (History and Physical Exam)	1° infection: asymptomatic or primary respiratory illness
	2° infection/reactivation: constitutional symptoms and site-dependent symptoms
	Pulmonary TB: chronic productive cough ± hemoptysis
	Miliary TB: widely disseminated spread especially to lungs, abdominal organs, marrow and CNS
	Extrapulmonary TB: lymphadenitis, pleurisy, pericarditis, peritonitis, osteomyelitis (affecting vertebrae is Pott's disease), adrenal infection (causing Addison's disease), renal, ovary

Investigations	PPD/Mantoux skin test: positive result only indicates latent infection, not active disease
	AM sputum on 3 consecutive days: for AFB, culture ± AMTD (TB rRNA assay)
	CXR features:
	Nodular/alveolar infiltrates with cavitation (middle/lower lobe lesions if primary, apical if secondary)
	Hilar/mediastinal adenopathy (90% are usually unilateral)
	Miliary TB: discrete nodules (2-4 mm in diameter) scattered throughout lungs
	Past disease: calcified lesions/lymph nodes
Management	Empiric Rx: INH + rifampin + pyrazinamide + ethambutol + pyridoxine
	Pulmonary TB: INH + rifampin + pyrazinamide + pyridoxine x 2 mos (initiation phase), then INH + rifampin + pyridoxine x 4 mos (continuation phase), total therapy for 6 mos
	Extrapulmonary TB: same regimen as pulmonary TB but increase to 9-12 mos for osteomyelitis and CNS disease, and add corticosteroids for meningitis and pericarditis

HIV/AIDS

Etiology	HIV-1 predominant in North America and most of world; HIV-2 in West Africa
Risk Factors	Unprotected anal or vaginal intercourse (rarely oral sex), sharing of contaminated needles or equipment, transfusion of contaminated blood/blood products, vertical transmission (mom to child), accidental needlestick to health care workers (0.3%)
Signs and symptoms	Acute seroconversion syndrome: 40-70% experience a mononucleosis-like acute seroconversion syndrome from 1-6 wks after initial infection, generally lasting 10-15 d. Symptoms: fever, pharyngitis, oral ulcers, lymphadenopathy, rash, myalgias, headaches, leukopenia, aseptic meningitis
	Highly transmissible because highest viral load at this point
	Asymptomatic Phase: CD4 counts usually greater than 200 cells/mm3 and persistent generalized lymphadenopathy occurs in 35-60% of asymptomatic patients. Progression of disease is highly variable, after rapid decrease in CD4 count in first year of infection, decline is approximately 50 cells/yr thereafter in untreated individuals
	Symptomatic Phase: CD4 counts <500 cells/mm^3 – constitutional symptoms, mucocutaneous lesions (seborrheic dermatitis, HSV, shingles, oral hairy leukoplakia (EBV), candidiasis (oral, esophageal, vaginal), Kaposi's sarcoma), recurrent bacterial pneumonia, TB, lymphoma
	CD4 counts <200 cells/mm^3 – PCP/PJP, visceral KS, local and/or disseminated fungal infections (Cryptococcus neoformans, Coccidioides immitis, Histoplasma capsulatum)
	CD4 counts <100 cells/mm^3 – progressive multifocal leukoencephalopathy (PML), CNS toxoplasmosis
	CD4 counts <50 cells/mm^3 – CMV infection (retinitis, colitis, cholangiopathy, CNS disease), Mycobacterium avium complex (MAC), bacillary angiomatosis (disseminated Bartonella), primary central nervous system lymphoma (PCNSL)
	AIDS: HIV-positive, AND one or more of: opportunistic infections (e.g. PCP, esophageal candidiasis, CMV, MAC, TB, toxoplasmosis); malignancy (Kaposi's sarcoma, invasive cervical cancer); wasting syndrome. NOT DEFINED BY CD4 COUNT! Now consider spectrum of HIV disease, rather than HIV with or without AIDS
Investigations	If they have seroconverted (i.e. have had disease for at least 3 months), then do ELISA to detect serum antibody to HIV and a Western blot confirmation by detecting antibodies to at least two different HIV protein bands (gp120/160, p24, gp41)
	If still in window period (i.e. recently exposed), do DNA PCR or p24 antigen detection and repeat ELISA at 6 wk and 3 months
	Once HIV confirmed, lab investigations needed are plasma HIV-RNA level and CD4 count q2-3 months; baseline tuberculin skin test (PPD) where induration greater than 5 mm is positive; baseline Toxoplasma antibody, syphilis serology (VDRL), hepatitis A, B and C antibodies, hep. B surface antigen, CMV antibody, liver enzymes, and CXR

Management   Confirm HIV+ by above tests, and then complete history and physical exam and f/u q3 months
Education: emphasize that most patients, even without antiviral therapy, survive for 10 to12 yrs after acquiring HIV infection and are asymptomatic during most of that time. Also, prevent further transmission through safer sex and clean needles for drug use. Assess ongoing counseling needs and refer for significant psychiatric or social problems. Give vaccines: influenza annually, 23-valent pneumococcal q5yrs, hepatitis B (if not immune), hepatitis A (if seronegative) and do annual PAP smear
Treatment is usually with three-drug HAART combinations to prevent development of HIV drug resistance (drugs include NNRTI, NRTI, protease inhibitors, fusion inhibitors and integrase inhibitors). HIV viral load should decrease 3-4 fold (0.5 log) within 2-8 wks and continue to decrease thereafter; goal is have undetectable viral load (i.e. <50 copies/mL) at 6 months, although may take longer if baseline viral load >100 000 copies/mL. Antiretrovirals are started when the CD4 count is <=350 (some suggest <= 500), the patient is symptomatic, or for prevention of mother-child transmission.

Complications   Immunocompromise and thus susceptible to many cancers and infections (as listed above in signs and symptoms)

Febrile Neutropenia

Definition   Fever: Single oral temperature of >38.3°C or temperature >38.0°C for >1 h
Neutropenia: ANC <0.5 or <1.0 and expected to decrease to <0.5
*ANC = [WBC x (%neut. + %bands)] / 100

Etiology   Immunocompromise due to:
Decreased neutrophil production
Iatrogenic (chemotherapy; neutrophils lowest 10 d post-chemotherapy), marrow infiltration (leukemia), vitamin deficiencies (folate, Vit. B_{12})
Increased neutrophil destruction
Autoimmune (SLE), splenic sequestration, etc.
Bacterial or fungal infection
60-70% due to Gram-positives
Fungal infections with prolonged neutropenia (Candida, Aspergillus)
Periodontium, the pharynx, lower esophagus, lung, perineum, eye and skin are most common sites

Physical Exam   Careful exam for any possible source of infection, including:
Catheter/lines sites, dentition, mucosal surfaces, perirectal and genital orifices (DO NOT do a DRE!)
Note that signs and symptoms will be greatly diminished as the patient is unable to mount an appropriate immune response to infection

Investigations   CBC with differential, BUN, Cr, transaminases
Gram stain and C&S of blood from EACH catheter lumen as well as from a peripheral vein
Gram stain and C&S of urine, and sputum
Gram stain and C&S of any pus from infected skin
Chest x-ray if respiratory symptoms or planned treatment as an outpatient

Management   Begin empiric therapy based on local patterns of infection and antibiotic susceptibility
Most hospitals have their own protocol. Example protocol below:
Low risk if: <60 yo, solid tumour, clinically well, no mucositis, normal CXR, no comorbidities, no change in level of consciousness, neutropenia expected for <10 d - PO ciprofloxacin + cephalexin
High risk if: mucositis, leukemia, bone marrow transplant, ANC <0.1, unlikely to recover in <10 d - cefazolin 1g IV q8h + tobramycin 7mg/kg IV q24h
Use vancomycin 1g IV q12h instead of cefazolin if MRSA positive, severe mucositis, line associated infection, or recent fluoroquinolone prophylaxis
If still febrile Day 3 add Pip-tazo 4.5 g IV q6h
If still febrile Day 7-10 add antifungal therapy
If specific organism is identified though investigations, optimize treatment, but continue
Stop antibiotics when afebrile for >48 h AND recovery of ANC x48 h if no source found
Neupogen (G-CSF): decreases hospital d, decreases cost of antibiotics but expensive → usually give to patients with repeated febrile neutropenia

Fever of Unknown Origin

Etiology	Infectious causes (15-25%):

Etiology

Infectious causes (15-25%):
- Abscess – usually in abdomen or pelvis; risk factors include cirrhosis, steroid or immunosuppressive medications, recent surgery, diabetes
- Osteomyelitis
- Bacterial endocarditis – cultures negative in 2-5%, especially in *Coxiella burnetii, Tropheryma whipplei, Brucella, Mycoplasma, Chlamydia, Histoplasma, Legionella, Bartonella,* HACEK organisms which require either special media or longer than usual incubation
- Prostatitis, dental abscesses, sinusitis, and cholangitis are sources of occult fever
- Returned travellers/new immigrants: TB, HIV/AIDS, CMV, EBV, malaria, typhoid fever, dengue fever, hepatitis A, Lyme disease, syphilis, psittacosis (bird exposure), rat-bite fever
- Uncommonly toxoplasmosis, Leishmania, amoebiasis, histoplasmosis, Cryptococcus

Neoplastic causes (<20%)
- Most commonly lymphomas (especially non-Hodgkin's) and leukemias
- Solid tumours: renal cell carcinoma most common, also breast, liver, colon, pancreas or liver metastases
- Malignant histiocytosis: rare but rapidly progressive with high fever, weight loss, lymphadenopathy, hepatosplenomegaly

Collagen vascular diseases (15-25% of cases):
- SLE, RA
- Rheumatic fever
- Vasculitis, especially temporal (giant cell) arteritis
- JRA, Still's disease

Miscellaneous (15-20% of cases)
- Drug fever: commonly antibiotics, antihistamines, antiarrhythmics, methyldopa, phenytoin, dilantin, NSAIDs
- Sarcoidosis
- Inherited Familial Mediterranean Fever and other febrile syndromes (i.e. Kikuchi's disease)
- Factitious disorder
- Pulmonary embolus

Unknown despite investigations

History

Enquire about travel, environmental/occupational exposures, infectious contacts, drug/medication history, immunizations, TB history, sexual history, PMHx

Thorough review of systems including complaints that disappeared before interview

Physical Exam

Perform a complete initial physical and neurological exam looking for any signs of possible infection

Daily physical exam to assess fever pattern, paying attention to rashes, murmurs, arthritic signs, lymphadenopathy

Investigations

Initial investigations

Bloodwork: CBC with differential and film, electrolytes, BUN, Cr, calcium profile, LFTs, ESR, CRP, muscle enzymes, RF, ANA, TSH, serum protein electrophoresis, Fe, transferrin, TIBC, vitamin B_{12}

Cultures: blood (x 2 sets), urine, sputum, stool C&S O&P, other fluids as appropriate

VDRL/RPR, heterophile Ab (mononucleosis), CMV antigenemia/serology, HIV serology, Viral hepatitis serology

CXR

If no diagnostic clues from the above, proceed with further investigations including: CT chest, abdomen and pelvis with contrast

If no diagnostic clue from the above, may proceed with further investigations including: 67Ga scan, 111In PMN scan, FDG PET scan

If diagnostic clues from any of the above steps, proceed with directed exam, biopsies or invasive

Testing as required followed by directed treatment once a diagnosis is established

Management

Treatment is directed at the specific cause found from the above investigations

If no diagnosis with the above consider empiric therapy vs. watchful waiting

Prognosis for most patients with FUO persisting without a diagnosis is very good without intervention

Therapeutic trials are rarely indicated without a strongly suspected source/organism

Common Nosocomial Infectious Agents

Bacteria	Characteristics	Manifestation	Investigations	Management
Methicillin-resistant *Staphylococcus aureus* (MRSA)	Gram-positive cocci	Skin and soft tissue infection Bacteremia Pneumonia	Admission screening culture from nares and peri-anal region identifies colonization Culture of infection site CXR	Contact precautions For infection: Vancomycin or linezolid To decolonize: 2% chlorhexidine wash OD x 7 d + rifampin 300mg PO bid x 7 d + doxycyline 100mg PO OD x 7 d + mucopirocin cream bid to nares x 7 d
Vancomycin-resistant *Enterococcus* (VRE)	Majority are *E. faecium* Resistant if minimum inhibitory concentration of vancomycin is ≥ 32 μg/mL	Rarely causes disease in healthy people UTI Bacteremia Endocarditis	Rectal or perirectal swab OR stool culture for colonization Culture of infected site	Contact precautions Ampicillin if susceptible Otherwise, linezolid, tigecycline, or daptomycin depending on site of infection No effective decolonization methods identified
Clostridium difficile (C. diff)	Releases exotoxins A and B; Hypervirulent strain has been responsible for increase in incidence and severity	Fever, nausea, anorexia Watery diarrhea $\pm$ occult blood Severe: toxic megacolon Risk bowel perforation Associated with antibiotic leukocytosis	Stool PCR, endoscopy (if not suspect fulminant colitis) AXR (may see colonic dilatation)	Contact precautions Stop culprit antibiotic therapy Supportive therapy (IV fluids) Mild-moderate disease: metronidazole 500 mg PO tid x 10-14 d Severe disease: vancomycin 125 mg PO qid x 10 - 14 d Toxic megacolon: metronidzole IV + vancomycin PO (as above) and gen. surg. consult
Extended spectrum β-lactamases (ESBL e.g. *Escherichia coli, Klebsiella pneumoniae*)	Resistant to most β-lactam producing antibiotics e.g. penicillins, aztreonam and cephalosporins	UTI Pulmonary infection Bacteremia Liver abscess in susceptible patients Meningitis	Blood, sputum, urine, or aspirated body fluid culture Imaging at infection site (CXR, CT, U/S)	Droplet or contact precautions depending on site of infection and institutional policies Dependent on culture and sensitivity results, carbapenems can be used for empiric therapy

Fever in the Returned Traveller

Illness	Pathogen	Incubation Period	Clinical Manifestations	Diagnosis	Treatment
Malaria	*Plasmodium falciparum* *Plasmodium vivax* *P. malaraie* *P. ovale* *P. knowlesi*	10 d to 40 yrs	Fever and flu-like illness, (shaking chills, headache, muscle aches, and fatigue) Nausea, vomiting, and diarrhea Anemia and jaundice *Plasmodium falciparum*: (severe) kidney failure, seizures, mental confusion, prostration, coma, death, respiratory failure	Blood smear (thick and thin) x3 Antigen detection PCR (mostly a research tool)	Artesunate (for severe disease) + malarone, doxycycline, or clindamycin Quinine sulfate + doxycycline or clindamycin Chloroquine + primaquine
Dengue	Dengue viruses (4)	3 d to 2 wks	Sudden onset of fever Headache Retro-orbital pain Myalgias and arthralgias Leukopenia Thrombocytopenia Hemorrhagic manifestations (rare in travelers)	Anti-dengue IgM positivity	Symptom relief: Acetaminophen (avoid using NSAIDs because of anticoagulant properties)
Typhoid (enteric fever)	*Salmonella Typhi* *Salmonella Paratyphi*	3 to 60 d	Sustained fever 103° to 104° F (39° to 40° C) Stomach pains, headache, loss of appetite Cough Constipation	Stool, urine or blood sample positive for *S. Typhi* or *S. Paratyphi*	Quinolone antibiotic (e.g. ciprofloxacin), ceftriaxone or macrolide
Tick typhus	*Rickettsia*	1 to 2 wks	Fever Headache Fatigue Muscle aches Occasionally rash Eschar at site of tick bite Thrombocytopenia Elevated liver enzymes	Serology Presence of classic tick eschar	Doxycycline
TB	*M. tuberculosis*	Variable	Fever Cough Hemoptysis	Tuberculin skin test CXR Sputum culture and AFB	Ethambutol, isoniazid, pyrazinamide, rifampin, pyridoxine
Mononucleosis	EBV or CMV	30 to 50 d	Malaise, fatigue, pharyngitis, lymphadenopathy, splenomegaly	Atypical lymphocytes on blood smear and positive heterophilic antibody (monospot) test	Acetaminophen or NSAIDs, fluids

Nephrology

Essential History, Physical Exam and Investigations

History and Physical Exam

- See *Individual Presentations*

Investigations

ASSESMENT OF RENAL FUNCTION: Methods to estimate the GFR
- **Creatinine Clearance (CrCl)**
  - Requires 24-h urine volume, Urine [Cr], Serum [Cr]
  - Change in GFR: GFR α 1 / Plasma [Cr]
- **Cockcroft-Gault Formula**
  - CrCl (ml/min) = (weight in kg) (140-age) x1.23 /(serum creatinine (umol/L or mg/dL)
    - Multiply by 0.85 for females.
  - Normal range is >90 mL/min (1.5 mL/s)
- **MDRD (Modification of Diet in Renal Disease) formula**
  - Most common way in which GFR estimated (MDRD 7 equation) (ml/min/1.73m^2)
  - Complex formula which includes: age, gender, serum Cr, African descent
- **Limitations of use of serum creatinine measurements**
  - MUST BE IN STEADY STATE
  - GFR must fall substantially before plasma [Cr] rises above normal ranges
  - Plasma [Cr] is influenced by the rate of creatinine production
  - Contribution of tubular secretion to Cr excretion is increased when GFR is low
  - Errors in creatinine measurement
  - Variations in Cr estimate depending on type of assay

URINALYSIS
- Measured by dipstick or automated sample processor in freshly-voided urine specimen
- **pH**: normally between 4.5-7.0; if persistently alkaline consider renal tubular acidosis or a UTI with a urease-producing organism (e.g. *Proteus* species)
- **Glucose**: freely filtered at the glomerulus and completely reabsorbed in the proximal tubule; if present, causes may include hyperglycemia
  (>9-11 mM) exceeding the tubular resorption capacity, increased GFR (e.g. pregnancy) or proximal tubule dysfunction (e.g. Fanconi's syndrome)
- **Protein**: only detects albumin and does not quantify other proteins
  (e.g. Bence-Jones, Tamm-Horsfall, IgG); sulfosalicylic acid precipitation is able to detect all proteins in urine
- **Leukocyte esterase**: WBC enzyme that indicates infection (e.g. UTI) or inflammation (e.g. AIN); when combined with nitrites is 94% sensitive for UTI diagnosis
- **Nitrites**: converted from nitrates by bacteria in urine; specific but low sensitivity for UTI (enterococcus does not metabolize nitrates)
- **Ketones**: positive in alcoholic, diabetic or starvation ketoacidosis
- **Hemoglobin**: positive in hemoglobinuria (e.g. hemolysis), myoglobinuria (e.g. Rhabdomyolysis) and true hematuria (RBCs on microscope); see section on Hematuria
- **Specific gravity**: ratio of mass of urine:water; dilute urine <1.010 and concentrated urine >1.020

URINE MICROSCOPY
• Centrifuge a urine specimen for 3-5 min, discard supernatant, resuspend sediment then plate on microscope slide, examine under light microscope

Cell Type/Sediment	Number	Pathology
Erythrocytes	Up to 2-3 RBCs/high-powered field (HPF) with >5 RBCs/HPF representing hematuria	Dysmorphic RBCs suggest glomerulonephritis while isomorphic RBCs suggest bleeding (e.g. bladder carcinoma)
Leukocytes	Normal <3 WBCs/HPF with >3 WBCs/HPF representing pyuria	Indicates inflammation or infection; if persistently sterile pyuria consider chronic urethritis, prostatitis, interstitial nephritis, papillary necrosis, renal TB, viral infection
Eosinophils	--------------------	Detected using Wright's or Hansel's stains; consider allergic interstitial nephritis or atheroembolic disease
Oval fat bodies	--------------------	Renal tubular cells filled with lipid droplets, seen with heavy proteinuria (e.g. nephrotic syndrome)
Crystals	--------------------	Uric acid crystals → acidic urine and hyperuricosemia/gout Calcium phosphate crystals → alkaline urine Sulphur crystals → sulfa drugs Calcium oxalate crystals → hyperoxaluria and ethylene glycol poisoning
Casts	--------------------	Cylindrical structures formed by intratubular precipitation of Tamm-Horsfall mucoprotein trapping cells

Active vs. Bland Sediment

	Active Sediment	Bland Sediment
Any one or more of the following seen on microscopy	Red cell casts White cell casts Muddy-brown granular or epithelial cell casts >2 red cells per high power field (HPF) >4 white cells per HPF Large quantities of uric acid, calcium	Hyaline casts <2 red cells per HPF <4 white cells per HPF Small quantities of crystals Small amount of bacteria Oxalate, or calcium phosphate crystals
Significance	Highly suggestive of significant pathology, casts specifically suggest renal pathology	Reduced likelihood of significant pathology, but not ruled out; more suggestive of pre-renal cause for acute kidney injury

Interpretation of Casts

Hyaline casts	Physiologic (concentrated urine, fever, exercise)
Red blood cell casts	Glomerular bleeding (glomerulonephritis, vasculitis)
White blood cell casts	Infection (pyelonephritis) Inflammation (interstitial nephritis)
Pigmented granular casts	Acute tubular necrosis (heme granular casts, muddy brown) Glomerulonephritis, interstitial nephritis
Fatty casts	Heavy proteinuria (>3.5 g/d)

Common Presentations

Proteinuria

Definitions
- 24 h urine protein excretion is gold standard to assess degree of proteinuria
- Albumin to creatinine ratio (ACR) is used to screen for diabetic nephropathy
- Microalbuminuria
    - Defined as ACR $\geq$2.8 mg/mmol (female) or $\geq$2.0 mg/mmol (male)
        - Marker of vascular endothelial function and important prognostic marker for kidney disease in diabetes and hypertension (elevated ACR is the earliest sign of diabetic nephropathy)

Daily Excretion of Protein

Daily Excretion	Interpretation
<150 mg total protein (and <30 mg albumin)	Normal
30-300 mg albumin	Microalbuminuria
>3500 mg total protein	Nephrotic range proteinuria
Variable amount of proteinuria	Can be seen with glomerular disease; i.e. mild glomerular disease can lead to a mild degree of proteinuria, proliferative lesions may also be associated with some degree of proteinuria
Up to 2000 mg per day	Possible with tubular disease because of failure to reabsorb filtered proteins

History and Physical Exam
- Signs and symptoms of transient physiologic or secondary causes (fever, CHF, collagen vascular diseases, malignancy, chronic infections, medications)

Investigations
- Urine R&M, C&S, Urea, Cr
- Further workup (proteinuria >0.5 g/d, casts and/or hematuria): CBC, glucose, electrolytes, 24h urine protein and Cr, urine and serum immunoelectrophoresis, abdo/pelvic U/S, serology (ANA, RF, p-ANCA, c-ANCA, Hep B, Hep C, HIV)
- Indications for referral:
    - Heavy proteinuria = ACR >30-1000 mg/mmoL
    - Nephritic syndrome: marked proteinuria >3.5 mg/1.73 m^2/d with hypoalbuminemia (<35 g/L)

Classification

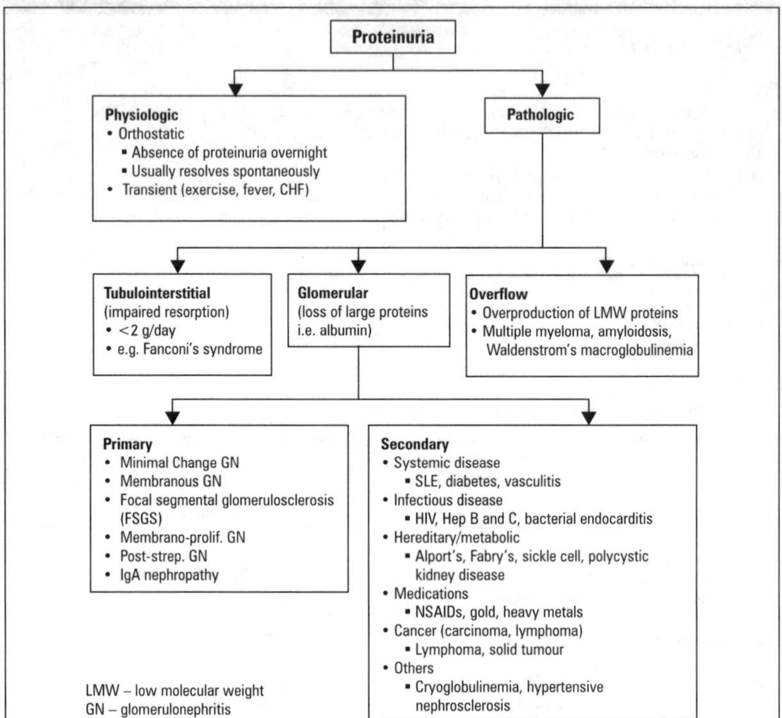

Hematuria

Definition
• Presence of blood or RBCs in urine
  ▪ Gross hematuria: pink, red, or tea-coloured urine
  ▪ Microscopic hematuria: normal coloured urine + >2-3 RBCs/HPF

History and Physical Exam
• FHx nephrolithiasis, hearing loss (Alport's), cerebral aneurysm (PCKD), diet, recent URTI, irritative and obstructive urinary symptoms (UTI)

Investigations
• 24h urine stone workup: calcium, oxalate, citrate, magnesium, uric acid, cysteine
• Further workup (if casts and/or proteinuria): CBC, electrolytes, 24h urine protein and Cr, serology (ANA, RF, C3, C4, p-ANCA, c-ANCA, anti-GBM), abdo/pelvic U/S, cystoscopy ± urology consult

Approach

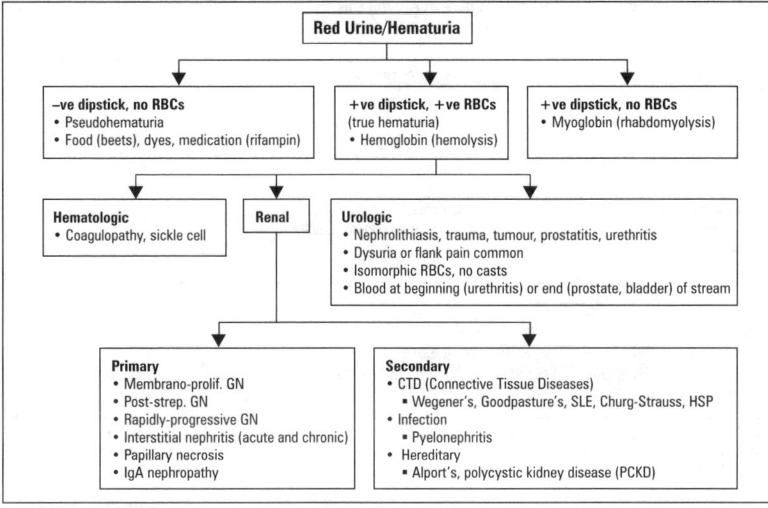

Acid-Base Disorders

GENERAL APPROACH TO ACID BASE DISORDERS

1. Identify the main disturbance from pH level: acidemic or alkalemic?
   - Acidemia – low pH (pH <7.40)
   - Alkalemia – high pH (pH >7.40)
2. Identify if it is a respiratory or metabolic process by changes in PCO_2 and HCO_3^-
   - Low pH + Low HCO_3^- = Metabolic acidosis
   - Low pH + High pCO_2 = Respiratory acidosis
   - High pH + High HCO_3^- = Metabolic alkalosis
   - High pH + Low pCO_2 = Respiratory alkalosis
3. Predict the compensatory response: the compensation response is always in the same direction as the primary disorder in an attempt to restore pH

Expected Compensation for Specific Acid-Base Disorders

Disturbance	$PaCO_2$ (mmHg)	HCO_3^- (mmHg)
Respiratory Acidosis		
Acute	Increase 10	Increase 1
Chronic	Increase 10	Increase 3
Respiratory Alkalosis		
Acute	Decrease 10	Decrease 2
Chronic	Decrease 10	Decrease 5
Metabolic Acidosis	Decrease 1	Decrease 1
Metabolic Alkalosis	Increase 5-7	Increase 10

4. Compare the predicted to observed compensation
5. Calculate the Anion Gap (AG): $AG = Na^+ - Cl^- - HCO_3^-$ (normal range of 10-14; baseline is 12)
   - Adjust for albumin: each decrease in albumin by 10 g/L, lowers baseline AG by 3

6. Compare increase in AG with the decrease in HCO_3^- (should be similar)
  - If decrease in HCO_3^- is larger than increase in AG, then secondary normal AG metabolic acidosis
  - If decrease in HCO_3^- is smaller than increase in AG, then secondary metabolic alkalosis

Causes of Increased Anion Gap	Causes of non-Anion Gap
Metabolic Acidosis: MUDPILES	**Metabolic Acidosis: HARDUP**
Methanol	**H**yperalimentation
Uremia	**A**cetazolamide
Diabetic/alcohol/starvation ketoacidosis	**R**TA
Paraldehyde	**D**iarrhea
Isopropyl alcohol/iron	**U**reteroenteric fistula
Lactic acidosis	**P**ancreaticoduodenal fistula
Ethylene glycol	
Salicylates	

7. Calculate the Osmolar Gap (OG):
- OG = measured osmolality – calculated osmolality
- Calculated osmolality = $2 \times Na^+ + urea + glucose$
- Normal OG is <10; if OG >10 consider: formaldehyde, methanol, ethylene glycol, alcoholic ketoacidosis, end stage renal disease

> **3 Clinical scenarios that produce a mixed metabolic disorder with near normal pH: (increased AG metabolic acidosis + resp. alkalosis)**
> - Cirrhosis, ASA overdose, sepsis

Common Conditions

Disorders of Sodium Homeostasis

Clinical Assessment of ECF Volume (Total Body Na^+)

Fluid Compartment	Hypovolemic	Hypervolemic
Intravascular		
JVP	Decreased	Increased
Blood pressure	Orthostatic drop	Normal to increased
Auscultation of heart	Tachycardia	S3
Auscultation of lungs	Normal	Inspiratory crackles
Interstitial		
Skin turgor	Decreased	Normal/increased
Edema (dependent)	Absent	Present
Other		
Urine output	Decreased	Variable
Body weight	Decreased	Increased
Hct, serum protein	Increased	Decreased

Hyponatremia

Definition
- Serum $[Na^+]$ <135 mmol/L, associated with normal, decreased or increased serum osmolality

Signs and Symptoms
- Depends on degree of hyponatremia and the rapidity of its onset
- Acute hyponatremia (<48 h) more likely to be symptomatic

- Chronic hyponatremia (>48 h) adapts to tonicity through loss of cellular electrolytes (hours) and organic osmoles (days) but is prone to complications of overly rapid correction
- Neurologic symptoms, secondary to cerebral edema predominate, including headache, nausea, malaise, lethargy, weakness, muscle cramps, anorexia, disorientation, personality changes, depressed reflexes, decreased LOC

Approach to Hyponatremia

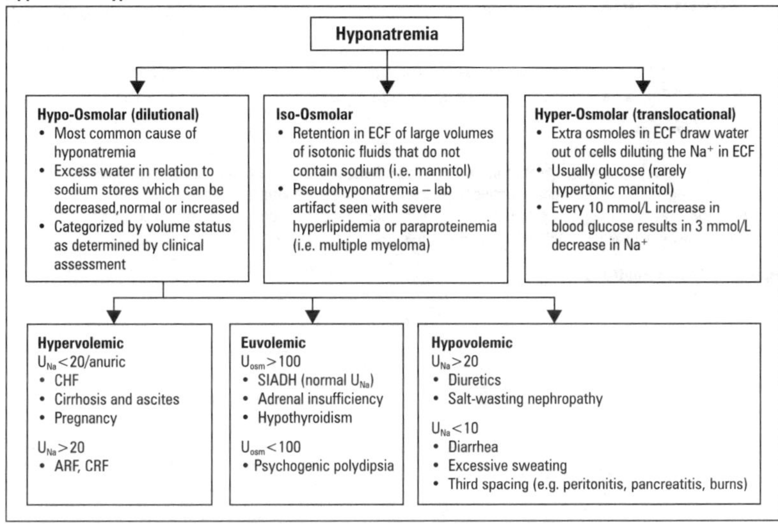

Complications
- Include seizures, coma, respiratory arrest, permanent brain damage, brain stem herniation and death
- Risk of Central Pontine Myelinolysis (CPN; CN palsies, quadriplegia, and decreased LOC) due to brain cell shrinkage and osmotic demyelination of pontine and extrapontine neurons with rapid correction of hyponatremia
- Particularly with correction of >8 mmol/d if chronic hyponatremia, malnutrition, hypokalemia and chronic alcohol use

Investigations
- ECF volume assessment, serum electrolytes, creatinine, BUN, glucose, osmolality
- Urine osmolality and electrolytes; Na^+ <10-20 mmol/L suggests volume depletion
- Assess for causes of SIADH (consider CT thorax, thyroid function tests and cortisol levels)

Treatment
- All patients: water restriction (<1 L/d), treat underlying cause, monitor serum $[Na^+]$ frequently to avoid rapid over-correction, monitor urine output closely as high U/O of dilute urine is a first sign of overly-rapid correction
- Known acute hyponatremia (reduced risk for CPM): if symptomatic correct rapidly with 3% NaCl 1-2cc/kg/h up to serum $[Na^+]$ of 125-130 mM, may need loop diuretic (e.g. furosemide) if volume overloaded; if asymptomatic and marked drop in serum Na^+, treat as if symptomatic
- Chronic hyponatremia or uncertain of acuity: if severe symptoms treat with hypertonic NaCl and/or furosemide to target a rise in serum $[Na^+]$ of 1-2 mM for 4-6 h and a total rise of 8 mM in 24 h; if asymptomatic consider normal saline and furosemide; if refractory consider furosemide, normal saline, demeclocycline (ADH antagonist) 300-600 mg PO bid, extra osmoles in the form of oral urea, very slow rate of 3% NaCl ($\sim$10 cc/h)
- Overly rapid correction: switch infusate to D5W, give DDAVP 5 mcg SC to stop water diuresis

> **To estimate the change in serum [Na$^+$] for 1L of a fluid bolus (assuming no losses of water or electrolytes)**
>
> $$[Na^+] = \frac{\text{infusate } [Na^+] - \text{serum } [Na^+]}{TBW + 1}$$
>
> TBW = 0.6xwt (kg) for males and 0.5xwt (kg) for females

Hypernatremia

Definition
- Serum [Na$^+$] >145 mmol/L usually because of a net water loss; less common than hyponatremia because of protective mechanisms of thirst and ADH secretion

Signs and Symptoms
- Usually occurs in the hospital setting
- Acute hypernatremia is more likely to be symptomatic because there is no time for cells to adapt by importing or generating osmotically active particles to normalize cell size
- Symptoms related to brain cell shrinkage and include altered mental status, weakness, neuromuscular irritability, focal neurological deficits, seizures, coma and death

Approach to Hypernatremia

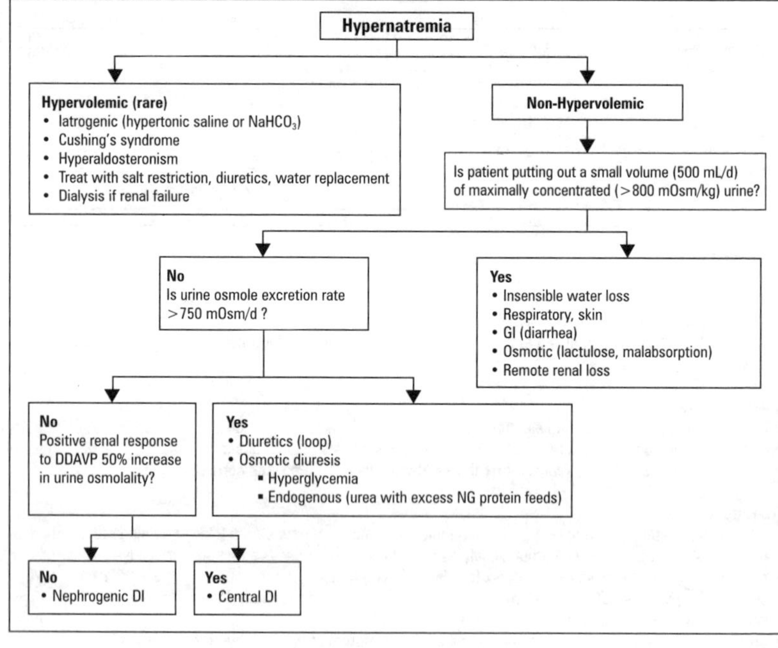

Complications
- Increased risk of vascular rupture resulting in intracranial hemorrhage; overly rapid correction may lead to cerebral edema

Investigations
- ECF volume assessment, serum electrolytes, creatinine, BUN, glucose
- Urine osmolality (DI likely if urine osmolality <600 mOsm/d)
- Dehydration test: 12-18 h without water, if fail to concentrate urine, most likely DI
- DDAVP administration (10 mcg intranasally or 4 mcg SC)
  - If central DI: increased urine osmolality and decreased urine volume
  - If nephrogenic DI: kidneys do not respond to exogenous ADH, no changes in osmolality or volume of urine

Treatment
- All patients: salt restriction and give free water orally or IV, treat underlying cause, monitor serum $[Na^+]$ frequently to avoid over-rapid correction
- Hypovolemic hypernatremia: if evidence of hemodynamic instability, first correct volume depletion with bolus of normal saline; replace water deficit (formula below) with water via oral route (PO/NG) or alternatively use IV hypotonic infusates; target maximum 12 mM (8 mM practically) decrease of $[Na^+]$ in 24 h

$$H_2O \text{ deficit} = \frac{TBW \times (serum\ [Na^+] - 140)}{140}$$

TBW = 0.6xwt (kg) for males and 0.5xwt (kg) for females

- **Hypervolemic hypernatremia**: remove excess total body Na^+ via diuresis or dialysis (renal failure); replace water deficit with D5W

Disorders of Potassium Homeostasis

- K^+ excretion = (urine flow rate) x (urine K^+ concentration)
- Factors which increase renal K^+ loss: hyperkalemia, increased distal tubular urine flow rate and Na^+ delivery (thiazides and loop diuretics), increased aldosterone (causes Na^+ reabsorption and K^+ excretion), metabolic alkalosis, hypomagnesemia, increased non-reabsorbable anions in tubule lumen (HCO_3^-, penicillin, salicylate)

Hypokalemia

Definition
- Serum $[K^+]$ <3.5 mmol/L (<3.5 mEq/L)

Approach
- ECG (emergent): if potentially life-threatening begin treatment immediately (see below)
- Rule out intracellular shift of K^+ as a cause
- Assess dietary intake (uncommon as a cause without additional K^+ loss)
- 24-hour K^+ excretion or spot urine K^+
- Transtubular potassium gradient (TTKG) = $(U_K/P_K)/(U_{osm}/P_{osm})$
- If renal losses, check BP and acid-base status
- Assess serum renin and aldosterone levels, serum $[Mg^{2+}]$

Signs and Symptoms
- Usually asymptomatic especially when mild ($[K^+]$ 3-3.5 mM)
- Nausea, vomiting, fatigue, generalized weakness, myalgias, muscle cramps, constipation
- If severe: arrhythmias, muscle necrosis, paralysis with respiratory impairment
- Arrhythmias occur at any K^+ level and more common if digoxin use, hypomagnesia, coronary artery disease
- ECG changes are more predictive of clinical picture than K^+ levels; U waves most important, flattened or inverted T waves, depressed ST segments and prolongation of QT interval; if severe hypokalemia PT prolongation, widened QRS complex and arrhythmias

ECG Changes in Hypokalemia

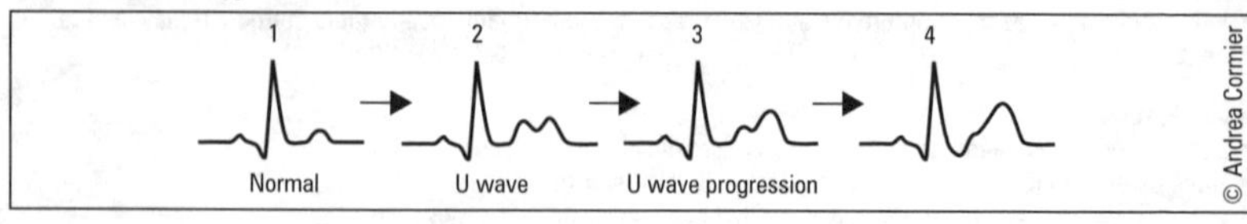

Management

- Treat underlying cause
- Replace K^+ deficit with extreme caution, especially if decreased U/O, impaired renal function, hypokalemia caused by transcellular shift, elderly or diabetic
- 100-200 mEq of K^+ raises serum $[K^+]$ approximately 1 mEq/L
- Maximum IV concentrations are 40 mEq/L in peripheral veins or 60 mEq/L in central lines
- For non-emergent cases, give K^+-Dur (20 mEq K^+ each) 2 tablets PO BID
- Replace with extreme caution if there is renal dysfunction
- If there is concomitant hypomagnesemia this must also be corrected in order to be able to correct hypokalemia

Hyperkalemia

Definition

- Serum $[K^+]$ >5.0 mmol/Ln (>5.0 mEq/L)

Approach

- ECG (emergent): if potentially life-threatening begin treatment immediately
- Rule out factitious hyperkalemia (e.g. sample hemolysis), repeat blood test
- Hold all exogenous K^+ and K^+-retaining medications
- Assess potential causes of extracellular shift
- Estimate GFR (see CrCl or Cockcroft-Gault)
- Calculate TTKG (see Hypokalemia)
- TTKG <7: decreased effective aldosterone
- TTKG ≥7: normal aldosterone function

Signs and Symptoms

- Usually asymptomatic but may develop nausea, palpitations, muscle weakness, muscle stiffness, parasthesias, areflexia, ascending paralysis and hypoventilation
- Impaired renal ammoniagenesis and metabolic acidosis
- ECG changes and cardiotoxicity do not correlate with $[K^+]$ level: peaked and narrow T waves, decreased amplitude and loss of P waves, prolonged PR interval, widened QRS complex approaching a sine wave pattern, AV block, ventricular fibrillation and asystole

Causes of Hyperkalemia

Factitious	Increased Intake	Cellular Release	Decreased Excretion
Prolonged use of tourniquet	Diet	Intravascular hemolysis	Decreased GFR
Sample taken from vein	KCl tabs	Rhabdomyolysis	Renal failure
where IV KCl is running	IV KCl	Insulin deficiency	Low effective circulating volume
Sample hemolysis		Hyperosmolar states	NSAIDs in renal insufficiency
Leukocytosis (extreme)		(e.g. hyperglycemia)	Normal GFR but
Thrombocytosis (extreme)		Metabolic acidosis (except for keto- and	hypoaldosteronism (see below)
		lactic acidosis)	
		Tumour lysis syndrome	
		Drugs	
		β-blockers	
		Digitalis overdose (blocks Na^+/K^+ ATPase)	
		Succinylcholine	

Causes of Hyperkalemia with Normal GFR

Decreased Aldosterone Stimulus (low renin, low aldosterone)	Decreased Aldosterone Production (normal renin, low aldosterone)	Aldosterone Resistance (decreased tubular response)
Hyporeninemic, hypoaldosteronism Associated with DM2, NSAIDs, chronic interstitial nephritis, HIV	Adrenal insufficiency of any cause (e.g. Addison's disease, AIDS, metastatic cancer) ACE inhibitors Angiotensin II receptor blockers Heparin Congenital adrenal hyperplasia with 21-hydroxylase deficiency	K^+-sparing diuretics Spironolactone Amiloride Triamterene Drugs mimicking K^+-sparing diuretics Pentamidine Trimethoprim Cyclosporine, tacrolimus Pseudohypoaldosteronism (rare inherited tubular disorders)

ECG Changes in Hyperkalemia

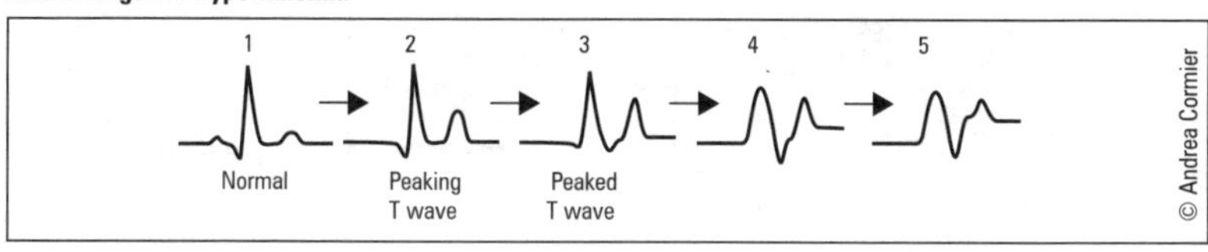

Management
- Acute therapy if ECG changes, $[K^+]$ >6.5 mM or symptoms
- Protect the heart: calcium gluconate 1-2 amps (10 mL of 10% solution) IV works within minutes and lasts 30-60 min (repeat if necessary)
- Shift K^+ into cells
  - 10-20 units of insulin R IV preceded by 1 amp of D50W IV acts within 15-30 min and lasts 1-2 h, repeat blood glucose with $[K^+]$ every hour, may repeat or infuse at 1 unit/h
  - 1-3 amps $NaHCO_3^-$ (as 3 amps 7.5% $NaHCO_3^-$ in 1L D5W) acts within 15-30 min exchanging K^+ for H^+
  - Nebulized β2-agonist (e.g. salbutamol) acts within 30-90 min by stimulating Na^+/K^+ ATPase; caution in heart disease because of resulting tachycardia
- Enhance K^+ removal
  - Furosemide (40 mg IV) ± IV NS to prevent hypovolemia
  - Fludrocortisone (synthetic mineralocorticoid) if suspected aldosterone deficiency
  - Cation exchange resins: calcium resonium or sodium kaexylate with sorbitol (use tap water if administered as enema)
- Dialysis if renal failure, life-threatening hyperkalemia, or unresponsive to therapy

Acute Kidney Injury

Definition
- Elevated urea and Cr in the blood usually caused by inability of the kidney to excrete urea, Cr and other nitrogen-containing compounds

> - 2 most common causes of acute kidney injury in hospitalized patients: **pre-renal azotemia** and **ATN**
> - Remember that prerenal failure can lead to ATN (analogous to TIA and stroke).

Chief Complaints
- Decreased urine volume – anuria, oliguria, polyuria, and voiding difficulty; headache, lethargy, somnolence, confusion, anorexia, nausea/vomiting, muscle cramps and muscle weakness

Approach to Acute Kidney Injury

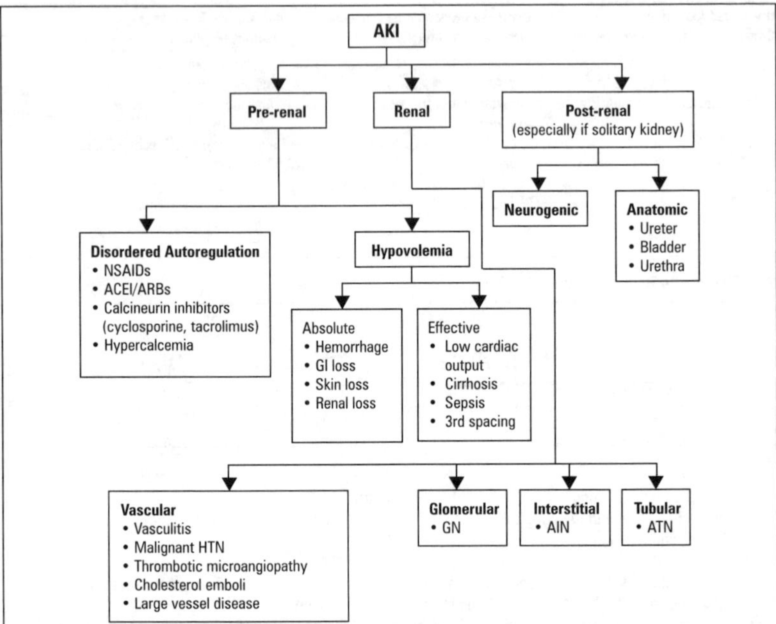

History
• Voiding difficulty, recent surgical or radiographic procedure, recent or recurrent infection/UTI, volume loss (burns, diarrhea, vomiting), medications and allergies, family history, associated symptoms including fever and rash (allergic interstitial nephritis) or arthralgias and rash (collagen vascular disease)

Complications
• Multi-organ failure, especially in pre-renal AKI

Physical Examination
• Vitals especially BP for orthostatic changes, body weight, volume status (pulse, skin turgor, JVP, mucous membranes, urine output), cardiorespiratory especially pulmonary edema and S3, uremia (asterixis, encephalopathy, pericarditis), abdominal examination for flank tenderness, distended abdomen, organomegaly, ascites

Investigations
• CBC, electrolytes, Cr, BUN (think pre-renal if BUN to Cr ratio is greater than 1:10), Ca^{2+}, PO_4^{3-}
• Urine: volume, R&M, ± C&S, osmolality and electrolytes (especially Na^+)
• ECG
• Foley to rule out bladder outlet obstruction
• Abdominal U/S to assess kidney size, hydronephrosis, post-renal obstruction
• Renal biopsy if diagnosis is uncertain and pre-renal azotemia or ATN is unlikely and if oliguria persists beyond 4 wks

Distinguishing Pre-Renal from Intra-Renal Disease in Acute Kidney Injury

Index	Pre-Renal	Intra-Renal (e.g. ATN)
Urine Osmolality	>500	<350
Urine Sodium (mmol/L)	<20	>40
FE_{Na}	<1%	3-6%
Plasma BUN/Cr (SI Units)	>80:1	<40:1
Urinalysis	Blond	RBC, pigmented granular casts

Management
- Definitive therapy depends on etiology, mainly supportive in nature
- Dialysis if indicated (see below):

INDICATIONS FOR DIALYSIS IN AKI (HAVE PEE)
Hyperkalemia (refractory)　　　**P**ericarditis
Acidosis (refractory)　　　**E**ncephalopathy
Volume overload (refractory)　　**E**dema (pulmonary)
Elevated BUN (>35 mM)

Glomerular Disease

The Spectrum of Glomerular Pathology

Nephrotic	Intermediate	Nephritic
		Hematuria, ↓ GFR
Proteinura →		
FSGS	Membranoproliferative GN	Diffuse proliferative GN
Membranous glomerulopathy	Focal proliferative GN	Crescentic GN
Minimal change	• IgA nephropathy	
	• Idiopathic membranoproliferative GN	
	• HBV, HCV	
	• SLE	
	• Cryoglobulinemia	

Investigations
- Bloodwork
    - First presentation: electrolytes, creatinine, urea, albumin, fasting lipids
    - Determining etiology: CBC, ESR, serum immune electrophoresis, anti-GBM, C3, C4, ANA, p-ANCA, c-ANCA, cryoglobulins, HBV, HCV serology, ASOT, VDRL, HIV
- Urine: R&M (RBCs, WBCs, casts, protein), 24h urine for protein and creatinine clearance, immunoelectrophoresis for Bence-Jones proteins if proteinuria present
- Radiology: CXR (infiltrates, CHF, pleural effusions), renal ultrasound
- Renal biopsy: percutaneous or open

ACUTE NEPHRITIC SYNDROME

Clinical and Lab Features of Nephritic Syndome (PHAROH):
- **P**roteinuria (<3.5 g/1.73 m²/d), **H**ematuria (abrupt onset, micro/macroscopic), **A**zotemia, **R**BC casts and/or dysmorphic RBCs in urine, **O**liguria, **H**ypertension (salt and water retention)
- Other: periorbital edema, smoky urine

Etiology of Nephritic Syndrome

	Low Complement Level	Normal Complement Level
Primary Causes	Postinfectious GN Membranoprolif. GN	IgA nephropathy Anti-GBM disease
Secondary Causes	SLE Endocarditis Abscess or shunt nephritis Cryoglobulinemia	Polyarteritis nodosa Wegener's granulomatosis Henoch-Schonlein purpura Goodpasture's syndrome

NEPHROTIC SYNDROME

Presentation of Nephrotic Syndrome
- Severe proteinuria (>3.5 g/d), hypoalbuminemia, edema, hyperlipidemia, lipiduria, oval fat bodies (microscopy), hypercoagulable state (antithrombin III, protein C and protein S loss in urine)

Etiology of Nephrotic Syndrome

	Minimal Change	Membranous Glomerulopathy	Focal Segmental Glomerulosclerosis	Membranoproliferative Glomerulonephritis
Secondary Causes	Lymphoma, bee stings	HBV, SLE, malignancy (lung, breast, GI)	Reflux nephropathy, HIV, HBV	HCV, malaria, SLE, leukemia, lymphoma
Drug Causes	NSAIDs	Gold, penicillamine	Heroin	
Therapy	Steroids	Reduce BP, ACEI, steroids	Steroids, ACEI/ARB for proteinuria	Aspirin, ACEI, dipyridamole (Persantine®) – controversial

RAPIDLY PROGRESSIVE GLOMERULONEPHRITIS (RPGN)

Features
- This is a clinical, not a histopathological diagnosis
  - A subset of nephritic syndrome in which renal failure progresses in weeks to months
  - Usually crescent formation seen on renal biopsy
  - RBC casts and/or dysmorphic RBC's in urine
  - Classification by immunofluorescence staining
  - Treatment: corticosteroids + cyclophosphamide or other cytotoxic agent
  - Prognosis: 50% recovery with early treatment, depends on underlying cause

SECONDARY CAUSES OF GLOMERULAR DISEASE
- Amyloidosis, SLE, Henoch-Schönlein Purpura, Goodpasture's disease, Wegener's granulomatosis, cryoglobulinemia, shunt nephritis, HIV-associated nephropathy (HIV-AN), infective endocarditis, hepatitis B, hepatitis C, syphilis, malaria

Tubulointerstitial Disease

Definition
- Cellular infiltrates affecting primarily the renal interstitium and tubule cells; functional tubule defects are disproportionately greater than the decrease in GFR; classified as acute or chronic

ACUTE TUBULAR NECROSIS (ATN)

Definition
- Abrupt and sustained decline in GFR within minutes-days of an ischemic or nephrotoxic insult

Etiology of ATN

Clinical Presentation
- Abrupt rise in BUN and creatinine following a hypotensive episode, sepsis, rhabdomyolysis or administration of a nephrotoxic drug

Complications
- Hyperkalemia, metabolic acidosis, decreased Ca^{2+}, decreased Na^+, increased PO_4^{3-}, low albumin

Investigations
- Blood: CBC, electrolytes, Cr, BUN, urea, Ca^{2+}, PO_4^{3-}, blood gases
- Urine: R&M (hemegranular casts), high FE_{Na}
- ECG

Treatment
- Largely supportive while correcting underlying etiology, may consider loop diuretics to help manage volume overload or early dialysis in severe cases for uremic syndromes

Prevention
- Correct fluid balance before surgical procedures, N-acetylcysteine (Mucomyst®) 1200 mg PO bid before and after radiocontrast in patients with chronic renal disease, renal-adjusted dosing of nephrotoxic drugs

ACUTE TUBULOINTERSTITIAL NEPHRITIS

Definition
- Rapid (days-weeks) decline in renal function representing 10-20% of all cases of acute renal failure

Etiology
- Hypersensitivity: antibiotics (β-lactams, sulfonamides, rifampin, quinolones, cephalosporins), NSAIDs, allopurinol, furosemide
- Infection: bacterial pyelonephritis, streptococcal infection, brucellosis, legionellosis, CMV, EBV, toxoplasmosis, leptospirosis
- Immune: SLE, acute allograft rejection, Sjögren's syndrome, sarcoidosis, mixed essential cryoglobulinemia

Pathophysiology
- Acute inflammatory cell infiltrates into renal interstitium

Signs and Symptoms
- Based upon underlying etiology
- Acute renal failure
- If hypersensitivity reaction: may see fever, skin rash, arthralgia, serum sickness-like syndrome
- If pyelonephritis: flank pain and CVA tenderness
- Hypertension and edema are uncommon

Investigations
- Urine: sterile pyuria, WBC casts, mild proteinuria, hematuria, eosinophils
- Blood: increased creatinine and urea, eosinophilia (if drug reaction), non-AG metabolic acidosis (i.e. renal tubular acidosis), hypophosphatemia, hyperkalemia, hyponatremia
- Radiographic: gallium scan shows intense signal from inflammatory infiltrate
- Renal biopsy: definitive diagnosis
- Treatment: treat underlying cause (i.e. stop offending medications, antibiotics if pyelonephritis), corticosteroids may be indicated in allergic or immune disease

Vascular Diseases of the Kidney

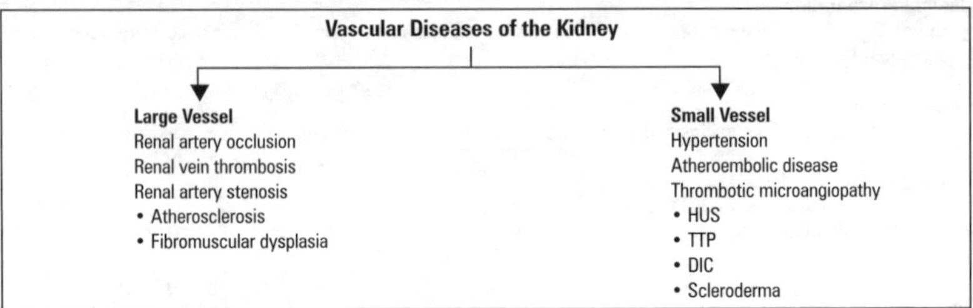

Large Vessel Disease

RENAL INFARCTION (ACUTE RENAL ARTERY OCCLUSION)
• Important, potentially reversible cause of renal failure

Etiology
• Abdominal trauma, surgery, embolism, vasculitis, extrarenal compression, hypercoaguable state, aortic dissection
• Kidney transplant more vulnerable

Signs and Symptoms (depend on presence of collateral circulation)
• Fever, nausea, vomiting, flank pain
• Leukocytosis, elevated AST, ALP and markedly elevated LDH
• Acute onset hypertension (activation of RAAS) or sudden worsening of long-standing hypertension
• Renal dysfunction (if bilateral or solitary functioning kidney)

Investigations
• Renal arteriography (more reliable but risk of atheroembolic renal disease)
• Contrast-enhanced CT or magnetic resonance angiography, duplex Doppler studies (operator dependent)

Treatment
• Prompt localization of occlusion and restoration of blood flow
• Anticoagulation, thrombolysis, percutaneous angioplasty or clot extraction, surgical thrombectomy
• Medical therapy in the long-term to reduce risk (e.g. antihypertensives)

ISCHEMIC RENAL DISEASE (RENAL ARTERY STENOSIS)
• Chronic renal impairment secondary to hemodynamically significant renal artery stenosis or microvascular disease
• Significant cause of ESRD: 15% in patients over 50 yrs old (higher prevalence if significant vascular disease)
• Usually associated with large vessel disease elsewhere
• Causes
  1. Atherosclerotic plaques (90%) – proximal 1/3 renal artery, usually males >55 yrs, smokers
  2. Fibromuscular dysplasia (10%) – distal 2/3 renal artery or segmental branches, usually young females (typical onset < age 30)
• Most common cause of secondary hypertension ("renovascular hypertension"), 1-2% of all hypertensive patients
  ▪ Decreased renal perfusion of one or both kidneys leads to increased renin release and subsequent angiotensin production
  ▪ Increased angiotensin raises blood pressure in 2 ways
    ◆ Causes generalized arteriolar constriction
    ◆ Release of aldosterone increases Na^+ and water retention
  ▪ Elevated blood pressure can in turn lead to further damage of kidneys and worsening HTN

Risk Factors
- >50 yrs old
- Smoking
- Other atherosclerotic disease
- Severe/refractory HTN and/or hypertensive crises
- Asymmetrical renal size
- Epigastric or flank bruits
- Spontaneous hypokalemia (renin activation in under-perfused kidney)
- Increasing Cr with ACEI/ARB
- Flash pulmonary edema with normal LV function

Investigations
- Must establish presence of renal vessel stenosis and prove it is responsible for renal dysfunction
- Duplex Doppler U/S (kidney size, blood flow): good screening test (operator dependent)
- Digital subtraction angiography (risk of contrast nephropathy)
- CT or MR angiography (effective noninvasive tests to establish presence of stenosis)
- ACE inhibitor renography (i.e. captopril renal scan)
- Renal arteriography (gold standard)

Treatment
- Medical therapy, percutaneous angioplasty + stent, surgical revascularization
- Little or no benefit if therapy is late

RENAL VEIN THROMBOSIS

Etiology
- Hypercoagulable states (e.g. nephrotic syndrome, especially membranous), ECF volume depletion, extrinsic compression of renal vein, significant trauma, malignancy (i.e. RCC), sickle cell
- Clinical presentation determined by rapidity of occlusion and formation of collateral circulation
- Acute: nausea/vomiting, flank pain, hematuria, elevated plasma LDH, ± rise in Cr, sudden rise in proteinuria
- Chronic: PE (typical first presenting symptom), increasing proteinuria and/or tubular dysfunction

Investigations
- Renal venography (gold standard), CT or MR angiography, duplex Doppler U/S

Treatment
- Thrombolytic therapy ± percutaneous thrombectomy for acute RVT
- Anticoagulation with heparin then warfarin (1 yr or indefinitely, depending on risk factors)

Small Vessel Disease

HYPERTENSIVE NEPHROSCLEROSIS
- See *Hypertension*

ATHEROEMBOLIC RENAL DISEASE
- Progressive renal insufficiency due to embolic obstruction of small and medium-sized renal vessels by atheromatous emboli
- Spontaneous or after renal artery manipulation such as surgery, angiography, or percutaneous angioplasty
- Anticoagulants and thrombolytics interfere with ulcerated plaque healing and can worsen disease
- Presentation: acute or chronic, progressive renal dysfunction, labile hypertension, extrarenal atheroembolic disease support diagnosis (livedo reticularis is a classic sign)
- Labwork: eosinophilia and/or eosinophiluria may be seen
- Renal biopsy: needle-shaped cholesterol clefts (due to tissue-processing artifacts) with surrounding tissue reaction in small/medium-sized vessels
- No effective treatment; avoid angiographic and surgical procedures in patients with diffuse atherosclerosis

THROMBOTIC MICROANGIOPATHY
- A spectrum which includes HUS, TTP, DIC and post-partum renal failure
- Renal involvement more common in HUS than TTP
- Renal involvement characterized by fibrin thrombi in glomerular capillary loops ± arterioles
- Treatment:
    - Depends on cause
    - supportive therapy always
    - TTP-HUS: plasma exchange, corticosteroids (splenectomy and rituximab if refractory)
    - Avoid platelet transfusions and ASA

SCLERODERMA
- 50% of scleroderma patients have renal involvement (mild proteinuria, high Cr, HTN)
- Histology: media thickened, "onion skin" hypertrophy of small renal arteries, fibrinoid necrosis of afferent arterioles and glomeruli
- 10-15% scleroderma patients have a "scleroderma renal crisis" (occurs in first few years of disease): malignant HTN, ARF, microangiopathy, volume overload, visual changes, HTN encephalopathy
- Renal involvement usually occurs early in the course of illness
- Treatment: BP control with ACEI slows progression of renal disease

CALCINEURIN INHIBITOR NEPHROPATHY
- Cyclosporine and tacrolimus
- Causes both acute reversible and chronic, largely irreversible nephrotoxicity
- Acute: due to afferent and efferent glomerular capillary constriction leading to decreased GFR (tubular vacuolization)
    - Pre-renal azotemia
    - Treatment: calcium channel blockers or prostaglandin analogs, reduce dose of cyclosporine/tacrolimus or switch to another immunosuppressive drug (e.g. sirolimus)
- Chronic: result of obliterative arteriolopathy causing interstitial nephritis and CRF (striped fibrosis)

Chronic Kidney Disease

Definition
- Evidence of structural or functional kidney abnormalities (abnormal urinalysis, imaging studies, or histology) that persist for at least three months, with or without a decreased GFR (as defined by a GFR of less than 60 mL/min per 1.73 m^2)

Etiology
- Diabetes (43%), hypertension (26%), glomerulonephritis (10%), unknown (8%), interstitial nephritis/ pyelonephritis (4%), cystic/hereditary/congenital (3%), secondary GN/vasculitis (2%)

Management
- Diet: restriction of protein, potassium (40 mmol/d), Na$^+$, water, PO$_4^{3-}$, Mg^{2+}
- Medical: renal adjusted medications, avoid nephrotoxins, erythropoietin for anemia, DDAVP for prolonged bleeding, ACEI for hypertension (target 125/75), loop diuretics when GFR <25 mL/min, statins for dyslipidemia, calcium supplementation, phosphate binders (e.g. sevelamer, lanthanum carbonate)
- Dialysis (in-centre or at home)
- Renal transplantation

INDICATIONS FOR DIALYSIS IN CHRONIC RF
- **Absolute indications**: volume overload unresponsive to medication, hyperkalemia unresponsive to medication, severe metabolic acidosis unresponsive to medication, neurologic signs or symptoms of uremia (encephalopathy, neuropathy, seizures), uremic pericarditis, refractory accelerated hypertension, clinically significant bleeding diathesis, persistent severe nausea and vomiting, plasma Cr >1060 μmol/L or BUN >36 mmol/L
- **Relative indications**: anorexia, decreased cognitive functioning, profound fatigue and weakness, severe anemia unresponsive to erythropoietin, persistent severe pruritus, restless leg syndrome

Peritoneal Dialysis vs. Hemodialysis

	Peritoneal Dialysis	Hemodialysis
Rate	Slow	Fast
Location	Home	Hospital (usually)
Ultrafiltration	Osmotic pressure via dextrose dialysate	Hydrostatic pressure
Solute Removal	Concentration gradient and convection	Concentration gradient and convection
Membrane	Peritoneum	Semi-permeable artificial membrane
Method	Indwelling catheter in peritoneal cavity	Line from vessel to artificial kidney
Complications	Infection at catheter site Bacterial peritonitis Metabolic effects of glucose Difficult to achieve adequate clearance in patients with large body mass	Vascular access (clots, collapse) Bacteremia Bleeding due to heparin Hemodynamic stress of extracorporeal circuit Disequilibrium syndrome (hypotension, nausea, muscle cramps related to solute/water flux over short time)
Preferred when	Young, high functioning, residual renal function, small body size, need to socialize	Bed-bound, co-morbidities, no renal function

Systemic Diseases of the Kidney

HYPERTENSION

Definition
- Diseases of renal parenchyma or renal vasculature can cause secondary hypertension. Conversely, hypertension due to other factors can cause renal disease (hypertensive nephrosclerosis) or worsen pre-existing renal disease

Hypertensive Nephrosclerosis

Chronic vs. Malignant Nephrosclerosis

	Chronic Nephrosclerosis	Malignant Nephrosclerosis
Histology	Slow vascular sclerosis with ischemic changes affecting intralobular and afferent arterioles	Fibrinoid necrosis of arterioles, disruption of vascular endothelium
Clinical Picture	African American, underlying chronic kidney disease, chronic hypertensive disease	Acute elevation in BP (dBP >120 mmHg) HTN encephalopathy
Urinalysis	Mild proteinuria, normal urine sediment	Proteinuria and hematuria
Therapy	Blood pressure control, frequent follow-up	Lower dBP to 100-110 mmHg within 6 h More aggressive treatment can cause ischemic event Identify and treat underlying cause of HTN
Prognosis	Can progress to renal failure despite patient adherence	Lower survival if renal insufficiency develops

RENOVASCULAR HYPERTENSION
- See *Ischemic Renal Disease* for details

RENAL PARENCHYMAL HYPERTENSION

Definition
- HTN caused secondary to GN, AIN, diabetic nephropathy, or any other chronic renal disease

MULTIPLE MYELOMA (see <u>Hematology</u>)

Presentation
• Patients may present with severe bone disease and renal failure

Etiology
• Kidney damage can occur due to: hypercalcemia, light chain cast nephropathy (LCCN), hyperuricemia, infection, secondary amyloidosis, monoclonal Ig deposition disease (MIDD), diffuse tubular obstruction

Investigations
• Increased Cr and BUN, urine protein immunoelectrophroesis positive for Bence-Jones protein, proteinuria and large tubular casts composed of light chains + Tamm-Horsfall protein (LCCN)

Fluid Resuscitation

Fluid Balance
• TBW = 60% total body weight = 2/3 ICF + 1/3 ECF where ECF = 3/4 interstitial + 1/4 intravascular
• Fluid requirements = maintenance fluids + replacing deficits + replacing ongoing losses

Maintenance Fluids
• Healthy adult requires ~2500 ml water/d to offset losses
• Requirements increase with fever, sweating, GI losses, adrenal insufficiency, hyperventilation, and polyuric renal disease
• Requirements decrease with anuria/oliguria, SIADH, highly humidified atmospheric pressures, CHF, cirrhosis and nephrotic syndrome

---

Determining maintenance fluid requirement – the 4:2:1 rule
4 mL/kg/h for the first 10 kg of a patient's body weight
2 mL/kg/h for the second 10 kg of patient's weight
1 mL/kg/h for the patient's remaining weight >20 kg

Determining maintenance electrolytes
Na^+: 3 mEq/kg/d
K^+: 1 mEq/kg/d

Concentration of Na^+ in Common Infusates
Na^+ in 0.45% NaCl = 77 mmol/L
Na^+ in 0.9% NaCl = 154 mmol/L
Na^+ in 3% NaCl = 513 mmol/L
Na^+ in 5% NaCl = 855 mmol/L
Na^+ in Ringers lactate = 130 mmol/L
Na^+ in D5W = 0

Neurology

Where is the Lesion and Essential Physical Exam

Where is the Lesion?

Anatomic Approach to Neurological Disorders, Symptoms and Signs

Location of the Lesion	General Symptoms	Common Disorders
Cortex and Internal Capsule	• Contralateral sensory and motor deficits • Cortical lesions: associated with aphasia, neglect, extinction, agraphesthesia, astereognosia, visual loss (higher level dysfunctions) • Internal capsule lesions: associated with pure motor, pure sensory losses, incoordination, absence of cortical features	Seizure disorder (cortex only) Coma Stroke
Internal Capsule	• Internal capsule lesions: associated with pure motor, pure sensory losses, incoordination, absence of cortical features	Stroke
Cerebellum and Basal Ganglia	• Incoordination • Abnormal intentional movements for cerebellar lesions (ipsilateral) → tremor, bradykinesia, involuntary movements for basal ganglia lesions	Cerebellar degeneration Parkinson's disease Stroke
Basal Ganglia	• Tremor, bradykinesia, involuntary movements	Parkinson's disease
Brainstem (unilateral) (midbrain CN 3-4; pons CN 6-7; medulla CN 8-10)	• Contralateral UMN paralysis, contralateral proprioceptive and pain-temperature loss below the head and ipsilateral CN defects. CN defects and sensory/motor deficits are on opposite sides in brain stem lesions – "crossed-signs" • MIDBRAIN: vertical diplopia, ptosis, pupillary change • PONS: LMN facial weakness, quadriparesis in bilateral pontine lesions, pinpoint pupils, horizontal diplopia • MEDULLA: lateral or medial medullary syndromes	Cranial nerve palsies Stroke
Spinal Cord (unilateral)	• Ipsilateral paralysis and proprioceptive loss, contralateral pain-temperature loss below the level of the lesion – "crossed-signs" • Sensory level, bowel/bladder dysfunction paraparesis • Brown-Sequard syndrome	Spinal cord syndromes
Nerve Root	• Radicular pain + sensory/motor deficits or absent reflex	Nerve root compression Disk herniation
Peripheral Nerve	• Ipsilateral motor and sensory deficits along a nerve distribution • Presence of LMN signs	Neuropathies
Neuromuscular Junction	• Proximal and symmetrical muscle weakness without sensory loss, fatigability or fasciculations • Diplopia, ptosis, bulbar weakness	Myasthenia gravis Lambert-Eaton syndrome Botulism
Muscle	• Proximal and symmetrical muscle weakness without sensory loss	Muscular dystrophies Myopathies including polymyositis Dermatomyositis

Physical Exam

CRANIAL NERVE EXAM

CN I (olfactory) – avoid noxious stimuli

CN II (optic)
- Visual acuity – best corrected vision or pinhole; visual fields; pupil (direct and consensual response + RAPD – afferent limb); fundoscopy

CN III, IV and VI (EOM)
- CNIII (oculomotor) – levator palpebrae superioris, MR, SR, IR, IO; CNIV (trochlear) – SO; CNVI (abducens) – LR

CN V (trigeminal)
- Sensory: V1-V3, corneal reflex; Corneal reflex: afferent (VI); Motor: temporalis, masseter, pterygoids

CN VII (facial)
- Sensorimotor: muscles of facial expression, jaw jerk, hyperacusis, corneal reflex efferent; Visceral sensory: taste to anterior 2/3 of tongue; Visceral motor: salivary and lacrimal gland

CN VIII (vestibulocochlear)
- Vestibular: nystagmus, caloric reflexes; Cochlear: Rinne, Weber

CN IX (glossopharyngeal) and X (vagus)
- Palatal elevation, gag reflex, vocal cord function, swallowing, taste to posterior 1/3 of tongue

CN XI (accessory)
- Trapezius and sternocleidomastoid

CN XII (hypoglossal)
- Tongue muscle bulk + deviation, fasciculations

Peripheral Nerve Exam

Root	Movement	Peripheral Nerve	Muscle
C5	Shoulder abduction	Axillary	Deltoid
C6	Elbow flexion	Musculocutaneous (C5/6) Radial (C6)	Biceps Brachioradialis
	Wrist extension	Radial	Extensor carpi radialis longus
C7	Elbow extension Finger extension	Radial Posterior interosseus	Triceps Extensor digitorum communis
C8	Finger flexion	Anterior interosseus Ulnar	Flexor pollicis longus and flexor digitorum longus Flexor digitorum profundus
T1	Finger abduction	Ulnar Median	First dorsal interosseus Abductor pollicis brevis

Peripheral Nerve Exam (continued)

Root	Movement	Peripheral Nerve	Muscle
L1/2	Hip flexion	N/A	Iliopsoas
L2/3	Hip adduction	Obturator	Adductor muscles
L3/4	Knee extension (L3/4) Ankle dorsiflexion (L4)	Femoral Deep peroneal	Quadriceps Tibialis anterior
L5	Hip extension (L5/S1) Ankle eversion (L5/S1) Big toe extension (L5)	Sciatic Superficial peroneal Deep peroneal	Gluteus maximus Peroneal muscles Extensor hallucis longus
S1	Knee flexion (S1) Ankle plantar flexion (S1/S2)	Sciatic Tibial	Hamstring muscles Gastrocnemius and soleus

MOTOR EXAM
- Posture
- Bulk
- Tone
- Abnormal movements
- Power
- Reflexes

SENSORY EXAM
- Primary sensation – pain and temperature (spinothalamic tract), proprioception and vibration (dorsal columns)
- Cortical function – discrimination: graphesthesia, stereognosis, extinction, 2-point discrimination

COORDINATION
- Finger-to-nose, heel-to-shin, rapid alternating movements

GAIT
- Tandem gait, toe-to-heel walk, Romberg, pull test for retropulsion

SOME HELPFUL FINDINGS ON PHYSICAL EXAMINATION

Cranial Nerve Lesions
- CNI: unilateral loss of smell suggests frontal lobe lesion (avoid irritative stimuli which stimulate CNV)
- CNII: look at optic discs for edema and optic atrophy
- CNIII/IV/VI: look for pupillary abnormalities, ptosis, abnormal eye movements
  - Pupil sparing: ischemic lesion (i.e. diabetes); pupil involved: compressive lesion (e.g. mass, aneurysm)
  - CNIII palsy = ptosis, eye down and out, with impaired pupillary response (pupil may be dilated)
- CN VII: frontalis sparing is an UMN lesion on the contralateral side
- Absent corneal reflex may be CNV (sensory deficit) or CNVII (motor deficit)
- CNIX/X: Dysarthria
- CNXII: tongue naturally deviates to weak side
- Horner's syndrome = ptosis, miosis, anhydrosis due to interrupted sympathetic nerve supply

Drug Reactions
- Bilaterally dilated and fixed pupils observed with anticholinergics (e.g. atropine, "mushrooms") and herniation
- Bilaterally small fixed pupils with opioids (not meperidine) and pontine hemorrhage

Motor System

Rating Power				
0	No muscle contraction	3	Complete ROM against gravity, without resistance
1	Muscle flicker	4	Submaximal power against resistance (4–, 4, 4+)
2	Complete ROM with gravity eliminated	5	Full power

- Postural instability with eyes closed is a positive Romberg's sign, suggesting a loss of proprioception or impaired coordination
- Postural instability with eyes open or closed suggests cerebellar disease/vestibular syndrome
- Pronator drift suggests hemiparesis
- Symmetrical weakness of proximal muscles suggests myopathy; of distal muscles suggests polyneuropathy

Sensory System
- Sensory level suggests a spinal cord lesion
- Symmetrical distal sensory loss suggests polyneuropathy
- Loss of vibration sense or proprioception suggests peripheral neuropathy or posterior column lesion
- Impaired graphesthesia and stereognosis with intact primary sensation suggests a parietal lesion

Reflexes
- Decreased/absent in lower motor neuron disease, myopathies or neuromuscular junction disorders
- Slow relaxation of ankle reflex is seen in hypothyroidism ("hung reflexes")
- Babinski sign suggests an upper motor neuron lesion, but may be seen in drug/alcohol intoxication or following a seizure
  - Other ways to elicit plantar reflex: tap on the foot dorsum; press on tibial tuberosity in inferior direction

Other
- "Doll's eye" movement, if absent, suggests pons or midbrain lesion or very deep coma
- Loss of vestibulo-ocular reflex with caloric stimulation suggests brainstem lesion or drug toxicity
- Absence seizures can be precipitated by hyperventilation
- Characteristic skin lesions are seen in neurocutaneous syndromes (e.g. neurofibromatosis, tuberous sclerosis, Sturge-Weber syndrome), non-blanching petechiae may be seen in meningococcal meningitis and thrombotic thrombocytopenic purpura (TTP)

Localization of Motor Deficits

	LMN	UMN	Extrapyramidal
Tone	Reduced	Spastic	Rigid
Involuntary Movements	Fasciculations	None	Present
Reflexes	Decreased	Increased	Normal
Babinski	Absent	Present	Absent
Weakness	Present	Present	Absent

Common Presentations

WEAKNESS AND PARASTHESIAS
- Stroke, tumour, Parkinson's disease, Wilson's disease, multiple sclerosis, myasthenia gravis, Guillain-Barré syndrome, amyotrophic lateral sclerosis, peripheral neuropathies, myopathies

NUMBNESS AND PARASTHESIAS
- Stroke, tumour, multiple sclerosis, peripheral neuropathies, B_{12} deficiency

FACIAL PAIN
- Sinusitis, dental disease, tic douloureux (trigeminal neuralgia = compression of trigeminal roots from tumours or aberrant vessels), trigeminal neuropathic pain ($2°$ to trigeminal nerve injury or disease), glossopharyngeal neuralgia, post-herpetic neuralgia, atypical facial pain, MS, compression of trigeminal roots from tumours or aberrant vessels

FACIAL WEAKNESS
- Upper motor neuron: TIA/stroke, post-ictal hemiparesis, tumour; infection (otitis media), mastoiditis, Epstein-Barr virus (EBV), herpes zoster/shingles (VZV), Lyme disease, HIV
- Lower motor neuron: idiopathic (Bell's palsy), sarcoid, neuropathy (e.g. DM), parotid gland

ALTERED MENTAL STATUS

	Etiology	Key Clinical Features	Investigations
INTRACRANIAL			
Vascular	Subarachnoid hemorrhage	Thunderclap headache Increased ICP Meningismus	CT (non-contrast) LP
	Stroke/TIA	Focal neurological signs	CT (non-contrast)
Infectious	Meningitis	Fever, headache, nausea, photophobia Meningismus	LP once ruled out mass lesion with CT
	Encephalitis	Focal neurological signs Fever, headache, ± seizure	CT LP MRI
	Abscess	Increased ICP Focal neurological signs	CT with contrast (often ring enhancing lesion)
Traumatic	Diffuse axonal shear, epidural hematoma, subdural hematoma	Trauma Hx Increased ICP Focal neurological signs Signs of basilar skull fracture (hemotympanum, raccoon eyes, Battle's sign)	CT (non-contrast) MRI
Autoimmune	Acute CNS vasculitis	Skin rash, active joints	ANA, ANCA, RF MRI Angiography
Neoplastic	Mass effect/edema, hemorrhage, seizure	Increased ICP Focal neurological signs Papilledema	CT (non-contrast) MRI
Seizure	Status epilepticus Post-ictal state	See *Seizure Disorders*	EEG
1° Psychiatric	Psychosis, mood/anxiety disorder	No organic signs or symptoms	Mental Status Exam

EXTRACRANIAL

Metabolic	Systemic
Diabetic ketoacidosis	Liver failure
Hypoglycemia	Renal failures
Electrolyte disturbance	Sepsis
Acid-base disturbance	
Thiamine deficiency	

ACUTE LOSS OF VISION

Painful	Minimal Pain
Angle closure glaucoma	Retinal detachment
Uveitis	Central retinal artery occlusion
Optic neuritis	TIA/stroke
Temporal arteritis	Pseudotumour cerebri
Trauma	

DIPLOPIA
- Neuromuscular
  - Cranial nerve III/IV/VI palsies (DM, tumour, trauma, aneurysm, ischemia)
  - Brainstem pathology (stroke, tumour, MS)
  - Myasthenia gravis
  - Wernicke encephalopathy
  - Leptomeningeal disease (e.g. meningitis)
  - Gullain-Barré syndrome (e.g. Miller-Fisher Variant)
- Mechanical
  - Thyroid ophthalmopathy
  - Cavernous sinus pathology
  - Trauma (e.g. orbital fracture)

PTOSIS
- Cranial nerve III palsy, myasthenia gravis (uni/bilateral), Horner's syndrome, congenital/idiopathic, myotonic dystrophy (bilateral)

VERTIGO
- Brainstem lesions, cerebellar lesions, vertebrobasilar insufficiency, multiple sclerosis, neurosyphilis, drugs/alcohol, peripheral causes (see Otolaryngology)

ATAXIA
- Acquired: vascular (infarction/TIA, hemorrhage, basilar migraine), infectious (bacterial abscess, viral encephalitis), toxins/medications (anticonvulsants, alcohol), autoimmune (multiple sclerosis, Miller-Fisher GBS), metabolic (hypothyroid, Wilson's disease, thiamine deficiency), neoplastic (medulloblastoma, astrocytoma, hemangioblastoma, paraneoplastic)
- Hereditary: Friedreich's ataxia, ataxia-telangiectasia, olivopontocerebellar atrophy, spinocerebellar ataxia

Common Conditions

Stroke/TIA

Definition
- A non-traumatic brain injury caused by occlusion or rupture of cerebral blood vessels that results in sudden neurological deficit characterized by loss of motor control, altered sensation, cognitive or language impairment, dysequilibrium, or coma

History
- Onset of symptoms – timing is crucial to the treatment of stroke
- N/V, headache, change in level of consciousness, facial droop, drooling, dysphagia, language disturbance
- Visual changes i.e. double vision, focal weakness, clumsiness/ataxia/incoordination, unsteady gait/posture, sensory loss
- Neglect of body parts
- Vertigo, dizziness, change of memory
- Seizure activity, urinary/fecal incontinence, aura, photophobia, constitutional symptoms, fever, trauma/falls

Predisposing Factors
- Age, hypertension, smoking, diabetes mellitus, hypercholesterolemia, previous MI/stroke, atrial fibrillation, obesity, family hx, hypercoagulable states, oral contraceptive pill

ABCD^2 Score
- The ABCD^2 score is a reliable predictor of short-term (2-d, 5-d, and 90-d) risk of stroke after presentation with a TIA. Specific cutpoints likely vary between settings and regions, but patients classified as high risk (score >5) are likely to benefit from urgent evaluation, treatment, and observation. A score of <4 was classified as low risk, and scores of 4 and 5 as medium risk (Johnston et al., 2007)

Factor	Criteria (points)
Age	>60 (1)
Blood pressure (first assessment after TIA)	SBP >140 mmHg or DBP >90 mmHg (1)
Clinical features of TIA	Unilateral weakness (2); speech impairment without weakness (1)
Duration of TIA	>59 min (2); 10-59 min (1)
Diabetes mellitus	Positive diagnosis (1)

Lancet. 2007; 369:283-92

Physical Exam

- Determine the location of the lesion in the CNS and relate to a stroke syndrome (below)
  - Vitals
  - Mental status examination
  - Neurological exam (i.e. cranial nerves, motor examination, sensory examination, coordination and gait, plantar response)
  - Cardiovascular examination (i.e. precordial examination, JVP, auscultate for murmurs, arrhythmias and carotid bruit)

TOAST Classification of Ischemic Stroke
1. Large artery atherosclerosis
2. Cardioembolism
3. Small vessel occlusion (lacunar)
4. Other determined etiology
5. Undetermined etiology

Stroke Syndromes

- Cerebral cortex
  - Anterior cerebral artery (**ACA**): contralateral leg paresis and sensory loss
  - Middle cerebral artery (**MCA**): contralateral weakness and sensory loss of face and arm greater than the leg, cortical sensory loss, aphasia if left hemisphere, neglect if right hemisphere, eye deviation towards the side of the lesion, may have contralateral homonymous hemianopia or quadrantanopia
  - Posterior cerebral artery (**PCA**): contralateral homonymous hemianopia or quadrantanopia, alexia without agraphia if left PCA, hemiballismus, midbrain signs (CN III and IV palsy, hemiparesis)
- Cerebellum (**SCA/AICA**): truncal ataxia, incoordination, nystagmus, cerebellar dysarthria
- **Lacunar infarction**: common in HTN, DM and with increasing age
  - Posterior internal capsule: most common; dense contralateral hemiplegia, pure motor, no neglect nor aphasia
  - Internal capsule, cerebellum: ataxic hemiparesis – ipsilateral ataxia and leg paresis
  - Thalamus: pure sensory deficit
  - Anterior pons (dysarthria-clumsy hand syndrome): dysarthria, facial weakness, dysphagia, mild hand weakness and clumsiness
- Brainstem
  - **Basilar artery** (locked-in syndrome): quadriparesis or quadriplegia, anarthria or dysarthria, impaired horizontal eye movements, spared vertical eye movements
  - **PICA** (lateral medullary, Wallenberg syndrome): ipsilateral ataxia, ipsilateral Horner's, ipsilateral facial sensory loss, contralateral limb impairment of pain and temperature, nystagmus, vertigo, N/V, dysphagia, dysarthria, hiccups
  - **Vertebral artery** (medial medullary syndrome): contralateral hemiparesis (facial sparing), contralateral impaired proprioception and vibration and ipsilateral tongue weakness

Management of Stroke
- Assess
  - Airway, breathing, circulation
  - Vitals and neurovitals q4h x 24h and then reassess
  - Monitors, i.e. HR, BP, pulse oximetry, consider telemetry
- Investigations
  - Imaging: urgent non-contrast CT to rule out hemorrhage, consider MR angiography and CT angiogram, carotid dopplers, echocardiogram
  - ECG
  - Labs: CBC, electrolytes, creatinine, INR/PTT, blood glucose, lipids (following am), HbA1c
- Other
  - Lower BP if sBP >220 or dBP >120 (values different for hemorrhagic stroke)
  - Foley catheterization if required
  - NPO until swallowing assessment by SLP
  - Implement fall risk protocol, OT/PT to see for mobility and ADLs/IADLs
- Acute Treatment of Ischemic Stroke
  - Thrombolysis: IV tPA if within 4.5 h of ischemic stroke, as per hospital protocol
    - Contraindication: hemorrhage on CT; high INR or aPTT; recent major surgery or trauma; recent hemorrhage; sBP >185, dBP >110; past history of intracranial hemorrhage
  - Antipyretics: acetaminophen 650 mg PO q4h PRN for temperature >37.5°C
  - Antiplatelet therapy: ASA 81 or 325 mg PO daily (Clopidogrel or Aggrenox are alternative options if ASA not tolerated by patient)
  - Anticoagulation: consider dabigatran (110 or 150 mg BID) or warfarin (titrate INR to 2-3) if suspected/known cardioembolic stroke
  - DVT Prophlyaxis: heparin or LMWH
  - Statin therapy
  - ACE Inhibitors
- Acute Treatment of Hemorrhagic Stroke
  - Prevent further bleeding: blood pressure control (most important), bed rest, analgesics for pain control, mild sedation, laxatives to reduce straining
- Consults
  - Consult Internal Medicine or Neurology for admission, Stroke Team for further assessment, possibly Neurosurgery

Seizure

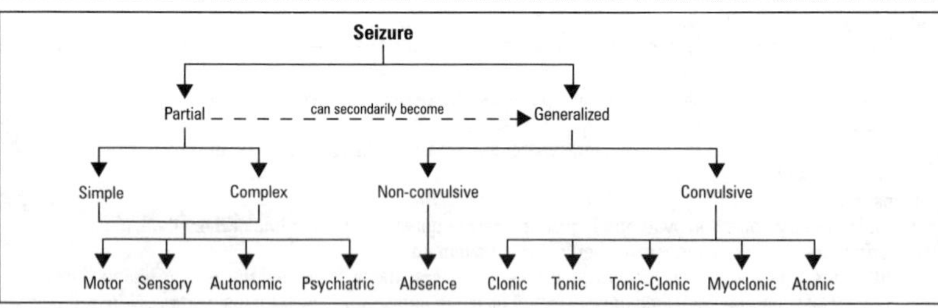

Differential Diagnosis
- Stroke, syncope, migraine headache, TIA, alcohol withdrawal/intoxication, hypoglycemia, sleep disorder (e.g. narcolepsy, cataplexy), movement disorder (e.g. paroxysmal dyskinesias), psychiatric conditions (e.g. conversion disorder, pseudoseizures, panic attacks), delirium and confusional states, life threatening diagnoses that must be ruled out: stroke/TIA, cardiogenic syncope

Characteristic	Seizure	Syncope
Position	Any	Upright, not recumbent
Aura	Possible specific aura	Dizzy, blurred vision, lightheaded
Colour	Normal or cyanotic	Pallor
Autonomic	Uncommon	Common; diaphoresis
Duration	Brief or prolonged	Brief
Incontinence	Common	Possible but rare
Post-ictal	Occurs in tonic-clonic or complex partial	Rare
Motor activity	Common	Occasional brief jerks
Injury	Common, tongue biting	Rare unless from fall
Automatisms	Common in absence or complex partial	None
EEG	Normal/Abnormal	Normal

Definitions
- Partial: aura implies focal onset
  - Simple partial seizure – focal onset and no impairment of consciousness
  - Complex partial seizure – focal onset and impaired consciousness
- Generalized
  - Seizure involving both hemispheres of the brain with impaired consciousness

Etiology
- Generalized
  - Infectious/Inflammatory: encephalitis, meningitis, neurocysticercosis
  - Toxic: medications (TCAs, MAOIs, neuroleptics, cyclosporine, theophylline, isoniazid), drugs (alcohol withdrawal, cocaine, amphetamines)
  - Anatomic: diffuse cerebral damage (anoxia, storage diseases)
  - Metabolic: hypoxia, electrolytes (hypocalcemia, hypoglycemia, hyponatremia, hypernatremia, hyperosmolality), end-stage organ failure (renal, hepatic), other (porphyria)
  - Vascular: late-onset epilepsy (>50 yrs old) is due to stroke until proven otherwise

History
- General
  - Frequency of seizures, status of driver's license
- History of event: may require collateral history from witness
  - Identifiable precipitants (see below), fever, aura
  - Duration, unresponsiveness, impaired level of consciousness, nature of neurological features (motor, visual hallucinations, olfactory hallucinations, gustatory hallucinations, Jacksonian march), salivation, cyanosis, tongue biting, incontinence, loud cry, automatisms (chewing, walking, lip-smacking), forcible head/eye turning, forced eye closure (pseudoseizure/malingering)
- Post-ictal: duration, confusion, limb pains, tongue soreness/injury, headache, drowsiness, Todd's paralysis (paresis)

Predisposing Factors and Precipitants
- Previous personal or family history of seizures, previous stroke/TIA or risk factors, past history of neurological insult (e.g. hypoxic birth injury, head trauma, CNS infection, drug use/abuse), headaches/migraines
- Precipitants: sleep deprivation, drugs, alcohol, TV screen, strobe lights, emotional upset, fever (infants)

Complications
- All seizures – mechanical injury
- Status epilepticus (see below)

Physical Exam
- Vitals (including temperature)
- Complete neurological exam (cranial nerves including fundoscopy, motor, sensory, co-ordination and gait) – look for any focal neurological deficits or neck stiffness (r/o meningismus)
- Precordial exam
- Abdominal exam – stigmata of liver diseases, small liver span, asterixis
- Dermatologic – rash (meningitis)

Management of Partial and Generalized Seizures in the Emergency Department
- ABCs
- Monitors – pulse oximetry, HR, BP, RR and temperature, consider telemetry
- Investigations:
    - CBC, Accucheck or glucose level, extended electrolytes including Ca^{2+}, liver tests, BUN, Cr, ABG, serum or urine drug screen, levels of anticonvulsant medications, EEG, ECG
    - Consider urgent CT, MRI, LP (only after initial CT), CXR
    - Prolactin level is elevated after generalized seizures and is useful in differentiating seizures from pseudoseizures/non-seizure but uncommonly ordered
    - LP to evaluate for infection and subarachnoid hemorrhage if CT normal
- Treat the underlying cause if known, i.e. correct metabolic disturbances, antibiotics for suspected CNS infections, etc.

STATUS EPILEPTICUS
- A life-threatening state (5-10% of epileptics) with either a continuous seizure lasting over 5-10 min or a series of seizures occurring without the patient regaining full consciousness between attacks
- Complications: repetitive grand mal seizures impair ventilation, resulting in anoxia, cerebral ischemia and cerebral edema; sustained muscle contraction can lead to rhabdomyolysis and renal failure
- Most common cause is abrupt discontinuation of anticonvulsants in a patient with epilepsy

Management of Status Epilepticus in the Emergency Department
- 0-5 min: ABCs
    - Give O_2, ensure adequate ventilation, monitor vitals, ECG, oximetry, start IV lines, blood samples (see above)
    - Give 50 mL 50% glucose IV preceded by thiamine 100 mg IM
    - Lorazepam 0.1 mg/kg IV at 2 mg/min to a max dose of 1 mg/kg (midazolam and diazepam (also PR) are alternatives)
- >5 min: if status persists
    - Phenytoin 15-20 mg/kg IV at maximum of 50 mg/min (maximum phenytoin 30 mg/kg) or fosphenytoin 20 mg/kg PE IV at 150 mg/min
    - Monitor cardiac rhythm and BP
- If status does not stop after 20 mg/kg phenytoin
    - Consult Neurology, Anaesthesia, ICU
    - Phenobarbital 20 mg/kg IV at 50 mg/min; watch for hypotension and respiratory depression – requires central line to monitor CVP, ventilatory assistance may be required
    - Anesthesia with midazolam or propofol in ICU: vasopressors or fluid volume usually necessary, EEG should be monitored and neuromuscular blockade may be needed
- Once seizure activity has stopped, ALWAYS get a follow-up EEG to ensure that the patient is not in non-convulsive status

Headache

History
- Onset, frequency, intensity and duration of attacks
- Location, radiation and quality of pain
- Associated symptoms: aura or prodome, visual changes
- Personal or family history of headaches
- Precipitating factors including food, alcohol, stress, sleep
- Relieving factors including response to treatments
- Relation to menstrual cycle or use of OCP

Red Flags
- History
  - Sudden onset
  - New type of headache, "worst headache of life"
  - Associated with altered mental status or seizure
  - Headache with exercise, cough, Valsalva or in early morning
  - Age over 50 with new or progressive headache
  - Immunosuppression or known active infection
  - Visual disturbances
  - Pain that radiates to the neck or shoulders
- Physical Examination
  - New focal or non-focal neurologic finding
  - Decreased level of consciousness
  - Meningeal signs: jolt accentuation, Kernig and Brudzinski
  - Abnormal vital signs
  - Toxic appearance
  - Papilledema, decreased vision, sluggish pupils
  - Signs of trauma

Headaches – Selected Primary Causes

	Tension-Type	Migraine	Cluster
Prevalence	70%	12%	<1%
Age of Onset	15-40	10-30	20-40
Sex Bias	F > M	F > M	M > F
Family History	None	+++	+
Location	Bilateral frontal Nucho-occipital	Unilateral>bilateral Fronto-temporal	Retro-orbital
Duration	Minutes-days	Hours-days	10 min-2 h
Onset/Course	Gradual; worse in PM	Gradual; worse in PM	Daily headache for weeks, months, nocturnal
Quality	Band-like; constant	Throbbing	Constant, aching, stabbing
Severity	Mild-moderate	Moderate-severe	Severe (wakes from sleep)
Provoking	Depression Anxiety Noise Hunger Sleep deprivation	Noise Light Straining Coughing Activity	Light EtOH
Palliating	Rest	Rest	Walking around

Headaches – Selected Primary Causes (continued)

	Tension-Type	Migraine	Cluster
Associated Sx	No vomiting No photophobia	Nausea/vomiting Photo/phonophobia Aura	Red watery eye Nasal congestion or rhinorrhea Unilateral Horner's
Physical Signs	Muscle tension in scalp/neck	Muscle tension in scalp/neck Tender scalp arteries	Red watery eye, rhinorrhea Eyelid droop
Management	Non-pharmacological 　Psychological counseling 　Physical modalities (e.g. heat, 　massage) Pharmacological 　Simple analgesics 　Tricyclic antidepressants	Acute Rx 　NSAIDS 　Triptans 　Ergotamine Prophylaxis 　TCA 　Anticonvulsants 　Propranolol	Acute Rx 　O_2 　Sumatriptan (nasal or injection) Prophylaxis 　Verapamil 　Lithium 　Methylsergide 　Prednisolone

Headaches – Selected Secondary Causes

	Meningial Irritation	Increased Intracranial Pressure	Temporal Arteritis
Etiology	Meningitis, SAH	Tumour, IIH, malignant hypertension	Vasculitis (GCA)
Incidence	<1%	<1%	<<1%
Age of Onset	Any age	Any age	>60
Gender Bias	No bias	No bias	No bias
Location	Generalized; stiff neck	Any location	Temporal
Duration	Variable	Chronic	Variable
Onset/Course	Meningitis: hours-days SAH: thunderclap onset	Gradual; worse in AM	Variable
Quality	Variable	Unlike any previous headache	Throbbing
Severity	Severe	Severe	Variable; can be severe
Provoking	Head movement	Lying down Valsalva Head low Exertion	
Palliating	Rest and immobility	Standing/sitting	
Associated Sx	Neck stiffness Photophobia Focal deficits (e.g. CN palsies)	Nausea/vomiting Focal neuro Sx Decreased level of consciousness	Polymyalgia rheumatica Jaw/tongue claudication Visual loss
Physical Signs	Kernig's sign Brudzinski's sign Jolt accentuation of h/a	Focal neuro Sx Papilledema	Temporal artery changes: Firm, nodular, incompressible Tender
Management	CT/LP	CT/MRI and treat appropriately See also Neurosurgery	Prednisone See also Rheumatology

SAH – subarachnoid hemorrhage; IIH – idiopathic intracranial hypertension; GCA – giant cell arteritis

Interpretation of Lumbar Puncture

Condition	Colour	Protein	Glucose	Cells	Other
Normal	Clear	<0.45 g/L	60% of serum glucose >3 mmol/L	0-5 WBC/ul or x10^6/L 0 RBC 0 neutrophils	
Infectious					
Viral infection	Clear or opalescent	Normal or slightly increased <0.45-1 g/L	Normal	Elevated mostly lymphocytes, some PMNs	
Bacterial infection	Opalescent yellow, may clot	>1 g/L	Decreased (<25% serum glucose or <2 mmol/L)	Markedly elevated PMNs	
Granulomatous infection (tuberculosis, fungal)	Clear or opalescent	Increased but usually <5 g/L	Decreased <2-4 mmol/L	Elevated lymphocytes	Opening pressure important in cryptococcal meningitis
Neurologic					
Guillain-Barré syndrome	Clear or cloudy	Markedly increased	Normal	Normal	Albuminocytologic dissociation
Multiple sclerosis	Clear	Normal or increased	Normal	0-20 x 10^6/L lymphocytes	Oligoclonal banding on protein electrophoresis
Pseudotumour cerebri	Clear	Normal	Normal	Normal	Elevated opening pressure
Other					
Neoplasm (neoplastic meningitis)	Clear or xanthochromic	Normal or increased	Normal or decreased	Normal or increased lymphocytes	Cytology positive
Traumatic tap	Bloody, no xanthochromia	Normal	Slightly increased	RBCs from peripheral blood Fewer RBCs in tube 4/5 than tube 1	
Subarachnoid hemorrhage	Bloody, or xanthochromia after 2-8 h	Increased	Normal	WBC/RBC ratio same as blood Same number of RBCs in tubes 1 and 4/5	

Neurosurgery

Common Presentations

Increased Intracranial Pressure

Definition
- Intracranial hypertension is defined as:
  - ICP >15 mmHg for older children and adults
  - ICP >7 mmHg for young children
  - ICP >6 mmHg for term infants
  - Cut off values to treat intracranial hypertension: ICP >20-25 mmHg, in adults

History
- **HPI**
  - Headache (location, quality, intensity, radiation, sudden or gradual onset, duration, frequency, progression, comparison to previous headaches, worsened by coughing/straining/bending over, worse in morning)
  - Seizure (first episode or recurrent, quality, side of onset, duration, treatment, prior investigations)
  - Nausea/vomiting
  - Diplopia (abnormal extra-ocular movements)
  - Decreased visual acuity, blindness
  - Mental status change (decreased LOC, confusion, dementia, personality change)
  - Focal deficits (onset, duration, progression)
  - History of trauma (mechanism of injury, head protection, associated loss of consciousness, skull fracture)
- **PMHx**
  - Medication History – anticoagulants, oral contraceptives
  - Medical History – handedness, malignancy (breast, colorectal, lung, renal cell, melanoma, sarcoma), severe sinus or ear infection, hypertension, diabetes, hyperlipidemia, CAD, SLE
  - Substance use – smoking, EtOH, drugs (including IV)
  - Surgical History – shunt, recent cranial or spinal surgery
- **Family History**
  - Ruptured and unruptured aneurysms in first degree relatives, colorectal cancer, breast cancer, kidney disease (PCKD), stroke, MI

Physical Exam
- ABCs
- *Vital Signs*
  - Cushing's Triad (1/3 of cases) – hypertension, bradycardia, abnormal respiratory pattern
- *HEENT*
  - Trauma to the skull and face (laceration, ecchymosis, Battle's sign, periorbital ecchymosis ("raccoon eyes"), hemotympanum, otorrhea, rhinorrhea, bony facial pain)
  - Abnormal EOM: CN III palsy (= aneurysm, uncal herniation), CN VI palsy or upward gaze palsy
  - Fundoscopy for papilledema, subhyaloid hemorrhages, optic atrophy ± retinal hemorrhages
  - Lymphadenopathy
- *Neurological Exam*
  - Mental Status (GCS, orientation), cranial nerves, motor, pronator drift, reflexes, sensory, coordination, gait

Differential Diagnosis
• Tumour (primary, secondary)
• Pus (infectious, inflammatory)
• Blood (ischemia, hemorrhage, hypertension)
• Hydrocephalus (obstructive, communicating)
• Tension pneumocephalus
• Status epilepticus

Complications
• Herniation syndromes, death

Management

ER
• Ensure iIntubate and ventilate if GCS ≤8 or respiratory distress
• Ensure adequate airway/C-spine precautions if trauma
• 2 large bore IVs, central line, arterial line
• Stat CBC, electrolytes, creatinine, INR, PTT, cross & type, serum osmolarity
• Avoid hyperventilation during the first 24 h after injury if possible; however, if acute neurologic deterioration then hyperventilate to pCO_2 = 30-35 mmHg
• Avoid hypoxia
• Avoid hypotension (SBP <90 mmHg): normalize intravascular volume, support with pressors if needed
• Head of bed up 30-45°, keep head midline
• Light sedation (Codeine 30-60 mg IM q4h PRN)
• Heavy sedation (Fentanyl 1-2 ml IV q1h) or paralysis (vecuronium 8-10 mg IV q2-3h) if intubated and ventilated, or severely increased ICP
• Mannitol 1-1.5 g/kg IV rapid infusion, then 0.25 g/kg IV q6h, hold if serum osmolarity >320 mOsm/L
• Non-contrast head CT
• Reverse anticoagulation if hemorrhage (e.g. octaplex if on warfarin)

Hospital/Inpatient
• Admission Orders
  ▪ Admit to Neurosurgery under Dr. X (ICU if patient requires intubation/ventilation)
  ▪ Diagnosis: Intracranial Hypertension secondary to ____________
  ▪ NPO
  ▪ Bed rest, head of bed 30-45°, keep head midline
  ▪ Vital signs q4h, Call MD if sBP <90 or >140, if HR <60 or >100
  ▪ Neurovitals q1h
  ▪ O_2 to keep SaO_2 >92%
  ▪ Foley to urometer
  ▪ TEDS
  ▪ IV NS + 20 mEq KCl @ maintenance rate (keep patient euvolemic to slightly hypovolemic)
  ▪ Arterial line monitor
  ▪ Previous medications as required
  ▪ Codeine 30-60 mg IM q4h PRN OR Lorazepam (Ativan®) 1-2 mg IV q4-6h PRN
  ▪ Ranitidine 50 mg IV q8h, if on corticosteroids
  ▪ Mannitol 1-1.5 g/kg IV rapid infusion, then 0.25 g/kg (over 20 min) q6h
    ◆ May alternate with Furosemide (Lasix®) 10-20 mg IV q6h (temporizing measure only)
  ▪ Note: Corticosteroids may be used when elevated ICP due to edema from an intracranial neoplasm. Dexamethasone 10-20 mg IV, then 1-1.5 mg IV/PO q6h
• Acetaminophen 325-650 mg PO q4-6h PRN for fever
• CBC, electrolytes, BUN, creatinine, serum osmolarity, INR, PTT, cross and type, ABG

- ICP monitoring with an intraventricular catheter required in patients with GCS ≤8 and either an abnormal admitting brain CT or 2 or more of: age >40, sBP <90 mmHg, decorticate or decerebrate posturing (unilateral or bilateral)
- Once intraventricular catheter is in place, treatment for elevated ICP should be initiated for ICP >25 mmHg lasting ≥5 min, which includes:
  - General measures as above
  - Heavy sedation and/or paralysis
  - CSF drainage, with external ventricular drain
  - Osmotic therapy
    - If ICP remains refractory to mannitol, consider hypertonic saline
    - Hold osmotic therapy if serum osmolarity >320 mOsm/L
  - Hyperventilate to $PaCO_2$: 30-35 mmHg (if above fails)

Surgical Treatment (if indicated, usually precedes above measures. If ICP remains refractory – rescan to rule out reaccumulation or new intracranial mass lesion)
1. Evacuation of any subdural or epidural hematoma >1 cm maximal thickness
2. Evacuation of hemorrhagic contusions when there is progressive deterioration
3. Decompressive craniectomy for elevated ICP that cannot be controlled medically

Neurotrauma

NEUROLOGICAL ASSESSMENT

Mini-History
- Period of LOC, post traumatic amnesia, loss of sensation/function, type of injury/accident

Signs of Basal Skull Fracture
- Raccoon eyes
- Battle's sign (ecchymosis over mastoid process)
- Otorrhea (CSF)
- Rhinorrhea (CSF)
- Hemotympanum
- CN injury possible to I (anterior fossa), II (optic canal), VI (clivus fracture), VII and VIII (temporal bone fracture)

Neurological Exam
- Mental status: GCS, orientation
- Head and neck (lacerations, bruises, basal skull fracture signs, facial fractures, foreign bodies)
- Spine (palpable deformity, midline pain/tenderness)
- Brainstem (breathing pattern)
- Cranial nerve exam
- Motor exam, sensory exam, reflexes
- Sphincter tone, sacral reflexes (bulbocavernosus, anal wink) if spinal trauma
- Record and repeat neurological exam at regular intervals

ADMITTING ORDERS FOR MINOR HEAD INJURY (GCS 13)
1. Admit to ICU for GCS <13
2. Activity: bed rest with head of bed elevated to 30-45°
3. Neurovitals q1-2h
4. NPO until alert; then clear liquids
5. Isotonic IVF (e.g. NS with 20 mEq KCl) run at maintenance (e.g. 75-100 cc/h)
6. Mild analgesics: acetaminophen (PO or PR if NPO), codeine if necessary
7. Anti-emetic: give infrequently to avoid excessive sedation (avoid phenothiazine anti-emetics as they can lower seizure threshold)

Key Points
- Suspected increased ICP is a relative contraindication for doing an LP because of the risk of cerebral herniation
- All patients with head injury have C-spine injury until proven otherwise
- Do not blame coma on alcohol – there may also be a hematoma
- Must clear spine both radiologically AND clinically (will require re-assessment if/when patient improves clinically)

Assessment of Spine CT/X-ray (parasagittal view) – "ABCDS"
- **A**lignment (columns: anterior vertebral line, posterior vertebral line, spinolaminar line, posterior spinous line)
- **B**one (vertebral bodies, facets, spinous processes)
- **C**artilage
- **D**isc (disc space and interspinous space)
- **S**oft tissues

Indications for CT Head in Acute Injury
- Drug or alcohol intoxication
- Physical findings of trauma above clavicle
- Seizure
- Coagulopathy
- Focal neurological deficit
- Mild head injury (GCS <13)

Canadian CT Head Rules [Stiell (2001) Lancet 357 for minor head injury (GCS 13-15)]
- High risk indications for head CT
    - Glasgow Coma Scale <15 at 2 h post injury
    - Open or depressed skull fracture
    - Vomiting (two or more episodes)
    - Age 65 yrs or over (other studies suggest age 60)
    - Basal skull fracture signs (see below)
- Moderate risk indications for head CT
    - Pre-trauma amnesia $\geq$30 min
    - High risk mechanism of injury
    - Pedestrian in motor vehicle accident
    - Passenger ejected from vehicle
    - Fall from height over 3 feet or 5 stairs

Skull Fractures
- Depressed fractures → double density on skull x-ray (outer table of depressed segment below inner table of skull), CT with bone windows is gold standard
- Simple fractures (closed injury) → no need for antibiotics, no surgery
- Compound fractures (open injury) → increased risk of infection, surgical debridement within 24 h is necessary
    - Internal fractures into sinus → meningitis, pneumocephalus, risk of operative bleed may limit treatment to antibiotics
- Basal skull fractures → not readily seen on x-ray, rely on clinical signs
    - Retroauricular ecchymoses (Battle's sign)
    - Periorbital ecchymoses (raccoon eyes)
    - Hemotympanum
    - CSF rhinorrhea, otorrhea (suspect CSF if halo or target sign present) suspect with Lefort II or III midface fracture (seen on imaging)

Mechanisms of Brain Injury
- Coup (damage at site of blow)
- Contrecoup (damage at opposite site of blow)
- Contusion (hemorrhagic)
    - High density areas on CT ± mass effect
    - Commonly occurs with brain impact on bony prominences

- Diffuse axonal injury/shearing
    - May tear blood vessels, with hemorrhagic foci
    - All brain injury causes shear
    - Often the cause of decreased LOC if no space occupying lesion on CT
- Delayed and progressive injury to the brain due to:
    - High glutamate release NMDA cytotoxic cascade
    - Cerebral edema
    - Intracranial hemorrhages
    - Ischemia/infarction
    - Raised ICP, intracranial HTN
    - Hydrocephalus

Common Conditions

Cord Syndromes

Syndrome	Motor	Sensory
Brown-Séquard	Ipsilateral weakness with UMN signs; LMN at level of lesion	Ipsilateral loss of vibration and proprioception below level of lesion Contralateral loss of pain and temperature 2-3 levels below level of lesion
Anterior Cord	Bilateral paraplegia (UMN below the level of lesion) Sphincter dysfunction (urinary retention)	Bilateral loss of pain and temperature below level of lesion
Central Cord	Bilateral motor weakness; upper > lower extremities	Intact sensation above and below affected dermatomes. If large central lesion, bilateral loss of pain and temperature below level of lesion
Posterior Cord	Preserved motor function	Bilateral loss of vibration, proprioception and light touch below level of lesion

CAUDA EQUINA SYNDROME

Etiology
- Compression of lumbosacral nerve roots below conus medullaris (~L1-2)
- Large central herniated disc (most commonly L4-5 or L5-S1) ± spinal stenosis, extrinsic mass

Clinical Features
- Motor (LMN signs)
    - Weakness/paraparesis in multiple root distribution
    - Reduced deep tendon reflexes (knee and ankle)
    - Sphincter disturbance (urinary retention and fecal incontinence due to loss of anal sphincter tone)
- Sensory
    - Pain in back radiating to legs
    - Bilateral sensory loss or pain: involving multiple dermatomes
    - Saddle anesthesia (most common sensory deficit)
    - Sexual dysfunction (late finding)

Treatment
- Requires **urgent** investigation and decompression (<48 h) to preserve bowel, bladder and motor function

Pus/Infection

- **Types**: epidural abscess, subdural empyema, meningitis/encephalitis, cerebral abscess
- **Routes of spread**: hematogenous spread (most common, often from lungs), direct implantation (dural disruption: trauma, iatrogenic, congenital), contiguous spread (adjacent infection), spread from PNS (e.g. viruses: rabies, VZV)

Types	Epidural Abscess	Subdural Empyema	Cerebral Abscess
Site	Epidural space (cranial and spinal)	Between dura and arachnoid	In brain substance, encapsulated
Causative Organisms	*S. aureus*, GN Enterics (*E. coli*)	*S. aureus*, *H. influenzae*, *S. pneumoniae*, Bacteroides, fungal	*S. pneumoniae*, *S. aureus* Bacteroides, Fungi Children: Proteus + Citrobacter
Clinical Features	Spinal: Classic triad – fever (variable), back pain, neurologic deficits. With progression: motor weakness, sphincter incontinence, sensory changes, paralysis Cranial: Fever, H/A, N/V, lethargy, encephalopathy, seizure	Fever, H/A, recent H+N infection, decreased LOC, hemiparesis, seizure, N/V, blurred vision, slurred speech	Focal neuro signs, H/A, seizures, decreased LOC, mass effect, increased ICP signs, hemiparesis and seizures, systemic infection (low-grade fever, leukocytosis)
Investigations	1. B/W: CBC-d, blood cultures 2. Imaging: MRI with gadolinium 3. CT-guided needle aspirate 4. LP contraindicated 5. Abscess fluid: Gram stain, cultures	1. CBC-d, blood cultures 2. MRI with gadolinium 3. LP contraindicated	1. CBC-d, blood cultures 2. MRI with gadolinium 3. LP contraindicated 4. Aspiration – investigate fluid for Gram stain, C+S, AFB, fungal culture
Treatment	1. Emergency surgical decompression and drainage 2. Abx for 4-8 wks: vanco, flagyl, ceftazidime 3. Seizure prophylaxis	1. Emergency surgical drainage via craniotomy 2. Abx for 3-6 wks, depending on source 3. Seizure prophylaxis	1. Surgical: excision if good location 2. Abx for 6-8 wks: vanco + ceftriaxone + flagyl, or chloramphenicol or rifampin 3. Seizure prophylaxis (2 yrs) 4. F/U CT (weekly)
Prognosis	Morbidity and mortality Increased with delayed surgical intervention	20% mortality	10% mortality, 50% permanent deficits

Hydrocephalus

Definition
- Increased CSF volume (usual etiology is obstruction of ventricular outflow, rarely increased CSF production)
- Clinical features similar to those of raised ICP (see above)

Classification

A. Obstructive (Non-Communicating) Hydrocephalus
- Acquired aqueductal stenosis (adhesions following infection, hemorrhage)
- Intraventricular lesions (tumours, hematoma)
- Mass causing tentorial herniation, aqueduct/4th ventricle compression
- Congenital: Dandy-Walker malformation, Chiari malformation
- CT findings: ventricular enlargement proximal to block

B. Non-Obstructive (Communicating) Hydrocephalus
- CSF absorption blocked at extraventricular site (arachnoid granulations)
- Post-infectious: meningitis, cysticercosis
- Post-hemorrhagic: SAH, IVH, traumatic
- Choroid plexus papilloma (rare, causes increased CSF production)
- Idiopathic: normal pressure hydrocephalus
- CT findings: all ventricles dilated without clear obstruction

C. Normal Pressure Hydrocephalus (NPH)
- Gradual onset of classic triad developing over weeks-months: gait disturbance (ataxia), urinary incontinence, dementia ("AID")
- Idiopathic: CSF pressure within clinically "normal" range, but symptoms resolve with ventricular shunting
- CT findings: enlarged ventricles without increased prominence of sulci

D. Hydrocephalus Ex Vacuo
- Enlargement of ventricles and sulci secondary to cerebral atrophy, not increased pressure

Investigations
- CT/MRI
  - Ventricular enlargement, may see prominent temporal horns
  - Periventricular hypodensity (transependymal migration of CSF)
  - Narrow/absent sulci
- Ultrasound (through anterior fontanelle in infants)
- ICP monitoring (e.g. LP)

Treatment
- Surgical removal of obstruction or excision of choroid plexus papilloma
- Ventricular shunting to drain excess CSF (e.g. ventriculo-peritoneal shunt)
  - Beware of shunt complications in previously shunted individuals including shunt blockage, infection and overshunting (slit ventricle syndrome)
- Third ventriculostomy (for obstructive hydrocephalus) via ventriculoscopy – treatment of choice for aqueductal stenosis
- LP/EVD (e.g. for transient IVH in premature infants)

Intracranial Hemorrhage

EXTRADURAL HEMATOMA
- Etiology
  - Most commonly due to ruptured middle meningeal artery (usually a history of trauma)
- Clinical Features
  - In <30% there is a classic sequence of post-traumatic reduced LOC, a lucid interval of several hours between trauma and coma, then obtundation, hemiparesis, ipsilateral pupillary dilatation
  - H/A, N/V, amnesia, altered LOC, HTN and respiratory distress depending on severity
- Investigations
  - CT without contrast: high density biconvex mass against skull, limited by suture lines
- Treatment
  - Head elevation, mannitol pre-op, craniotomy to evacuate clot, follow up CT
- Prognosis
  - Good with prompt management, as the brain often is not damaged

ACUTE SUBDURAL HEMATOMA
- Etiology
  - Rupture of vessels that bridge the subarachnoid space
  - Contused brain that ruptures and bleeds into subdural space
- Risk Factors
  - Anticoagulants, EtOH, cerebral atrophy
- Clinical Features
  - No lucid interval, signs and symptoms can include altered LOC, pupillary irregularity, hemiparesis
- Investigations
  - CT – high density concave "crescentic" mass crossing suture lines; usually less uniform, less dense and more diffuse than extradural hematoma
- Treatment
  - Craniotomy for subdurals greater than 1 cm or midline shift >5 mm, optimal if surgery <4 h from onset
- Prognosis
  - Poor overall since the brain is often injured

CHRONIC SUBDURAL HEMATOMA

- Etiology
  - May begin as an acute SDH. Over time the clot remodels/liquefies, neomembranes form, and a combination of bleeding from neomembranes and fluid resorption determines the size and shape of the SDH
- Risk Factors
  - Older, alcoholics, patients with CSF shunts, anticoagulants, coagulopathies
- Clinical Features
  - Often minor/no history of injury
  - May present with minor H/A, confusion, language difficulties, TIA-like symptoms
  - Sometimes raised ICP ± seizures, progressive dementia, gait disturbance (ataxia)
  - Obtundation disproportionate to focal deficit; mistaken for dementia/tumour
- Investigations
  - CT – hypodense (liquefied clot), crescentic mass
- Treatment
  - Burr hole drainage of liquefied clot indicated if symptomatic or thickness >1 cm, craniotomy if recurrent
- Prognosis
  - Good overall as brain usually undamaged, but may require repeat drainage

SUBARACHNOID HEMORRHAGE

Definition
- Bleeding into subarachnoid space (intracranial vessels between arachnoid and pia)

Etiology
- Trauma
- Spontaneous
- Aneurysms
- AVMs
- Coagulopathies (iatrogenic or primary), vasculitides, tumours (<5%)

Risk Factors
- Hypertension
- Pregnancy/parturition in patients with pre-existing AVMs, eclampsia
- Oral contraceptive pill
- Substance abuse [cigarette smoking, cocaine, alcohol (controversial)]
- Conditions associated with high incidence of aneurysms (e.g. PCKD)

Clinical Features
- Sudden onset (seconds) of severe/thunderclap headache, often described as the "worst headache of my life"
  - Sentinel bleeds [SAH-like symptoms lasting <1 d ("thunderclap H/A")]
- N/V, photophobia
- Meningismus (neck pain/stiffness, positive Kernig's and Brudzinski's sign)
- Decreased LOC (due to raised ICP, ischemia, seizure)
- Focal deficits: cranial nerve palsy (e.g. III, IV), hemiparesis
- Ocular hemorrhage in 20-40% (due to sudden raised ICP compressing central retinal vein); subhyaloid/pre-retinal hemorrhages
- Reactive hypertension

Investigations
- Non-contrast CT to look for acute blood in the subarachnoid space
- CT may suggest site of aneurysm but CTA/MRA/angio needed for localization
- Positive history for SAH with negative CT requires LP to look for blood or xanthochromia (may be negative <12 h)

Treatment
- Admit to ICU or NICU
- Oxygen/ventilation prn

- NPO, bed rest, elevate head of bed 30°, minimal external stimulation, neurological vitals q1h, IV fluids (>3 L/d)
- Maintain sBP = 120-150 (balance of vasospasm prophylaxis, risk of re-bleed, risk of hypotension since CBF autoregulation impaired by SAH)
- Keppra if seizure or temporal lobe clot
- Analgesia
- Nimodipine for vasospasm neuroprotection (continue x21d)
- Cardiac rhythm monitor
- Foley prn, strict ins and outs
- 4 vessel angiography, early surgery or coiling to prevent re-bleed (if aneurysm)

Complications
- Vasospasm = vasoconstriction and permanent pathologic vascular changes in response to irritating arterial blood clot outside vessels at the base of the brain
    - Clinical features: progressively decreasing LOC, focal deficit (speech or motor)
    - Onset: 4-14 d post SAH (if deterioration within first 3 d, MUST look for other cause)
    - Detect clinically and/or with angiogram or transcranial Doppler (increased velocity of blood flow), CBC/electrolytes/CT urgently to r/o other causes
    - Treatment: "Triple H" therapy (hypertension, hypervolemia, hemodilution) using fluids and pressors (norepinephrine, phenylephrine) or angioplasty/intraarterial verapamil for refractory cases
- Hydrocephalus (15-20%) – due to blood obstructing CSF drainage or subarachnoid space
- Hyponatremia – (due to cerebral salt wasting)
- Diabetes insipidus
- Cardiac – arrhythmia (>50% have ECG changes), MI, CHF
- Neurogenic pulmonary edema

Prognosis
- 10-15% mortality before reaching hospital, overall 50% mortality (majority within first 2-3 wks)
- 30% of survivors have moderate to severe disability
- Major cause of mortality is rebleeding and vasospams

CNS Tumours

Classification
- Primary vs. metastatic, intra-axial (parenchymal) vs. extra-axial, supratentorial vs. infratentorial, adult vs. pediatric, benign vs. malignant

Types
- **Glioma**: astrocytomas, oligodendrogliomas, ependymomas
- **Neuronal**: ganglion cell tumours, cerebral neurocytomas
- **Meningeal**: meningioma
- **Poorly differentiated neoplasms**: medulloblastoma, atypical teratoid/rhabdoid
- **Other**: primary CNS lymphoma, primary brain germ cell tumours, pineal tumours

Epidemiology
- Age <15: 60% infratentorial
- Age >15: 80% supratentorial

Clinical Features
- **Progressive neurological deficit:** motor > sensory, cognitive, personality, endocrine, increased ICP, H/A, N/V, seizures, papilledema, visual change

Investigations
- **Imaging**: CT/MRI – single (1°) vs. multiple (mets) lesions
- **Ring-enhancing lesion**
    - **DDx: MAGICAL DR** – **M**etastases, **A**bscess, **G**lioblastoma, **I**nfarct, **C**ontusion, **A**IDS, **L**ymphoma, **D**emyelination, **R**esolving hematoma
- **Stereotactic biopsy**: tissue diagnosis

Treatment
- Conservative: serial Hx, Px, imaging for slow growing/benign lesions
- Medical: corticosteroids (reduce vasogenic edema)
- Surgical: total or partial excision (decompressive, palliative), shunt (if hydrocephalus)
- Radiotherapy: conventional fractionated radiotherapy (XRT), stereotactic radiosurgery (Gamma Knife®)
- Chemotherapy: e.g. alkylating agents (temozolomide for glioblastoma)

Tumour Type	Epidemiology	Features	Investigations	Treatment	Prognosis
Metastatic	Most common overall sources: lung > breast > kidney (RCC) > GI > melanoma	At MCA territory in cerebral hemispheres	MRI W/u to locate primary Stereotactic biopsy	Seizure prophylaxis Corticosteroids ± chemo Tx Whole brain radiation therapy (WBRT) Surgery for single/solitary lesions	Without treatment, 1 month survival With treatment, 6-9 month survival
Astrocytoma	Most common primary 4th – 6th decades	Hemispheres >> cerebellum, brainstem, spinal cord	CT/MRI: appearance proportional to grade Stereotactic biopsy: grade correlates to prognosis	Low-grade: surgery (± curative), radiation, chemo Tx High-grade: gross, total surgical removal, then WBRT	Grade 1 – >10 yrs Grade 4 – 8-10 months
Pituitary adenoma	3rd – 4th decades M = F Incidence at autopsy = 20%	Micro- (<1 cm) vs. macro- (>1 cm) adenoma Functional/secretory vs. non- Symptoms: H/A, bitemporal hemianopsia, CN III, IV, V1, V2, VI palsies, paraneoplastic syndromes (especially hyperprolactinemia)	Px: careful CN and visual field testing Endocrine tests (PRL, TSH, cortisol, fasting glucose, FSH, LH, IGF-1) MRI with gadolinium	Corticosteroids Bromocriptine for prolactinoma Surgical resection (trans-sphenoidal, trans-ethmoidal, or trans-cranial)	
Meningioma	F:M = 3:2 Middle-aged	99% are benign Slow-growing, solitary Extra-axial (arise from arachnoid) at falx, sphenoid, tuberculum sellae, foramen magnum, olfactory groove Progesterone-R (increase with pregnancy)	MRI/CT with contrast: homogeneous, dense Angiography: assess vascularity	Non-progressive, asymptomatic conservative Progressive ± symptomatic/ asymptomatic: surgery ± pre-op embolization	5-yr survival: >90% Recurrence 10-20%
Acoustic Neuroma (vestibular schwannoma)	All age groups Peak age: 4th – 6th decades	Progressive unilateral/ assymetrical sensorineural hearing loss, tinnitus, disequilibrium Slow-growing, from vestibular branch of CN VIII Bilateral = NF2	MRI with gadolinium Audiogram Brainstem auditory evoked potentials	First line: stereotactic radiosurgery Surgery if: >3 cm, brainstem compression, edema, hydrocephalus	Almost always curable with complete resection

Primary Sources of Metastatic Brain Tumours

Lung	44%
Breast	10%
Kidney (RCC)	7%
GI	6%
Melanoma	3%

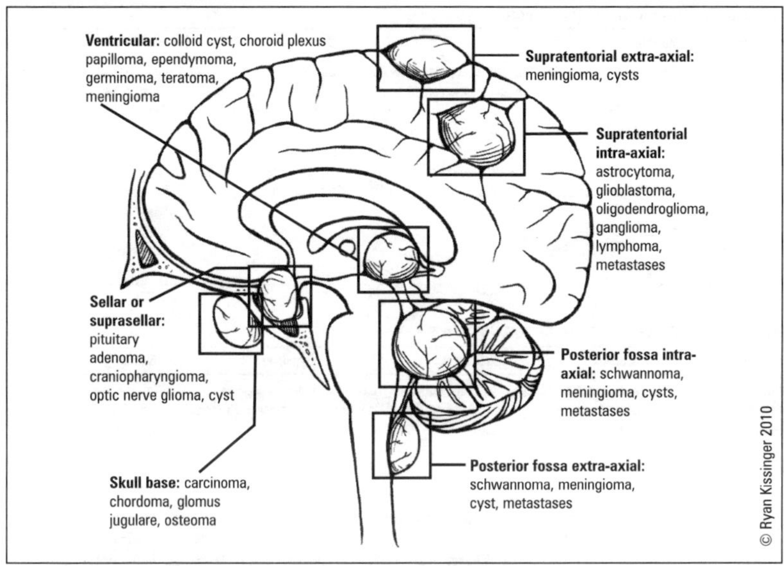

Functional Neurosurgery

Surgical Targets for Movement Disorders

Disorder	Indications	Procedures	Outcomes	Morbidity
Parkinson's Disease	Intractable contralateral bradykinesia/tremor Failure of medical management (advanced disease) Drug-induced dyskinesias (see dystonia, below)	Simultaneous, bilateral surgery/stimulation is most comon Preferred target: anterodorsal subthalamic nucleus (STN) Other targets: stereotactic ablation (pallidotomy)/stimulation of posteroventral globus pallidus interna (GPi) Caudal zona incerta Parkinsonian tremor: stereotactic ablation (thalamotomy)/stimulation of ventral intermediate (Vim) nucleus of thalamus	39-48% improvement in Unified Parkinson's Disease Rating Scale (UPDRS) scores Reduced dosage of medications (STN) More effective than medical management in advanced PD Early intervention may reduce severity, course, and progression of disease Of little benefit for patients with atypical presentations	Intracerebral hemorrhage, infection, seizure (1%-4%) Paresthesias Involuntary movements Cognitive functioning: decreased lexical fluency, impaired executive function (STN > GPi) Psychiatric: depression, mania, anxiety, apathy (STN > GPi)
Dystonia	Contralateral primary (generalized) dystonias; cervical and tardive dystonias (GPi) Contralateral secondary dyskinesia (i.e. drug-induced: L-dopa, neuroleptics; STN)	Preferred target (primary dystonia): stereotactic ablation (pallidotomy/stimulation of posteroventral GPi Secondary dystonia: stimulation of anterodorsal STN Stimulation of ventral posterior lateral thalamic nucleus (VPL)	Primary dystonia: 51% reduction in Burke-Fahn-Marsden Dystonia Scale (BFMDS) score Secondary dystonia: 62-89% improvement in dystonias Delayed effects: weeks → months	Intracerebral hemorrhage, infection, seizure (1%-4%) Minor effects on cognitive functioning (esp. decreased lexical fluency; STN > GPi)

Surgical Targets for Movement Disorders (continued)

Disorder	Indications	Procedures	Outcomes	Morbidity
Tremor	Contralateral appendicular ET (first disorder to be treated by DBS; DBS is viable alternative to Rx) Intention (cerebellar) tremor (IT) resulting from demyelination of cerebellar outflow tracts (i.e. in multiple sclerosis) Brainstem tremor (Holmes tremor)	Preferred target: stereotactic ablation (thalamotomy)/ stimulation of Vim nucleus of thalamus Other targets: stimulation of caudal zona incerta Parkinsonian tremor: stimulation of anterodorsal STN	Durable reductions in essential tremor rating scale (ETRS) scores Reduced dosage of medications Conflicting data on vocal/ facial tremor	Intracerebral hemorrhage, infection, seizure (1%–4%) Paresthesias/pain Dysarthria Ataxia Minor effects on cognitive functioning (esp. decreased lexical fluency) Tolerance may develop over time

Surgical Targets for Neuropsychiatric Disorders

Disorder	Indications	Procedures	Outcomes	Morbidity
Obsessive Compulsive Disorder (OCD)	Severe symptoms refractory to medical management	Anterior capsulotomy/stimulation of the anterior limb of the internal capsule (IC)	Currently under investigation Reportedly 25-75% response rate	Intracerebral hemorrhages (1%-2%) Mild effects on cognitive functioning Anxiety ± panic disorder (case report)
Tourette's Syndrome	Severe symptoms refractory to medical management	Stimulation of midline intralaminar nuclei of the thalamus Stimulation of motor and limbic portions of GPi Stimulation of the anterior limb of the IC	Currently under investigation Reportedly >70% reduction in vocal or motor tics + urge	Intracerebral hemorrhages (1%-2%) Mild sexual dysfunction
Major Depressive Disorder (MDD)	Severe depression refractory to medical management and ECT	Stimulation of the subgenual cingulate cortex	Currently under investigation Reportedly 60% response rate; 35% remission rate	Intracerebral hemorrhages (1%-2%) Pain, headache Worsening mood, irritability

Surgical Targets for Chronic Pain

Disorder	Indications	Procedures	Outcomes	Morbidity
Neuropathic Pain	Severe, intractable, organic neuropathic pain (i.e. post-stroke pain, phantom limb pain, trigeminal neuralgia, chronic low-back pain, complex regional pain syndrome)	Preferred target: stimulation of the contralateral ventral posterior lateral (VPL) and medial (VPM) thalamic nuclei ± periventricular/periaqueductal grey matter (PVG/PAG) Other targets: stimulation of the contralateral IC Stimulation of the contralateral motor cortex	47% improvement in perception of pain intensity Less favourable results in central pain syndromes and poorly localized pain	Intracerebral hemorrhages (1%-2%) Paraesthesia Anxiety ± panic disorder
Nociceptive Pain	Severe, intractable, organic nociceptive pain	Bilateral (most common) stimulation of the PVG/PAG	Reportedly 63% improvement in perception of pain intensity	Intracerebral hemorrhages (1%-2%) Paraesthesia Anxiety ± panic disorder

Surgical Management of Epilepsy

Indications
- Seizures resistant to two first line anti-seizure medications used in succession (medically refractory)
- Identification of a distinct epileptogenic region through clinical history, EEG, MRI, and neuropsychological testing.
- If a distinct epileptogenic region cannot be identified, the patient may be a candidate for a palliative procedure such as corpus callosotomy

Procedure
- Most commonly
    - Adults: resection of the hippocampus and parahippocampal gyrus for mesial temporal lobe epilepsy arising from mesial temporal sclerosis
    - Children: resection of an epileptogenic space-occupying lesion
- Hemispherectomy and corpus callosotomy are less common

Outcomes and Goals
- Freedom from seizures
- 41-79% of adult patients are seizure free for 5 years after temporal lobe resection
- 58-78% of children are seizure free after surgery
- Improvements in preexisting psychiatric conditions (i.e. depression and anxiety), as well as improvement in quality of life measures

Morbidity
- 0.4-4% of surgical patients will have partial hemianopsia, aphasia, motor deficit, sensory deficit, or cranial nerve palsy following anterior mesial temporal lobectomies
- Most patients will have some decline in verbal memory following dominant temporal lobectomy and in visuospatial memory in non-dominant temporal resection
- The degree of memory decline stabilizes after 1-2 years

Predictors
- Positive predictive factors for seizure freedom following anteromedial temporal lobe resection
    - Hippocampal sclerosis (unilateral)
    - Focal localization of interictal epileptiform discharges
    - Absence of preoperative generalized seizures
    - Tumoural cause
    - Complete resection of the lesion

Obstetrics

Essential History and Physical Exam

History

- **Gravidity (G)** = total number of pregnancies at any gestation
  - Includes current pregnancies, abortions, ectopic pregnancies and hydatidiform moles (twins=1 pregnancy)
- **Parity (TPAL):**
  T = number of term infants delivered (>37 wks)
  P = number of premature infants delivered (20-37 wks)
  A = number of abortions (loss of intrauterine pregnancy with fetus <20 wks and/or <500 g fetal weight – can be induced or spontaneous)
  L = number of live children
- **Naegle's Rule** = estimated date of confinement (EDC):
  - 1st day of LMP + 7 d – 3 months
- **Symptoms associated with pregnancy**: amenorrhea, nausea and vomiting, breast tenderness, urinary frequency, fatigue

Physical Exam

- Chadwick's sign: bluish discoloration of the cervix and vagina due to pelvic vasculature engorgement (6 wks)
- Hegar's sign: softening of the cervical isthmus (6-8 wks)
- Uterine enlargement
- Leopold's maneuver: used to determine the baby's position
- Goodell's sign: softening of the cervix (4-6 wks)

Leopold's Maneuvers (T3)

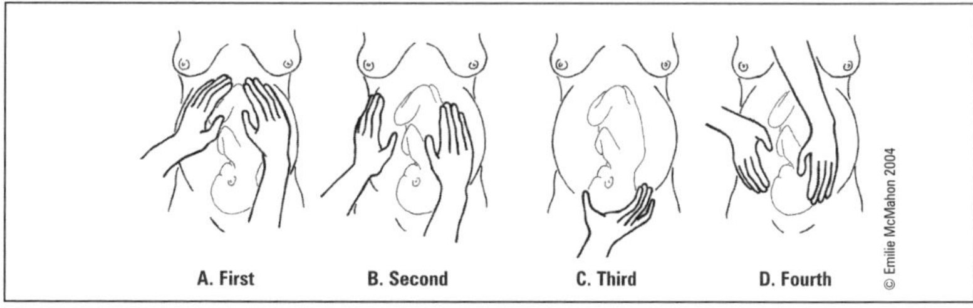

Reprinted with permission from *Essentials of Clinical Examination Handbook*, 6th ed.

Investigations
- β-hCG: positive in serum 7 d post-conception, positive in urine 28 d after last menstrual period
  - Plasma levels double every 1-2 d, peak at 8-10 wks, then fall to a plateau until delivery
  - Levels less than expected = ectopic, abortion or wrong dates
  - Levels higher than expected = multiple gestation, molar pregnancy, trisomy 21 or wrong dates
- Transabdominal U/S: intrauterine pregnancy visible at 6-8 wks (β-hCG >6500 mIU/ml)
- Biophysical profile: 30 min U/S assessment of the fetus ± NST

Scoring of the Biophysical Profile

Parameter	Reassuring (2 points)	Non-Reassuring (0 points)
AFV*	Fluid pocket of 2 cm in 2 axes	Oligohydramnios
Breathing	At least one episode of breathing lasting at least 30 sec	No breathing
Limb Movement	Three discrete movements	Two or less
Fetal Tone	At least one episode of limb extension followed by flexion	No movement

*Amniotic fluid volume (AFV) is a marker of chronic hypoxia, all other parameters indicate acute hypoxia

Classification of Antepartum Non-Stress Test

Parameter	Normal NST (Previously "Reactive")	Atypical NST (Previously "Non-Reactive")	Abnormal NST (Previously "Non-Reactive")
Baseline	110-160 bpm	100-110 bpm or >160 bpm for <30 min Rising baseline	Bradycardia <100 bpm Tachycardia >160 for >30 min Erratic baseline
Variability	6-25 bpm (moderate) ≤5 bpm (absent or minimal) for <40 min	5 bpm (absent or minimal) for 40-80 min 25 bpm for >10 min	≤5 bpm for 80 min Sinusoidal
Decelerations	None or occasional variable <30 s	Variable decelerations 30-60 s duration	Variable decelerations >60 s Late deceleration(s)
Accelerations in Term Fetus	2 accelerations with acme of ≥15 bpm, lasting 15 s over <40 min of testing	2 accelerations with acme of ≥15 bpm, lasting 15 s in 40-80 min	<2 accelerations with acme of ≥15 bpm, lasting 15 s in >80 min
Accelerations in Preterm Fetus (<32 wks)	>2 accelerations with acme of >10 bpm, lasting 10 s in <40 min	<2 accelerations with acme of >10 bpm, lasting 10 s in 40-80 min	<2 accelerations with acme of >10 bpm, lasting 10 s in >80 min
Action	FURTHER ASSESSMENT OPTIONAL, based on total clinical picture	FURTHER ASSESSMENT REQUIRED	URGENT ACTION REQUIRED An overall assessment of the situation and further investigation with U/S or BPP is required. Some situations will require delivery

Adapted from SOGC, Fetal Health Surveillance: Antepartum and Intrapartum Consensus Guideline, September 2007.

• Other screening investigations:

Gestation-Dependent Screening Investigations

Gestational Age (wks)	Investigations
8-12	Dating U/S
10-12	Chorionic Villus Sampling (CVS)
11-14	First Trimester Screening Integrated Prenatal Screening Part 1
11-13	Nuchal Translucency U/S
15-16 to term	Amniocentesis
15-18	Integrated Prenatal Screening Part 2
16-18	Maternal Serum Screen
18-20 to term	Fetal Movements (quickening)
18-20	U/S for dates, structural assessment
24-28	50 g oral glucose challenge test (OGCT)
28	Repeat CBC RhIG for all Rh negative women
36	Rh antibody screen if indicated Group *B Streptococcus* (GBS) Screen
6 wks postpartum	Discuss contraception, menses, breast feeding, depression, mental health supports P/E: breast, pelvic (including Pap)

Comparison of FTS, MSS and IPS

First Trimester Screen (FTS)	Maternal Serum Screen (MSS)	Integrated Prematal Screen
11-14 wks Measures 1. Nuchal translucency on U/S 2. β-hCG 3. Pregnancy-associated plasma protein A (PAPP-A)	15-18 wks Measures 1. Maternal serum α-fetoprotein (MSAFP) 2. β-hCG 3. Unconjugated estrogen (estriol or μE3)	Nuchal transparency on 12 wks U/S FTS at 11-14 wks MSS at 15-18 wks+ inhibin A at 15-18 wks
Risk estimate for 1. Down syndrome (Trisomy 21): increased NT, increased β-hCG, decreased PAPP-A	Risk estimate for 1. Open neural tube defect (oNTD) MSAFP (sensitivity 80-90%) 2. Trisomy 21: $\downarrow$ MSAFP, $\uparrow$ β-hCG, $\downarrow$ μE3 (sensitivity 65%) 3. Trisomy 18: $\downarrow$ MSAFP, $\downarrow$ β-hCG, $\downarrow$ μE3 (sensitivity 80%)	Risk estimate for oNTD, Trisomy 18 and 21
Useful when patient wants results within the first trimester More accurate estimate of Down syndrome risk than MSS, sensitivity ~85% (when combined with age) 5% false positive rate Patients with positive screen should be offered CVS or amniocentesis	Only offered alone if patient missed the time window for IPS or FTS 8% baseline false positive rate for t21, lower for oNTD and t18 Patients with positive screen should be offered U/S or amniocentesis	Sensitivity ~85-90% 2% false-positive rate Patients with positive screen should be offered U/S and/or amniocentesis

Maternal Triage Assessment

- **ID**: Age, GPTA, EDC, GA, GBS status, Rh status, Serology

- **CC**:

- **HPI: 4 key questions**
  - Contractions: since when, how close (qxmin), how long (xsec), how painful
  - Bleeding (PVB): since when, how much (# of pads), colour (pinky mucous= show vs. brown vs. bright red ± clots), pain, trauma/intercourse
  - Fluid (ROM): since when, large gush vs. trickle, soaked pants, clear vs. green vs. red
- Fetal movement (FM): as much as usual? last movement? kick counts

- **Hx of pregnancy**: Any complications (HTN, GDM, infections), PPS/FTS screening, last ultrasound (BPP score, growth/estimated fetal weight, position), last vaginal exam

- **POBHx**: Every previous pregnancy and outcome: year, SVD/CS/Miscarriage/Abortion, baby size, length of labour, use of vacuum or forceps, complications

- **PMHx, Meds, Allergies, SHx**

- **O/E**: Maternal vitals, fetal heart tracing, Leopold's maneuvers, vaginal exam, U/S

Common Presentations

First and Second Trimester Bleeding

Differential Diagnosis
- Physiological: implantation bleed
- Abortion: threatened, inevitable, incomplete, complete
- Abnormal pregnancy: ectopic, molar
- Trauma: post-coital
- Genital lesions: cervical polyps or neoplasm
- Placental: placenta previa
- Coagulopathy
- Other: bleeding from urethra or rectum

History
- LMP, GTPAL, contraception use
- Onset, amount, timing, continuous vs. intermittent, clots
- Constitutional symptoms (e.g. wt loss, decreased appetite, fever, night sweats)
- Recent trauma/intercourse
- Pain, N/V, syncope, bruising

Risk Factors/Predisposing/Precipitants
- Hx ectopic or spontaneous abortion
- Hx PID or STD
- IUD use
- Infertility or in vitro fertilization

Complications/PMHx/FmHx
- Hx abortion, ectopic, molar, neoplasm, bleeding disorder, hypothyroid
- Gyne Hx (fibroids, # prev uterine surgeries, PID, STD, infertility treatment, endometritis, endometriosis)
- Medications

Physical Exam
- Vitals (with postural change to assess amount of blood loss)
- Abdominal exam
- Gyne exam (inspection, speculum and bimanual)

Management
- ABCs: ensure hemodynamically stable
- Lines: 2 large bore IV (16 gauge) with normal saline ± blood
- Investigations: β-hCG, CBC, group and screen (Rh status), U/S
- Give Rhogam if Rh negative
- Definitive treatment: based on etiology – expectant vs medical vs surgical

ANTEPARTUM HEMORRHAGE

Definition
- Vaginal bleeding from 20 wks to term

Differential Diagnosis
- Bloody show (shedding of cervical mucus plug) – most common etiology in T3
- Placenta previa
- Abruptio placentae – most common pathological etiology in T3
- Vasa previa
- Marginal sinus bleeding
- Cervical lesion (cervicitis, polyp, ectropion, cervical cancer)
- Uterine rupture
- Other: bleeding from bowel or bladder, placenta accreta, abnormal coagulation

PLACENTA PREVIA

Definition
- Abnormal location of the placenta near, partially or completely over the cervical os

Classification
- Total: placenta completely covers the internal os
- Partial: placenta partially covers the internal os
- Marginal: within 2 cm of os but does not cover any part of os
- Risk of hemorrhage during cervical effacement and dilatation
- Low lying (NOT a previa): placenta in lower segment but clear of os (can also bleed, but usually in labour)

Risk Factors
- History of placenta previa (4-8% recurrence risk)
- Multiparity
- Increased maternal age
- Multiple gestation
- Uterine tumour (e.g. fibroids) or other uterine anomalies
- Uterine scar due to previous abortion, C/S, D&C, myomectomy

Clinical Presentation
- PAINLESS
- NO tenderness
- Uterus SOFT
- No uterine irritability/contractions
- Malpresentation and/or high presenting part

- Fetal heart usually NORMAL
- Shock and anemia CORRESPOND to apparent blood loss
- Coagulopathy very UNCOMMON initially

Physical Exam
- Uterus soft and non-tender
- Presenting part high or displaced
- Do **NOT** perform a vaginal exam until placenta previa has been ruled out by U/S

Complications
- Fetal
    - Perinatal mortality low but still higher than with a normal pregnancy
    - Prematurity (bleeding often dictates early C/S)
    - Intrauterine hypoxia (acute or IUGR)
    - Fetal malpresentation
    - PPROM
    - Risk of fetal blood loss from placenta, especially if incised during C/S
- Maternal
    - <1% maternal mortality
    - Hemorrhage and hypovolemic shock, anemia, acute renal failure, pituitary necrosis (Sheehan syndrome)
    - Placenta accreta – especially in previous uterine surgery; anterior placenta previa
    - Hysterectomy

Investigations
- Ultrasound diagnosis (transabdominal ultrasound has 95% accuracy)
- Due to development of lower uterine segment, 90-95% of previas diagnosed in T2 resolve by T3 – (repeat U/S at 30-32 wks for partial or total previas, repeat U/S for low-lying not indicated unless recurrent bleeding)

Management
- Goal: keep pregnancy intrauterine until the risk of delivery < risk of not delivering
- Stabilize and monitor
- CBC, INR/PTT, platelets, fibrinogen, FDP, type and cross match
- Electronic fetal monitoring
- U/S assessment: when fetal and maternal condition permit, determine fetal viability, gestational age and placental status/position
- Rhogam® if mother is Rh negative
- Kleihauer-Betke test to determine extent of fetomaternal transfusion so that appropriate dose of Rhogam® can be given
- GA <36 wks and minimal bleeding – expectant management
    - Admit to hospital
    - Limited physical activity, no douches, enemas, or sexual intercourse
    - Consider corticosteroids for fetal lung maturity if <34 wks
    - Delivery when fetus is mature or hemorrhage dictates
- GA >36 wks, profuse bleeding or L/S ratio is >2:1 – deliver by C/S

ABRUPTIO PLACENTAE

Definition
- Premature separation of a normally implanted placenta after 20 wks gestation

Risk Factors
- Previous abruption (recurrence rate 5-16%)
- Maternal hypertension (chronic or gestational in 50% of abruptions) or vascular disease
- Cigarette smoking (>1 ppd), excessive alcohol consumption, cocaine
- Multiparity and/or maternal age >35 (felt to reflect parity)
- PPROM
- Rapid decompression of a distended uterus (polyhydramnios, multiple gestation)
- Uterine anomaly, fibroids
- Trauma (e.g. motor vehicle collision, maternal battery)

Clinical Features
- Abdominal pain and/or backache
- Uterine tenderness
- Increased uterine tone
- Uterine irritability/contractions
- Usually normal fetal presentation
- FHR may be absent or non-reassuring
- Shock and anemia out of proportion to apparent blood loss
- May have coagulopathy

Classification
- Total (fetal death inevitable) vs. partial
- External/revealed/apparent: blood dissects downward toward cervix
- Internal/concealed (20%): blood dissects upward toward fetus
- Most are mixed

Complications
- Fetal complications:
  - Perinatal mortality 25-60%
  - Prematurity
  - Intrauterine hypoxia
- Maternal complications:
  - <1% maternal mortality, DIC (in 20% of abruptions); placental abruption is the most common cause of DIC in pregnancy
  - Acute renal failure
  - Anemia
  - Hemorrhagic shock
  - Pituitary necrosis (Sheehan syndrome)
  - Amniotic fluid embolus

Investigations
- A clinical diagnosis: ultrasound not sensitive for abruption (sensitivity = 15%) – may see clot

Management
- Maternal stabilization: large bore IV with hydration; O_2 for hypotensive patients
- Electronic fetal monitoring
- Maternal monitoring: vitals, urine output, blood loss, bloodwork (hematocrit, CBC, PTT/PT, platelets, fibrinogen, FDP, type and cross match)
- Blood products on hand (red cells, platelets, cryoprecipitate) because of DIC risk
- Rhogam® if Rh negative
- Kleihauer-Betke test may confirm abruption

- Mild Abruption
  - GA <36 wks: use serial Hct to assess concealed bleeding, if <34 wks administer celestone, deliver when fetus is mature or hemorrhage dictates
  - GA >36 wks: stabilize and deliver
- Moderate to Severe Abruption
  - Hydrate and restore blood loss and correct coagulation defect if present
  - Vaginal delivery if no evidence of fetal or maternal distress and if cephalic presentation OR with fetal demise
- C/S if live fetus and fetal or maternal distress develops with fluid/blood replacement, labour fails to progress or non-cephalic fetal presentation

VASA PREVIA

Definition
- Unprotected fetal vessels pass over the cervical os; associated with velamentous insertion of cord into membranes of placenta or succenturiate lobe

Clinical Features
- PAINLESS vaginal bleeding and fetal distress (tachy- to bradyarrhythmia)
- 50% perinatal mortality, increasing to 75% if membranes rupture (most infants die of exsanguination)

Investigations
- Apt test (NaOH mixed with the blood) can be done immediately to determine if the source of the bleeding is fetal (supernatant turns pink) or maternal (supernatant turns yellow)
- Wright stain on blood smear and look for nucleated red blood cells (in cord, not maternal blood)

Management
- Emergency C/S (since bleeding is from fetus, a small amount of blood loss can have catastrophic consequences)

Spontaneous Abortion

Type	History	Clinical	Management (± Rhogam®)
Threatened	Vaginal bleeding ± cramping	Cervix closed and soft U/S shows viable fetus	Watch and wait <5% go on to abort
Inevitable	Increased bleeding and cramps ± rupture of membranes	Cervix closed until products start to expel, then external os opens	Watch and wait Misoprostol D&C ± oxytocin
Incomplete	Extremely heavy bleeding and cramps ± passage of tissue noticed	Cervix open	Watch and wait Misoprostol D&C ± oxytocin
Complete	Bleeding and complete passage of sac and placenta	Cervix open	No D&C – expectant management
Missed	No bleeding (fetal death in utero)	Cervix closed U/S may show SGA	Watch and wait Misoprostol D&C ± oxytocin
Habitual	3+ consecutive spontaneous abortions		Evaluate mechanical, genetic, environmental and other risk factors
Septic	Contents of uterus infected – infrequent		D&C IV broad spectrum antibiotics

Postpartum Hemorrhage

Definition
- Loss of >500 mL of blood with vaginal delivery, or >1000 mL with C/S
- Early – within first 24 h postpartum
- Late – after 24 h but within first 6 wks

Differential Diagnosis: Early
- **Tone**: Atony- Overdistended uterus, uterine muscle exhaustion, intra-amniotic infection, functional/anatomic distortion
- **Tissue**: Retained placental tissues- abnormal placentaion, retained cotyledone or succenturiate lobe, retained blood clot
- **Trauma**: Uterine, cervical or vaginal injury; uterine rupture or inversion
- **Thrombin**: Coagulopathy- ITP, DIC, anticoagulation

Differential Diagnosis: Late
- Retained products, endometritis, subinvolution of uterus

Investigations
- Clinical exam to assess degree of blood loss
- Explore uterus and lower genital tract for evidence of tone, tissue, or trauma

Management
- ABC, cross and type 4 units pRBCs
- 2 large bore IV + crystalloids
- CBC, coagulation profile
- Treat underlying cause
- Medical therapy
    - Oxytocin 20U/L IV infusion – in addition can give 10 U intramyometrial (IMM) after delivery of placenta
    - Ergotamine 0.25 mg IM/IMM q5min up to 1.25 mg – can be given as IV bolus of 0.125 mg
    - Carboprost (Hemabate) 0.25 mg IM/IMM q15min up to 2 mg
    - Misoprostal PR 800-1000 µg
- Local control
    - Bimanual compression
    - Uterine compression
- Surgical therapy for intractable PPH
    - D&C
    - Laparotomy with bilateral ligation of uterine artery, internal iliac artery, ovarian artery, or hypogastric artery

Labour and Delivery

Contractions

- **Labour**: regular, become more frequent with time, increasing intensity, do not subside, associated with dilatation and effacement of cervix
- **Braxton-Hicks**: irregular, varying intensity, may be related to position, paroxysmal, not associated with cervical change

Preterm Labour

Etiology
- Idiopathic (most common)
- Maternal: infection (recurrent pyelonephritis, untreated bacteriuria, chorioamnionitis), genital infection (bacterial vaginosis is associated with a twofold increase in relative risk of preterm birth), HTN, DM, chronic illness, mechanical factors, previous obstetric, gynecological and abdominal surgeries, socio-environmental (poor nutrition, smoking, drugs, alcohol, stress)
- Maternal-fetal: PPROM (a common cause), polyhydramnios, placenta previa or abruption, placental insufficiency
- Fetal: multiple gestation, congenital abnormalities of fetus, fetal hydrops
- Uterine: incompetent cervix, excessive enlargement (hydramnios), malformations (leiomyomas, septate)

MANAGEMENT

A. Initial
- Transfer to appropriate facility if stable
- Hydration (NS @ 150 mL/h)
- Bed rest in LLDP
- Sedation (morphine)
- Avoid repeated pelvic exams (increased infection risk)
- U/S examination of fetus (for GA, BPP, position, placenta location, estimated fetal weight (EFW))
- Prophylactic antibiotics; controversial but may help delay delivery, important to consider if PPROM

B. Suppression of Labour – Tocolysis
- Does not inhibit preterm labour completely, but may buy time to allow Celestone® use/transfer to appropriate centre
- Requirements – all must be satisfied: preterm labour, live immature fetus, intact membranes, cervical dilatation of <4 cm, absence of maternal or fetal contraindications
- Contraindications: maternal bleeding (placenta previa or abruption), maternal disease (hypertension, diabetes, heart disease), preeclampsia or eclampsia, chorioamnionitis, erythroblastosis fetalis, severe congenital anomalies, fetal distress/demise, IUGR, multiple gestation (relative)
- Tocolytic procedure
  - Calcium channel blockers: nifedipine
  - Prostaglandin synthesis inhibitors : indomethacin
  - Magnesium Sulfate
- Should be used only for <48 h, and/or transfer to an appropriate facility

C. Enhancement of Fetal Pulmonary Maturity (<34 weeks)
- Betamethasone valerate (Celestone®) 12 mg IM q24h x 2 or dexamethasone 6 mg IM q12h x 4
- 28-34 wks GA: reduces incidence of respiratory distress syndrome (RDS)
- 24-28 wks GA: reduces severity of RDS, overall mortality and rate of intraventricular hemorrhage (IVH)
- Specific maternal contraindications: active TB, viral keratosis, maternal DM

D. Cervical Cerclage (<24 weeks)
- Indications: cervical incompetence – cervical dilation and effacement in the absence of increased uterine contractility
- Proven benefit in the prevention of PTL in women with primary structural abnormality of the cervix (e.g. conization of the cervix, connective tissue disorders)
- Benefit is variable in those with secondary cervical incompetence causing premature ripening of the cervix (e.g. infection, abnormal placentation)

Prognosis
- Prematurity is the leading cause of perinatal morbidity and mortality
  - 30 wks or 1500 g (3.3 lb) = 90% survival
  - 33 wks or 2000 g (4.4 lb) = 99% survival
- Morbidity due to asphyxia (may lead to cerebral hemorrhage), hypoxia (may lead to necrotizing enterocolitis), sepsis, respiratory distress syndrome (RDS), intraventricular hemorrhage, thermal instability, retinopathy of prematurity, bronchopulmonary dysplasia

Prevention of Preterm Labour
- Currently there are no agents approved by Health Canada to arrest preterm labour
- Preventative measures: good prenatal care, identify pregnancies at risk, treat silent vaginal infection or UTI, patient education
- Transvaginal ultrasound of cervical length is not supported for routine prenatal care; however, it is recommended for high-risk pregnancies: cervical length of >30 mm has a high negative predictive value for delivery before 34 wks (this measurement can be used to avoid unnecessary intervention)

Normal Labour and Delivery

1. **First Stage** (6-18 h nulliparous/2-10 h multiparous)
   a. Latent Phase: uterine contractions infrequent and irregular and cervical dilation to 3-4 cm with effacement
   b. Active Phases: rapid cervical dilation to full dilation (1.2-1.5 cm/h), painful regular contractions (q2min for 45-60 s)
2. **Second Stage** (full dilation to delivery of baby 30 min-3 h nulliparous/5-30 min multiparous)
   a. Desire to bear down and push with contractions
   b. Progress measured by descent
3. **Third Stage** (separation and expulsion of placenta)
   a. Can last up to 30 min
   b. Gush of blood, lengthening of cord, uterus firms and fundus rises
   c. Start oxytocin drip after delivery of anterior shoulder
4. **Fourth Stage** (first postpartum hour)
   a. Monitor vital signs and bleeding
   b. Repair lacerations
   c. Ensure uterus is contracted
   d. Placenta inspected for completeness

Labour Monitors
- Uterine activity measured by tocometer
  - 20 s = 1 small square
  - 1 min = 3 small squares (may vary with machine)
- Fetal heart rate described in terms of baseline, variability (short term, long term), and periodicity (accelerations, decelerations)
- While widely used, studies have shown that continuous FHM does not significantly improve infant mortality or other standards of infant well-being. It increases the incidence of C-section and instrument-assisted vaginal delivery.

Approach
- Is the **uterine activity** acceptable?
- What is the **baseline** of the fetal heart (FH)?
- Is the **variability** of the FH reassuring?
- Are there **accelerations**?
- Are there **decelerations**? If so, what kind?
- What interventions or management steps should be taken?

Uterine Activity
- Frequency of contractions
- Duration of contractions
- Increased intensity of contractions

Baseline
- Average fetal heart rate excluding accelerations or decelerations
- Normal range considered to be between 110-160 bpm
- Baseline evaluated over 20 min
- Variability is evaluated when there is no contraction
- Bradycardia: <110 bpm (R/O fetal hypoxia)
- Tachycardia: >160 bpm (R/O maternal fever or drug effect)

Variability
- Powerful predictor of fetal health
- If absent for >40 min, need to assess fetal well being (e.g. biophysical profile)
- Causes of minimal variability (<5 bpm):
    - Persistent hypoxia
    - Fetal sleep
    - Maternal smoking
    - Drugs – narcotics, sedatives, β-blockers, $MgSO_4$
    - Preterm fetus
    - Fetal tachycardia
    - Congenital anomalies

Accelerations
- Abrupt increase of fetal heart rate of at least 15 bpm persisting for at least
  15 sec and lasting less than 2 min
- Must have minimum of 2 in 20 min for a reassuring fetal heart strip
- Most important indicator of fetal well being

Decelerations
- Early: mirror image of contraction – normal variability
- Variable: V, U, W shaped – often due to umbilical cord compression
- Late: begins with contraction, lowest depth at peak of contraction – associated with minimal variability and
  uteroplacental insufficiency

Management of a Non-Reassuring Fetal Heart Strip
- Document findings and plan on progress note
- Notify patient
- Consult obs/pediatrics
- Maximize fetal oxygenation
- Consider further evaluation: fetal spiral electrode, fetal scalp blood sampling, biophysical profile, umbilical
  cord sampling
- Prepare for delivery or transfer of care

Comparison of Decelerations

Early Decelerations

- Uniform shape with onset early in contraction; returns to baseline by end of contraction
- Gradual deceleration
- Often repetitive; no effect on baseline FHR or variability
- Due to vagal response to head compression
- Benign, usually seen with cervical dilatation of 4-7 cm
- **Management**
  No action (normal response)

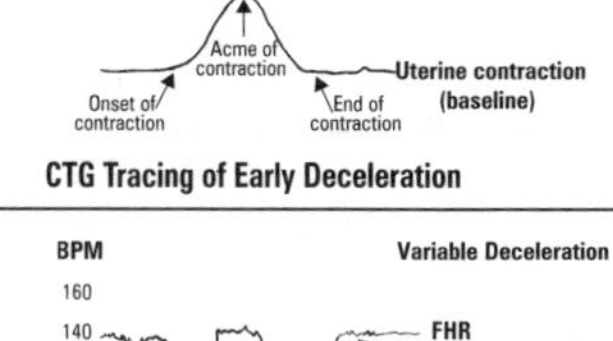

CTG Tracing of Early Deceleration

Variable Decelerations

- Variable in shape, onset, and duration
- Most common type of periodicity seen during labour
- May or may not be repetitive
- Often with abrupt drop in FHR; usually no effect on baseline FHR or variability
- Due to cord compression or, in second stage, forceful pushing with contractions
- Benign unless repetitive, with slow recovery, or when associated with other abnormalities of FHR
- **Management if non-reassuring**:
  Intrauterine resuscitation
  Confirm fetal well being
  Amnioinfusion
  Consider operative delivery (vacuum, forceps, C/S)

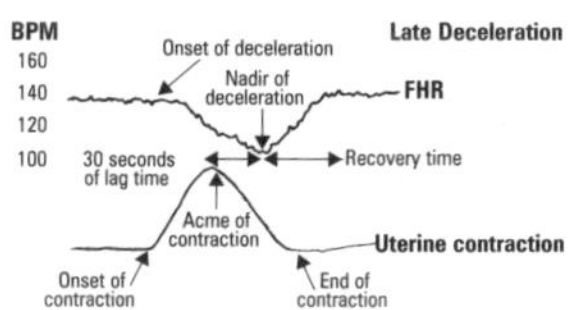

CTG Tracing of Variable Deceleration

Late Decelerations

- Uniform shape with onset late in contraction, lowest depth after peak of contraction, and return to baseline after end of contraction
- May cause decreased variability and change in baseline FHR
- Must see 3 in a row, all with the same shape to define a late deceleration
- Due to fetal hypoxia and acidemia, maternal hypotension or uterine hypertonus
- Usually a sign of uteroplacental insufficiency (an ominous sign)
- **Management if persistent**:
  Intrauterine resuscitation
  Consider operative delivery
  Confirm fetal well being
  See fetal blood sampling

CTG Tracing of Late Deceleration

Operative Vaginal Delivery

- Definition: forceps or vacuum delivery
- RCTs indicate that forceps delivery is associated with more maternal perineal and vaginal trauma while vacuum extraction causes more neonatal injury

Prerequisites for Operative Vaginal Delivery: ABCDEFGHIJK

Anesthesia
Bladder empty
Cervix fully dilated and effaced with ROM
Determine position of fetal head
Equipment ready (including facilities for emergent C/S)
Fontanelle (posterior fontanelle midway between thighs, fenestration barely palpable)
Gentle traction
Handle elevated
Incision (episiotomy)
Once **J**aw visible remove forceps
Knowledgeable operator

Caesarean Delivery

Epidemiology
• Incidence 20-25%

Indications
• Maternal: obstruction, active herpetic lesion on vulva, invasive cervical cancer, previous uterine surgery, underlying maternal illness (eclampsia, HELLP syndrome, heart disease)
• Maternal-fetal: failure to progress, placental abruption or previa
• Fetal: NRFHR, malpresentation, cord prolapse, certain congenital anomalies

Types of Caesarean Incisions
• Skin
  ▪ Vertical midline
    ♦ Rapid peritoneal entry and increased exposure
    ♦ Increased dehiscence
  ▪ Transverse
    ♦ Decreased exposure and slower entry
    ♦ Improved strength and cosmesis
• Uterine
  ▪ Low transverse (most common) – in noncontractile segment – decreased chance for rupture in subsequent pregnancies
  ▪ Low vertical – used for very preterm infants, poorly developed maternal lower uterine segment
  ▪ Classical (rare) – in thick, contractile segment – used for transverse lie, fetal anomaly, >2 fetuses, lower segment adhesions, obstructing fibroid

Risks/Complications
• Anesthesia
• Hemorrhage (average blood loss ~1000 cc)
• Infection (UTI, wound, endometritis)
• Injury to surrounding structures (bowel, bladder, uterus)
• Thromboembolic phenomena
• Increased recovery time/hospital stay
• Maternal mortality (<0.1%)

Common Conditions

Infections During Pregnancy   * indicates TORCH infection

Infection	Agent	Source of Transmission	Greatest Transmission Risk to Fetus	Effects on Fetus	Effects on Mother	Diagnosis	Management
Chicken Pox	Varicella zoster virus (herpes family)	Direct, respiratory, transplacental	13-30 wks GA, and 5d pre- to 2d post-delivery	Congenital varicella syndrome (limb aplasia, chorioretinitis, cataracts, cutaneous scars, cortical atrophy, IUGR, hydrops), preterm labour (PTL)	Fever, malaise, vesicular pruritic lesions	Clinical, ± vesicle fluid culture, ± serology	VZIG for mother decreases CVS Note: Do not administer vaccine during pregnancy (live attenuated)
***CMV**	DNA virus (herpes family)	Blood/organ transfusion, sexual contact, breast milk, transplacental, hydrocephalus, microcephaly	T1-T3	5-10% develop CNS involvement (mental retardation, cerebral calcification, deafness, chorioretinitis)	Asymptomatic or flu-like	Serologic screen; isolate virus from urine or secretion culture	No specific treatment; maintain good hygiene and avoid high risk situations during delivery
Erythema Infectiosum (Fifth Disease)	Parvovirus B19	Respiratory, infected blood products, transplacental	10-20 wks GA	Spontaneous abortion (SA), stillbirth, hydrops in utero	Flu-like, rash, arthritis; often asymptomatic	Serology, viral PCR, maternal AFP; if IgM present, follow fetus with U/S for hydrops	If hydrops occurs, consider fetal transfusion
Hepatitis B	DNA virus	Blood, saliva, semen, vaginal secretions, breast milk, transplacental	T3 10% vertical transmission if asymptomatic HBsAg +ve; 85-90% if HBsAg and HBeAg +ve	Prematurity, low birth weight, neonatal death	Fever, N/V, fatigue, jaundice, elevated liver enzymes	Serologic screening for all pregnancies	Rx neonate with HBIG and vaccine (at birth, 1, 6 months); 90% effective

Infections During Pregnancy   * indicates TORCH infection (continued)

Infection	Agent	Source of Transmission	Greatest Transmission Risk to Fetus	Effects on Fetus	Effects on Mother	Diagnosis	Management
HIV	RNA retrovirus	Blood, semen, vaginal secretions, breast milk, during delivery, in utero	1/3 in utero, 1/3 at delivery, 1/3 breastfeeding	IUGR, preterm labour, premature rupture of membranes	See Infectious Diseases	Serology, viral PCR All pregnant women are offered screening	Triple antiretroviral therapy decreases transmission to <1%, elective C/S: no previous ANTI-RETROVIRAL Rx or monotherapy only, viral load unknown or >500 RNA copies/mL, unknown prenatal care, patient request
*Rubella	ssRNA togavirus	Respiratory droplets (highly contagious), transplacental	T1	SA or congenital rubella syndrome (hearing loss, cataracts, CV lesions, MR, IUGR, hepatitis, CNS defects, osseous changes)	Rash (50%), fever, posterior auricular or occipital lymphadenopathy, arthralgia	Serologic testing; all pregnant women screened (immune if titre >1:16); infection if IgM present or >4x increase in IgG	No specific treatment; offer vaccine following pregnancy Do not administer VACCINE during pregnancy (live attenuated)
Syphilis	Spirochete (*Treponema pallidum*)	Transplacental	T1-T3	Risk of PTL, multisystem involvement, fetal death	See Infectious Diseases	VDRL screening for all pregnancies; confirm with TPHA or FTA-ABS	Pen G 2.4 M U IM 1 dose if early syphilis 3 doses if late syphilis monitor VDRL monthly
*Toxoplasmosis	Protozoa (*Toxoplasma gondii*)	Raw meat, unpasteurized goat's milk, cat feces/urine, transplacental	T3 (but most severe if infected in T1); only concern if primary infection during pregnancy	Congenital toxoplasmosis (chorioretinitis, hydrocephaly, intracranial calcification, MR, microcephaly) NB: 75% initially asymptomatic at birth	Majority subclinical; may have flu-like symptoms	IgM and IgG serology PCR of amniotic fluid	Self-limiting in mother; spiramycin decreases fetal morbidity, not rate of transmission

Ectopic Pregnancy

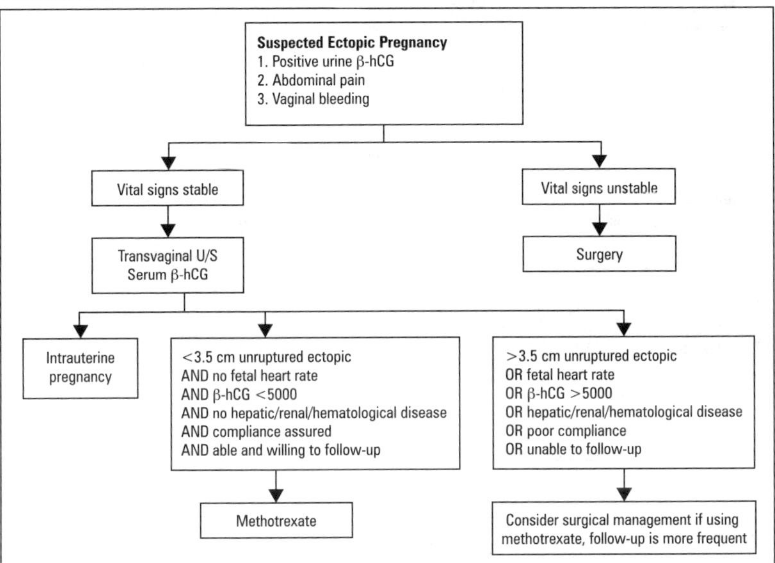

Hypertensive Emergencies in Pregnancy

There are four hypertensive disorders that can affect pregnant women:

1. Preexisting HTN
- HTN (>140/90) prior to 20 wks GA [except in a gestational trophoblastic neoplasia (GTN)], persisting postpartum
- Essential hypertension is associated with an increased risk of gestational HTN, abruptio placenta, IUGR and intrauterine fetal demise (IUFD)

2. Preeclampsia Superimposed on Preexisting HTN
- Pre-existing hypertension with new onset proteinuria or adverse conditions or resistant hypertension
- 2-7 fold increased likelihood of developing preeclampsia/eclampsia if pre-existing maternal hypertension
- Occurs early, tends to be severe (often with IUGR) and to recur with subsequent pregnancies

3. Gestational HTN
- sBP>140 or dBP >90 AND no proteinuria, developing after 20th wk GA in a woman known to be normotensive before pregnancy
- BP should be elevated on at least 2 occasions at least 6 h apart.

RFs for Gestational HTN
- Maternal factors
  - Primigravida (80-90% of gestational HTN)
  - First conception with a new partner
  - PMHx or FHx of gestational HTN
  - DM, chronic HTN, or renal insufficiency
  - Antiphospholipid antibody syndrome (APLA)
  - Extremes of maternal age (<18 or >35 yrs)
- Fetal factors
  - IUGR or oligohydramnios, GTN, multiple gestation, fetal hydrops

4. Preeclampsia
- Gestational hypertension with new onset proteinuria after 20 wks GA in a previously normotensive woman

RFs for Preeclampsia
- Nulliparity
- Preeclampsia in a previous pregnancy
- Age >40 yrs or <18 yrs
- Fhx of preeclampsia
- Chronic HTN
- Chronic renal disease
- Antiphospholipid antibody syndrome or inherited thrombophilia
- Vascular or connective tissue disease
- Diabetes mellitus (pregestational and gestational)
- High BMI
- Hydrops fetalis
- Unexplained fetal growth restriction
- Woman small for gestational age
- Abruptio placentae

- Untreated preeclampsia can progress to eclampsia, which presents with the occurrence of one or more generalized convulsions and/or coma in the setting of preeclampsia and in the absence of other neurologic conditions. The diagnosis of eclampsia is made clinically, and the definitive treatment is DELIVERY irrespective of GA to reduce morbidity and mortality from complications associated with eclampsia

Clinical Evaluation of HTN in Pregnancy
1. Evaluation of Mother
- On history: RUQ pain, headache, and visual disturbances are potentially ominous symptoms requiring immediate assessment
- Central nervous system: presence and severity of headache, visual disturbances – blurring, scotoma, tremulousness, irritability, somnolence, hyperreflexia
- Hematologic: bleeding, petechiae
- Hepatic: RUQ or epigastric pain, severe nausea and vomiting
- Renal: urine output, urine colour
- Non-dependent edema (i.e. hands and face)
- Bloodwork and labs: CBC, LFTs, INR and aPTT, creatinine, uric acid, LDH, albumin, bilirubin, urine dip and 24 h collection

2. Evaluation of Fetus
- Fetal movement
- Fetal heart rate tracing – NST
- Ultrasound for growth
- Biophysical profile (BPP)
- Doppler flow studies

Management of HTN in Pregnancy with Adverse Conditions (i.e. HELLP, cerebral hemorrhage, eclampsia, etc.) (This is SEVERE PREECLAMPSIA)
- Stabilize and deliver; only "cure" is delivery, independent of gestational age (vaginal delivery preferred)
- Increased maternal monitoring to hourly input and output, urine dip q12h and neurological vitals q1h
- Increased fetal evaluation to include continuous monitoring
- Anticonvulsant therapy to raise seizure threshold: Mg^{2+} sulfate (4 g IV bolus over 20 min followed by maintenance of 2-4 g/h)
- Monitor for signs of Mg^{2+} toxicity: depressed deep tendon reflexes, decreased RR, anuric, hypotonic, CNS or cardiac depression antagonist to Mg^{2+} sulfate: calcium gluconate (10%) 10 mL (1 g) IV over 2 min
- Antihypertensive therapy to decrease the risk of stroke: 1st line: hydralazine 5-10 mg IV bolus over 5 min q15-30 min as necessary, labetalol 20-50 mg IV q10 min; 2nd line: nifedipine 10-20 mg PO q20-60 min; ACEi are contraindicated
- Postpartum management: risk of seizure highest in first 24 h postpartum, thus continue Mg^{2+} sulfate for 12-24 h, vitals q1h, consider HELLP syndrome in toxic patients, most return to a normotensive BP within 2 wks

Gestational Diabetes

Screening
- 1-hour 50 g oral glucose challenge test at 24-28 wks GA
  - Plasma glucose <7.8 mmol/L (140 mg/dL)= no GDM
  - 7.8 (140) >PG <10.3 mmol/L (185 mg/dL) = do 2-hour 75 g oral glucose tolerance test
  - PG >10.3 mmol/L (185 mg/dL) = diagnosis of GDM

Diagnosis
- Evaluate fasting plasma glucose and 2-hour 75 g OGTT
- FPG >5.3 mmol/L (95 mg/dL)
- PG 1-hour, 75 g OGTT >10.6 (191 mg/dL)
- PG 2-hour, 75 g OGTT >8.9 (160 mg/dL)
  - If 2/3 criteria met = diagnosis of GDM
  - If 1 of the following criteria met = impaired glucose tolerance

Management
- Treat both impaired glucose tolerance and GDM
- Diet management ± insulin
- Avoid oral hypoglycemics
- Monitor 24 h urine protein, Cr, retinal exam, HbA1c
- Regular fetal surveillance (NST, BPP)
- Type of delivery dependent on fetal and maternal health
  - Induce by 40 wks
  - Monitor blood sugars during labour, avoid blood sugars below 3.5 mmol/L (63 mg/dL)to reduce risk of neonatal hypoglycemia
  - Increased risk of CPD and shoulder dystocia
- Stop insulin and diabetic diet postpartum
- Follow up with 2-h 75 g OGTT 6 months postpartum

Common Medications

Drug Name (Brand Name)	Dosing Schedule	Indications/Comments
betamethasone valerate (Celestone®)	12 mg IM q24h x 2 doses	Enhancement of fetal pulmonary maturity for PTL
carboprost (Hemabate®)	0.25 mg IM/IMM q15min; max 2 mg	Treatment of uterine atony
dexamethasone	6 mg IM q12h x 4 doses	Enhancement of fetal pulmonary maturity for PTL
dinoprostone (Cervidil®- PGE_2 impregnated thread)	10 mg PV (remove after 12h) max of 3 doses	Induction of labour Advantage: can remove if uterine hyperstimulation
doxylamine succinate (Diclectin®)	2 tabs qhs + 1 tab qAM + 1 tab qPM max of 8 tabs/d	Each tablet contains 10 mg doxylamine succinate with vitamin B_6 Used for hyperemesis gravidarum
folic acid	0.4-1.0 mg PO OD x 1-3 months preconception and T1 4.0 mg PO OD with past Hx of NTD	Prevention of oNTD
methotrexate	50 mg/m^2 IM or 50 mg po x 1 dose	For ectopic pregnancy or medical abortion
methylergonavine maleate (Ergotamine®)	0.25 mg IM/IMM q5min up to 1.25 mg or IV bolus 0.125 mg	Treatment of uterine atony
misoprostol (Cytotec®)	800-1000 µg pr x 1 dose 400 µg po x 1 dose or 800 µg pv x 1 dose, 3 to 7 d after methotrexate	For treatment of PPH For medical abortion Also used for NSAID-induced ulcers (warn patients of contraindications)
oxytocin (Pitocin®)	0.5-2.0 mU/min IV, or 10 U/L N/S incr. by 1-2 mU/min q20-60min max of 36-48 mU/min 10 U IM @ delivery of ant shoulder 20 U/L NS or RL IV continuous infusion	Augmentation of labour (also induction of labour) Prevention of uterine atony Treatment of uterine atony
Penicillin G	5 million U IV then 2.5 million U IV q4h until delivery	GBS prophylaxis
PGE_2 gel (Prostin® gel)	0.5 mg PV q6-12h; max of 3 doses	Induction of labour
Rh IgG (Rhogam®)	300 µg IM x 1 dose	Given to Rh negative women • Routinely at 28 wks GA • Within 72 h of birth of Rh +ve fetus • Positive Kleihauer-Betke test • With any invasive procedure in pregnancy • Ectopic pregnancy • Antepartum hemorrhage • Miscarriage or TA (dose: 50 µg IM only)

Ophthalmology

Essential History, Physical Exam and Investigations

Ocular Examination

- Note: Sometimes vision may be blurry secondary to eye drops/ointment/mucus, applying too much pressure; when testing visual acuity ask patient to blink a few times

VISION ASSESSMENT
- Always test visual acuity first, especially in emergency room
- Test best corrected vision (with corrective lenses) whenever possible
- Assess both distance (Snellen chart) and near vision (Rosenbaum pocket screener)
- Test right eye first, then left. Cover eye not being tested
- Improvement of visual acuity using a "pinhole test" indicates an uncorrected refractive error
- OD = oculus dexter = right eye; OS = oculus sinister = left eye; OU = oculus uterque = both eyes

Ophthalmology Nomenclature for Visual Acuity

Example 1 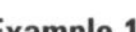 20/40 -1 20/80 +2 → 20/25 PH	**Note:** RIGHT EYE visual acuity always listed on top. **V** — Vision **SC** — Without correction **CC** — With correction **20/40 -1** — All except one letter of 20/40 **20/80 +2** — All of 20/80 plus two letters of 20/70
Example 2 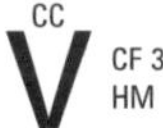 CF 3' HM	**PH** — Visual acuity with pinhole correction **CF3'** — Counting fingers at 3 feet **HM** — Hand motion

VISUAL ACUITY

Distance
- Snellen Fraction = testing distance (usually 20 feet or 6 metres) / smallest line patient can read on the chart
- e.g. 20/40 = what the patient can see at 20 feet (numerator), a "normal" person can see at 40 feet (denominator)
- Testing hierarchy for low vision: Snellen acuity (20/x) → counting fingers at x distance (CF) → hand motion (HM) → light perception with projection (LP with projection) → light perception (LP) → no light perception (NLP)
- Legal blindness is best corrected visual acuity that is worse or equal to 20/200 in the better eye, or a limit to the binocular central field of vision of <20 degrees

Near
- Use pocket vision chart (e.g. Rosenbaum Pocket Vision Screener)
- Record Jaeger (J) or Point number and testing distance (usually 30 cm), e.g. J2 @ 30 cm

- Conversion to distance visual acuity can be made when distance vision cannot be tested (e.g. immobile patient, no distance chart available)

Visual Acuity for Infants, Children, Non-English Speakers, and Patients with Dysphasia
- Newborns
  - Visual acuity cannot be tested
- 3 mo-3 y.o. (can only assess visual function, not acuity)
  - Test each eye for fixation and maintaining fixation using an interesting object, such as a toy
  - Noted as "CSM" = central, steady and maintained
- 3 y.o. until alphabet known
  - Picture chart/card (child names simple objects presented at different sizes)
  - Tumbling "E" chart (child indicates direction of "E")
  - Sheridan-Gardiner matching test

Colour Vision
- Important for testing optic nerve function (e.g. optic neuritis, chloroquine use, thyroid ophthalmopathy)
- Test with Ishihara Plates
- Record number correct out of total plates presented to each eye individually. Compare incorrect plate number with reference provided by Ishihara manual

Visual Fields
- Test "visual fields by confrontation" (4 quadrants, each eye tested separately) for estimate of visual field loss
- Accurate, quantifiable assessment done with automated visual field testing (Humphrey or Goldmann) or Tangent Screen
- Use Amsler grid (each eye individually) to test for central or paracentral scotomas (island-like gaps in vision), especially for patients with AMD

Ophthalmology Nomenclature for Visual Fields by Confrontation

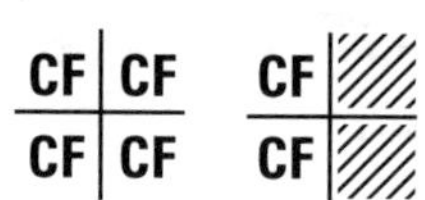

Pupils
- Use reduced room illumination with patient focusing on distant object to prevent "near reflex"
- For patients with dark irides, test the pupils using an ophthalmoscope focused on the red reflex (vs. a penlight)
- Examine pupils for shape, size, symmetry and reactivity to light (both direct and consensual response)
- Test for relative afferent pupillary defect (RAPD) with swinging flashlight test
- Test pupillary constriction portion of near reflex by bringing object close to patient's nose
- "Normal" pupil testing often noted as "PERRLA" = pupils equal, round, and reactive to light and accommodation

Anterior Chamber Depth
- Shine light tangentially from temporal side
- Shallow anterior chamber (AC): >2/3 of nasal side of iris in shadow (see Figure below)

Estimator of Anterior Chamber Depth

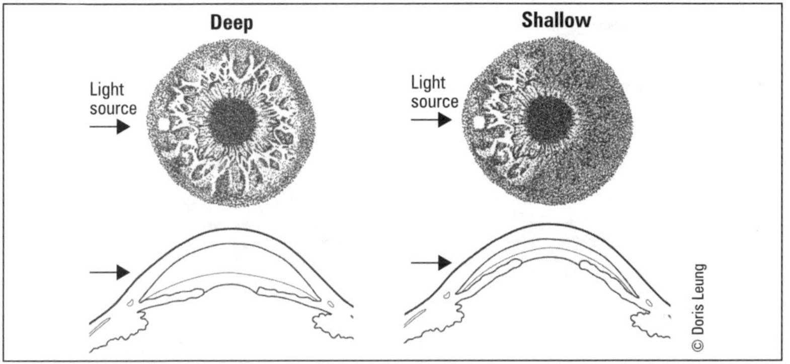

EXTRAOCULAR MUSCLES

Alignment
- Hirschberg corneal reflex test
  - Examine in primary position of gaze (i.e. straight ahead) with patient focusing on distant object (to eliminate accommodative convergence)
  - Shine light into patient's eyes from ~30 cm away
  - Corneal light reflex should be symmetric and at same position on each cornea
- Strabismus testing as indicated (cover test, cover-uncover test, prism testing)

Movement
- Examine movement of eyeball through six cardinal positions of gaze (with six muscles responsible for extra-ocular movement)
- Ask patient if diplopia is present in any position of gaze
- Observe for horizontal, vertical or rotatory nystagmus (rhythmic, oscillating movements of the eye)
- Resolving horizontal nystagmus at end gaze is usually normal
- Cranial nerve III: superior rectus (SR), medial rectus (MR), inferior rectus (IR), inferior oblique (IO)
- Cranial nerve IV: superior oblique (SO)
- Cranial nerve VI: lateral rectus (LR)

EXTERNAL EXAMINATION
- The four L's: Lymph nodes (preauricular, submandibular), Lids, Lashes, Lacrimal system

Investigations

Slit-Lamp Examination
- Lids (including upper lid eversion if necessary), lashes, and lacrimal system
- Conjunctiva and sclera
- Cornea
- Iris
- Anterior chamber (for depth, cells, and flare)
  - To observe cells and flare: 1. Dark room, 2. High power beam, 3. 1 mm beam height, 4. Thin beam, 5. Highest magnification, 6. Approach at angle and focus on anterior chamber (space between cornea and lens)
- Lens
- Anterior vitreous
- When necessary use fluorescein dye (stains Bowman's membrane in de-epithelialized cornea, appearing green with cobalt blue filtered light), Rose Bengal dye (stains devitalized corneal epithelium)

Slit-Lamp

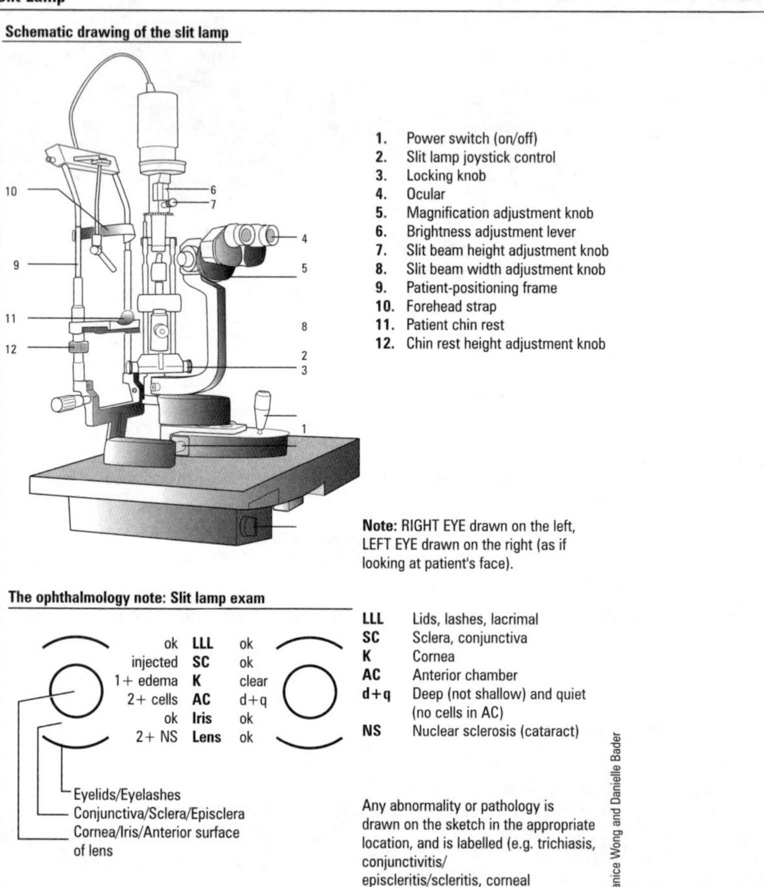

TONOMETRY

- Measurement of intraocular pressure (IOP)
- Normal range is 10-21 mmHg, with a mean of 15 mmHg
- Commonly measured by:
  - Goldmann applanation tonometry (GAT): gold standard, performed using slit-lamp with special tip (prism)
  - Tono-Pen®: use when cornea scarred/asymmetric
  - Air puff (least reliable)

OPHTHALMOSCOPY/FUNDOSCOPY
- Can be performed with direct ophthalmoscope (monocular with small field of view, only posterior pole visualized)
- Assess red reflex: anything that interferes with the passage of light will diminish the red reflex (e.g. large vitreous hemorrhage, cataract)
- Examine the posterior segment of the eye (see Figure below), vitreous, optic disc (colour, cup/disc ratio, sharpness of disc margin), macula, fovea, retinal vessels, retinal background (best performed with pupils fully dilated)

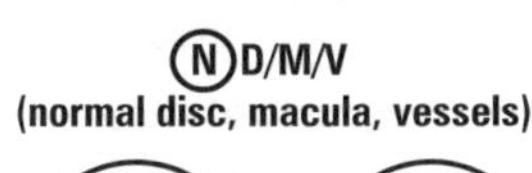
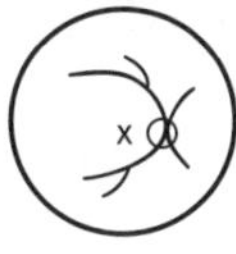
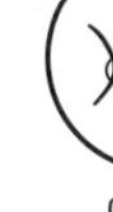

Documentation of Posterior Segment Exam

CONTRAINDICATIONS TO PUPILLARY DILATION
- Shallow anterior chamber – can precipitate acute angle closure glaucoma
- Iris-supported anterior chamber lens implant
- Potential neurologic abnormality requiring pupil evaluation
- Use caution with cardiovascular disease – mydriatics may cause tachycardia

Differential Diagnoses of Common Presentations

Transient Loss of Vision (lasting seconds to hours)

- Transient ischemic attack (TIA), migraine with aura

Acute Loss of Vision (occurring in seconds to days)

Top 3 DDx
1. trauma/foreign body 2. retinal artery/vein occlusion 3. retinal detachment

- **Corneal/Anterior Segment**
  - Trauma/foreign body, corneal edema, hyphema, acute angle-closure glaucoma
- **Vitreous/Retina/Optic Nerve**
  - Retinal artery/vein occlusion, vitreous hemorrhage, retinal detachment, acute macular lesion, optic neuritis, temporal arteritis, anterior ischemic optic neuropathy (AION)
- **Cortical/Other**
  - Occipital infarction/hemorrhage, cortical blindness, functional (non-organic, diagnosis of exclusion)

Chronic Loss of Vision (occurring over weeks to months)

Top 3 DDx
- Reversible: 1. cataract, 2. refractive error, 3. corneal dystrophy
- Irreversible: 1. ARMD, 2. glaucoma, 3. diabetic retinopathy

- **Corneal/Anterior Segment**
  - Corneal dystrophy, scarring, edema, refractive error, cataract, glaucoma
- **Vitreous/Fundus/Optic Nerve**
  - Age-related macular degeneration (ARMD), diabetic retinopathy, retinal vascular insufficiency, compressive optic neuropathy (intracranial mass), intraocular neoplasm, retinitis pigmentosa (RP)
- **Cortical/Other**
  - Pituitary adenoma, medication-induced (sildenafil, amiodarone), nutritional deficiency, papilledema

The Red Eye

Common Differential Diagnosis of Red Eye

	Conjunctivitis	Acute Iritis	Acute Angle Closure Glaucoma	Keratitis
Discharge	Bacteria: purulent Virus: serous Allergy: mucous	No	No	Profuse tearing
Pain	No	+ + (tender globe)	+ + + (nauseating)	+ + (on blinking)
Photophobia	No	+ + +	+	+ +
Blurred Vision	No	+ +	+ + +	Varies
Pupil	Normal	Smaller	Fixed in mid-dilation	Same or smaller
Injection	Conjunctiva with limbal pallor	Ciliary flush	Diffuse	Diffuse
Cornea	Normal or opacified	Keratic precipitates	Cloudy	Infiltrate, edema, epithelial defects
Intraocular pressure	Normal	Varies	Increased markedly	Normal or increased
Anterior chamber	Normal	Cells + flare	Shallow	Cells + flare or normal
Other	Large, tender preauricular node if viral	Posterior synechiae	Coloured halos Nausea and vomiting	

Ocular Pain

- Differentiate from ocular ache: eye fatigue (asthenopia)
- Herpes zoster prodrome, trauma/foreign body, keratitis, corneal abrasion, corneal ulcer, acute angle-closure glaucoma, acute uveitis, scleritis, episcleritis, optic neuritis, ocular migraine

Floaters

- Vitreous syneresis (shrinkage and collapse of vitreous gel), posterior vitreous detachment (PVD), vitreous hemorrhage, retinal tear/detachment, posterior uveitis
- Must rule out retinal detachment

Flashes of Light (photopsia)

- Posterior vitreous detachment (PVD), retinal tear/detachment, migraine with aura

Photophobia (severe light sensitivity)

- Corneal abrasion, corneal ulcer, keratitis, acute angle-closure glaucoma, iritis, meningitis, encephalitis, migraine

Diplopia (double vision)

- Binocular diplopia: strabismus, CN palsy (III, IV, VI) secondary to ischemia, diabetes, tumour, trauma, myasthenia gravis, muscle restriction/entrapment, thyroid ophthalmopathy, internuclear ophthalmologia (INO) secondary to multiple sclerosis, brainstem infarct
- Monocular diplopia: refractive error, strands of mucus in tear film, keratoconus, cataract, dislocated lens, peripheral iridotomy

Ocular Problems in the Elderly

- Blepharitis, ptosis, entropion, ectropion, dry eyes, epiphora, presbyopia, cataracts, glaucoma, age-related macular degeneration, retinal artery/vein occlusion, temporal arteritis (arteritic ischemic optic neuropathy)

Ocular Problems in the Contact Lens Wearer

- Superficial punctate keratitis (SPK)/dry eyes, solution hypersensitivity, tight lens syndrome, corneal abrasion, giant papillary conjunctivitis, sterile corneal infiltrates (immunologic), infected ulcers (*Pseudomonas, Acanthamoeba*)

Ocular Emergencies

- ***Require urgent consultation to an ophthalmologist for management***

SIGHT THREATENING
- Lid/globe lacerations, corneal ulcer, gonococcal conjunctivitis, acute iritis, acute angle-closure glaucoma, central retinal artery occlusion (CRAO), intraocular foreign body, retinal detachment, endophthalmitis

LIFE THREATENING
- Proptosis (rule out cavernous sinus fistula or thrombosis), CN III palsy with dilated pupil (intracranial aneurysm or neoplastic lesion), papilledema (must rule out intracranial mass lesion), orbital cellulitis, giant cell (temporal) arteritis, leukocoria – white pupil (must rule out retinoblastoma)

Common Presentations

Red Eye

Differential Diagnosis
- Use an anatomical approach (from outside to in):
  - **Lids Lacrimal System**: hordeolum/chalazion, blepharitis, foreign body/laceration, dacryocystitis/dacryadenitis
  - **Conjunctiva/Sclera**: acute conjunctivitis (allergic, viral, bacterial, chlamydial), subconjunctival hemorrhage, scleritis/episcleritis, pterygium/pinguecula
  - **Cornea**: foreign body, keratitis (abrasion, ulcer, dry eye, contact lens wear, UV burn)

- **Anterior chamber**: acute angle closure glaucoma (ACG), hyphema, hypopyon
- **Iris**: acute iritis
- **Intraorbital**: endophthalmitis

History
- Unilateral or bilateral
- Has there been any injury to the eye? Hammering of metal? Recent eye surgery?
- Any history of contact lens wear?
- Have you had any associated eye pain?
- Have you had any eye discharge? Describe it (mucoid vs. watery vs. mucopurulent).
- Have you had contact with anyone else with a red eye? Recent URTI?
- Have you had any recent coughing spells, vomiting, or straining?

Associated Signs and Symptoms
- Conjunctivitis
- Keratitis: profuse tearing, pain (worse on blinking), photophobia, ± blurred vision
- Acute angle closure glaucoma (ACG): intense pain, headache, nausea and vomiting, blurred vision, coloured halos around lights, fixed mid-dilated pupil
- Iritis: pain, intense photophobia, blurred vision

Risk Factors
- Viral conjunctivitis: sick contacts
- Corneal abrasion/ulcer: contact lens wearer
- Angle closure glaucoma: hyperopia, female, elderly (age >70), FHx, Inuit or Asian, shallow anterior chamber, pupil dilation (topical and systemic anticholinergics, stress, darkness)
- Endophthalmitis: recent eye surgery

PMHx/FHx
- Always ask about previous episodes of presenting complaint (e.g. HSV keratitis)
- Coagulation abnormalities may underlie recurrent subconjunctival hemorrhage
- Connective tissue disease in scleritis
- 1st degree relative with angle closure glaucoma
- Autoimmune disease in iritis

Physical Exam
- **Visual acuity**: blurred vision in ACG and iritis, varying in keratitis
- **External inspection** (pattern of injection/redness: conjunctiva with limbal pallor in conjunctivitis, ciliary/ perilimbal flush in iritis, diffuse in ACG and keratitis)
- **Pupils**: fixed in mid-dilation in ACG, smaller in iritis and keratitis
- **Visual fields**
- **Extra-ocular movements**
- **Slit-Lamp Exam (SLE)**
    - Conjunctivitis: injection, ± subepithelial infiltrates
    - Keratitis: infiltrate (ulcer), corneal edema, epithelial defects with fluorescein staining and use of cobalt blue filter (HSV keratitis can be recognized on the basis of dendritic epithelial defect), ± cells and flare
    - ACG: injection, cloudy (edematous) cornea, shallow AC, cells and flare
    - Iritis: injection, keratic precipitates, cells and flare ± hypopyon, posterior synechia (adhesions b/w iris and lens), eye will be tender to palpation through upper eyelid
- **Intra-ocular pressure (IOP)**
    - Applanation, Tono-Pen®, palpation (eye will feel firm relative to other eye on palpation of globe through upper eyelid in ACG)
- **Fundoscopy**

MANAGEMENT (ER/outpatient)

Conjunctivitis

- *Allergic conjunctivitis*: cool compresses and antihistamines
- *Viral conjunctivitis*: very contagious for 7-10 d but usually self-limiting (2-3 wks), cool compresses, topical lubrication, arrange F/U with phthalmology as patient may develop subepithelial infiltrates requiring specific treatment
- *Bacterial conjunctivitis*: usually self-limiting but resolves quicker with treatment, topical broad-spectrum antibiotic (e.g. moxifloxacin [Vigamox®] for 2-5 d) ± systemic antibiotics, especially in children (e.g. erythromycin 50 mg/kg/d PO divided qid for 2 wks)
- Conjunctivitis occurring in the setting of GU infection: suspect chlamydial conjunctivitis and treat with topical (e.g. tetracycline ointment qid) and systemic antibiotics (e.g. erythromycin 50 mg/kg/d PO divided qid for 2 wks in children or doxycycline 100 mg PO bid for 7-21 d in adults), refer to ophthalmology
- *Hyperpurulent conjunctivitis*: suspect infection with gonococcus and refer urgently to ophthalmology for intensive systemic (e.g. penicillin G 100 U/kg/d IV divided qid for 1 wk) and topical treatment (e.g. tetracycline ointment q4h to both eyes) Note: risk of perforation

Iritis

- Consult ophthalmology urgently
- Topical mydriatics – cycloplegia (Homatropine 1% 1 gtt tid) to prevent posterior synechiae and relieve pain
- Topical steroids (prednisolone 1% [PredForte] 1 gtt q1-6h)
- Recurrent iritis warrants a full medical work up to r/o systemic disorders

Keratitis

- *Corneal abrasion*: topical antibiotic, consider patch (AVOID patching if patient has history of contact lens wear), usually resolve within 24-48 h
- *Corneal ulcer*: urgent referral to ophthalmology, culture first, topical antibiotics hourly
- *HSV keratitis*: refer to ophthalmology, topical antiviral (e.g. trifluridine 1% (Viroptic®) 1 gtt into affected eye q2h while awake; max. of 9 gtt/d, followed by 1 gtt q4h for another 7d; not to exceed 21d) ± oral antiviral (acyclovir 400 mg tab PO 5 times/d for 10 d). AVOID steroids initially as they will promote viral replication
- *HZV keratitis*: oral antiviral (e.g. acyclovir 800 mg q4h PO 5 times/d for 7 d acutely and 400 mg bid up to 12 months for recurrent disease), lubrication, erythromycin ointment if conjunctival involvement, topical antivirals not indicated, refer to ophthalmology for management of complications

MANAGEMENT (Hospital/Inpatient)

Acute Angle Closure Glaucoma

- Ocular emergency – refer to ophthalmology urgently
- Immediate treatment to 1) preserve vision 2) prevent adhesions of peripheral iris to trabecular meshwork resulting in permanent closure of angle
- Reverse pupillary block with miotic drops (e.g. pilocarpine 1-10% 1 or 2 gtt tid/qid)
- Decrease IOP with topical β-blockers (e.g. timolol 0.25-0.5% 1 gtt bid), topical adrenergics (e.g. brimonidine [Alphagan®] 1 gtt OU bid), topical miotics (dose as above), systemic carbonic anhydrase inhibitors (e.g. acetazolamide [Diamox®] 250 mg to 1 g PO/IV q24h), systemic hyperosmotic agents (e.g. mannitol 1.0-1.5 mg/kg IV – caution with history of heart disease)
- Definitive treatment with laser iridotomy. The medical therapy of acute ACG is directed toward preparing the patient for laser or surgical iridotomy
- A short admission may be needed

Endophthalmitis

- Ocular emergency – refer to ophthalmology urgently
- Emergency admission to prevent loss of eye
- Light perception or worse: immediate vitrectomy
- Hand motion or better: vitreous tap and intravitreal antibiotics (e.g. vancomycin 1 mg in 0.1 mL, ceftazidine 2.2 mg in 0.1 ml)
- Topical fortified antibiotics (e.g. vancomycin 50 mg/mL gtt, tobramycin 14 mg/ml gtt)

> **Helpful Hints**
> - Not every red eye is conjunctivitis
> - Pre-auricular and submandibular lymphadenopathy support a diagnosis of viral or chlamydial conjunctivitis
> - An abrasion appears clear while an ulcer will have an opaque base
> - In patients with abrasions, NEVER send home with anesthetic drops
> - NEVER prescribe steroids in a red eye, this should be done by an ophthalmologist

Foreign Body

Differential Diagnosis
- **Corneal Foreign Body (FB):** foreign body in or on the cornea
- **Intraorbital Foreign Body:** foreign body within the orbit but outside the globe
- **Intraocular Foreign Body:** foreign body within the globe

Etiology
- Generally accidental trauma caused by small pieces of wood, metal, plastic, or sand

History
- Timing; type of exposure (e.g. metal vs. wood); past ocular disease
- Occupational exposure to metal or wood (e.g. working with power tools), windy weather, risky recreational activities, firearms exposure

Associated Signs and Symptoms
- Symptoms: tearing, photophobia, pain, blurred vision, foreign body sensation, redness
- Signs: visible foreign body, conjunctival injection, epithelial defect that stains with fluorescein, corneal edema, anterior chamber cells/flare, rust ring (if metallic foreign body)

PMHx
- Corneal FB: abrasion, infection, scarring, rust ring, secondary iritis

Physical Exam
- Visual acuity
- External inspection: lid edema, conjunctival injection
- Pupils
- Visual fields
- Extraocular movements
- Slit-lamp exam (SLE): conjunctival and corneal edema, visible corneal FB, fluorescein staining (Note: FB behind lid may cause multiple vertical corneal abrasions due to blinking), rust ring, cells and flare
- Intraocular pressure (IOP)
- Fundoscopy

Investigations
- Whenever a FB injury is suspected on history, get x-ray/CT scan to help r/o intraorbital or intraocular FB
- If you suspect a globe rupture, protect the eye and call ophthalmology immediately

MANAGEMENT (ER and Outpatient)

Corneal Foreign Body
- SLE to rule out corneal perforation
- For more subtle perforations, use fluorescein to inspect for aqueous leakage through the wound (Seidel's sign)
- If there is no penetration, remove the object under topical anesthesia (e.g. proparacaine 0.5% 1-2 gtt)
- A direct stream of sterile irrigating solution may be sufficient to dislodge some small foreign bodies. If this is not successful, use a flexible-loop foreign body spud or 25-gauge needle to remove the object under the slit lamp

MANAGEMENT (Hospital/Inpatient)
- For both, consult ophthalmology

Ocular Trauma

BLUNT TRAUMA

Etiology
- Caused by blunt object (e.g. fist, squash ball)

History
- Injury, ocular history, drug allergy, tetanus status

Physical Exam
- Visual acuity (VA) first, pupil size and reaction, EOM (diplopia), external and slit lamp exam, fundoscopy
- If VA normal or slightly reduced, globe less likely to be perforated
- If VA reduced, may be perforated globe, corneal abrasion, lens dislocation, retinal tear
- Bone fractures
  - Blow out fracture: restricted EOM, diplopia, enophthalmos (sunken eye)
  - Ethmoid fracture: subcutaneous emphysema of lid
- Lids: swelling, laceration, emphysema
- Conjunctiva: subconjunctival hemorrhage
- Cornea: abrasions – detect with fluorescein staining and cobalt blue filter in ophthalmoscope or slit lamp
- Anterior chamber: assess depth, hyphema, hypopyon
- Iris: prolapse, iritis
- Lens: cataract, dislocation
- Retinal tear/detachment

PENETRATING TRAUMA

Etiology
- Includes ruptured globe ± prolapsed iris, intraocular foreign body

Investigations
- CT of orbit (rule out intraocular foreign body, especially if history of "metal striking metal")

Initial Management: Refer Immediately!!
- ABCs, **do not press on eyeball**, do not check IOP if possibility of globe rupture, check vision, diplopia, apply rigid eye shield to minimize further trauma, keep head elevated 30-45° to keep IOP down, keep NPO, tetanus status, give IV antibiotics

HYPHEMA
- Blood in anterior chamber often due to damage to root of the iris
- May occur with blunt trauma

Treatment
- Refer to ophthalmology
- Shield and bedrest x 5 d or as determined by ophthalmologist
- Sleep with head upright
- May need surgical drainage if hyphema persists or if re-bleed occurs

Complications
- Risk of re-bleed highest on days 2-5, can result in secondary glaucoma, corneal staining, and iris necrosis
- Never prescribe aspirin as it will increase the risk of a re-bleed

BLOW-OUT FRACTURE (see Plastic Surgery)

Definition and Etiology
- Blunt trauma causing fracture of orbital floor and herniation of orbital contents into maxillary sinus
- Orbital rim remains intact
- Inferior rectus and/or inferior oblique muscles may be incarcerated at fracture site
- Infraorbital nerve courses along the floor of the orbit and may be damaged

Clinical Features
- Classic signs of "Blow-Out"
    - Enopthalmos, decreased upgaze (inferior rectus trapped), cheek anesthetized (infraorbital nerve trapped)
- Pain and nausea at time of injury
- Diplopia, restriction of EOM
- Infraorbital and upper lip paresthesia (CN V2)
- Periorbital ecchymoses

Investigations
- Plain films: Waters' view and lateral
- CT: anteroposterior and coronal view of orbits

Treatment
- Refrain from coughing or blowing nose
- Systemic antibiotics may be indicated
- Surgery if fracture >50% orbital floor, diplopia not improving, or enophthalmos >2 mm
- May delay surgery if the diplopia improves

Chemical Burns

Treatment
- Irrigate at site of accident immediately, with water or buffered solution
    - Flush eye for at least 20-30 min with eyelids retracted in emergency department using sterile solution
    - Swab upper and lower fornices to remove possible particulate matter
- Do not attempt to neutralize because the heat produced by the reaction will damage the cornea
- Cycloplegic drops to decrease iris spasm (pain) and prevent secondary glaucoma (due to posterior synechiae formation)
- Topical antibiotics and patching
- Topical steroids (not in primary care) to decrease inflammation, use for less than two wks (in the case of a persistent epithelial defect)

Prognosis
- Alkali burns have a worse prognosis vs. acid burns because acids coagulate tissue and inhibit further corneal penetration
- Poor prognosis if cornea is opaque, likely irreversible stromal damage
- Even with a clear cornea initially, alkali burns can progress for weeks

Common Conditions

Pupils

Approach to Anisocoria

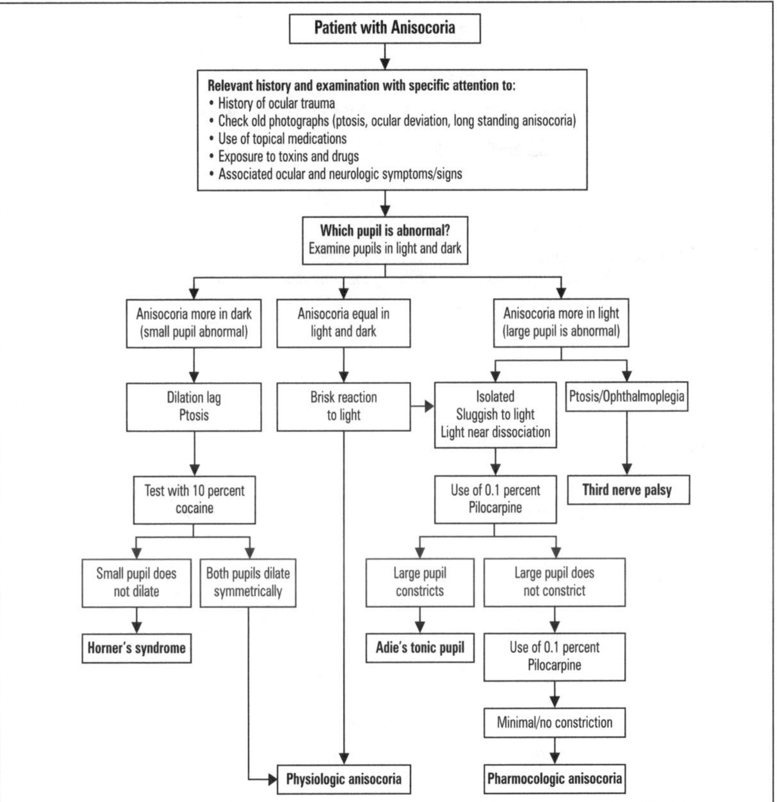

Reproduced with permission from: Kedar S, Biousse V, Newman NJ. Approach to the patient with anisocoria. In: UpToDate, Rose, BD (ed), UpToDate, Waltham, MA, 2011. Copyright 2011 UpToDate, Inc. For more information visit www.uptodate.com.

The Orbit

PRESEPTAL CELLULITIS
- Infection of soft tissue anterior to orbital septum

Etiology
- Usually follows periorbital trauma or dermal infection

Treatment
- Warm compresses
- Systemic antibiotics such as Amox-Clav (suspect *H. influenzae* in children; S. aureus or Streptococcus in adults)
- If severe or child <1 yr treat as orbital cellulitis

ORBITAL CELLULITIS
- OCULAR and MEDICAL EMERGENCY
- Inflammation of orbital contents posterior to orbital septum
- Common in children, but also in the elderly and immunocompromised

Etiology
- Usually secondary to sinus/facial/tooth infections or trauma

Treatment
- Admit, blood cultures x 2, orbital CT, IV antibiotics, commonly ceftriaxone + vancomycin or equivalent for 1 wk
- Surgical drainage of abscess and follow closely

Complications
- Optic nerve inflammation, cavernous sinus thrombosis, meningitis, brain abscess with possible loss of vision, death

Differentiating between Preseptal and Orbital Cellulitis

Finding	Preseptal Cellulitis	Orbital Cellulitis
Fever	May be present	Present
Lid edema	Moderate to severe	Severe
Chemosis	Absent or mild	Marked
Proptosis	Absent	Present
Pain on eye movement	Absent	Present
Ocular mobility	Normal	Decreased
Vision	Normal	Diminished ± diplopia
RAPD	Absent	May be seen
Leukocytosis	Moderate	Marked
ESR	Normal or elevated	Elevated
Additional findings	Skin infection	Sinusitis, dental abscess

Conjunctiva

CONJUNCTIVITIS

Etiology
- Infectious: bacterial, viral, chlamydial, fungal, parasitic
- Non-infectious:
  - Allergic: atopic, seasonal, giant papillary conjunctivitis (in contact lens wearers)
  - Toxic: irritants, dust, smoke, irradiation
  - Secondary to another disorder such as dacryocystitis, dacryoadenitis, cellulitis, Kawasaki's disease

Clinical Features
- Red eye, conjunctival injection often with limbal pallor, itching, foreign body sensation, chemosis (conjunctival edema), tearing, discharge, crusting of lashes in the morning, lid edema, preauricular node, subepithelial infiltrates
- Follicles: pale lymphoid elevations of the conjunctiva
- Papillae: fibrovascular elevations of the conjunctiva with central network of finely branching vessels (cobblestone appearance)

Treatment
- Varies depending on etiology
- Bacterial and chlamydial generally require topical antibiotics ± systemic antibiotics

Cornea

CORNEAL ABRASION

Definition
- Epithelial defect usually due to trauma (e.g. fingernails, paper, twigs, contact lens)

Clinical Features
- Pain, redness, tearing, photophobia, foreign body sensation
- De-epithelialized area stains with fluorescein dye
- Pain relieved with topical anesthetic

Complications
- Infection, ulceration, recurrent erosion, secondary iritis

Treatment
- Topical antibiotic (drops or ointment)
- Consider topical NSAID, cycloplegic (relieves pain and photophobia by paralyzing ciliary muscle), tight patch
- Pressure patch alone is not effective
  - NEVER patch abrasion if patient wears contact lenses (prone to *Pseudomonas* infection)
- Most abrasions clear spontaneously within 24-48 h

CORNEAL ULCER

Etiology
- Local necrosis of corneal tissue due to infection, usually bacterial in origin
- Secondary to corneal exposure, abrasion, foreign body, contact lens use (50% of ulcers)
- Also associated with conjunctivitis, blepharitis, keratitis, vitamin A deficiency

OPHTHALMOLOGY

Clinical Features
- Pain, photophobia, tearing, foreign body sensation, decreased visual acuity (if central ulcer)
- Corneal opacity that necroses and forms an excavated ulcer with infiltrative base
- Overlying corneal epithelial defect that stains with fluorescein
- May develop corneal edema, conjunctival injection, anterior chamber cell/flare, hypopyon, corneal hypoesthesia (in viral keratitis)
- Bacterial ulcers may have purulent discharge, viral ulcers may have watery discharge

Complications
- Decreased vision, corneal perforation, iritis, endophthalmitis

Treatment
- Urgent referral to ophthalmology
- Culture before antibiotics
- Topical antibiotics every hour
- Must treat vigorously to avoid complications

Corneal Abrasion vs. Corneal Ulcer

	Abrasion	Ulcer
Time course	Acute (instantaneous)	Subacute (days)
History of trauma	Yes	Not usually
Cornea	Clear	White, necrotic area
Iris detail	Clear	Obscured
Corneal thickness	Normal	May have crater defect/thinning
Extent of lesion	Limited to epithelium	Extension into stroma

Retina

RETINAL DETACHMENT (RD)

Etiology
- Cleavage in the plane between the neurosensory retina and the retinal pigment epithelium (RPE)

Classification
- Rhegmatogenous
    - Most common type of RD
    - Caused by a tear or hole in the neurosensory retina, allowing fluid from the vitreous to pass into the subretinal space
    - Tears may be caused by posterior vitreous detachment (PVD), degenerative retinal changes, trauma, or iatrogenically
    - Incidence increases with advancing age, and more likely to occur spontaneously in high myopes, or after ocular surgery/trauma
- Tractional
    - Caused by traction (due to vitreal, epiretinal or subretinal membrane) pulling the neurosensory retina away from the underlying RPE
    - Found in conditions such as diabetic retinopathy, CRVO, sickle cell disease, retinopathy of prematurity (ROP), and ocular trauma
- Exudative
    - Caused by damage to the RPE resulting in fluid accumulation in the subretinal space
    - Main causes are intraocular tumours, posterior uveitis, central serous retinopathy

> Superotemporal retina is the most common site for horseshoe tears

History
- Sudden onset
- Flashes of light (mechanical stimulation of retinal photoreceptors)
- Many floaters (hazy spots in the line of vision which move with eye position due to blood in vitreous)
- Curtain of darkness/peripheral field loss (retinal detachment)
- Loss of central vision (if macula becomes detached)

Physical Exam
- Decreased IOP (usually 4-5 mmHg lower than the other, normal eye)
- ± relative afferent pupillary defect (RAPD)
- Fundoscopy: detached retina is grey with surface blood vessels, loss of red reflex

Treatment
- Prophylactic (flashes or floaters): laser cryotherapy to prevent progression to detachment
- Therapeutic: depends on type, includes scleral buckle, pneumatic retinopexy, vitrectomy, and/or treatment of underlying cause
- Refer to ophthalmology

Complications
- Loss of vision, vitreous hemorrhage, recurrent retinal detachment
- A retinal detachment should be considered an emergency, especially if the macula is still attached
- Prognosis for visual recovery varies inversely with the amount of time the retina is detached and whether the macula is attached or not

CENTRAL RETINAL ARTERY OCCLUSION (CRAO)

Etiology
- Emboli (carotid arteries or heart), thrombus, temporal/giant cell arteritis

History
- Sudden, PAINLESS (except temporal arteritis), severe monocular loss of vision
- Previous history of amaurosis fugax (transient episodes in the past)

Physical Exam
- RAPD
- Fundoscopy: "cherry-red spot", retinal pallor, narrowed arterioles/boxcarring, cotton-wool spots (retinal infarcts), Hollenhorst plaques (cholesterol emboli)

Treatment
- OCULAR EMERGENCY: attempt to restore blood flow within 2 h
- Massage globe, decrease IOP (topical β-blockers, inhaled oxygen-carbon dioxide mixture, IV acetazolamide, IV mannitol), drain aqueous fluid
- Treat underlying cause to prevent CRAO in the other eye
- Follow-up 1 month to rule out neovascularization

BRANCH RETINAL ARTERY OCCLUSION (BRAO)

Etiology
- Only part of the retina becomes ischemic resulting in visual field loss
- More likely to be of embolic etiology than CRAO; need to search for source

Treatment
- Ocular massage to dislodge embolus if visual acuity is affected

CENTRAL/BRANCH RETINAL VEIN OCCLUSION (CRVO/BRVO)

Etiology
- Thrombus within lumen of blood vessel
- Usually a manifestation of systemic disease (HTN, DM)
- Predisposing factors: arteriosclerotic vascular disease, HTN, DM, glaucoma, hyperviscosity, drugs (OCP, diuretics)

Classification
- Venous stasis/non-ischemic retinopathy: no RAPD, VA 20/80, mild hemorrhage, few cotton wool spots; spontaneous resolution (weeks to months), may regain normal vision
- Hemorrhagic/ischemic retinopathy (usually older patient with deficient arterial supply): RAPD, VA 20/200, reduced peripheral vision, more hemorrhages, cotton wool spots, congestion; poor visual prognosis

History
- Painless, monocular, gradual or sudden visual loss

Physical Exam
- $\pm$ RAPD
- Fundoscopy: "blood and thunder" appearance, diffuse retinal hemorrhages, cotton-wool spots, venous engorgement, swollen optic disc, macular edema

Complications
- Degeneration of RPE, neovascularisation, vitreous hemorrhage, macular edema

Treatment
- No treatment available to restore vision in CRVO
- Identify underlying cause/contributing factors
- Retinal laser photocoagulation, intravitreal corticosteroid or anti-VEGF injection to reduce neovascularization and prevent neovascular glaucoma

---

Shaken Baby Syndrome
Syndrome of findings characterized by no external signs of abuse and respiratory arrest, seizures, and coma. Ocular exam findings are important diagnostically for Shaken Baby Syndrome. These findings include extensive retinal and vitreous hemorrhages that occur during the shaking process and are extremely rare in accidental trauma. A detailed fundoscopic exam or an ophthalmology referral should be conducted for all infants in whom abuse is suspected.

Ocular Manifestations of Systemic Disease

Diabetes

DIABETIC RETINOPATHY (DR)
- Most common cause of blindness in young people in North America

Etiology
- Altered vascular permeability (loss of pericytes, breakdown of blood-retinal barrier, thickening of basement membrane)
- Predisposition to retinal vessel obstruction

Classification
- Non-proliferative: increased vascular permeability and retinal ischemia
  - Dot and blot hemorrhages, microaneurysms, hard exudates (lipid deposits), macular edema
- Advanced non-proliferative (or pre-proliferative): non-proliferative findings PLUS
  - Venous beading (in $\geq$2 of 4 retinal quadrants), intraretinal microvascular anomalies (IRMA – dilated leaky vessels within the retina) in $\geq$1 of 4 retinal quadrants, cotton wool spots (nerve fibre layer infarcts)
- Proliferative
  - 5% of patients with diabetes will reach this stage
  - Neovascularization: iris, disc, retina
  - Neovascularization of iris (rubeosis iridis) can lead to neovascular glaucoma
  - Vitreous hemorrhage from bleeding fragile new vessels, fibrous tissue can contract causing tractional retinal detachment
  - Increased risk of severe visual loss

Screening Guidelines for Diabetic Retinopathy
- Type 1 DM
  - Screen for retinopathy beginning annually 5 yrs after diagnosis
  - Screening not indicated before the onset of puberty
- Type 2 DM
  - Initial examination shortly after diagnosis, then repeat annually
  - Ocular exam in 1st trimester, close follow-up throughout as pregnancy can exacerbate DR
  - Gestational diabetics not at risk for retinopathy

Treatment
- Tight control of blood sugar decreases frequency and severity of microvascular complications
- Blood pressure control
- Focal laser for clinically significant macular edema
- Panretinal laser photocoagulation, for proliferative diabetic retinopathy
- Vitrectomy for vitreous hemorrhage and retinal detachment in proliferative diabetic retinopathy which is complicated by non-clearing vitreous hemorrhage or retinal detachment

LENS CHANGES IN DIABETES
- Earlier onset of senile nuclear sclerosis and cortical cataract
- May get hyperglycemic cataract due to sorbitol accumulation (rare)
- Sudden changes in refraction of lens: changes in blood glucose levels (poor control) may cause refractive changes of 3-4 diopters

EXTRA OCULAR MUSCLE PALSY IN DIABETES
- Usually CN III infarct
- Pupil usually spared in diabetic CN III palsy, but get ptosis
- May involve CN IV and VI
- Usually recover within few months

OPTIC NEUROPATHY
- Visual acuity loss due to infarction of optic disc/nerve

Hypertension

- Retinopathy is the most common ocular manifestation of hypertension
- Key features of **chronic** HTN retinopathy: AV nicking, blot retinal hemorrhages, microaneurysms, cotton-wool spots
- Key features of **acute** HTN retinopathy: retinal arteriolar spasm, superficial retinal hemorrhage, cotton wool spots, optic disc edema

Keith-Wagener-Barker Classification

Group 1	Mild narrowing of the arterioles
Group 2	Moderate to marked narrowing of the arterioles and focal irregularities (e.g. AV nicking)
Group 3	Group 2 plus:
	Cotton-wool spots
	Hemorrhages and/or exudates
Group 4	Group 3 plus papilledema

TIA/Amaurosis Fugax

- Sudden, transient blindness from intermittent vascular compromise; ipsilateral carotid most frequent embolic source
- Usually monocular, lasting <5-10 min
- Hollenhorst plaques (glistening microemboli seen at branch points of retinal arterioles)

Giant Cell/Temporal Arteritis (GCA)

Clinical Features
- Common in women >60 yrs
- Abrupt monocular loss of vision, pain over temporal artery, jaw claudication, scalp tenderness, constitutional symptoms
- Ischemic optic atrophy – 50% lose vision in other eye if untreated
- Associated with polymyalgia rheumatica

Diagnosis
- Temporal arterial biopsy + increased ESR, if biopsy on one side is negative, biopsy other side

Treatment
- High dose corticosteroid to relieve pain and prevent further ischemic episodes
- If diagnosis of GCA is suspected clinically: start treatment + perform temporal artery biopsy to confirm diagnosis (**DO NOT WAIT TO START TREATMENT**)

HIV/AIDS

- Up to 75% of patients with AIDS have ocular manifestations
- HIV retinopathy (most common)
  - Cotton wool spots, intraretinal hemorrhage
- Other retinal complications include: CMV retinitis, necrotizing retinitis, disseminated choroiditis
- External ocular signs: Kaposi's sarcoma, multiple molluscum contagiosum, herpes simplex keratitis, herpes zoster

Multiple Sclerosis

Clinical Features
- Optic neuritis: blurred vision, decreased colour vision
- Central scotoma, diplopia, RAPD, ptosis, nystagmus, uveitis, optic atrophy
- Internuclear ophthalmoplegia: MLF affected, causes impaired adduction on ipsilateral side with contralateral lateral gaze
- White matter demyelinating lesions of optic nerve on MRI

Treatment
- IV steroids for optic neuritis
  - NOT oral steroids (increased likelihood of developing MS later)

Graves' Disease

Clinical Features (Progression of signs and symptoms: "**NO SPECS**")
- **N**o signs/sx → **O**nly signs (lid retraction, lid lag, impaired convergence) → **S**oft tissue swelling (periorbital edema) → **P**roptosis → **E**xtraocular muscle weakness (diplopia)/decreased movements → **C**orneal exposure → **S**ight loss
- Graves ophthalmopathy can precede/occur concurrently/follow presentation of hyperthyroidism

Treatment
- Treat hyperthyroidism (β-blocker, PTU, methimazole)
- Monitor for corneal exposure and maintain corneal hydration
- Manage diplopia, proptosis and compressive optic neuropathy with:
  - Steroids (acute phase), orbital bony decompression, external beam radiation
- Consider strabismus and/or eyelid surgical procedures once acute phase subsides

Topical Ocular Diagnostic Drugs

FLUORESCEIN DYE
- Water soluble orange-yellow dye
- Green under cobalt blue light – ophthalmoscope or slit lamp
- Absorbed in areas of epithelial loss (ulcer or abrasion)
- Also stains mucus and contact lenses

Rose Bengal Stain
- Stain devitalized epithelial cells and mucus

ANESTHETICS
- e.g. proparacaine HCl 0.5%, tetracaine 0.5%
- Indications: removal of foreign body and sutures, tonometry, examination of painful cornea
- Toxic to corneal epithelium (inhibit mitosis and migration) and can lead to corneal ulceration and scarring with prolonged use, therefore **NEVER** prescribe

MYDRIATICS
- Dilate pupils
- **Cholinergic blocking**: dilation plus cycloplegia (loss of accommodation) by paralysis of iris sphincter and the ciliary body, e.g. tropicamide (Mydriacyl®)
  - Indications: refraction, fundoscopy, therapy for iritis
- **Adrenergic stimulating**: stimulate pupillary dilator muscles, no effect on accommodation, e.g. phenylephrine HCl 2.5% (duration: 30-40 min)
  - Usually used with tropicamide for additive effects
  - Side effects: hypertension, tachycardia, arrhythmias

Mydriatic Cycloplegic Drugs and Duration of Action

Drugs	Duration of action
Tropicamide (Mydriacyl®) 0.5%, 1%	4-5 h
Cyclopentolate HCL 0.5%, 1%	3-6 h
Homatropine HBr 1%, 2%	3-7 d
Atropine sulfate 0.5%, 1%	1-2 wks
Scopolamine HBr 0.25%, 5%	1-2 wks

Drugs With Ocular Toxicity

Amiodarone	Corneal microdeposits and superficial keratopathy (vortex keratopathy) Rare: ischemic optic neuropathy
Atropine, benztropine	Pupillary dilation (risk of angle closure glaucoma)
Bisphosphonates (Fosamax®, Actonel®)	Inflammatory eye disease (iritis, scleritis, episcleritis)
Chloroquine, hydroxychloroquine	Bull's eye maculopathy Vortex keratopathy
Chlorpromazine	Anterior subcapsular cataract
Contraceptive pills	Decreased tolerance to contact lenses Migraine Optic neuritis Central vein occlusion
Digitalis	Yellow vision Blurred vision
Ethambutol	Optic neuropathy
Haloperidol (Haldol®)	Oculogyric crises Blurred vision
Indomethacin	Superficial keratopathy
Isoniazid	Optic neuropathy
Nalidixic acid	Papilledema
Steroids	Posterior subcapsular cataracts Glaucoma Papilledema (systemic steroids) Increased severity of HSV infections (geographic ulcers) Predisposition to fungal infections
Tamsulosin (Flomax®)	Intraoperative Floppy Iris Syndrome (IFIS), which can complicate cataract surgery
Tetracycline	Papilledema (associated with pseudotumour cerebri)
Thioridazine	Pigmentary degeneration of retina
Vigabatrin	Retinal deposition with macular sparing, peripheral visual field loss
Vitamin A intoxication	Papilledema
Vitamin D intoxication	Band keratopathy

Orthopedics

Essential Anatomy, History, Physical Exam and Investigations

Anatomy

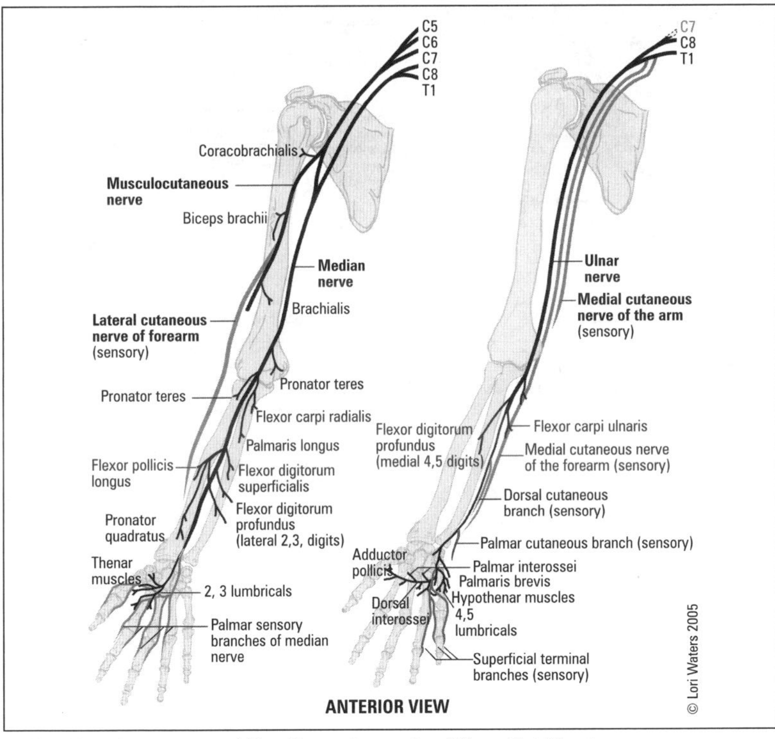

Median, Musculocutaneous and Ulnar Nerves: Innervation of Upper Limb Muscles

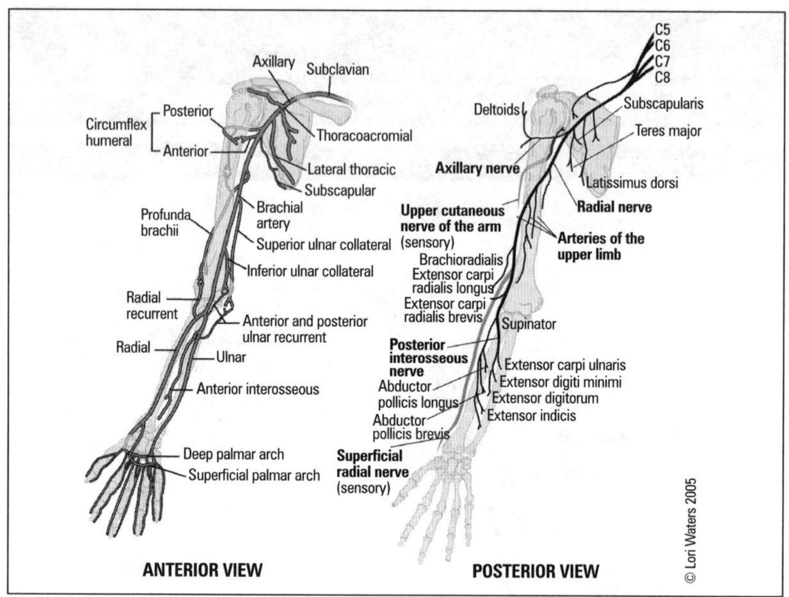

(Left) Blood Supply to the Upper Limb
(Right) Axillary and Radial Nerves: Innervation of Upper Limb

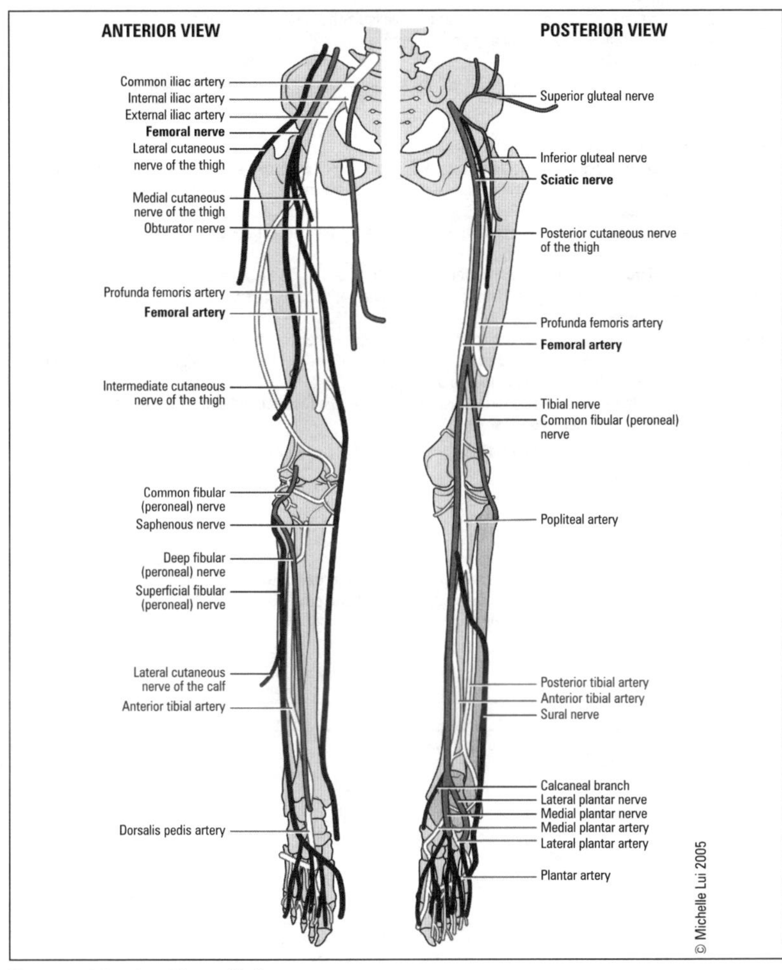

Nerves and Arteries of Lower Limbs

History

Key Points
- Pain characteristics: acute vs. chronic, intermittent vs. constant, ask patient to localize the pain
- Ability to weight bear/severe antalgic gait
- Trauma, mechanism of injury
- Potential for head injury
- Pain in other joints, abnormal gait, anesthesia/paresthesia

- Corticosteroid use, excessive EtOH, back or neck sx, vascular disease
- Osteoporosis and osteoporosis RFs (see <u>Endocrinology</u>)
- Last meal (if preparing for OR)
- In the elderly with suspected hip #: decreased vision/balance/sensation, environmental hazards, use of long-acting benzodiazepines

The Basic Orthopedic Consult Note
1. **ID** – Age, occupation, residence (including specifics regarding type of residence, accessibility and assistance at home), handedness or baseline ambulation (depending on the injury – upper extremity versus lower extremity, respectively)
2. **HPI** – As per usual requirements but ensure one asks specifically about mechanism, pain and potential head injury
3. **Past Medical History** – As per usual requirements, with emphasis on those medical conditions, past surgeries, medications and allergies that may be contraindications to surgery
4. **Social/Family History**
5. **Physical Exam** – As per usual requirements but ensure assessment of neurovascular status is done; moreover, rule out any other injury and assess joints above and below the site of injury. Ensure subsection that includes results of any investigations, including imaging
6. **Impression and Plan** – As per usual requirements, with specific recommendations for admission, surgical interventions and future disposition

Physical Exam

General Approach: "Look, Feel, Move"
- Vitals: BP, HR, RR, oxygen saturation, ABCs
- Inspection: deformity, hematoma/bruising, asymmetry
  - For lower extremity: weight bearing ability/antalgic gait, shortened, externally rotated leg
- Palpation: tenderness along bone or joint line, edema, peripheral pulses
- ROM: passive and active, limitations/pain with movement
- Special tests

NEUROVASCULAR

Upper Extremity

1. Sensation	Medial aspect of 5th digit – Ulnar Nerve Lateral aspect of 2nd digit – Median Nerve Dorsal aspect of thumb and snuff box – Radial Nerve (PIN)
2. Motor	"Spread Fingers" – Ulnar Nerve "Thumbs Up" – Radial Nerve (PIN) "OK Sign" – Median Nerve (AIN)
3. Vascular	Radial/Ulnar pulses, Capillary refill

Lower Extremity

1. Sensation	Medial aspect of calf/foot – Saphenous Nerve (branch of Femoral) Lateral aspect of calf – Lat. Cut. Nerve of Calf (br. of Sciatic) Lateral aspect of foot (dorsum) – Sural Nerve (br. of Sciatic) Middle aspect of foot (dorsum) – Superficial Per. Nerve (Sciatic) 1st webspace (dorsum) – Deep Peroneal Nerve (br. of Sciatic) Plantar surface of foot – Tibial Nerve branches
2. Motor	Dorsiflex/Eversion – Deep Peroneal Nerve (br. of Sciatic) Plantar Flex/Inversion – Tibial Nerve (br. of Sciatic)
3. Vascular	Dorsalis Pedis/Tibialis Posterior Pulses, Capillary refill

Note: Neurovascular exam should be done pre and post reduction

Investigations

IMAGING
- X-ray: be sure to image the joints above and below
- Others: CT, MRI, Dopplers, etc.

PRE-OPERATIVE
- Bloodwork: CBC, electrolytes, Cr, BUN, INR, PTT, cross and type 2 units
- ECG

Common Presentations

Orthopedic Emergencies ("VON CHOP")

Beware of Orthopedic Emergencies
VON CHOP
Vascular compromise
Open fracture
Neurological compromise or cauda equina syndrome
Compartment syndrome
Hip dislocation
Osteomyelitis/septic arthritis
Unstable **P**elvic fracture

KEY POINTS
- Pelvis fracture: possible spine #, obtain AP inlet and outlet films, Judet if acetabular # suspected, assess GU injury (more common in males; examine for blood at penile meatus, scrotal/perineal hematoma or high-riding prostate)
- Open fracture: prep for OR for operative debridement with repeat I&D likely; IV Abx
- Septic joint and osteomyelitis: see <u>Infectious Diseases</u>
- **Compartment syndrome**
  - Long bone fractures account for the vast majority of cases (tibia #, supracondylar # in children)
  - Most common site affected is lower (lower) limb, followed by forearm
  - Pain with active contraction or passive stretch of compartment (5 P's are a late sign)
  - If clinical exam unreliable, measure compartment pressure with intra-compartment catheter
  - Compartment syndrome progresses rapidly, serial clinical exams are essential
  - If compartment syndrome suspected, remove constrictive dressings (splints, casts) and elevate limb
    - Prep patient for OR – urgent fasciotomy required

Compartment Syndrome: The 5 P's

- **Pain**
  - Out of proportion for injury
  - Not relieved by analgesics
  - Increased with passive stretch of compartment muscles (most specific)
- **Pallor**: late finding
- **Paresthesia**
- **Paralysis**: late finding
- **Pulselessness**: late finding

Fascial Compartments of the Lower Limb

Compartment	Major Muscles and Function	Neurovascular Structures
Anterior*	Tibialis Anterior – dorsiflexes ankle, inverts foot Extensor Hallucis Longus – extends big toe Extensor Digitorum Longus – extends 2nd-5th digits	Deep Peroneal Nerve Anterior Tibial Artery (becomes Dorsalis Pedis)
Lateral	Peroneus Longus – everts foot Peroneus Brevis – everts foot	Superficical Peroneal Nerve (loss of function results in foot drop
Superficial Posterior	Gastrocnemius - plantarflexes ankle, raises heel Soleus – plantarflexes ankle	Tibial Nerve Posterior Tibial Artery
Deep Posterior	Tibialis Posterior – platar flexes ankle, inverts foot Flexor Hallucis Longus – flexes big toe Flexor digitorum longus – flexes 2nd-5th digits Popliteus – unlocks fully extended knee	

*Anterior compartment most susceptible, all four compartments should be decompressed in urgent fasciotomy

Joint Pain

Differential Diagnosis
- Extrinsic: neurologic (nerve root compression, herpes zoster, etc.), generalized (fibromyalgia, PMR, sickle cell [ischemic], dermato/polymyositis), referred pain, pain originating from surrounding organs
- Intrinsic: articular arthritis (degenerative, rheumatoid, crystal-induced, septic, avascular necrosis), neoplastic, traumatic (fracture, soft tissue damage, neuropathic arthropathy), non-articular
- Bursa, tendons, ligaments, muscle (bursitis, tendonitis, myositis)

Fractures

BASIC APPROACH

Description
- Integrity of skin: open vs. closed
- Location: epiphysis, diaphysis, metaphysic, physis
- Orientation: comminuted, transverse, oblique, butterfly, segmental, spiral, intra-articular, torus, greenstick, pathologic (definitive classification requires additional testing)
- Displacement: nondisplaced, displaced, distracted, angulated (varus vs. valgus), translated

Management
- ABCs, **AMPLE** history (**A**llergies, **M**eds, **P**ast med Hx, **L**ast meal, **E**vents around #), baseline function, occupation, mechanism of #, neurovascular status, analgesia, imaging, obtain reduction (repeat imaging and neurovascular exam), maintain reduction, rehab

Complications
- Compartment syndrome, neurovascular injury, AVN, infection, mal/nonunion, heterotopic ossification, post-traumatic arthritis, sepsis, DVT/PE, ARDS, hemorrhagic shock

Gustilo and Anderson Classification of Open Fractures

Type	Description	Antibiotics
I	Clean wound <1 cm, minimal soft tissue injury	Cefazolin (Ancef®) 1 g IV q8h x 3 d
II	Wound >1 cm, moderate contamination, moderate soft tissue injury	Cefazolin (Ancef®) 1 g IV q8h x 3 d
III	Wound >10 cm, high contamination	Cefazolin plus gentamycin 1.5 mg/kg q8h x 5 d Add penicillin 4 million units q6h for clostridium prophylaxis if farm/lake/stream contamination

DESCRIPTION OF FRACTURE
- **Who?** – Age and Sex
- **How?** – Mechanism of Injury (low/high energy)
- **When?** – Time of Injury
- **Where?**
  - Which bone?
  - Segment? (proximal, middle, distal)
    - Proximal/distal – epiphysis/metaphysis
    - Middle – diaphysis
- **What is the Pattern?**
  - Diaphysis: simple, wedge, complex, spiral, oblique (>30 degrees), tranverse (<30 degrees)
  - Epiphysis/metaphysic: extra-articular, partial articular, complete articular, involvement of the growth plate (Salter-Harris classification)
- **Is there Displacement?** – Describe distal fragment relative to proximal fragment
  - Three possible translations:
    - Anterior or posterior (use sagittal plane)
    - Medial or lateral (use coronal plane)
    - Superior or inferior
  - Three possible angulations/rotations
    - Apex anterior or posterior (sagittal plane angulation)
    - Apex medial or lateral (coronal plane angulation)
    - Internal or external rotation (axial or transverse plane rotation)
- **Is there Injury to Soft Tissue?**
  - Closed (skin intact)
  - Open (open wound communicates with fracture)
  - Compartment syndrome
- **What is the Neurovascular Status?**
  - Circulation (pulses/cap refill)
  - Neurological status; motor and sensory

EVALUATION AND MANAGEMENT

CLOSED FRACTURES

ABCs, Primary Survey and Secondary Survey, AMPLE History

Analgesia

Imaging
- X-ray rule of 2's: 2 sides (bilateral), 2 views (AP + lateral), 2 joints (above + below), 2 times (before + after reduction)

Obtain the Reduction
- Closed reduction – reverse mechanism that produced the fracture
- Open reduction – indications for open reduction: "NO CAST"

Indications for Open Reduction
NO CAST:
Non-union
Open fracture
Neurovascular **C**ompromise
Intra-**A**rticular fracture
Salter-Harris 3, 4, 5
Poly**T**rauma

Maintain the Reduction
- External stabilization – splints, casts, traction, external fixator
- Internal stabilization – percutaneous pinning, extramedullary (screws, plates, wires), intramedullary (rods)

Post-Reduction Imaging

Rehabilitate
- To regain functioning and avoid joint stiffness

OPEN FRACTURE
(fractured bone in communication with the external environment)
- In addition to above:
  - Remove debris and irrigate the wound
  - Cover wound with sterile dressing and splint fracture
  - Tetanus status
  - IV antibiotics
    - 1st generation cephalosporin (cefazolin), consider gram negative coverage (gentamicin)
  - NPO and prepare for OR (bloodwork, consent, ECG)

Common Conditions

Upper Extremity

ANTERIOR SHOULDER DISLOCATION
- >90% shoulder dislocations
- Symptoms: pain, arm in abduction and external rotation, loss of internal rotation, squared shoulder; signs: +apprehension, relocation tests, sulcus sign

> **Radiographic findings:**
> Trans-scapular view: humeral head ant. to Mercedes-Benz sign
> Axillary view: bony Bankart lesion (anteroinferior glenoid rim)
> AP view: Hill-Sachs lesion (posterolateral humeral head #)

- Management: 1) radiography (AP, trans-scapular, axillary views); 2) closed reduction with IV sedation and muscle relaxation
- Reduction methods:
  - Traction-counter traction
  - Stimson (prone, arm hanging with weight at wrist)
- Immobilization: shoulder sling x3 wks
- Remember to check axillary nerve function post-reduction

ROTATOR CUFF INJURY
- Pathology: impingement, tendonitis/bursitis, micro and macro tears (partial/full tears)
- Symptoms: pain sleeping on affected side, on palpation, and trouble with overhand activities; signs: ±Jobe's, lift-off, Neer's, Hawkin's, painful arc
  - Ruling IN rotator cuff tear: supraspinatus weakness + weakness in ER + positive impingement sign(s) = 98% probability
- Management: mild-moderate – NSAIDs, PT, steroid injections; severe – may require arthroscopic/surgical repair
- Surgical anatomy:
  - Anterior approach: deltopectoral line → deltoid, pectoralis major, cephalic vein → biceps short head, coracobrachialis, coracoid process → subscapularis → joint capsule
  - Watch for musculocutaneous nerve and cephalic vein

Shoulder injection sites	Description
Glenohumeral Joint	Inject glenohumeral joint from posterior aspect, approx. 2cm inferior and 1cm medial of posteriolateral acromion
Acromioclavicular Joint	Palpate AC joint; inject at 45° to skin (lat to med).
Subacromial Space	Palpate acromial arch; inject under arch from anterior to posterior

CLAVICLE FRACTURE
- FOOSH
- middle third >> distal third > proximal third
- Presentation: pain, tenting of skin, arm clasped to chest to prevent movement
- Management: mandatory neurovascular exam of affected arm
  - Proximal and mid third #: figure-of-eight sling 1-2 wks, early ROM, consider ORIF if ends overlap (i.e. longitudinally) >2 cm
  - Distal third: undisplaced, sling 1-2 wks; displaced (CC ligament injury), ORIF

PROXIMAL HUMERUS
- Mechanism: high energy trauma in the young, FOOSH in older pts
- Imaging: AP, trans-scap, axillary, CT if complex
- Neer classification (2-,3-,4-part fracture combination of: 1) anatomical neck, 2) surgical neck, 3) greater tuberosity, 4) lesser tuberosity)
- Management:
  - Nondisplaced – sling immobilization, ROM in 7-10 d
  - Minimal displacement – closed reduction with sling immobilization x 2 wks
  - Displaced/dislocated – ORIF
- Key complications: AVN, axillary nerve injury, malunion, PT arthritis

HUMERAL SHAFT
- Mechanism: FOOSH, direct trauma, twisting (elderly)
- Presentation: pain, swelling ± shortening
- TEST RADIAL NERVE FUNCTION BEFORE AND AFTER TREATMENT – look for drop wrist, sensory impairment dorsum of hand
- Imaging: AP and lateral full views of humerus
- Management: usually conservative (reduction, hanging cast with collar and cuff sling until swelling subsides, sling 7-10 d, brace). ORIF if open #, NV injury, poly trauma, floating elbow, etc.
- Options include: compression plate, intramedullary rod, external fixation
- Key complications: radial nerve injury (most resolve within 3 months), brachial artery injury

SUPRACONDYLAR
- Most commonly found in paediatric age group
- Mechanism: FOOSH – transverse # distal 1/3 of humerus
- Presentation: pain, swelling, point tenderness, NV injury (especially AIN in extension type)
- Imaging: AP and lateral x-rays of elbow
  - Lateral view: posterior fat pad sign
- Management: Undisplaced – cast in flexion x 3 wks. Displaced – percutaneous pinning with elbow flexed >90 degrees, ORIF in adults
- Key complications: compartment syndrome (can lead to Volkmann's contracture), brachial a. injury, median and/or ulnar nerve injury, malignant cubitus varus
- Do not immobilize elbow joint >2-3 wks to avoid stiffness

RADIAL HEAD FRACTURE
- Common in young patients
- FOOSH, elbow extended, forearm in pronation
- Presentation: local tenderness, pin/mechanical block to supination/pronation
- Mason classification (undisplaced/displaced/comminuted/comminuted+dislocation)
- Management: Depends on displacement/comminution (Mason classification 1-4). Can range from elbow slab/sling to ORIF to radial head excision + prosthesis

EPICONDYLITIS
- Lateral epicondylitis: "tennis elbow" – inflammation of common extensor tendon as it inserts into lateral
EPICONDYLITIS
- Lateral epicondylitis: "tennis elbow" – inflammation of common extensor tendon as it inserts into lateral
  epicondyle
- DDx: PIN syndrome, C6/C7 entrapment, radial head arthritis
- Maudsley's test: +pain at lateral epicondyle with resisted extension of the 3rd digit
- Medial epicondylitis "golfer's elbow": inflammation of common flexor tendon as it inserts into medial epicondyle
- +pain with resisted pronation, flexion
- Management: reduce strenuous activities x >6wks, steroid injection, ±surgical debridement
- Elbow joint steroid injection: inject at the center of the triangle formed by the lateral epicondyle, radial head and olecranon

FOREARM FRACTURES

RADIUS AND ULNAR FRACTURE
- FOOSH / direct trauma
- Imaging: AP and lateral forearm; AP, lateral, oblique of wrist and elbow; CT if close to joint
- Management: ORIF with plate and screws with goal of anatomic reduction

MONTEGGIA FRACTURE
- Definition: proximal ulna #, radial head dislocation (proximal RU joint disruption)
- Ulna angled apex anterior and radial head dislocated anteriorly (rarely the reverse deformity occurs)
- Management: ORIF of ulna with indirect radius reduction in 90%. Splint and early post-op ROM if elbow completely stable; otherwise, immobilization in plaster with elbow flexed x 6 wks.
- Key complication: radial nerve/PIN injury

GALEAZZI FRACTURE
- Definition: distal radial shaft # with disruption of distal radioulnar joint (DRUJ)
- Imaging: shortening of distal radius >5 mm relative to distal ulna. Dislocation of radius with respect to ulna on true lateral
- Management: ORIF distal radius. If DRUJ stable, splint with early ROM. If DRUJ unstable, DRUJ pinning and long arm cast in supination x 6 wks

WRIST FRACTURES

COLLE'S FRACTURE
- Definition: transverse distal radius fracture with dorsal displacement ± ulnar styloid fracture
- Mechanism: FOOSH
- Presentation: dinner fork deformity, swelling, ecchymosis

> **Radiologic description of Colles' # (distal radius #) – comment on:**
> 1. Distal fragment:
>   Degree of dorsal tilt and displacement (lat. view)
>   Degree of radial tilt and displacement (AP view)
> 2. Presence of an ulnar styloid # (AP view)
> 3. Amount of radial shortening (AP view)

- Management:
  - Pre- and post-reduction x-rays – restore radial height (12mm), radial inclination (22°) and volar tilt (11°); repeat reduction if necessary + consider ORIF
  - Closed reduction
    - Hematoma block (sterile prep and drape, local anesthetic injection directly into # site)
    - Traction with extension, then traction with ulnar deviation, pronation, flexion of distal fragment
  - Dorsal slab/below elbow cast x 5-6 wks
  - X-ray q1wk to ensure maintenance of reduction
    - Surgical anatomy:
      - Volar approach: flexor retinaculum → tendons of palmaris longus, flexor carpi radialis, median nerve flexor digitorum superficialis → volar capsule of wrist joint
      - Structures to watch for: median nerve (esp. palmar cutaneous branch)

SMITH'S FRACTURE (reverse Colle's)
- Definition: volar displacement of distal radius
- Mechanism: fall onto back of flexed hand
- Management: unstable thus usually req. ORIF. Long-arm cast in supination x 6 wks

SCAPHOID FRACTURE
- Common in young men. NOT common in children or in patients beyond middle age
- Mechanism: FOOSH resulting most commonly in transverse # through middle (waist) of bone
- Presentation: pain on movement, snuff box tenderness
- Scaphoid fracture special tests
  - Tender snuff box (100% sensitivity, 29% specific)
  - Tenderness also at scaphoid tubercle and with compression along axis of thumb
- Imaging: PA/lat/scaphoid x-rays with wrist extended in ulnar deviation q2wks, + CT or MRI, bone scan rarely used
  - Fracture may not be evident on x-ray for up to 2 wks
- Management
  - Non-displaced: long-arm thumb spica cast x 4 wks then short arm cast until radiographic evidence of healing
  - Displaced: open or percutaneous screw fixation
- Complications: delayed/non-union, AVN, OA
- Prognosis: distal # near 100% healing, waist # 80-90% rate of healing, proximal # have >40% rate of nonunion or AVN
- Surgical anatomy:
  - Volar approach – radial artery, flexor carpi radialis → volar radiocarpal joint capsule

Axial Skeleton

Spine Columns

Anterior column	Anterior longitudinal ligament Anterior aspect of vertebral body Anterior aspect of annulus fibrosis
Middle column	Posterior longitudinal ligament Posterior aspect of vertebral body Posterior aspect of annulus fibrosis
Posterior column	Pedicle Facet joint Neural arch Ligamentum flavum Interspinous ligament Supraspinous ligament

Spine Fracture Types

Fracture Type	Column Failure	Stable/Unstable	Mechanism
Compression	Anterior	Stable	Compression
Burst	Anterior, middle	± unstable	High energy axial loading + flexion
Flexion-distraction (Chance fracture)	Middle, posterior	± unstable	MVA (lap belt only) causing flexion and distraction
Fracture-dislocation	Anterior, middle, posterior	Unstable	Significant force applied to spine (flexion, extension, distraction, rotation, shear or axial load)

Classification of Nerve Lesions

Neuropraxis	Localized myelin damage (compression injury)
Axontmesis	Loss of axonal continuity ± endoneurial, perineural continutiy
Neurotmesis	Complete nerve lesion

Cervical Radiculopthy/Neuropathy

Root	C5	C6	C7	C8
Motor	Deltoid Biceps Wrist extension	Biceps Brachioradialis	Triceps Wrist flexion Finger extension	Interossei Digital flexors
Sensory	Axillary nerve (patch over lateral deltoid)	Thumb and index finger	Middle finger	Ring and little finger
Reflex	Biceps	Biceps Brachioradialis	Triceps	Finger jerk

C-SPINE X-RAYS (See Emergency Medicine for Canadian C-Spine Rules)

- AP: alignment
- AP odontoid: atlantoaxial articulation
- Lateral:
  - Vertebral alignment: posterior vertebral bodies should be aligned (translation >3.5 mm is abnormal)
  - Angulation: between adjacent vertebral bodies (>11° is abnormal)
  - Disc or facet joint widening
  - Anterior soft tissue space (at C3 should be <3 mm; at C4 should be <8-10 mm)
- Oblique: evaluate pedicles and intervertebral foramen
- ± swimmer's view: lateral view with arm abducted 180° to evaluate C7-T1 junction if lateral view is inadequate (must see C7-T1 in all trauma situations)
- ± lateral flexion/extension view: evaluate subluxation of cervical vertebrae

Lumbar Radiculopathy/Neuropathy

Root	L4	L5	S1
Motor	Quadriceps (knee extension, hip adduction) Tibialis anterior (ankle inversion + dorsiflexion)	EHL (extensor hallucis longus) Gluteus medius (hip abductor)	Peroneus longus + brevis (ankle eversion) Gastrocnemius, soleus (plantarflexion)
Sensory	Medial leg	1st dorsal webspace and lateral leg	Lateral foot
Reflex	Knee	Medial hamstring	Ankle
Test	Femoral stretch	Straight leg raise	

Lower Back Pain

	Mechanical Back Pain (Disc Origin)	Mechanical Back Pain (Facet Origin)	Direct Nerve Root Compression (Spinal Stenosis)	Direct Nerve Root Compression (Root Compression)
Pain Dominance	Back	Back	Leg	Leg
Aggravation	Flexion	Extension Standing, walking	Exercise, extension, walking, standing	Flexion
Onset	Gradual	More sudden	Congenital or acquired	Acute leg ± back pain
Duration	Long (weeks, months)	Shorter (days, weeks)	Acute or chronic history (weeks to months)	Short episodes Attacks (minutes)
Treatment	Relief of strain, exercise	Relief of strain, exercise	Relief of strain, exercise	Relief of strain, exercise + surgical progressive or severe deficit

Management of Acute Low Back Pain

- Rule out red flags
- Good prognosis: majority of patients improve in 1-3wks
- Avoid prolonged bed rest, start walking and return to normal activity as soon as possible
- Analgesics: NSAIDs or acetaminophen, opioids should be limited or avoided
- Muscle relaxant: cyclobenzaprine, caution patient about sedation
- Physiotherapy and injections are not indicated in the short-term
- Spinal manipulation may be effective; use should be guided by patient preference

---

Flags for BACK PAIN

Bowel or bladder dysfunction	**P**aresthesias
Anesthesia (saddle)	**A**ge >50
Constitutional symptoms/malignancy	**I**V drug use
Khronic disease	**N**euromotor deficits

Common Lower Extremity Injuries

PELVIC FRACTURES
- Mechanism: high energy trauma, either direct or axial load, lateral compression (most common), vertical shear, or anteroposterior compression fractures
- Presentation: local swelling and tenderness; inability to weight bear; painful ROM; possible deformity, instability, and signs/symptoms of hemorrhage
- Imaging: x-rays → AP pelvis, inlet and outlet views, and Judet views
- Retroperitoneal space can accommodate up to 4L of blood before tamponade effect
- Most blood loss due to low pressure cancellous or venous bleed – 80%
- High pressure bleed most often from superior gluteal artery which is most often severed in AP compression fractures

---

Possible radiological findings:
- Pubic rami fractures – superior/inferior
- Pubic symphysis diastasis – common in AP compression (N=5mm)
- Sacral fractures - common in lateral compression
- SI joint diastasis – common in AP compression (N=1-4mm)
- Disrupted anterior column (iliopectineal line) or posterior column (ilioischial line)
- "Teardrop" displacement – acetabular fracture
- Iliac, ischial avulsion fractures
- Displacement of the major fragment – superior (VC), open book (APC), bucket handle (LC)

Classification of Pelvic Fractures

Type	Stability	Description
A	Rotationally stable Vertically stable	A1: fracture not involving pelvic ring A2: minimally displaced fracture of pelvic ring (e.g. ramus fracture)
B	Rotationally unstable Vertically stable	B1: open book B2: lateral compression – ipsilateral B3: lateral compression – contralateral
C	Rotationally unstable Vertically unstable (complete disruption of posterior sacroiliac complex)	C1: unilateral C2: bilateral C3: associated acetabular fracture

Management
- ABCs – ± pelvic binder, emergent angiography/embolization, external fixation
- Assess GU injury (rectal, vaginal exam) – if present, fracture considered open
- Type A – bedrest, mobilize with walking aids
- Type B, C – ORIF or external fixation

HIP FRACTURES

Femoral Neck (Subcapital) Fracture
- Definition: intracapsular fracture of the femoral neck
- Mechanism: young → high energy trauma; older → minimal trauma
- Clinical features: acute onset of hip pain following injury; inability to weight bear; shortened and externally rotated ipsilateral leg; painful ROM
- Investigations: x-ray → AP and lateral hip; AP pelvis
- Classification: Garden classification; main issue is to assess displacement [Garden I, II (undisplaced) vs. III, IV (displaced) as it alters management]

- Treatment:
    - If undisplaced, reduction with internal fixation
    - If displaced, treatment is dependent on age and function:
        - Young patient: reduction with internal fixation
        - Older, high function: bipolar hemiarthroplasty
        - Older, low function: total hip arthroplasty
- Complications: AVN of femoral head; DVT/PE; nonunion

Intertrochanteric Hip Fracture
- Definition: extracapsular fracture including the greater and lesser trochanters, along with the transitional bone between the femoral neck and shaft
- Mechanism: direct or indirect force transmitted to the intertrochanteric area
- Clinical features: acute onset of hip pain following injury; inability to weight bear; shortened and externally rotated ipsilateral leg; painful ROM;
- Investigations: x-ray → AP and lateral hip; AP pelvis
- Classification: assess stability by determining if the posteromedial cortex is intact on x-ray. If intact, fracture is stable; if not intact, fracture is unstable
- Treatment: reduction and internal fixation with dynamic hip screw or IM nail
- Complications: DVT/PE, displacement, malrotation, non-union, failure of fixation device

Subtrochanteric Hip Fracture
- Definition: fracture of the femur at or just below the lesser trochanter
- Mechanism: young → high energy trauma; older → minimal trauma
- Clinical features: acute onset of hip pain following injury; inability to weight bear; shortened and externally rotated ipsilateral leg; painful ROM
- Investigations: x-ray → AP and lateral hip; AP pelvis; AP and lateral femur
- Classification: Seinsheimer classification - Type I: nondisplaced; Type II: 2 parts, subtypes based on displacement and pattern; Type III: 3 parts, subtypes based on displacement and pattern; Type IV: comminuted; Type V: intertrochanteric extension
- Treatment: reduction and internal fixation with IM nail or plate
- Complications: malalignment, nonunion, DVT/PE

FEMORAL SHAFT FRACTURE
- Mechanism: high energy trauma
- Clinical features: acute onset of ipsilateral thigh pain following injury; inability to weight bear; shortened and externally rotated ipsilateral leg if displaced; painful ROM; often open injury, Gustilo III
- Investigations: x-ray → AP/lateral hip; AP/lateral femur; AP/lateral knee
- Winquist classification – Type I: no comminution or fragment less than 25% than width of bone; Type II: comminuted with fragment 50% or less; Type III: comminution with fragment greater than 50% of bone width; Type IV: severe comminution of entire bone segment; Type V: segmental bone loss
- AO/OTA classification – Type A: simple pattern; Type B: small butterfly or wedge fragment; Type C: segmental comminution
- Treatment: immobilize leg and apply traction; reduction and internal fixation with an intramedullary nail (if comminuted, may require plate fixation); early mobilization and strengthening
- Complications: hemorrhage, fat embolism, neurovascular injury, malunion, nonunion, knee and hip stiffness

KNEE COMPLAINTS
- General orthopedic history including presence or absence of clicking, locking, instability, pain, or swelling (CLIPS)
- General orthopedic physical exam (do not forget to evaluate hip); anterior and posterior drawer tests, Lachmann test, posterior sag sign, pivot shift sign, crouch compression test, McMurray's test, collateral ligament stress test
- Investigations: AP standing and lateral, skyline, 3 foot standing

ANTERIOR CRUCIATE LIGAMENT INJURIES
- Mechanism: sudden deceleration
- Clinical features: audible "pop" on Hx, effusion, posterolateral joint line tenderness, positive anterior drawer, Lachmann, and pivot shift tests
- Investigations: MRI
- Treatment: If stable - immobilization 2-4 wks with early ROM; if high demand lifestyle – ligament reconstruction
- Composite assessment: 25.0 positive likelihood ratio, 0.04 negative likelihood ratio

POSTERIOR CRUCIATE LIGAMENT INJURIES
- Mechanism: sudden posterior displacement of tibia when knee isflexed or hyperextended
- Clinical features: audible "pop" on Hx, effusion, anteromedial joint line tenderness, positive posterior drawer and reverse pivot shift tests
- Investigations: MRI
- Treatment: If unstable/high demand lifestyle - ligament reconstruction
- Composite assessment: 21.0 positive likelihood ratio, 0.05 negative likelihood ratio

COLLATERAL LIGAMENT INJURIES
- Mechanism: valgus force to knee = medial collateral ligament; varus force to knee = lateral collateral ligament
- Clinical features: swelling/effusion, tenderness below joint line medially (MCL) or laterally (LCL), joint laxity with varus/valgus force - no endpoint suggests complete tear; endpoint suggests incomplete tear; investigate other possible concomitant injuries
- Investigations: MRI
- Treatment: partial tear - immobilization 2-4 wks with early ROM and strengthening; complete tear - surgical repair of ligaments if multiple ligamentous injuries

MENISCAL INJURIES
- Mechanism: twisting force on knee when partially flexed
- Clinical features: acute onset of pain, difficulty weight bearing, instability, clicking, increased pain with squatting/twisting, effusion with insidious onset, joint line tenderness, locking
- Investigations: MRI, arthroscopy
- Treatment: not locked – ROM and strengthening, NSAIDs; locked or failed – arthroscopic repair/partial meniscectomy
- Composite assessment: 2.7 positive likelihood ratio, 0.4 negative likelihood ratio

ANKLE FRACTURES
- Definition: fracture of the distal tibia and/or distal fibula
- Mechanism: variable; fracture pattern depends on direction of force and position of foot and ankle
- Clinical Features: acute onset of ankle pain following injury; inability of weight bear on ipsilateral ankle; deformity
- Investigations: x-ray → AP/lateral ankle with mortise views; consider CT
- Follow the Ottawa Ankle Rules to determine need for x-ray
- Danis-Weber Classification:
  - Type A (infra-syndesmotic): Inversion injury causing a lateral malleolus avulsion fracture (below the plafond) with or without a shear fracture of the medial malleolus. Possible torn calcaneofibular ligament
  - Type B (trans-syndesmotic): external rotation and eversion injury causing a spiral fracture of the lateral malleolus (starting at the level of the plafond) and possibly a medial malleolus avulsion fracture. Possible deltoid ligament tear
  - Type C (supra-syndesmotic): pure external rotation injury causing an avulsion fracture of the medial malleolus, fibula fracture (above the level of the plafond) and possibly a posterior malleolus avulsion fracture. Frequently disrupts the syndesmosis. Possible torn deltoid ligament
- Treatment: if undisplaced, then below knee cast; consider open reduction and internal fixation if the fracture is displaced, the fracture pattern mirrors a type C ankle fracture, if the fracture is trimalleolar, if there is a talar tilt of >10 degrees or any open fracture

Foot Injuries

TALAR FRACTURE
- Mechanism: axial load or hyperdorsiflexion
- Clinical findings: acute ipsilateral ankle pain; inability to weight bear; painful ROM; possible deformity
- Investigations: x-ray → AP/lateral ankle; CT if need to better visualize fracture; consider MRI if there is suspicion of talar avascular necrosis
- Hawkins classification – Type I: nondisplaced talar neck fracture; Type II: displaced with subtalar joint dislocation or subluxation; Type III: displaced with dislocation from ankle mortise; Type IV: displaced with talonavicular joint dislocation or subluxation
- Complications: important to note that most of talus (60%) is covered with articular cartilage and blood supply poor; as such, fractures of the talus carry substantial risk of AVN; nonunion

ACHILLES TENDON RUPTURE
- Mechanism: loading activity; occasionally 2° to chronic tendonitis
- Clinical features: pain with push off; apprehension on toe off during gait; weak plantar flexion; positive Thompson test; palpable gap over Achilles tendon; possibly an audible pop at time of injury
- Investigations: generally diagnosed clinically, but consider MRI
- Treatment: if low demand, cast foot in plantar flexion x 8-12 wks; if high demand, surgical intervention with post operative cast x 6-8 wks

METATARSAL FRACTURES

Fracture Type	Mechanism	Clinical	Treatment
Avulsion of base of 5th MT	Sudden inversion followed by contraction of peroneus brevis	Tender base of 5th MT X-ray foot	Requires ORIF if displaced
Midshaft 5th MT (Jones fracture)	Stress injury	Painful shaft of 5th MT	NWB BK cast x 6 wks ORIF if athlete
Shaft 2nd, 3rd MT (March fracture)	Stress injury	Painful shaft of 2nd or 3rd MT	Symptomatic
1st MT	Trauma	Painful 1st MT	ORIF if displaced otherwise NWB BK cast x3 wks then walking cast x2 wks
Tarso-MT fracture-dislocation (Lisfranc fracture)	Fall onto plantar flexed foot or direct crush injury	Shortened forefoot prominent base	ORIF

Pediatric Orthopedics

GENERAL PRINCIPLES
- Type – greenstick or buckle because periosteum is thicker and stronger
- Epiphyseal growth plate – plate often mistaken for fracture or vice versa
  - X-ray opposite limb for comparison
  - Mechanism which causes ligamentous injury in adults causes growth plate injury in children
  - Intra-articular fractures have worse consequences in children because they usually involve the growth plate
- Anatomic reduction
  - May cause limb length discrepancy in children
  - Accept greater angular deformity in children
- Time to heal – shorter in children
- Always be aware of the possibility of child abuse
  - Make sure mechanism compatible with injury
  - Look for other signs, including x-ray evidence of healing fractures at other sites

CLASSIFICATION

Salter-Harris Classification of Epiphyseal Injury

Type	Description
I	Transverse through growth plate
II	Through metaphysic and along growth plate
III	Through epiphysis to plate and along growth plate
IV	Through epiphysis and metaphysis
V	Crush injury of growth plate

Bone Tumours

Distinguishing Benign from Malignant Bone Lesions on X-ray

Benign	Malignant
No periosteal reaction	Acute periosteal reaction Codman's triangle "Onion skin" "Sunburst"
Thick endosteal reaction	Broad border between lesion and normal bone
Well developed bone formation	Varied bone formation
Intraosseous and even calcification	Extraosseous and irregular calcification

Most Common Malignant Tumour Types for Age

Age	Tumour
<1	Neuroblastoma
1-10	Ewing's of tubular bones
10-30	Osteosarcoma, Ewing's of flat bones
30-40	Reticulum cell sarcoma, fibrosarcoma, periosteal osteosarcoma, malignant giant cell tumour, lymphoma
>40	Metastatic carcinoma, multiple myeloma, chondrosarcoma

Common Medications

Drug Name	Dosing Schedule	Indications	Comments
cefazolin (Ancef®)	1-2 g IV q8h	Prophylactically before orthopedic surgery	First generation cephalosporin; do not use with penicillin allergy
heparin	5000 IU SC q12h	To prevent venous thombosis and pulmonary emboli	Monitor platelets, follow PTT which should rise 1.5-2x
LMWH dalteparin (Fragmin®) enoxaparin (Lovenox®) fondaparinux (Arixtra®)	5000 IU SC qid 30-40 mg SC bid 2.5 mg SC qid	DVT prophylaxis esp. in hip and knee surgery	Fixed dose, no monitoring, improved bioavailability, increased bleeding rates
triamcinolone (Aristocort®) – an injectable steroid	0.5-1 mL of 25 mg/mL	Suspension (injected into inflamed joint or bursa)	Potent anti-inflammatory effect Increased pain for 24 h, rarely causes fat necrosis and skin depigmentation
misoprostol (Cytotec®)	200 µg qid	Prophylaxis of heterotopic ossification after THA	Use with indomethacin
indomethacin (Indocid®)	25 mg PO tid	Prophylaxis of heterotopic ossification after THA	Use with misoprostol

Otolaryngology

Common Presentations

Vertigo/Dizziness

Differential Diagnosis of Dizziness

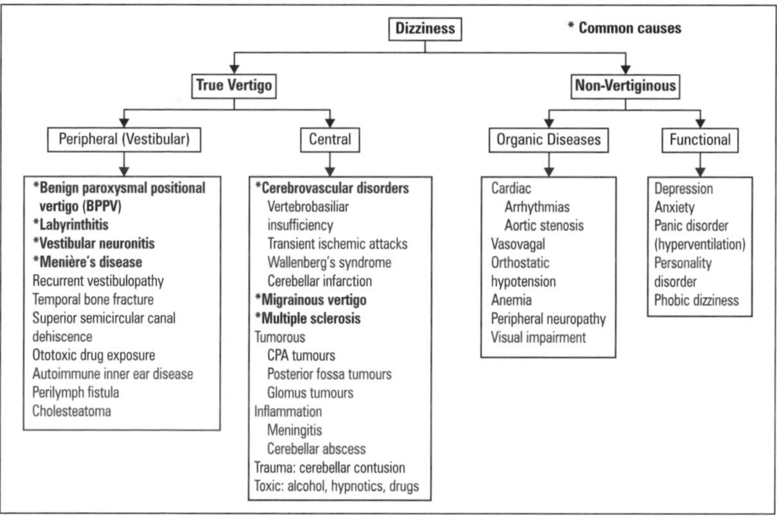

Differentiate from True vs. non-vertigo
• True vertigo = sensation of moving/spinning or of objects moving around patient

Differential Diagnosis of Vertigo Based on History

Condition	Duration	Hearing Loss	Tinnitus	Aural Fullness	Other Features
Benign Paroxysmal Positional Vertigo (BPPV)	Seconds	–	–	–	Brought on by positional changes
Menière's Disease	Minutes to hours	Uni/bilateral (low frequency)	+	Pressure/warmth	
Recurrent Vestibulopathy	Minutes to hours	–	–	None	
Vestibular Neuronitis	Hours to days	Unilateral	–	–	
Labyrinthitis	Days	Unilateral	Whistling	–	Recent AOM
Vestibular Schwannoma (acoustic neuroma)	Chronic	Progressive	–	–	Ataxia CN VII palsy

Peripheral vs. Central Vertigo

Symptoms	Peripheral	Central
Imbalance	Mild-Moderate	Severe
Nausea and Vomiting	Severe	Variable
Auditory Symptoms	Common	Rare
Neurologic Symptoms	Rare	Common
Compensation	Rapid	Slow
Nystagmus	Unidirectional Horizontal (only)	Bidirectional Horizontal or vertical

Otalgia

Differential Diagnosis of Otalgia – Local Causes

Etiology	External Ear Pain	Middle and Inner Ear Pain
Infection	a. Otitis externa b. Herpes simplex/Zoster c. Auricular cellulitis d. External canal abscess	a. Acute otitis media b. Otitis media with effusion c. Mastoiditis, myringitis, skull base infections (malignant otitis in diabetics)
Trauma	Frostbite, burns, hematoma, lacerations	Traumatic perforation, barotrauma
Other	Neoplasm of external canal, foreign body, cerumen impaction	Neoplasm, Wegener's, cholesteatoma

Referred Pain (from CN V, IX, & X) – Ten T's + 2
- Eustachian Tube
- TMJ Syndrome (pain in front of the ears)
- Trismus (spasm of masticator muscles; early symptom of tetanus)
- Teeth
- Tongue
- Tonsil (tonsillitis, tonsillar cancer, post-tonsillectomy)
- Tic (glossopharyngeal neuralgia)
- Throat (cancer of larynx)
- Trachea (foreign body; tracheitis)
- Thyroiditis
- Geniculate herpes and Ramsay Hunt syndrome
- ± CN VII palsy (Bell's palsy, Ramsay Hunt Syndrome)

Hearing Loss

Differential Diagnosis of Hearing Loss

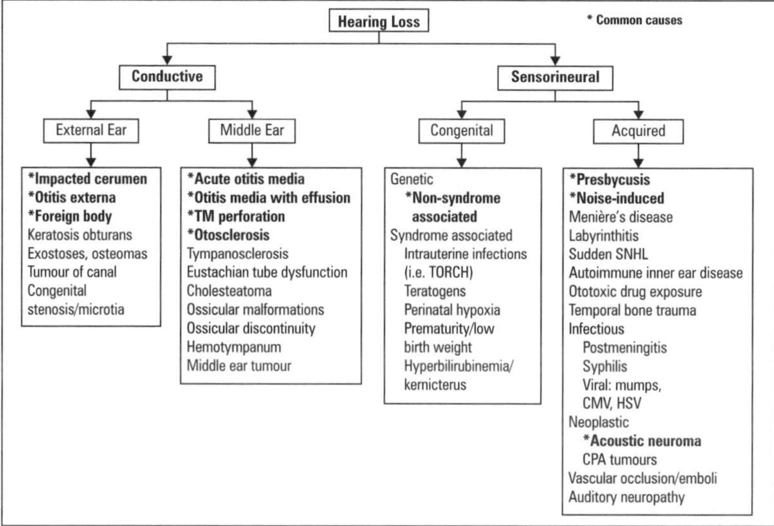

Types of Hearing Loss

1. Conductive Hearing Loss (CHL) – conduction of sound to the cochlea is impaired (external or middle ear disease)
2. Sensorineural Hearing Loss (SNHL) – a defect in the conversion of sound into neural signals or in the transmission of those signals to the cortex (caused by disease of the cochlea, acoustic nerve (CN VIII), brainstem, or cortex)
3. Mixed Hearing Loss – the conduction of sound to the cochlea is impaired, as well as transmission through the cochlea to the cortex

Interpretation of Tuning Fork Tests

Examples	Weber	Rinne
Normal or bilateral sensorineural hearing loss	Central	AC>BC (+) bilaterally
Right-sided conductive hearing loss, normal left ear	Lateralizes to Right	BC>AC (–) right
Right-sided sensorineural hearing loss, normal left ear	Lateralizes to Left	AC>BC (+) bilaterally
Right-sided severe sensorineural hearing loss or dead right ear, normal left ear	Lateralizes to Left	BC>AC (–) right *

* A vibrating tuning fork on the mastoid stimulates the cochlea bilaterally, therefore in this case, the left cochlea is stimulated by the Rinne test on the right, i.e. a false negative test
These tests are not valid if the ear canals are obstructed with cerumen (i.e. will create conductive loss)
The Rinne Test is sensitive to hearing loss that is a minimum of 20 dB in magnitude; the Weber Test is sensitive to hearing loss that is a minimum of 5 dB in magnitude; therefore, a patient with a lateralizing Weber Test but negative Rinne Test has a hearing loss between 5-20 dB.

Types of Hearing Loss and Associated Audiograms

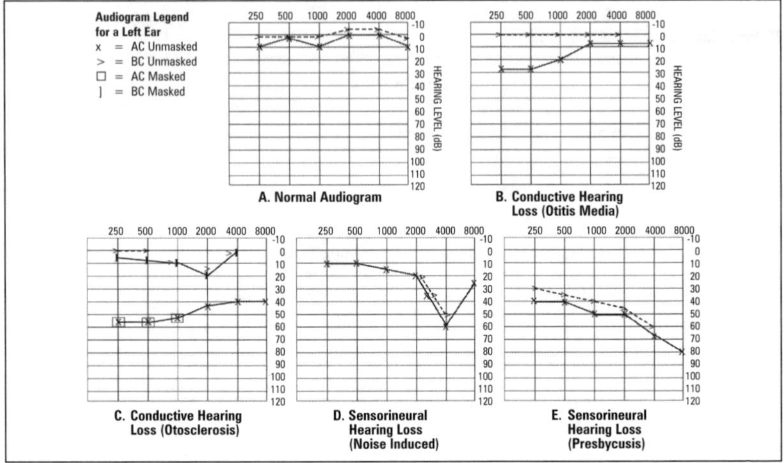

Pure Tone Audiometry Patterns

1. CHL – normal bone conduction but abnormal air conduction with a minimum 10 dB air-bone gap
2. SNHL – abnormal bone and air conduction with no air-bone gap (<10 dB difference between air and bone conduction thresholds)
3. Mixed Hearing Loss – abnormal bone and air conduction with a minimum 10 dB air-bone gap

Tympanograms

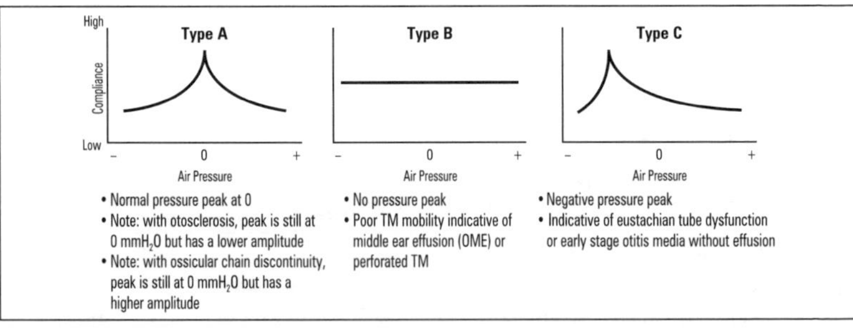

- Normal pressure peak at 0
- Note: with otosclerosis, peak is still at 0 mmH$_2$O but has a lower amplitude
- Note: with ossicular chain discontinuity, peak is still at 0 mmH$_2$O but has a higher amplitude

- No pressure peak
- Poor TM mobility indicative of middle ear effusion (OME) or perforated TM

- Negative pressure peak
- Indicative of eustachian tube dysfunction or early stage otitis media without effusion

Tinnitus

Differential Diagnosis of Tinnitus

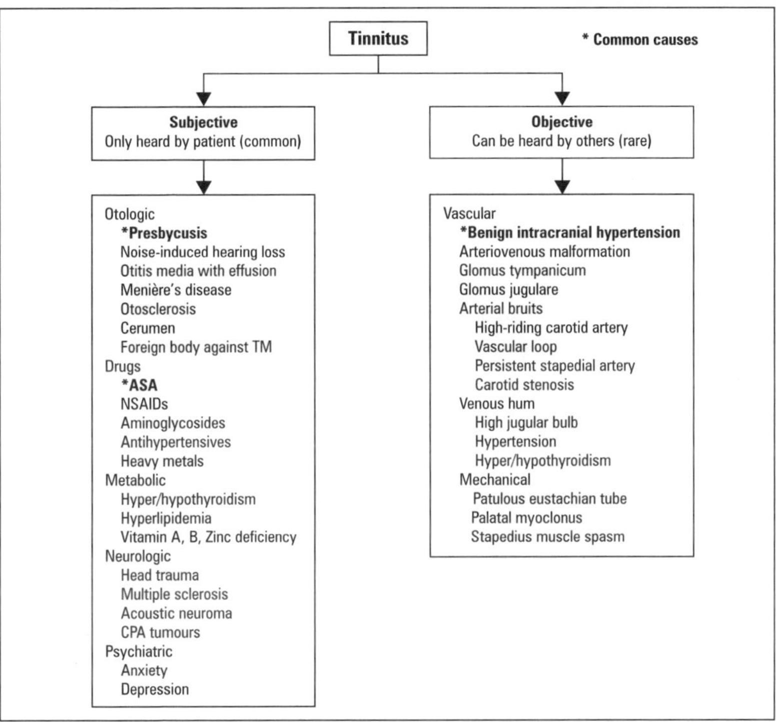

Hoarseness

Differential Diagnosis of Hoarseness

Infectious	Acute/chronic laryngitis Laryngotracheobronchitis (croup) Bacterial tracheitis
Inflammatory	Gastro-esophageal reflux (GERD), smoking, chronic sinusitis with PND or muscle tension, dystonia, overuse Vocal cord polyps Reinke's edema (polypoid corditis) Contact ulcers or granulomas Vocal cord nodules
Trauma	**External:** laryngeal trauma; **Iatrogenic:** endoscopy and endotracheal tube

Neoplasia

Benign tumours	**Malignant tumours**
Vocal cord polyps	Early leukoplakic lesions
Papillomas (HPV infection)	Squamous cell carcinoma (SCC)
Chondromas, lipomas, hemangiomas	Kaposi's sarcoma

Cysts	Retention cysts, Laryngoceles
Systemic	Endocrine (hypothyroidism, virilization); connective tissue (RA, SLE); Angioneurotic edema

Neurologic
(vocal cord paralysis due to superior ± recurrent laryngeal nerve injury)

Central lesions
- Cerebrovascular accident (CVA)
- Head injury
- Multiple sclerosis (MS)
- Arnold-Chiari
- Skull base tumours

Peripheral lesions

Unilateral
- Most common cause of vocal cord paralysis = lung malignancy
- Neck, chest, laryngeal trauma
- Thoracic aneurysm
- Neoplasms: glomus jugulare, thyroid, bronchogenic, esophageal, neural
- Iatrogenic injury – thyroid, parathyroid surgery, carotid endarterectomy
- Anterior approach to cervical spine disc surgery
- Radiation induced fibrosis
- Degenerative neural disorders: bulbar palsies (e.g. polio), demyelinating disease, vascular syndromes (Wallenberg's)
- Cardiac: left atrial enlargement, aneurysm of aortic arch

Bilateral
- Iatrogenic injury: bilateral thyroid surgery

Neuromuscular
- Myasthenia gravis
- Presbylaryngeus/presbyphonia (decreased tone of vocalis muscle with age)
- Spasmodic dysphonia

Functional	Psychogenic aphonia (hysterical aphonia) Habitual aphonia Ventricular dysphonias Catatonic state
Congenital	Webs, atresia, laryngomalacia

Neck Mass

Differential Diagnosis of a Neck Mass

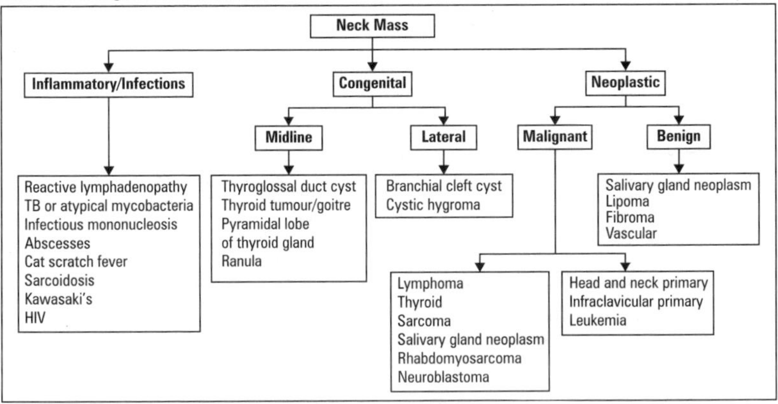

Rhinitis

Nasal Discharge: Character and Associated Conditions

Character	Associated Conditions
Watery/mucoid	Allergic, viral, vasomotor, CSF leak (halo sign)
Mucopurulent	Bacterial, foreign body
Serosanguinous	Neoplasia
Bloody	Trauma, neoplasia, bleeding disorder, hypertension/vascular disease

Classification of Rhinitis

Inflammatory	Non-Inflammatory

Perennial non-allergic
  Asthma, ASA sensitivity
  Allergic
  Seasonal, perennial
Atrophic
  Primary: *Klebsiella ozena* (especially in elderly)
  Acquired: post-surgery if too much mucosa or turbinate has been resected
Infectious
  Viral: e.g. rhinovirus, influenza, parainfluenza, etc.
  Bacterial: e.g. *S. aureus*
  Fungal
  Granulomatous: TB, syphilis, leprosy
Non-infectious
  Sarcoidosis, Wegener's granulomatosis
Irritant
  Dust, chemicals, pollution
	Rhinitis medicamentosa
	  Topical decongestants
	Hormonal
	  Pregnancy, estrogens, thyroid
	Idiopathic vasomotor

Epistaxis

Blood Supply to the Nasal Septum
1. Superior posterior septum
   - Internal carotid → ophthalmic → anterior/posterior ethmoidal
2. Posterior septum
   - External carotid → internal maxillary → sphenopalatine artery → nasopalatine
3. Lower anterior septum
   - External carotid → facial artery → superior labial artery → nasal branch
   - External carotid → internal maxillary → descending palatine → greater palatine
- These arteries anastomose to form Kiesselbach's plexus, located at Little's area (anterior portion of the cartilaginous septum), where 90% of nosebleeds occur
- Bleeding from above middle turbinate is internal carotid, and from below is external carotid

Etiology of Epistaxis

Type	Causes	

Local	Trauma (most common)
	  Fractures: facial, nasal
	  Self-induced: digital, foreign body
	  Iatrogenic: nasal, sinus, orbit surgery
	Barometric changes
	Nasal dryness: dry air, ± septal deformities
	Septal perforation
	Chemical: cocaine, nasal sprays, ammonia
		Tumours
		  Benign: polyps, inverting papilloma, angiofibroma
		  Malignant: squamous cell carcinoma,
		  esthesioneuroblastoma
		Inflammation
		  Rhinitis: allergic, non-allergic
		  Infections: bacterial, viral, fungal
		  Idiopathic

Systemic	Coagulopathies
	  Meds: anticoagulants, NSAIDs
	  Hemophilias, von Willebrand's
	  Hematological malignancies
	  Liver failure, uremia
	Vascular: hypertension, atherosclerosis, Osler-Weber-Rendu
	Others: Wegener's, SLE	

Common Conditions

Benign Paroxysmal Positional Vertigo

- **Definition**: acute attacks of transient vertigo lasting seconds to minutes initiated by certain head positions, accompanied by nystagmus
- **Etiology**: head injury, viral infection (URTI), degenerative disease, idiopathic
- **Diagnosis**: clinical and a positive Dix-Hallpike maneuver (see Figure)

Dix-Hallpike Maneuver
- The patient is rapidly moved from a sitting position to a supine position with the head hanging over the end of the table, turned to one side at 45° holding the position for 20 sec. Onset of vertigo is noted and the eyes are observed for nystagmus
- 5 signs of BPPV seen with the Dix-Hallpike maneuver:
  - Geotropic rotatory nystagmus
  - Fatigues with repeated maneuver
  - Reversal of nystagmus upon sitting
  - Latency of ~20 sec
  - Crescendo/decrescendo vertigo for ~20 sec

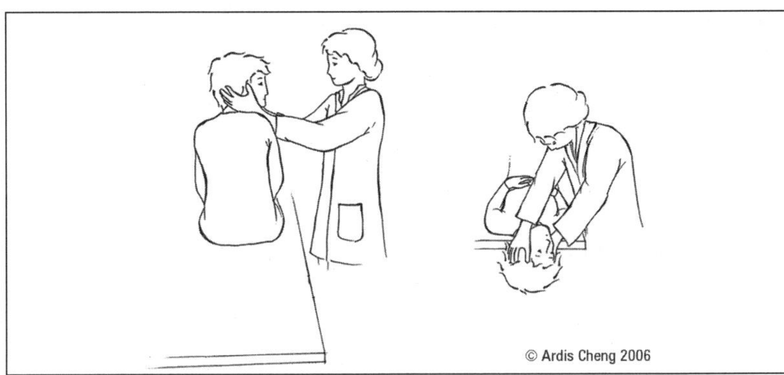

Sinusitis

Definition
- Acute infection and inflammation of the paranasal sinuses

Etiology
- Viral vs. bacterial
- Children are more prone to a bacterial etiology than adults, but viral is still more common overall
- Maxillary sinus most commonly affected
- Must rule out fungal causes (mucormycosis) in immunocompromised hosts
- Organisms
    - Viral (most common): rhinovirus, influenza, parainfluenza
    - Bacterial: *S. pneumoniae* (35%), *H. influenzae* (35%), *M. catarrhalis*, anaerobes (dental)

Clinical Features
- Sudden onset of:
    - Nasal blockage/congestion and/or
    - Nasal discharge/posterior nasal drip
- ± facial pain or pressure, hyposmia
- Signs more suggestive of a bacterial etiology are erythematous nasal mucosa, mucopurulent discharge, pus originating from the middle meatus and the presence of nasal polyps of a deviated septum
- Acute viral rhinosinusitis lasts <10 d. If symptoms increase after 5 d or last longer than 10 d, consider a bacterial etiology

Management
- Investigations: anterior rhinoscopy; X-ray/CT scan not recommended unless suspected complications
- Symptoms improving within 5 d: symptomatic relief and expectant management (saline rinse, steam, fluids, etc.)
- Moderate symptoms that worsen or persist beyond 5 d: institute an intranasal corticosteroid spray (INCS) and continue for 14 d if symptomatic relief is noted within 48 h
- Severe symptoms that worsen or persist beyond 5 d and refractory to INCS: amoxicillin therapy ± INCS ± referral to a specialist
- Surgery if medical therapy fails: FESS

Etiologies of Sinusitis

Ostial Obstruction	Inflammation:	URTI Allergy
	Mechanical:	Septal deviation Turbinate hypertrophy Polyps Tumours Adenoid hypertrophy Foreign body Congenital abnormalities i.e. cleft palate
Non-ostial Obstruction	Immune:	Wegener's granulomatosis Lymphoma, leukemia Immunosuppressed patients (e.g. neutropenics, diabetics, HIV)
	Systemic:	Cystic fibrosis Immotile cilia (Kartagener's)
Direct Extension	Dental:	Infection
	Trauma:	Facial fractures

Source: Dr. J. Chapnik. https://portal.utoronto.ca/webapps/portal/otolaryngology/OTI300/sinusitis.pdf

Head and Neck Malignancies

Quick Look-Up Summary of Head and Neck Malignancies – Diagnosis and Treatment

Clinical Features	Investigations	Treatment	Prognosis
Oral Cavity Cancers			

Asymptomatic neck mass (30%)
Non-healing ulcer ± bleeding
Dysphagia, sialorrhea, dysphonia
Oral fetor, otalgia leukoplakia or
erythroplakia (pre-malignant mouth)
	Biopsy
	CT
		1° surgery
		  local resection
		  ±neck dissection
		  ±reconstruction
		2° radiation
			5-yr: - T1/T2: 75%
			       - T3/T4: 30-35%
			Poor prognostic indicators: Depth of invasion,
			close surgical margins location (tongue worse
			than floor of changes or CIS)
			Cervical nodes, extra capsular spread

Nose and Paranasal Sinus Cancers			
Early symptoms: Unilateral nasal obstruction Epistaxis, rhinorrhea **Late symptoms:** 2° to invasion of nose, orbit, nerves, oral cavity, skin, skull base, cribriform plate	CT/MRI Biopsy	Surgery and radiation Chemoradiotherapy for unresectable disease	5-yr: 30 to 60% Poor prognosis 2° to late presentation
Carcinoma of the Pharynx – Subtypes **Nasopharynx**			
Cervical nodes (60-90%) Nasal obstruction, epistaxis Unilateral AOM ± hearing loss CN III to VI, IX to XII (25%) Proptosis, voice change, dysphagia	Nasopharyngoscopy Biopsy CT/MRI	1° radiation 2° surgery	5-yr survival: - I: 79% - II: 72% - III: 50-60% - IV: 36-42%

Clinical Features	Investigations	Treatment	Prognosis
Carcinoma of the Pharynx – Subtypes			
Oropharynx			
Odynophagia, otalgia Ulcerated/enlarged tonsil Fixed tongue/trismus/dysarthria Oral fetor, bloody sputum Cervical lymphadenopathy (60%) Distal mets: lung/bone/liver (7%)	Biopsy CT	1° radiation 2° local resection ± neck dissection ± reconstruction If advanced: chemo ± anti-EGFr	Base of tongue – control rates T1: >90% T4: 13 to 52% Tonsils – cure rate T1/T2: 90-100% T4: 15-33%
Hypopharynx Cancers			
Dysphagia, odynophagia Otalgia, hoarseness Cervical lymphadenopathy	Pharyngoscopy Biopsy CXR r/o lung mets CT	1° radiation 2° surgery	T2/T3 cure rate: 60% T4 5 yr survival: 25-40%
Larynx Cancers			
Dysphagia, odynophagia, globus Otalgia, hoarseness, Cough/hemoptysis Cervical nodes (rare w/ glottic CA)	Laryngoscopy CT/MRI	1° radiation 2° surgery	5-yr T4 >40% (surgery with radiation) Control rate early lesions >90% (radiation) Dyspnea/stridor 1° surgery for bulky T4 10-12% of small lesions fail radiotherapy
Salivary Gland Cancers			
Painless mass CN VII – parotid mass Cervical lymphadenopathy Rapid growth Invasion of skin Constitutional signs/symptoms	Fine needle aspirate CT	**Surgery** Benign and malignant Lymph node sampling Post-op radiotherapy Chemo if unresectable	Parotid 10-yr survival: 85, 69, 43, and 14% for stages I to IV Submandibular 2-yr: 82%, 5-yr: 69% Minor salivary gland 10-yr: 83, 52, 25, 23% for stages I to IV
Thyroid Cancers			
Thyroid mass, cervical nodes Vocal cord paralysis Hyper/hypothyroidism Dysphagia	FNA U/S	1° surgery ± I^{131} for mets suppression	Recurrences occur within 5 yrs Long-term f/u: clinical exam, post-op TSH stimulated thyroglobulin levels
Parathyroid Cancers			
Increased serum Ca^{2+} Neck mass Bone disease, renal disease Pancreatitis		Wide surgical excision Post-op monitoring of serum Ca^{2+}	Recurrence rates: 1-yr 27% 5-yr 82% 10-yr 91% Mean survival: 6 to 7 yrs

Thyroid Mass

Investigation of the Thyroid Nodule

Lab Tests	Imaging	Invasive Tests
TSH and T4	U/S	FNA
Thyroglobulin and anti-thyroid peroxidase antibody	Thyroid scan	

Management of the Thyroid Nodule

Treatment	Indications
Radioiodine therapy	Hyperthyroid with suspicious solid mass, that is "HOT" on thyroid scan
Chemotherapy and/or radiotherapy	Anaplastic CA or thyroid lymphoma
Surgical excision	Recurrent cyst that is "suspicious" on FNA or if patient is extremely anxious Malignancy other than anaplastic CA or thyroid lymphoma Solid "suspicious" mass that is "cold" on thyroid scan (excise to r/o capsular invasion) Hyperthyroid with suspicious solid mass, that is "HOT" on thyroid scan

Approach to the Thyroid Nodule
- All patients with thyroid nodules require evaluation of serum TSH and ultrasound
- Any nodule >5 mm with suspicious sonographic features (particularly microcalcifications) should undergo FNA
- Any nodule >1 cm should undergo FNA
- When performing repeat FNA on initially non-diagnostic nodules, U/S-guided FNA should be employed
- Nuclear scanning has minimal value in the investigation of the thyroid nodule

Thyroid Carcinoma

	Papillary	Follicular	Medullary	Anaplastic	Lymphoma
Incidence (% of all thyroid Ca)	80%	10%	3 to 5% (10% familial; 90% sporadic)	2 to 4%	<1% 2% of extranodal lymphomas
Route of Spread	Lymphatic	Hematogenous	Lymphatic and hematogenous		
Histology	Orphan Annie nuclei Psammoma bodies	Capsular/blood vessel invasion influences prognosis	Amyloid May secrete calcitonin, prostaglandins, ACTH, serotonin, kallikrein or bradykinin	Giant cells Spindle cells	
Other	**P**'s – papillary cancer **P**opular (most common) **P**alpable lymph nodes **P**ositive I131 uptake Positive prognosis **P**ost-op I131 scan to diagnose treatments	**F**'s – follicular cancer **F**ar away mets **F**emale (3:1) **F**NA, NOT (can't be diagnosed **F**avourable prognosis by FNA)	**M**ultiple endocrine neoplasia (MEN IIa or IIb) a**M**yloid **M**edian node dissection	More common in elderly 70% in women 20 to 30% have history of diff. thyroid Ca (mostly papillary) or nodular goitres Rapidly enlarging neck mass	Usually non-Hodgkin's rapidly enlarging goitre Hashimoto's thyroiditis increased risk 60x 4:1 female predominance Dysphagia, dyspnea, stridor, hoarseness, neck pain, facial edema accompanied by "B" symptoms *
Prognosis	98% at 10 yrs	92% at 10 yrs	50% at 10 yrs 20% at 10 yrs if detected when clinically palpable	Extremely high mortality 20 to 35% at 1 yr 13% at 10 yrs	5 yr survival Stage IE 55%-80% Stage IIE 20%-50% Stage IIE/IV 15%-35%
Treatment	All tumours: Near total/ Total thyroidectomy ±post-op I131	All tumours: Near total/ Total thyroidectomy ±post-op I131	Total thyroidectomy median lymph node dissection If lateral cervical nodes +ve modified neck dissection Post-op thyroxine Tracheostomy Screen asymptomatic relatives	Small tumours: Total thyroidectomy ± external beam radiation	Non-surgical Combined radiation chemotherapy (CHOP**)

*B symptoms = fever, night sweats, weight loss >10% in 6 months

** CHOP = cyclophosphamide, adriamycin, vincristine, prednisone

Pediatric Otolaryngology

Acute Otitis Media (AOM)

Definition
• Acute inflammation of middle ear

Epidemiology
• 60 to 70% of children have at least 1 episode of AOM before 3 yrs of age
• 18 months to 6 yrs most common age group
• Peak incidence January to April
• One third of children have had 3 or more episodes by age 3

Etiology
• *S. pneumoniae* – 35% of cases (incidence decreasing due to pneumococcus vaccine)
• *H. influenzae* – 25% of cases
• *M. catarrhalis* – 10% of cases
• *S. aureus* and *S. pyogenes* (all β-lactamase producing)
• Anaerobes (newborns)
• Gram negative enterics (infants)
• Viral

Risk Factors
• Bottle feeding, pacifier use
• Passive smoke
• Crowded living conditions (day care/group child care facilities)
• Sick contacts
• Male
• Family history (presumably due to eustachian tube or middle ear anatomy)

Pathogenesis
• Obstruction of eustachian tube → air absorbed in middle ear → negative pressure (an irritant to middle ear mucosa) → edema of mucosa with exudate/effusion → infection of exudate from nasopharyngeal secretions

Clinical Features
• Triad of otalgia, fever (especially in younger children), and conductive hearing loss
• Rarely tinnitus, vertigo, and/or facial nerve paralysis
• Otorrhea if tympanic membrane perforated
• Pain over mastoid
• Infants/toddlers
    ▪ Ear-tugging
    ▪ Hearing loss, balance disturbances (mild)
    ▪ Irritable, poor sleeping
    ▪ Vomiting and diarrhea
    ▪ Anorexia
• Otoscopy of tympanic membrane
    ▪ Hyperemia
    ▪ Bulging
    ▪ Loss of landmarks: handle and short process of malleus not visible

Treatment
- Antibiotic treatment: hastens resolution – 10 d course
  - 1st line:
    - Amoxicillin 80-90 mg/kg/d divided into two doses – safe, effective, and inexpensive
    - If penicillin allergic: macrolide (clarithromycin, azithromycin), trimethoprim-sulphamethoxazole (Bactrim®)
  - 2nd line (for amoxicillin failures):
    - amoxicillin-clavulinic acid (Clavulin®)
    - Cephalosporins: cefuroxime axetil (Ceftin®), ceftriaxone IM (Rocephin®), cefaclor (Ceclor®), cefixime (Suprax®)
  - AOM deemed unresponsive if clinical signs/symptoms and otoscopic findings persist beyond 48 h of antibiotic treatment
- Symptomatic therapy
  - Antipyretics/analgesics (e.g. acetaminophen)
  - Decongestants – may relieve nasal congestion but does not treat AOM
- Prevention
  - Parent education about risk factors (see above)
  - Antibiotic prophylaxis – amoxicillin or macrolide shown effective at half therapeutic dose
  - Pneumococcal and influenza vaccine
  - Surgery
    - Choice of surgical therapy for recurrent AOM depends on whether local factors (eustachian tube dysfunction) are responsible (use ventilation tubes), or regional disease factors (tonsillitis, adenoid hypertrophy, sinusitis) are responsible

Indications for Myringotomy and Tympanostomy Tubes in Recurrent AOM and OME (tubes are more commonly inserted for OME, rarely for AOM)
- Persistent effusion >3 months with conductive hearing loss
- Lack of response to >3 months of antibiotic therapy for recurring AOM
- Persistent effusion for >3 months after episode of AOM with conductive hearing loss
- Recurrent episodes of AOM (>7 episodes in 6 months)
- Bilateral conductive hearing loss of >20 dB
- Chronic retraction of the tympanic membrane or pars flaccida
- Bilateral OME lasting >4 to 6 months
- Craniofacial anomalies predisposing to middle ear infections (e.g. cleft palate)
- Complications of AOM

Complications of AOM
- Otologic
  - TM perforation, chronic suppurative OM, ossicular necrosis, cholesteatoma, persistent effusion (often leading to hearing loss)
- CNS
  - Meningitis, brain abscess, facial nerve paralysis, OTIC hydrocephalus
- Other
  - Mastoiditis, labyrinthitis, sigmoid sinus thrombophlebitis

Acute Tonsillitis

Etiology
- Group A β-hemolytic *streptococcus* and Group G *streptococcus*
- *S. pneumoniae, S. aureus, H. influenzae, M. catarrhalis*
- Epstein-Barr virus (EBV)

Clinical Features
- Symptoms
  - Sore throat, dysphagia, odynophagia, trismus, malaise, fever, otalgia (referred)
- Signs
  - Tender cervical lymphadenopathy especially submandibular, jugulodigastric
  - Tonsils enlarged, inflammation ± exudates/white follicles
  - Strawberry tongue, scarletiniform rash (scarlet fever)
  - Palatal petechiae (infectious mononucleosis)

Investigations
- CBC, swab for C&S, latex agglutination tests, Monospot – less reliable in children <2 yrs old

Treatment
- Bed rest, soft diet, ample fluid intake
- Gargle with warm saline solution
- Analgesics and antipyretics
- Antibiotics
  - Only after appropriate swab for C&S
  - 1st line penicillin or amoxicillin (erythromycin if penicillin allergic) x 10 d
  - Rheumatic fever risk emerges approximately 9 d after the onset of symptoms: antibiotics are utilized mainly to avoid this serious sequela and to provide earlier symptomatic relief
  - No evidence for the role of antibiotics in the avoidance of post-streptococcal glomerulonephritis

Complications
- Deep neck space infection, abscess: peritonsillar, intratonsillar, sepsis, glomerulonephritis

Peritonsillar Abscess (Quinsy)

Definition
- Cellulitis of space behind tonsillar capsule extending onto soft palate leading to abscess

Etiology
- Bacterial: Group A strep (GAS) (50% of cases), *S. pyogenes, S. aureus, H. influenzae,* and anaerobes

Epidemiology
- Can develop from acute tonsillitis with infection spreading into plane of tonsillar bed
- Unilateral, most common in 15 to 30 yr old age group

Clinical Features
- Fever and dehydration
- Sore throat, dysphagia and odynophagia
- Extensive peritonsillar swelling but tonsil may appear normal
- Edema of soft palate
- Uvular deviation
- Involvement of motor branch of CN V can lead to increased salivation and trismus
- Dysphonia with "hot potato" voice (edema failure to elevate palate) 2° to CN X involvement
- Unilateral referred otalgia
- Cervical lymphadenitis

Complications
- Aspiration pneumonia 2° to spontaneous rupture of abscess
- Airway obstruction
- Lateral dissection into parapharyngeal and/or carotid space
- Bacteremia

Treatment
- Secure airway
- Surgical drainage (incision or needle aspiration) with C&S
- Warm saline irrigation
- IV penicillin G x 10 d if cultures positive for GAS
- Add oral/IV metronidazole or clindamycin x 10 d if culture +ve for Bacteroides
- Possible tonsillectomy 6 wks later with interim oral antibiotic prophylaxis for high risk individuals

OTHER PARAPHARYNGEAL SPACE INFECTION
- Pharyngitis
- Parotitis
- Otitis
- Mastoiditis (Bezold's abscess)
- Odontogenic infection

Common Medications

Antibiotics

Generic Name (Brand Name)	Dose	Indications	Notes
amoxicillin (Amoxil®, Amoxi®, Amox®)	Adult: 500 mg PO tid Children: 80-90 mg/kg/d in 2 divided doses	*Streptococcus, Pneumococcus, H. influenzae*, Proteus coverage	In patients with infectious mononucleosis, may cause rash
piperacillin with tazobactam (Zosyn®)	3 g PO q6h	Gram-positive and negative aerobes and anaerobes plus Pseudomonas coverage	May cause pseudomembranous colitis
ciprofloxacin (Cipro®, Ciloxan®)	500 mg PO bid	*Pseudomonas, Streptococci*, MRSA, and most Gram-negative; no anaerobic coverage	Do not give quinolones to children
erythromycin (Erythrocin®, EryPed®, Staticin®, T-Stat®, Erybid®, Novorythro Encap®)	500 mg PO qid	Alternative to penicillin	Ototoxic

Otic Drops

Generic Name (Brand Name)	Dose	Indications / Notes
ciprofloxacin (Ciprodex®)	4 gtt in affected ear bid	For otitis externa and complications of otitis media Pseudomonas, Streptococci, MRSA, and most Gram-negative; no anaerobic coverage
neomycin, polymyxin B sulfate, and hydrocortisone (Cortisporin Otic®)	5 gtt in affected ear tid	For otitis externa Used for inflammatory conditions which are currently infected or at risk of bacterial infections May cause hearing loss if placed in inner ear
hydrocortisone and acetic acid (VoSol HC®)	5-10 gtt in affected ear tid	Bactericidal by lowering pH
tobramycin and dexamethasone (TobraDex®)	5-10 gtt in affected ear bid	For chronic suppurative otitis media Risk of vestibular or cochlear toxicity

Nasal Sprays

Generic Name (Brand Name)	Indications	Notes: General
Steroid		
flunisolide (Rhinalar®) budesonide (Rhinocort®) triamcinolonoe (Nasacort®) beclomethasone (Beconase®) mometasone furoate, monohydrate (Nasonex®) fluticasone furoate (Avamys®)	Allergic rhinitis Chronic sinusitis	Requires up to four wks of consistent use to have effect Long term use Dries nasal mucosa; get minor bleeding Patient should stop if epistaxis May sting Flonase® and Nasonex® not absorbed systemically
Antihistamine		
levocarbastine (Livostin®)	Allergic rhinitis	Immediate effect If no effect by 3 d then discontinue Use during allergy season
Decongestant		
xylometazoline (Otrivin®) oxymetazoline (Dristan®) phenylephrine (Neosynephrine®)	Acute sinusitis Rhinitis	Careful if patient has hypertension Short term use (<5 d) If long terrn use, can cause decongestant addiction (i.e. rhinitis medicamentosa)
Antibiotic / Decongestant		
framycetin, gramicidin, phenylephrine (Soframycin®)	Acute sinusitis	
Anticholinergic		
ipratropium bromide (Atrovent®)	Vasomotor rhinitis	Careful not to spray into eyes Increased rate of epistaxis when combined with topical nasal steroids
Lubricants		
saline, NeilMed®, Rhinaris®, Secaris®, Polysporin®, Vaseline®	Dry nasal mucosa	Use prn Rhinaris® and Secaris® may cause stinging

Source: Dr. M.M. Carr icarus.med.utoronto.ca/carr/manual/sprays.html

Pediatrics

Essential History, Physical Exam, Investigations and Immunizations

History and Physical Exam

- The pediatric history and physical exam is age-specific
- The order and depth of the physical exam will vary depending on the age and how cooperative the child is

PEDIATRIC HISTORY AND PHYSICAL EXAM

History	Physical Exam
ID Age, sex, gestational age at birth	**General** Overall appearance: well vs. toxic, vitals, height, weight, colour Relationship to caregiver Vitals (see next Table for ranges by age group)
CC/HPI OPQRST approach to complaint Previous episodes, sick contacts, and travel history	**H&N** Head: shape and symmetry, fontanelles, sutures, dysmorphism Ears: shape, hearing, otoscopic exam Eyes: acuity (>3 yrs), lids, pupils, fundus for red reflex Mouth: mucous membranes, teeth, uvula, tonsils, tongue, frenulum, palate Neck: stiffness, lymph nodes, thyroid
ROS Growth patterns, infections, breathing difficulties, cyanosis, abdominal pain, bowel movements, sexual activity, age of menarche, urinary problems, seizures, rashes, etc.	
PMHx Mother's pregnancy history (GPTAL, previous complications, substance abuse, TORCH infections, Rh and GBS status, mother's health and medications) Birth and labour including weight and APGARs (appearance, pulse, grimace, activity, respirations) Feeding history, development, immunizations, ongoing or previous medical problems or infections, medications, and allergies	**Resp** Inspect for respiratory rate and signs of distress Palpate and percuss chest if indicated Auscultate all lung fields **CVS** Inspect for distress, cyanosis (central and peripheral) and clubbing Palpate chest for thrills, heaves and peripheral pulses, comparing brachial and femoral Auscultate heart (features of pathologic murmurs: >3/6, pansystolic or continuous, associated with fixed, split or single S2; features of innocent murmurs: soft, SEM, changing with position)
FHx Childhood diseases, infant deaths, genetic abnormalities Age, health, and occupation of parents	**GU** Age appropriate exam for boys and girls Inspect genitalia of boys for urethral opening, descended testes Avoid vaginal exam unless absolutely necessary Tanner staging for pubertal syndromes
	GI Inspect abdomen – distension, scars Percuss and palpate for tenderness, masses, hepatosplenomegaly Auscultate for bowel sounds
	MSK Look, feel, and move all joints, spine Examine spine for scoliosis, spina bifida occulta Examine hips in babies: Barlow and Ortolani test

PEDIATRIC HISTORY AND PHYSICAL EXAM (continued)

History	Physical Exam
SHx Inhabitants at home, daycare, CAS involvement, abuse HEADSS screen for adolescents (Home, Education, Activities, Drugs, Sexuality, Suicide)	**CNS** Age appropriate exam for higher cortical function and development, cranial nerves, power, tone, reflexes, sensory, and cerebellar function **Derm** Full body inspection for rashes, bruises, café-au-lait spots, neurofibromas and hemangiomas

VITALS: RANGE BY AGE GROUP

Age	Pulse (bpm)	Resp. Rate (br/min)	sBP (mmHg)
Neonate	90 – 170	40 – 60	70 – 90
3-12 months	80 – 165	30 – 55	80 – 100
1-2 yrs	80 – 125	25 – 45	90 – 100
3-11 yrs	70 – 115	18 – 30	100 – 110
12-15 yrs	60 – 100	12 – 18	110 – 130

NEONATAL PHYSICAL EXAM

Physical Exam	
General Impression	Appears well/ill/septic, level of consciousness, size, colour, hydration Deformities or dysmorphic features Vitals, height, weight, head circumference
H&N	Head: size, shape, fontanelles, caput secundum ("cone head" from blood above periosteum, crosses suture lines) or cephalohematoma (subperiosteal blood, does not cross suture lines) Eyes: red reflex, conjunctivitis Ears and nose: size, shape, position – note any facial deformities Cleft lip and palate Neck: congenital neck masses, cystic hygroma, thyroglossal duct cysts
Resp	Inspect for respiratory rate and signs of distress Auscultate all lung fields
CVS	Inspect for distress, cyanosis (central and peripheral) Palpate chest for thrills, heaves and peripheral pulses Auscultate heart (features of pathologic murmurs: >3/6, pansystolic or continuous, associated with fixed, split or single S2; features of innocent murmurs: soft, SEM, changing with position)
GU	Males – cryptorchidism, hypospadias, scrotal hernia Females – look for ambiguous genitalia (agglutination of labia majora and/or minora)
GI	Inspect abdomen – size, shape, masses, skin changes Herniations – gastroschisis (herniated intestine with no covering sac), omphalocele (herniated bowel, stomach, and spleen covered with peritoneum), umbilical hernia Percuss and palpate for tenderness, masses, hepatosplenomegaly Auscultate for bowel sounds Anus – imperforate or prolapsed Examine spine for continuity and curvature
MSK	Barlow test – with the infant supine, stabilize the pelvis, flex knees, flex and slightly adduct the hips, and apply posterior pressure; positive if unstable or posteriorly dislocatable hip(s) Ortolani test – with patient supine, flex the knees and hips, abduct the hips and apply anterior pressure; positive if audible and palpable "clunk" indicating relocation of the hip(s)

NEONATAL PHYSICAL EXAM (continued)

Physical Exam	
CNS	Movements – symmetric bilaterally, non-choreic Tone – flaccid paralysis, hyperreflexive Power, deep tendon reflexes, primitive reflexes
Primitive Reflexes	Galant's – with the baby prone, stroke the back 1cm from midline; the trunk should curve toward the stroked side Placing – with the baby upright, gently touch the top of the foot to the table edge; the child will mimic walking on the table Rooting – stroke the baby's cheek and they will turn their head to the stroked side Palmar grasp – place a finger into the ulnar side of the palm and the baby will tightly grasp the finger Moro – startle the baby with loud noise or suddenly lower a supine baby; arms will extend and abduct with hands open and extended fingers, then come together Tonic neck – turn the baby's head to one side; the arm and leg on that side will extend and the opposite side will flex (fencing position)
Derm	Skin changes, rashes, lower back hair tuft or dimple indicating spina bifida occulta

DEVELOPMENTAL MILESTONES

Age	Gross Motor	Fine Motor	Speech and Language	Adaptive and Social Skills
6 wks	Prone – lifts chin intermittently			Social smile
1 month	Reacts to pain		Responds to noise	Looks at faces, makes eye contact
2 months	Prone – arms extended forward	Pulls at clothes	Coos	Recognizes parent
4 months	Prone – raises head and chest, rolls over, no head lag	Reach and grasp, objects to mouth	Responds to voice, laughs, squeals	
6 months	Prone – weight on hands, tripod sit, rolls back to front	Ulnar grasp	Begins to babble, responds to name	Stranger anxiety, beginning of object permanence
9 months	Pulls to stand, crawls	Finger-thumb grasp	"Mama, dada" – imitates 1 word	Separation/stranger anxiety, plays games
12 months	Walks with support	Pincer grasp, throws	2 words with meaning besides "mama, dada", follows 1-step command	Drinks with cup, waves bye-bye
15 months	Walks without support	Draws a line	Jargon	Points to needs
18 months	Up steps with help	Tower of 3 cubes, scribbling	10 words, follows simple commands	Uses spoon, points to body parts
24 months	Up 2 feet/step, runs, kicks ball, walks up and down steps	Tower of 6 cubes, undresses	2-3 words phrases, uses " I, me, you", 50% intelligible	Parallel play, helps to dress
3 yrs	Tricycle, up 1 foot/step and down 2 feet/step, stands on one foot, jumps	Copies a circle and and a cross, puts on shoes	Prepositions, plurals, counts to 10, 75% intelligible	Dress/undress fully except buttons, knows sex and age
4 yrs	Hops on 1 foot, down 1 foot/step	Copies a square, uses scissors	Tells story, knows 4 colours, normal fluency, speech intelligible, uses past tense	Cooperative play, toilet trained, buttons clothes
5 yrs	Skips, rides bicycle	Copies a triangle, prints name, ties shoelaces	Fluent speech, future tense, knows alphabet	
RED FLAGS	Not walking at 18 months	Handedness <10 months	<3 words at 18 months Loss/plateauing of language skills	Not smiling at 3 months

Investigations

AVERAGE BLOOD CHEMISTRY AT VARIOUS AGES

Test	Birth	Preschool	Adolescent
Sodium (mmol/L)	133 – 142	135 – 143	135 – 145
Potassium (mmol/L)	4.5 – 6.5	3.5 – 5.2	3.5 – 5.2
Chloride (mmol/L)	96 – 106	99 – 111	98 – 106
Serum Creatinine (μmol/L)	<441	<44	<106
BUN (mmol/L)	2.9 – 10	1.8 – 5.4	2.9 – 7.1
Glucose (fasting; mmol/L)	>2.5	2.8 – 6.1	3.3 – 6.1
Glucose (fasting; mg/dL)	>45	50 – 110	60 – 110
pH (arterial)	7.30 – 7.40	7.35 – 7.45	7.35 – 7.45
pCO_2 (mmHg)	30 – 50	30 – 42	33 – 46
pO_2 (mmHg)	50 – 60	80 – 100	80 – 100
Bicarbonate (mmol/L)	16 – 22	18 – 24	20 – 28
ALT (U/L)	<60	<40	<40
AST (U/L)	<110	<45	<36

AVERAGE HEMATOLOGICAL LABS AT VARIOUS AGES

Test	2 Days	1 Week	1 Month	1-5 Yrs	6-14 Yrs
Hemoglobin (g/L)	150–250		115–180	110–140	120–160
RBC count ($\times 10^{12}$/L)	3.5–6.0		3.5–5.5	4.0–5.0	4.5–5.5
Reticulocytes ($\times 10^9$/L)	<5.0		<5.0	10.0–100.0	10.0–100.0
WBC ($\times 10^9$/L)	20–40	5–21		5–12	4–10
Polymorphs ($\times 10^9$/L)	6–26	1.5–10		1.5–8.5	1.5–7.5
Bands ($\times 10^9$/L)	0–4.5	0–4.5		0	0
Lymphocytes ($\times 10^9$/L)	2.0–11.0	2.0–11.0		2.0–8.0	1.5–7.0
Platelets ($\times 10^9$/L)	150–450	150–450	150–450	150–450	150–450
INR	0.9–2.7	0.9–2.7	0.8–1.2	0.8–1.2	0.8–1.2
PTT (s)	25–60	25–60	25–60	25–40	25–40
TSH (mU/L)	1–38.9		1.7–9.1	0.7–6.4	0.7–6.4

Immunizations

- In Canada, each province and territory has an individual immunization schedule. This is a general guide based on recommendations from the National Advisory Council on Immunization (NACI)

General Principles of Immunization
- Two live vaccines (varicella, MMR) must be given either at the same visit or separated by 4 wks or more
- Refer to catch-up schedules for children with uncertain vaccination history
- Injection sites: anterolateral thigh if <12 months; deltoid in older children
- Children in high-risk groups (complement deficiency, immunosuppressed, functional or anatomic asplenia, prematurity) will require additional immunizations and may follow different immunization schedules
- Safety of MMR Vaccine: According to the CDC, the weight of current available scientific evidence does not support the hypothesis that MMR vaccine causes either autism or IBD

ROUTINE IMMUNIZATION SCHEDULES

Vaccine	Schedule	Route	Reaction
DTaP-IPV	2, 4, 6, 18 mos 4-6 yrs	IM	At 24-48 hrs Minor: fever, local redness, swelling, irritability Major: prolonged crying (1%), hypotonic unresponsive state (1:1750), seizure (1:1950) on day of vaccine Prophylaxis: acetaminophen 10-15 mg/kg given 4 hrs prior to injection and q4h afterwards
Hib	2, 4, 6, 18 mos	IM	Minor: fever, local redness, swelling, irritability
Pneu-C-13	2, 4, 12 mos	IM	Minor: fever, local redness, swelling, irritability
Rot-1	2, 4 mos or 4, 6 mos	PO	Minor: fever, cough, diarrhea, vomiting and irritability
MMR*	12, 18 mos	SC	At 7-14 d Fever, measle-like rash, lymphadenopathy, arthralgia, arthritis, parotitis (rare)
Men-C-C	12 mos	IM	Redness/swelling (<50%), fever (9%), irritability (<80%), rash (0.1%)
Var*	15 mos	SC	Mild local reaction (20% but higher in immunocompromised) Mild varicella-like papules or vesicles (5%) Low-grade fever (15%)
Hep B	3 doses: 0, 1, 6 mos; given in some provinces in grade 7 Given at birth if at increased risk i.e. from endemic country, given with HBIg if mother HBsAg +ve)	IM	Local redness, swelling
MMRV	4-6 yrs	SC	See above MMRV and Var
dTap	Start at 14-16 yrs	IM	Anaphylaxis (very rare)
Td	Adult yrs, q10 yrs	IM	Local erythema and swelling (70%)

ROUTINE IMMUNIZATION SCHEDULES (continued)

Vaccine	Schedule	Route	Reaction
Flu**	Start at 6-23 mos, every autumn	IM	Local tenderness at injection site Fever, malaise, myalgia, rash, febrile seizures Hypersensitivity reactions
Gardasil®	3 doses 0, 2, 6 mos for females between 9-26 (given in some provinces in grades 7 or 8)	IM	Local tenderness, redness, itching, swelling at injection site, fever

DTaP – IPV – diptheria, tetanus, acellular pertussis, inactivated polio vaccine (for children under 7 yrs)
MMR – measles, mumps, rubella
Hib – Hemophilus influenzae type b conjugate vaccine
Men-C – meningococcal C conjugate vaccine
Hep B – Hepatitis B vaccine
Flu – influenza vaccine
Flu – influenza vaccine

Vaccine/Pneu-C – pneumococcal 7-valent conjugate vaccine
Var – varicella vaccine
dTap – diphtheria, tetanus, acellular pertussis vaccine
(adolescent/adult formulation)
Td – tetanus and diphtheria adult type formulation
HPV – human papilloma virus vaccine

*If varicella vaccine and MMR vaccine not given during the same visit, they must be administered at least 28 d apart.
**For children with severe or chronic disease, e.g. cardiac, pulmonary, or renal disease, sickle cell disease, diabetes, endocrine disorders, HIV, immunosuppressed, long-term aspirin therapy, or those who visit residents of chronic care facilities
Adapted from: National Advisory Committee on Immunization. *Recommended Immunization Schedule for Infants, Children and Youth* (updated March 2005)

Common Presentations

Dehydration

ASSESSMENT OF DEHYDRATION

	Mild Dehydration	Moderate Dehydration	Severe Dehydration
Heart rate*	Normal	Rapid	Rapid and weak
Blood pressure	Normal	Normal-low	Shock
Urine output*	Decreased	Markedly decreased	Anuria
Oral mucosa*	Slightly dry	Dry	Parched
Anterior fontanelle	Normal	Sunken	Markedly sunken
Eyes	Normal	Sunken	Markedly sunken
Skin turgor	Normal	Decreased	Tenting
Capillary refill*	<3 sec		>3 sec
Weight loss (age <2)*	5%	10%	15%
Weight loss (age >2)*	3%	6%	9%

Assessment	Method
Volume deficit	History and physical examination
Osmolar disturbance	Serum Na^+
Acid-base disturbance	Blood pH, pCO_2, bicarbonate
Potassium	Serum K^+
Renal function	BUN, creatinine, urine specific gravity/sediment

* Better, earlier predictors of dehydration

Principles of Fluid and Electrolyte Therapy
- Maintenance of daily fluid and electrolyte requirements PLUS replacement of fluid and electrolyte deficit PLUS replacement of ongoing losses

MAINTENANCE FLUID REQUIREMENTS

Body Weight	100:50:20 Rule	4:2:1 Rule
1-10 kg	100 cc/kg/d	4 cc/kg/h
11-20 kg	50 cc/kg/d	2 cc/kg/h
>20 kg	20 cc/kg/d	1 cc/kg/h

Management
- Maintenance Electrolyte Requirements
  - Na^+: 3 mEq/kg/d
  - K^+: 2 mEq/kg/d
  - Cl^-: 3 mEq/kg/d
  - Give ½ of deficit therapy + maintenance over first 8 h
  - Give remaining ½ of deficit + maintenance over next 16 h
- Common IV Fluids
  - First month of life: D5W/0.2 NS + 20 mEq KCl/L (only add KCl if voiding well)
  - Children: D5W/0.9 NS + 20 mEq KCl/L or D5W/0.45 NS + 20 mEq KCl/L
  - NS: as bolus to restore circulation in dehydrated children (10-40 ml/kg over 30-60 min)

Normal Growth

AVERAGE GROWTH PARAMETERS

	Normal	Growth	Comments
Birth Weight	3.25 kg (7 lbs)	2 x birth wt by 4-5 months 3 x birth wt by 1 yr 4 x birth wt by 2 yrs	Wt. loss (up to 10% of birth wt) in first 7 d of life is normal Neonate should regain wt by ~14 d of age
Length/Height	50 cm (20 in)	25 cm in 1st yr 12 cm in 2nd yr 8 cm in 3rd yr then 4-7 cm/yr until puberty 1/2 adult height at 2 yrs	Measure supine length until 2 yrs of age, then measure standing height
Head Circumference	35 cm (14 in)	2 cm/month for 1st 3 months 1 cm/month at 3-6 months 0.5 cm/month at 6-12 months	Measure around occipital, parietal, and frontal prominences to obtain the greatest circumference

Short Stature

Definition
- Short stature = height <3rd percentile, height crossing 2 major percentile lines, growth velocity <25th percentile

History (4 questions to ask about short stature)
1) Was there IUGR?
2) Is the growth proportionate?
3) Is the growth velocity normal?
4) Is bone age delayed? (differentiate between familial short stature and constitutional delay)

Differential Diagnosis
- Short stature with normal growth velocity

- Familial short stature (most common) – normal bone age, family history of short stature
- Constitutional growth delay – delayed puberty, delayed bone age, often midparental height is normal
- Short stature with decreased growth velocity
  - Primordial (height, weight, and HC affected) – chromosome abnormalities, skeletal dysplasia, IUGR
  - Endocrine (short and fat) – growth hormone deficiency (rare), hypothyroidism, Cushing syndrome, hypopituitarism
  - Chronic disease (short and skinny) – cyanotic heart disease, celiac, IBD, CF, chronic infections, chronic renal failure
  - Psychosocial neglect – improves when the child is removed from their environment

Investigations
- Bone age (anteroposterior x-ray of left hand and wrist)
- Karyotype in girls to r/o Turner syndrome or if dysmorphic features present
- Other tests as indicated by history and physical exam

Management
- Depends on severity of problem as perceived by parents/child
- No treatment for non-pathological short stature
- GH therapy if meets criteria for growth hormone deficiency:
  - GH shown to be deficient by 2 different stimulation tests
  - Insufficient growth velocity, <3rd percentile
  - Bone age x-rays show unfused epiphyses
  - Turner syndrome, Noonan syndrome, chronic renal failure

Failure to Thrive (FTT)

Definition
- Weight <3rd percentile, falls across two major percentile curves, or <80% of expected weight for height and age

Etiology

CAUSES OF FTT

Growth Parameters	Suggestive Abnormality
Decreased weight, normal height, normal HC	Caloric insufficiency, decreased intake, hypermetabolic state, increased losses
Decreased weight, decreased height, normal HC	Structural dystrophies, endocrine disorder, familial short stature, constitutional delay
Decreased weight, decreased height, decreased HC	Intrauterine insult, genetic abnormality

HC = head circumference

Differential Diagnosis
- **Organic FTT**
  - Inability to feed – insufficiency breast milk, GERD, vomiting, neuromuscular, anorexia from chronic disease
  - Inadequate absorption – celiac disease, CF, chronic diarrhea or vomiting
  - Inappropriate utilization of nutrients – renal loss, inborn errors of metabolism, type 1 diabetes, diabetes insipidus, congenital hypothyroidism, hypopituitarism
  - Increased energy requirements – pulmonary disease (CF), cardiac disease, malignancy, chronic infections, hyperthyroidism, DI, hypopituitarism, SLE
  - Decreased growth potential – genetic syndromes, IUGR, FAS, TORCH infections
- **Non-Organic FTT**
  - Malnutrition, poor feeding techniques, inappropriately prepared formula, emotional deprivation, child abuse
  - These children may have delayed psychomotor, language, and/or social development

- FTT in the first year of life can lead to poor outcomes due to rapid brain growth during this time
- Assess child's temperament, child-parent interaction, feeding behaviour, and parental psychosocial stressors; consider observing child and caregiver during feeding

History
- Duration of problem, growth history
- Dietary and feeding history – inadequate caloric intake most common factor in poor weight gain, may have other nutritional deficiencies (e.g. protein, iron, vitamin D)
- Bowel habits
- Pregnancy, birth, and postpartum history
- Developmental, social, and family history (parental height, weight, growth pattern)

Physical Exam
- Height, weight, head circumference, arm span, upper-to-lower segment ratio
- Nutritional status, dysmorphism, Tanner stage, evidence of chronic disease
- Observation of a feeding session and parent-child interaction
- Signs of abuse or neglect

Investigations: as indicated by clinical presentation
- CBC, blood smear, electrolytes, urea, ESR, T4, TSH, urinalysis
- Bone age x-ray (left wrist – compared to standardized wrist x-rays)
- Karyotype in all short girls and in short boys where appropriate
- Any other tests indicated from history and physical exam: renal or liver function tests, venous blood gases, ferritin, immunoglobulins, sweat chloride, fecal fat

Fever

Approach to the Febrile Child

Common Conditions

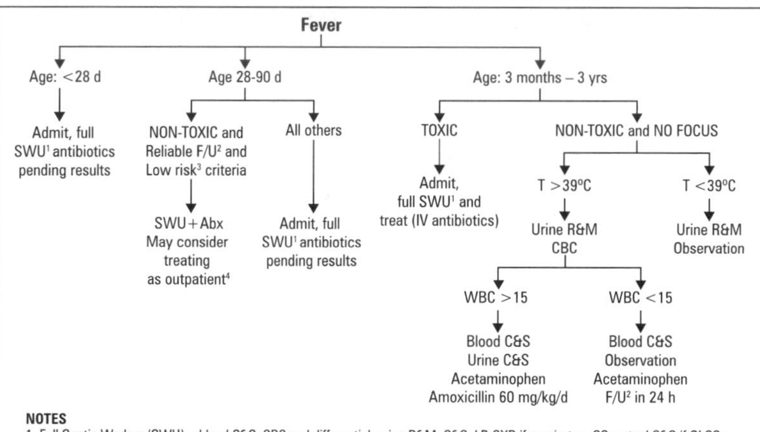

NOTES
1. Full Septic Workup (SWU) – blood C&S, CBC and differential, urine R&M, C&S, LP, CXR if respiratory SSx, stool C&S if GI SSx
2. Follow-up is crucial – if adequate F/U is not assured, a more aggressive diagnostic and therapeutic approach may be indicated
3. Low-Risk (Rochester) Criteria
4. Considerable practice variation exists in terms of empirical Abx treatment
5. Important Principles – the younger the child, the greater the difficulty to clinically assess the degree of illness

Upper Respiratory Tract Diseases

- Disease above the thoracic inlet characterized by inspiratory stridor, hoarseness, and suprasternal retractions

	Croup	Bacterial Tracheitis	Epiglottitis
Epidemiology	6 months to 4 yrs	Any pediatric age group	2-6 yr
Etiology	Parainfluenza (75%), influenza A and B, RSV, adenovirus	*S. aureus* (most common), Hib, α-hemolytic Strep *Pneumococcus*, *Moraxella catarrhalis*	HiB, β-hemolytic Strep
Clinical Presentation	Prodrome of URTI, hoarse voice, barking cough, stridor, worse at night, better with cold air	Initially similar to croup, but then rapid deterioration with high fever, toxic appearance	Toxic appearance, severe airway obstruction, drooling, dysphagia, distress, fever, sore throat, tripod position, sternal croup
Investigations	CXR – "steeple sign" from subglottic narrowing	Endoscopy for tracheal secretions for definitive diagnosis	Avoid examining the throat to prevent further respiratory exacerbation Neck XR – "thumb sign"
Treatment	Humidified O_2; for more severe cases: single-dose dexamethasone, racemic epinephrine 1-3 doses, q1-2h, intubation if unresponsive to treatment	Therapy as with croup, but requires intubation and antibiotics	Requires intubation and antibiotics Prevented with Hib vaccine

Asthma

ASTHMA ASSESSMENT AND MANAGEMENT

Classifications	History and Physical Examination	Management
Respiratory Arrest	Exhausted, confused, diaphoretic, cyanotic	100% O_2, cardiac monitor, IV access
Imminent	Silent chest, ineffective respiratory effort Decreased HR O_2 sat <90% despite supplemental O_2	Intubate β-agonist: MDI 4-8 puffs OR nebulizer 5 mg continually Anticholinergics: MDI 4-8 puffs q20min x 3 OR nebulizer 0.5 mg q20min x 3 IV steroids: methylprednisolone 125 mg, hydrocortisone 500 mg
Severe Asthma	Agitated, diaphoretic, laboured respirations Difficulty speaking in full sentences No relief from β-agonist O_2 sat <90%, FEV_1 <50%	Anticipate need for intubation Similar to above management β-agonist may be less frequent; q15-20min
Moderate Asthma	SOB at rest, cough, congestion, chest tightness Nocturnal symptoms Inadequate relief from β-agonist FEV_1 50-80%	O_2 to achieve O_2-sat >90% β-agonist: puffer of neb q1h Steroids: prednisone 40-60 mg PO Anticholinergics
Mild Asthma	Exertional SOB/cough with some nocturnal symptoms Good response to b-agonist FEV_1 >80%	β-agonist Monitor FEV_1 Consider steroids (nebulized or PO)

Considerations for Hospital Admission

- Previous ICU admission
- Poor response to corticosteroids after 4 h of initiation (i.e. persistent respiratory distress)

- Unable to tolerate inhaled β2-agonists at intervals <4 h
- Pre-treatment SaO_2 <92%
- Poor chronic asthma control, social issues
- Co-morbidities (e.g. co-existent cardiopulmonary disease, severe neuromuscular disease)

Discharge Treatment
- Salbutamol (metered-dose inhaler, 100 µg/puff)
  - Severe presentations: 0.3 puffs/kg/dose q4h prn x first 24 h, then 2-3 puffs q4h x 7 d
  - Mild presentations: 2-3 puffs/kg/dose x 7 d
- Prednisolone
  - 1 mg/kg/d x 4-5 d, followed by: Inhaled fluticasone (Flovent®)
  - 100-150 µg BID x 4-8 wks as prophylaxis

MANAGEMENT OF CHRONIC/PERSISTENT ASTHMA

Non-pharmacological Treatments
- Education + Environmental control

Pharmacological Treatments

Relievers (bronchodilators)	Controllers (anti-inflammatories)
Short-acting β2-agonist (salbutamol, terbutaline) – first line Long-acting β2-agonist (Serevat®, Oxeze®) – only use in conjunction with inhaled corticosteroids	Inhaled corticosteroids – first-line (Flovent®, Pulmicort®) Leukotriene antagonists (Singulair®) Oral corticosteroids (OCS) (Prednisone®) – severe cases

Acute Otitis Media

- See Otolaryngology section for surgical management of acute otitis media

Definitions
- Certain diagnosis: recent, usually abrupt, onset of signs and symptoms of middle ear inflammation and effusion
- Uncertain diagnosis: does not meet above criteria
- Severe illness: moderate to severe otalgia or fever >39°C
- Non-severe illness: mild otalgia and fever <39°C

History
- Otalgia, tugging at ears, otorrhea, decreased hearing
- Irritability, fever, URI symptoms
- Nausea, vomiting, diarrhea
- Risk factors: bottle feeding, passive smoking, daycare, low SES, cleft lip, Down syndrome, previous/recurrent AOM, family history of recurrent OM, prematurity, male gender, siblings in household
- Risk of drug resistance: previous antibiotic therapy in past month, history of AOM, daycare attendance, age 18-24 months, recent hospitalization
- Recurrent AOM – 3 episodes in 6 months or 4 episodes in 1 yr

Treatment of AOM

Age	Certain Diagnosis	Uncertain Diagnosis
<6 months	Antibacterial therapy x 10d	Antibacterial therapy x 10d
6 months to 2 yrs	Antibacterial therapy x 10d	Severe illness: antibacterial therapy x 10d Non-severe illness: observation option
≥2 yrs	Antibacterial therapy if severe illness x 5d; observation option if nonsevere illness	Observation option

Kawasaki Disease

Diagnostic Criteria
* Fever persisting 5 d or more AND 4 of the following features:
    1. Bilateral nonpurulent conjunctivitis
    2. Red fissured lips, strawberry tongue, erythema of oropharynx
    3. Changes of the peripheral extremities
        + Acute phase: erythema, edema of hands and feet
        + Subacute phase: peeling from tips of fingers and toes
    4. Polymorphous rash
    5. Cervical lymphadenopathy >1.5 cm in diameter
* Exclusion of other diseases (e.g. scarlet fever, measles)
* Atypical Kawasaki disease: less than 5 of 6 diagnostic features but coronary artery involvement

Management
* High (anti-inflammatory) dose of ASA while febrile
* Low (anti-platelet) dose of ASA in subacute phase until platelets normalize or longer if coronary artery involvement
* IV immunoglobulin (2 g/kg) preferably within 10 d of onset reduces risk of coronary aneurysm formation
* Baseline 2D-echo and follow up periodic 2D-echocardiograms (usually at 6 wks)

Limb/Joint Pain

Differential Diagnosis of Limb/Joint Pain

Investigations
* CBC, differential, blood smear, ESR
* X-rays of painful joints/limbs
* As indicated: blood C&S, ANA, RF, PTT, sickle cell prep, viral serology, immunoglobulins, complement, urinalysis, synovial analysis and culture, TB test, ASOT, slit lamp

Limb/Joint Pain

Cause	<3 yrs	3-10 yrs	>10 yrs
Trauma	X	X	X
Infectious			
Septic arthritis	X	X	X
Osteomyelitis	X	X	X
Inflammatory			
Transient synovitis	X	X	
JIA	X	X	X
Seronegative spondyloarthropathy		X	
SLE			X
Dermatomyositis			X
HSP		X	
Anatomic/Orthopedic			
Legg-Calve-Perthes disease		X	X
Slipped capital femoral epiphysis		X	
Osgood-Schlatter disease			X

Limb/Joint Pain (continued)

Cause	<3 yrs	3-10 yrs	>10 yrs
Trauma	X	X	X
Neoplastic			
Leukemia	X	X	X
Neuroblastoma	X	X	X
Bone tumour		X	X
Hematologic			
Hemophilia (hemarthosis)	X	X	X
Sickle cell anemia	X	X	X
Pain Syndromes			
Growing pains		X	X
Fibromyalgia			X
Reflex sympathetic dystrophy			X

Neonatology

Neonatal Resuscitation

Apgar Scores

Sign	0	1	2
Heart Rate	Absent	<100/min	>100/min
Respiratory Effort	Absent	Slow, irregular	Good, crying
Irritability	No response	Grimace	Cough/cry
Tone	Limp	Some flexion of extremities	Active motion
Colour	Blue, pale	Body pink, extremities blue	Completely pink

*Assess at 1 and 5 mins, if <7 at 5 min reassess q5min until >7; do not wait to assign Apgar score before initiating resuscitation

Neonatal Jaundice

CAUSES OF JAUNDICE BY AGE

<24 h	24-72 h	72-96 h	Prolonged (>1 wk)

ALWAYS PATHOLOGIC
Hemolytic
  Rh or AB
  incompatibility
Sepsis
  GBS
  Congenital infection
  (TORCH)
	Physiologic, polycythemia
	Dehydration (breastfeeding jaundice)
	Hemolysis
	  G6PD deficiency
	  Pyruvate kinase deficiency
	  Spherocytosis
	  Bruising, hemorrhage, hematoma
	Sepsis/congenital infection
		Physiologic ±
		breast feeding
		Sepsis
			Breast milk jaundice
			Prolonged physiologic jaundice in preterm
			Hypothyroidism
			Neonatal hepatitis
			Conjugation dysfunction
			  e.g. Gilbert syndrome, Crigler-Najjar syndrome
			Inborn errors of metabolism
			  e.g. galactosemia
			Biliary tract obstruction
			  e.g. biliary atresia

Common Infections

SUMMARY OF COMMON PEDIATRIC INFECTIONS

Infection	Important Signs and Symptoms	Causative Organisms	Treatment (1st and 2nd line)
Otitis media	Otalgia, decreased hearing, bulging tympanic membrane	*S. pneumoniae, H. influenzae, Moraxella catarrhalis*	Amoxicillin High-dose amoxicillin OR clavulin
Meningitis (neonate)	Sepsis, vomiting, bulging fontanelle, lethargy, irritability	GBS, *E. coli, Listeria*, Gram negative bacilli	Ampicillin + cefotaxime + vancomycin
Meningitis (1-3 months)	Sepsis, vomiting, bulging fontanelle, lethargy, irritability	Same pathogens as above and below	Ampicillin + cefotaxime + vancomycin
Meningitis (>3 months)	Toxic-looking, neck stiffness, vomiting, photophobia (rash in meningococcemia)	*S. pneumococcus, N. meningitidis, H. influenzae* type b (>5 y.o.)	Ceftriaxone + vancomycin
Streptococcal Pharyngitis	Sore throat with no cough, cervical lymphadenopathy	Group A β-hemolytic strep	Penicillin OR amoxicillin (erythromycin if penicillin allergy)
UTI	Dysuria, frequency, hematuria	*E. coli, Klebsiella, Proteus, H. influenzae, Pseudomonas, S. saprophyticus, Enterococcus*, GBS	Uncomplicated: oral cephalexin, cefixime Complicated (neonate, immunocompromised, vomiting): IV ampicillin+ gentamycin, or 3rd/4th generation cephalosporin (cefotaxime, ceftriaxone, cefepime)
Pneumonia (neonate)	Fever and dyspnea	GBS, GN bacilli (*E. coli*), *C. trachomatis, S. aureus, Listeria*	Ampicillin + gentamycin, add erythromycin if Chlamydia suspected
Pneumonia (1-3 months)	Fever and dyspnea	*S. pneumoniae, C. trachomatis, B. pertussis, S. aureus, H. influenzae*	Cefuroxime + macrolide (erythromycin) OR ampicillin + macrolide
Pneumonia (3 months-5 yrs)	Fever and dyspnea	*S. pneumoniae, S. aureus, H. influenzae, Mycoplasma*	Ampicillin/amoxicillin OR cefuroxime or clavulin
Pneumonia (>5 yrs)	Fever and dyspnea	*S. pneumoniae, S. aureus, H. influenzae, Mycoplasma*	Macrolide (1st line) OR cefuroxime OR ampicillin/amoxicillin OR clavulin
Infectious Mononucleosis	"The great imitator" – non-specific symptoms (sore throat, lymphadenopathy, arthritis, hepatitis, rash)	EBV	Supportive
Chickenpox	Fever and respiratory symptoms, characteristic rash	VZV/HHV3	Supportive – do NOT use ASA due to risk of Reye syndrome Acyclovir (for severe disease, immunocompromised patients, neonates)
Roseola	High fever with rash after the fever resolves	HHV-6	Supportive (acetaminophen)
Erythema infectiosum	Flu-like illness followed by "slapped-cheek" rash	Parvovirus B-19	Supportive; transfusion if aplastic crisis develops

Plastic Surgery

Diagrams and Terminology

Diagrams

Carpal Bone Mnemonic
(in order: proximal then distal row, radial to ulnar side)
Some – scaphoid
Lovers – lunate
Try – triquetrum
Positions – pisiform
That – trapezium
They – trapezoid
Cannot – capitate
Handle – hamate

Carpal Bones

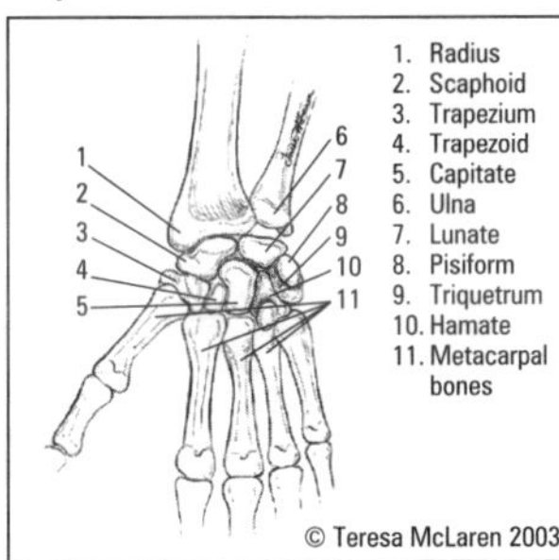

© Teresa McLaren 2003

Sensory Distribution in the Hand

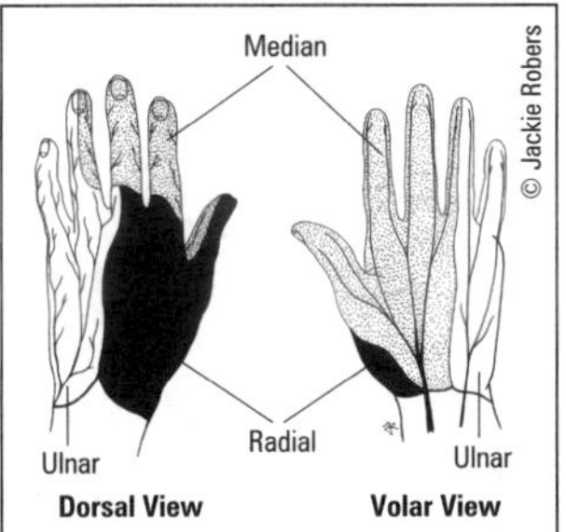

Testing Profundus (FDP)

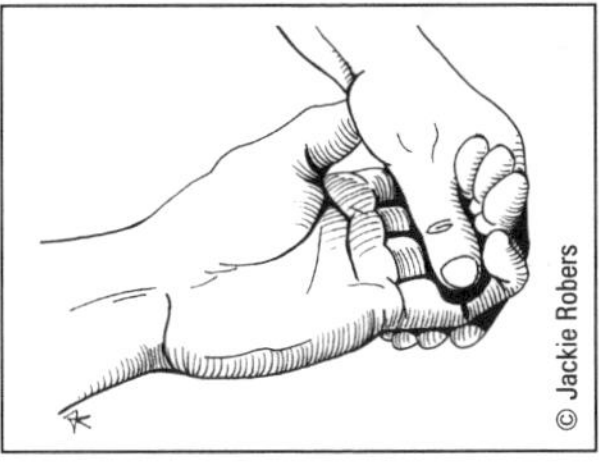

Testing Superficialis (FDS)

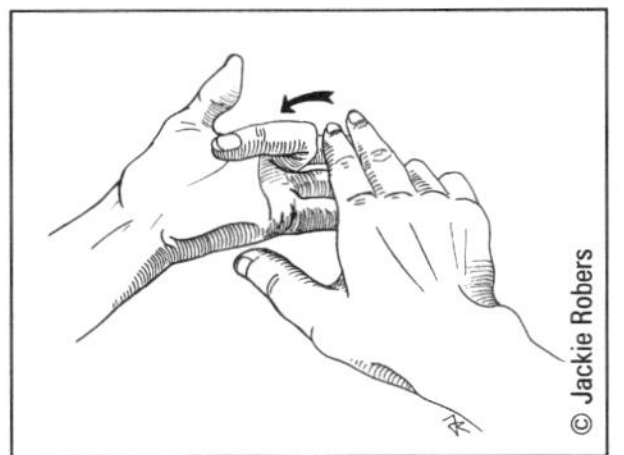

Extensor Compartments of the Wrist (dorsal view and cross-sectional view)

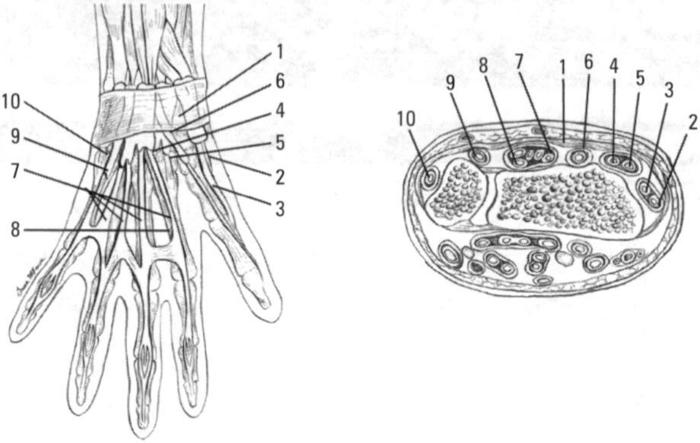

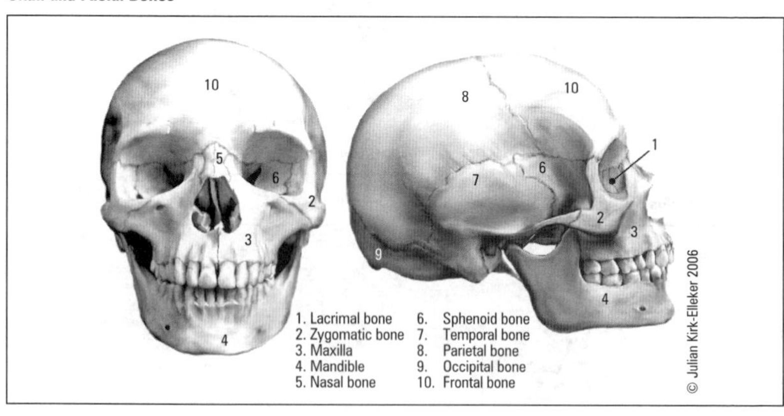

1. Extensor retinaculum

Compartment 1
2. Abductor pollicis longus
3. Extensor pollicis brevis

Compartment 2
4. Extensor carpi radialis brevis
5. Extensor carpi radialis longus

Compartment 3
6. Extensor pollicis longus
   (EPL tendon passes around Lister's tubercle)

Compartment 4
7. Extensor digitorum
8. Extensor indicis

Compartment 5
9. Extensor digiti minimi

Compartment 6
10. Extensor carpi ulnaris

Skull and Facial Bones

1. Lacrimal bone
2. Zygomatic bone
3. Maxilla
4. Mandible
5. Nasal bone
6. Sphenoid bone
7. Temporal bone
8. Parietal bone
9. Occipital bone
10. Frontal bone

© Julian Kirk-Elleker 2006

Terminology

BASIC SUTURE METHODS

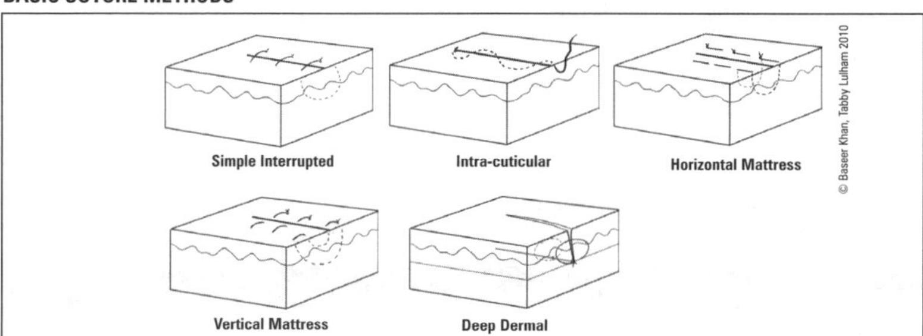

WOUND CLOSURE

- **Primary Closure (1st intention):** wound closure by direct approximation of edges within hours of wound creation (sutures, staples, skin graft, etc.)
  Indication: recent (<6 h), clean wounds
- **Secondary Closure/Spontaneous Healing (2nd intention):** wound closure left to heal spontaneously
  - Indication: when primary wound closure not indicated, such as animal/human bites, crush injuries, infection, long time lapse since injury, retained foreign body
- **Tertiary Closure/Delayed Primary Closure (3rd intention):** intentionally interrupting the healing process (e.g. with packing) then wound is closed 4-10 d post-injury after granulation tissue has formed
  - Indication: contamination, long time lapse since initial injury, severe crush component with significant tissue devitalization

PHASES OF WOUND HEALING

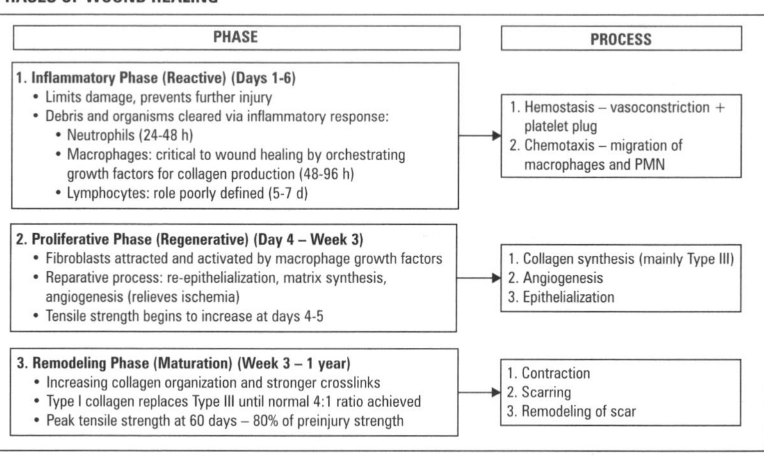

PHASE	PROCESS

1. Inflammatory Phase (Reactive) (Days 1-6)
• Limits damage, prevents further injury
• Debris and organisms cleared via inflammatory response:
  • Neutrophils (24-48 h)
  • Macrophages: critical to wound healing by orchestrating growth factors for collagen production (48-96 h)
  • Lymphocytes: role poorly defined (5-7 d)
	1. Hemostasis – vasoconstriction + platelet plug
	2. Chemotaxis – migration of macrophages and PMN

2. Proliferative Phase (Regenerative) (Day 4 – Week 3) • Fibroblasts attracted and activated by macrophage growth factors • Reparative process: re-epithelialization, matrix synthesis, angiogenesis (relieves ischemia) • Tensile strength begins to increase at days 4-5	1. Collagen synthesis (mainly Type III) 2. Angiogenesis 3. Epithelialization
3. Remodeling Phase (Maturation) (Week 3 – 1 year) • Increasing collagen organization and stronger crosslinks • Type I collagen replaces Type III until normal 4:1 ratio achieved • Peak tensile strength at 60 days – 80% of preinjury strength	1. Contraction 2. Scarring 3. Remodeling of scar

ABNORMAL WOUND HEALING
- **Hypertrophic Scar**
  - Scar remains roughly within the bounds of the initial injury
  - Red, raised, widened, frequently pruritic
  - Back, shoulder, sternum
- **Keloid Scar**
  - Scar extends beyond the boundaries of the initial injury
  - Pruritic, painful, collagen in whirls, more often in those with darker skin
  - Sternum, deltoid, earlobe
- **Chronic Wound**
  - Fails to heal within 6 wks
  - Diabetic, pressure and venous stasis ulcers
  - Marjolin's ulcer = squamous cell carcinoma arising in a chronic wound

Common Presentations

Non-Healing Wound

Differential Diagnosis
- Diabetic, arterial or venous ulcer
- Pressure ulcer
- Edema (compartment syndrome release)
- Loss of tissue (trauma, surgery)
- Malignancy (basal, squamous cell carcinoma; also metastases such as renal cell carcinoma)

History
- Mechanism, location, size
- Length of time open (chronic >6 wks)
- Factors impairing healing
  - Local factors – arterial insufficiency, venous insufficiency, edema, infection, pressure, radiation, foreign body, necrosis
  - Systemic factors – diabetes, malnutrition, vitamin deficiency, chemotherapy, smoking, advanced age, drug use
  - Ischemia – Reperfusion injury
- Assess risk of infection (mechanism, post-wound contamination, for operative wounds – breaks in sterile technique, contact with GI, GU or resp tracts)
- Treatment to date

Physical Exam
- Vitals – febrile?
- Inspection – erythema (blanchable vs. non-blanchable), purulent discharge, foul odour, edema, swelling, wound breakdown, friable granulation tissue
- Palpation – peripheral pulses, warmth, tenderness
- Special tests: e.g. ankle-brachial index

MANAGEMENT

ER
- Labs: routine medicine labs
- Swab the wound and take biopsy if necessary
- Consider consults – Plastic Surgery, Infectious Disease (if infection suspected), Wound Care

Inpatient
- Investigations:
  - Blood cultures, wound cultures (biopsy if possible, or swab)
  - If unusual, biopsy to rule out malignancy
- Special tests:
  - Doppler U/S
  - Transcutaneous O_2 pressure
  - Angiography – if vascular penetration suspected
- Treatment:
  - Risk factor modification
  - Pressure ulcer: prevention, relieve pressure, skin care, debridement of necrotic tissue, surgical intervention for complicated ulcers
  - Venous ulcer: leg elevation, compression therapy, may require moist dressings
  - Arterial ulcers: rest, no elevation/compression, moist dressings, vascular sugery consult, revascularization, debridement after vascular assessment, pain control

Outpatient
- Home-care nurse
  - Moist, not sopping wet
  - In contact with full wound but not surrounding tissue
  - Use gauze for packing – nothing with fillers like ABD pads
- Switch to moist wound dressings when wound bed is clean and granulation tissue present

Management Principles
1. Optimize healing (control systemic factors)
2. Debridement (when necessary)
   - Surgical
     - Uses scalpel/scissors
     - Indications: grossly infected wounds, presence of necrotic tissues
   - Mechanical
     - Uses irrigation or dressing changes (see wound care products below)
     - Indications: locally infected wounds, presence of necrotic tissue
     - Can interfere with healing in wounds that are clean with pink granulation tissue
   - Enzymatic (available in US)
3. Antimicrobials
   - Topical
     - Avoids development of resistance
     - Avoid common allergens (neomycin)
     - Silver compounds are favoured by some
   - Systemic antimicrobials
     - Appropriate if signs of systemic infection, or surrounding cellulitis
     - May also continue topical therapy as systemic antibiotics will not penetrate to necrotic tissue (which requires debridement)

Local Bacterial Load Reduction	Improves Epithelialization
1. Bacteriocidal Products containing iodized silver: ACTICOAT®, Aquacel Ag® Cadexamer Iodine: Iodosorb®, Iodoform Chlorhexidine: Bactigras®	**1. Moisture Balance** Foams: Allevyn® Hydrofibres: Aquacel® Alginates: Algisite® Hydrocolloids: CombiDERM® Films: Tegaderm® Gels: Intrasite®
2. Bacteriostatic Antibiotic creams/ointments Fusidic acid, Flamazine®, Bactigras®	

Helpful Hints
- Wound bed preparation – includes decreasing bacterial load, managing exudate, removing necrotic/fibrous tissue, maintaining adequate moisture, manage wound edge to facilitate reepithelialization
- Pressure ulcers – susceptible to fecal contamination (mixed aerobic and anaerobic)
- Venous ulcers – polymicrobial, often *S. aureus*, often heavily colonized but rarely infected
- Diabetic foot – polymicrobial, often *S. aureus* + anaerobes, increased susceptibility to infection

Complications
- Infection (cellulitis, osteomyelitis, necrotizing soft tissue infection, MSK infection)
- Malignant degeneration of chronic wound (classically squamous cell from old burn or trauma)
- Amputation

Burns

Burn Classification

BURN DEPTH	Layers	Erythema	Blanching	Sensation	Other Features Changes
First degree	Epidermis	+	+	Tender	
Second degree (superficial)	Epidermis and upper dermis	+	+	Painful	Blisters, hair follicle present
Second degree (deep)	Epidermis and deep dermis	+	–	± pain	Some hair
Third degree	Full thickness	Leathery eschar	–	Numb	No hair
Fourth degree	Underlying	Leathery eschar – exposed structures	–	Numb muscle, bone	No hair

BURN SIZE
- Burn size is quoted with respect to percent of Total Body Surface Area (TBSA) affected by second or third degree burns
- Can be estimated by the Rule of 9's in adults, TBSA involved for a given patient is a sum of the % TBSA for each patch of burns that one patient sustains
- For patchy burns, the size of the patient's palm is approximately 1% TBSA
- Use a Lund-Browder chart in children to estimate burn size

Rule of 9's for Total Body Surface Area (TBSA)

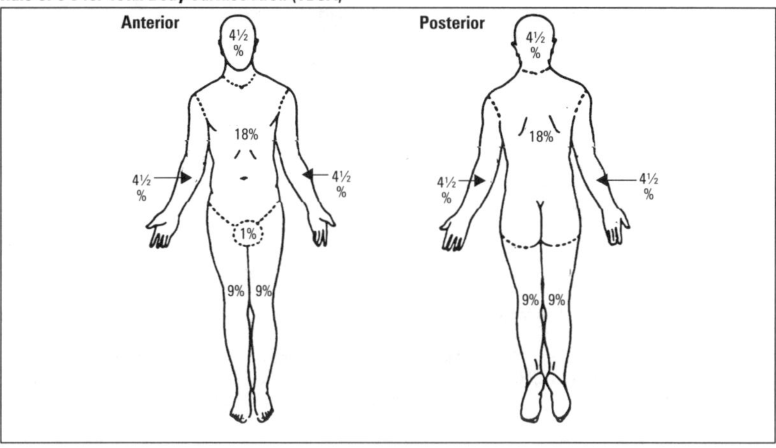

Lund-Browder Diagram

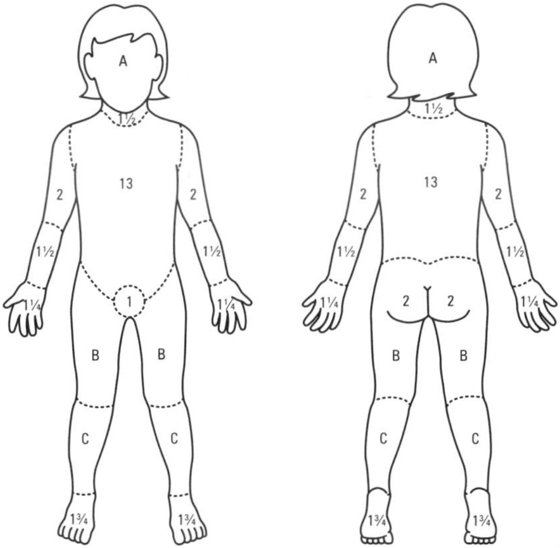

Area	Age 0	Age 1	Age 5	Age 10	Age 15	Adult
A = ½ head area	9 ½	8 ½	6 ½	5 ½	4 ½	3 ½
B = ½ thigh area	2 ¾	3 ¼	4 ¼	4 ¼	4 ½	4 ¾
C = ½ leg area	2 ½	2 ½	3	3	3 ¼	3 ½

CRITERIA FOR ADMISSION TO A BURN CENTRE
- 2° and 3° burns greater than 10% TBSA in patients aged under 10 or over 50
- 2° and 3° burns greater than 20% TBSA in any age group
- 2° and 3° burns threatening functional or cosmetic impairment (e.g. face, hands, genitalia, perineum, major joints)
- 3° burns greater than 5% TBSA in any age group
- Electrical burns
- Pediatric burn
- Chemical burns threatening functional or cosmetic impairment
- Inhalational injury
- Burns associated with major trauma

GENERAL MANAGEMENT
1. Follow general ATLS protocol with following special precautions in burns
2. 100% O_2 by face mask: to treat potential carbon monoxide poisoning
3. Intubation may be required for facial burns involving inhalation injury, >40% TBSA burns, or smoke inhalation injury
4. Assess for circumferential chest burns which may require escharotomy for respiratory distress
5. Circulation: 2 large bore IV's of Ringer's Lactate (RL) high rate over the first hour as assessment is done
6. Assess limbs for potential circumferential burns which require escharotomy to allow circulation to periphery
7. Assess burn depth and size
8. Estimate 1° vs 2°/3° vs. 4° in order to be able to determine the TBSA burns
9. Calculate burn size (rule of 9's)
10. Calculate fluid requirement using Parkland formula:
    - Over the first 24 h; give IV RL 4cc/kg/%TBSA
    - Divide total required over first 24 h with 1/2 given in 1st 8 h and 1/2 given in next 16 h
    - May require more fluid if >80% TBSA burns, 4° burns, associated traumatic injury, electrical burn, inhalation injury, delayed start of resuscitation, pediatric burns)
11. Monitor resuscitation via U/O (30-55 cc/h), MAP >70, clear sensorium, pulse <120, HCO_3 >18 mEq/L, CO >3.1 L/m^2
12. Burn excision (tangential excision) and would closure (autograft, allograft, xenograft, skin substitutes, cultured epithelial cells)

For a patient requiring admission to a Burn Unit (e.g. with TBSA >30%):
- General orders: do not apply to all patients and must be considered in context of burn size and degree, age of patients, presence of inhalational injury, etc.
1. Admit to Burn Centre under Dr. X
2. Activity: depending on location of burns: keep burned areas elevated
3. VSR q15min or continuous, temperature q2h
4. Check extremity circulation q30 min
5. Foley to closed drainage; closely monitor output
6. Ins and outs – call MD if U/O <30 cc/h
7. 100% O_2 by face mask ± intubation depending on the patient
8. NPO
9. NG to low suction
10. Group and Screen, cross-match 2 U pRBC, CBC, Electrolytes, Cr, BUN, Carboxyhemoglobin levels, ABG, U/A, CXR, ECG
11. Tetanus toxoid 0.5 cc IM
12. IV RL as per Parkland formula (above) for 1st 24 h then 0.35-0.5 cc plasma/kg/%TBSA then D5W to maintain normal serum Na^+
13. Cleanse, dress wounds and apply topical antibacterials (e.g. Flamazine)
14. Splint extremities as per PT if limbs involved

Hand Complaint

Differential Diagnosis
- Trauma (dislocations, fractures, sprain, lacerations)
- Arthritis (osteo vs. rheumatoid)
- Trigger finger, mallet finger, tendon cyst, Dupuytren's contracture, carpal tunnel syndrome
- Vascular, tumour, etc.

History
- OPQRST
- Age, hand dominance, occupation/hobbies
- Mechanism of injury (if traumatic e.g. crush, laceration, forced flexion/extension)
- Pain, stiffness, bony enlargement, range of motion, effect on function
- Other affected joints
- Neurological symptoms – numbness, tingling

Risk Factors/Predisposing/Precipitants
- Previous hand injury/surgery/infections
- Trauma: hazardous line of work/hobbies (farming, sports, construction, power tools)
- Arthritis: previously diagnosed autoimmune problems (SLE, psoriasis, IBD)
- Other: DM, pregnancy

Physical Exam
- Inspection – **S**welling, **E**rythema, **A**trophy, **D**eformity, **S**kin Changes
- Palpation
  - Assess joint stability – anterior, posterior, radial and ulnar stress to each IP and MCP joint in extension and flexion
  - Palpate all flexor tendons and palmar fascia, as well as over ulnar collateral ligament of the thumb (in 1st webspace over MCP, r/o gamekeeper's thumb)
- Active ROM – flexion and extension motion at each joint
  - For thumb include abduction, adduction and opposition
- Always check passive range of motion unless you suspect tendon injury
- Neurological
  - Power – grip and pinch strength
  - Sensation – inspect for areas of dryness (loss of sympathetic innervation); 2-point discrimination on palm/dorsum (compare to uninjured side); if unreliable history, can use immersion test – 5 min soaking in water (denervated skin wrinkles more)
- Circulation
  - Colour cap refill
  - Allen test – compress radial and ulnar artery, open and close hand, then release radial artery – normal is <5s refill; repeat with ulnar artery

MANAGEMENT

ER
- ABCs
- Assess for other injuries
- Consider tetanus immune status
- Immediate treatment required for: vascular injury causing hemorrhage or compromising perfusion, compartment syndrome, amputation with potential for replant, chemical burns (hydrofluoric acid), high pressure injuries
- For lacerations, first do full neurologic exam. Can then use local digital block. Begin with copious irrigation, then explore for foreign bodies, suture skin (if <6-8 h after injury and if "clean" wound; otherwise, use sterile dressing and recheck in 2-4 d with consideration for delayed primary closure)

- Bites are considered infected – do not close primarily and give antibiotics (esp. for human or cat bites)
- If suspected infection, consider clavulin 500 mg PO q8h or clindamycin 300 mg PO q6h + ciprofloxacin 500 mg PO q12h
- Dislocations: PIP + DIP may be reduced in the ER, MCP may be attempted, but often unsuccessful, immobilize after reduction
- Extensor tendon injury: partial tendon injury often do not require repair; close skin, splint, f/u with hand surgeon
- Flexor tendon injury: forms adhesions; **do not attempt repair – should be done in OR**
- Consults: hand surgeon (typically plastics or orthopedics)
- Emergent: vascular compromise
- Urgent: MCP dislocation (if cannot relocate), failed DIP reduction, finger requiring revascularization/ replacement
- Non-urgent: sprain, extensor tendon injury, flexor tendon injury, disrupted nerve

Inpatient
- Management depends on magnitude of problem, and etiology, as above

Outpatient
- Most hand surgery can be done on a short stay or outpatient basis. For replants or reconstructions using free flaps, several days admission may be necessary to monitor vascularity of flap/replanted part

Helpful Hints
- Superficial location predisposes tendons to injury from superficial lacerations, crushes and burns

Complications
- Tendon, ligament or nerve injury – pain/stiffness, loss of function
- Vascular compromise – loss of digit/hand (rare)
- Infection (abscess)
- Foreign body

Wrist Pain

Differential Diagnosis

Bony	Ligamentous	Tendonous	Neurologic
Fracture	Triangular fibrocartilage complex (TFCC) tear	Tendonitis (esp. with repetitive use)	Carpal tunnel syndrome
Osteoarthritis	Distal radioulnar joint (DRUJ)		Schwanomma
Rheumatoid arthritis	Instability	Stenosing tenosinovitis	Neuroma
Osteoma	Other intercarpal ligamentous injuries, e.g.		Intersection syndrome
Tumour	scapholunate ligament		
Keinbock's disease			

History
- OPQRST
- Trauma, association with repetitive motions or overuse
- Stiffness, range of motion
- Other affected joints, neurological status
- Constitutional symptoms – fever, weight loss, fatigue

Physical Examination
- Always start with non-affected side and then compare both sides
- Inspection – **S**welling, **E**rythema, **A**trophy, **D**eformity, **S**kin changes (SEADS)
- Palpation – note point of maximal tenderness, underlying masses or nodules
- Active range of motion – extension, flexion, radial deviation, ulnar deviation
- Check passive range of motion

- Neurological – check power of hand and forearm, check sensation of hand
- Special tests
  - TFCC load test – ulnar deviate the wrist, apply axial pressure, then passively flex and extend the wrist; test is positive and implies TFCC tear, if pain is reproduced
  - Phalen's test and Tinel's sign for carpal tunnel syndrome

Investigations
- Blood tests based on Hx and Px – CBC and differential, RF, ANA
- X-ray wrist
  - Posterioanterior and lateral views
- Bone scan if suspected tumour
- Ultrasonography – for evaluation of tendons and tendon sheaths
- Arthroscopy – if indicated

Management
- Treat underlying cause
- Consider use of splint, analgesia; refer accordingly

Facial Fractures

Initial Approach
- ATLS Protocol
- Wound I&D
- Palpate/explore wounds for damage to underlying structures
- Tetanus prophylaxis, antibiotics if indicated
- Visual and radiological assessment
- Repair when patient's general condition allows

History
- Nature of the injury
  - Low vs. high velocity
  - Lateral vs. anterior force
  - Time of injury (important consideration for repair)
- Bruising, tenderness, loss of function
- Associated neck pain – suspect C-spine injury in facial trauma
- Tetanus immunization status

Facial Fracture Classification

Fracture	Imaging	Clinical Features	Clinical Features	Complications
Mandibular	Panoramic CT	Pain, trismus, swelling Malocclusion Damaged, loose, lost teeth Mandibular "step" Numbness in V3 Intraoral laceration/hematoma	Maxillary/mandibular archbars or ORIF Antibiotics to cover *S. aureus* and anaerobes	Malocclusion Malunion Tooth loss Sensation loss TMJ ankylosis
Nasal	None req'd	Epistaxis Deviation, flattening Swelling, periorbital ecchymosis Subconjunctival hemorrhage Tenderness, crepitus Septal hematoma Respiratory obstruction	** Always drain septal hematoma ± reduction: closed reduction + anesthesia, pack nose w/ Adaptic®, splint X 7d Reduction best within 6 h or at 5-7d in OR	Saddle nose Residual deformity: rhinoplasty may be necessary

Facial Fracture Classification (continued)

Fracture	Imaging	Clinical Features	Clinical Features	Complications
Maxillary	CT scan: axial and coronal	**Classification: see Table below Dish pan/equine facies Periorbital hematoma/epistaxis Malocclusion Mobility of maxilla	Usually require ORIF	Malocclusion/facial deformity Airway comprimise Altered sensation
Zygomatic		**Classification: see below 3 pathognomonic features: 1. V2 numbness 2. Subconj. hemorrhage 3. Pain to palpation over fracture Flattening of malar prominence/ periorbital ecchymosis Orbital rim step deformity Ipsilateral epistaxis Enopthalmos, diplopia, proptosis, vertical dystrophia, inferior displacement of globe *Associated with orbital floor #	Undisplaced/ asymptomatic- no treament ± Ophtho assessment Elevate depressed #using a Gilles approach if isolated area Failed Gilles/Comminuted #: ORIF	Orbital floor # Ophthalmologic complications
Orbital Blow-out		Periorbital edema/bruising/ subconj. hemorrhage Ptosis/exophthalmos/exorbitism/ enophthalmos Diplopia/limited EOM **Check visual fields and acuity for injury to globe	Open reduction and reconstruction if: orbital floor, diplopia not improving, or enophthalmos **Ophtho consult ASAP	Superior Orbital Fissure Syndrome Orbital Apex Syndrome: # through optic canal with CNII injury Watch for: ptosis, proptosis, CN III, IV, VI paralysis, V1 anesthesia

Classification of Mandibular Fractures

	Areas/Boundaries
Symphysis	Midline of the mandible; between the central incisors from the alveolar process through the inferior border of the mandible
Body	From the symphysis to the distal alveolar border of the third molar
Angle	Triangular region between the anterior border of the masseter and the posterosuperior insertion of the masseter distal to the third molar
Ramus	Part of the mandible that extends posteriosuperiorly into the condylar and coronoid processes
Condylar	Area of condylar process of mandible
Subcondylar	Area below the condylar neck (i.e. sigmoid notch) of the mandible
Coronoid Process	Area of the coronoid process of mandible

Classification of Maxillary Fractures

	Le Fort I	Le Fort II	Le Fort III
Alternative Name	Guerin fracture	Pyramidal fracture	Craniofacial dysjunction
Type of fracture	Horizontal	Pyramidal	Transverse
Structures involved	Piriform aperture Maxillary sinus Pterygoid plates	Nasal bones Medial orbital wall Maxilla Pterygoid plates	Nasofrontal suture Zygomatofrontal suture Zygomatic arch Pterygoid plates
Anatomical result	Maxilla divided into 2 segments	Maxillary teeth separated from face	Detach entire midfacial skeleton from cranial base

© Rio Sakay 2007

Classification of Zygomatic Fractures

1. Fracture restricted to zygomatic arch
2. Depressed fracture of zygomatic complex (zygoma)
3. Unstable fracture of zygomatic complex (tripod fracture) – zygoma separates from maxilla, frontal, temporal bone

Signs of Basal Skull/Le Fort III Fracture

1. Battle sign (bruised mastoid process)
2. Hemotympanum
3. Raccoon eyes (periorbital bruising)
4. CSF otorrhea

Common Conditions

Skin Lesions

Differential Diagnosis, History, and Physical
• See Dermatology

MANAGEMENT

Benign Skin Lesion
• Step 1: Make an elliptical incision around the lesion that includes approximately 0.5 cm of tissue beyond the borders of the lesion margins (incision can extend to 1-2 mm if lesion is benign)
• Step 2: Make the incision along RSTL (relaxed skin tension line)
• Step 3: Extend incision, or dissect, down to the subcutaneous tissue but do not violate the fascia
• Step 4: Secure the tissue with forceps or instrument and release from underlying tissue. Place in clearly labeled specimen container
• Step 5: May close in two layers. To reduce tension across the wound, you may have to undermine around the incision margins (release surrounding tissue by dissection). Close dermis with 3-0 Vicryl (4-0 on face). Close epidermis with 4-0 Prolene/Ethilon (5-0 on face). May use other suture type, depending on area, amount of tension, and surgeon's preference

Malignant Skin Lesion (Excision performed by Oncologic surgeon)
• Follow Step 1-5 as above with the following excision guidelines:
• Basal Cell and Squamous Cell Carcinoma:
  ▪ Non-melanomatic skin lesions up to 20 mm can be excised with tissue margins of 5.0 mm. Biopsy should be obtained prior to definitive excision to rule out sclerosing subtype basal cell carcinoma
• Recommended Excision Margins Cutaneous Melanoma:

Tumour Thickness (mm)	Excision Margins (cm)
0-1	1
1-2	1-2
>2	2

Skin Infections

Differential Diagnosis
• Erysipelas, cellulitis, fasciitis, impetigo

History
• Redness, warmth, pain, tenderness, edema
• Onset, duration, and rapidity of progression of symptoms

Associated Symptoms
• Fever, chills, malaise

Risk Factors/Predisposing/Precipitants
• History of soft tissue injury/trauma/bug bite, recent surgery, PVD, diabetes mellitus, foreign bodies (IV, surgical pins, etc.)

Complications/PMHx/FHx
• PVD, diabetes mellitus, foreign bodies, recent trauma

Physical Exam
- Vitals: Temperature, BP, HR, RR, O_2 saturation
- Inspection: erythema (demarcate with a marker), swelling, bullae, ulcers, ascending lymphangitis (red streaks proximal to affected area), skin discolouration (blue/black = thrombosis/necrosis in necrotizing fasciitis), evidence of trauma/lacerations, previous surgical incisions, bug bites
- Palpation: warmth, tenderness and distribution relative to erythema, edema, blanching of erythema, regional lymph node exam (enlarged, tender, firm, mobile, nonmatted), soft tissue crepitus (subcutaneous gas from anaerobes in necrotizing fasciitis), fluctuant area indicating an abscess
- MSK joint exam including ROM if over a joint

Dressings
- Goals: protection, environment for healing (absorption), immobilization, cosmesis, compression
- Wet dressing: for healing uninfected wounds; does not debride wound
- 1st layer (contact layer)
    - Clean wounds (heal by re-epithelialization)
        - Protect new epithelium
        - Use "wet-to-wet" dressing, non-adherent (e.g. Mepitel) impregnated gauze (e.g. Jelonet, Bactigras®) or antibiotic ointment
    - Chronic/contaminated wounds:
        - Mechanically debride nonviable tissue
        - Use "wet-to-dry" dressing (e.g. adherent saline or betadine soaked gauze)
- 2nd layer (absorbent layer): saline soaked gauze, to encourage exudate into dressing by "wick" effect
- 3rd layer (protective layer): dry gauze held in place with roller gauze or tape

ERYSIPELAS

Definition
- Skin infection affecting the epidermis (more superficial than cellulites, sharply demarcated borders)

Etiology/DDx
- GABHS (Group A *Streptococcus*)

Management

ER
- ABCs
- Microbiology: wound swab for C&S
- No bloodwork required
- No investigations required
- Treatment: cloxacillin PO 500 mg qid
- If severe: IV penicillin G 1-2 million U q4h
- Demarcate border of erythema

Outpatient
- F/U with family MD if worsening or if not resolved in 7-10 d

Inpatient
- Discharge once symptoms have resolved
- F/U with family MD or plastic surgeon
- Return to ER if worsening pain or spreading erythema

CELLULITIS

Definition
• Nonsuppurative infection of skin and subcutaneous tissues

Etiology/DDx
• Usually skin flora: *S. aureus*, β-hemolytic *Streptococcus*
• Immunocompromised: GN bacilli, fungi

Management

ER
• ABC's
• Bloodwork: CBC, electrolytes, Cr
• Microbiology: wound swab for C&S (if open wound)
• If severe: IV cloxacillin 2 g q4h OR IV cefazolin (Ancef) 1-2 g q8h
• Otherwise: cephalexin (Keflex) 500 mg PO qid
• No investigations
• Trace border of erythema

Outpatient
• F/U with family MD if worsening or if not resolved in 2-3 d

Inpatient
• Discharge once symptoms have resolved, F/U with family MD, return to ER if worsening pain++ or spreading erythema

NECROTIZING FASCIITIS

Definition
• Necrotizing soft tissue infection that spreads along gangrenous fascia

Etiology/DDx
• Type I: β-hemolytic *Streptococcus*
• Type II: polymicrobial

Management
• ABCs
• Vitals: assess hemodynamic stability
• Bloodwork: CBC, electrolytes, Cr, INR, aPTT, blood cultures
• Microbiology: wound swab for Gram stain + C&S (if open wound)
• Blood: Gram stain + C&S
• Urgent Plastics referral for prompt surgical debridement and biopsy
• Infectious Disease referral
• Investigations
  ▪ Must do x-ray of affected area to look for presence of subcutaneous gas
• Trace border of erythema
• Inpatient management – never to be managed on outpatient basis

Helpful Hints
• If suspicious for necrotizing fasciitis, urgent Plastic Surgery consult is required for surgical debridement and biopsy
• Trace area of erythema to monitor spread/resolution
• Erysipelas has distinct borders to erythema while cellulitis does not
• Crepitus, vesicles, ulcers, and pain severity and distribution greater than area of erythema should raise suspicion of necrotizing faciitis

Common Operations

Skin Grafts

Split and Full (whole) Thickness Skin Grafts

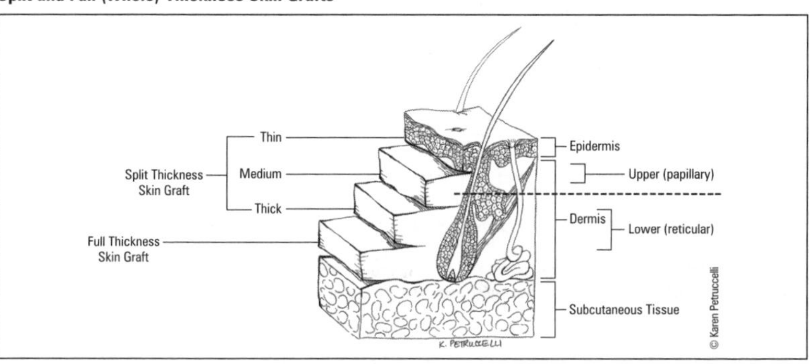

Definition
- Segment of skin detached from its blood supply at the donor site and dependent on revascularization from the recipient site

Donor Site Selection
- Must consider size, hair pattern, texture, thickness of skin, and colour (facial grafts best if taken from "blush zones" above clavicle e.g. pre/post auricular or neck)
- Partial thickness grafts usually taken from inconspicuous areas (e.g. buttocks, lateral thighs, etc.)

Partial Thickness Skin Graft Survival
- 3 phases of skin graft "take"
    1. Plasmatic imbibition – diffusion of nutrition from recipient site (first 48 h)
    2. Inosculation – vessels in graft connect with those in recipient bed
    3. Neovascular ingrowth – graft revascularization (day 3-5)
- Requirements for survival
    - Bed: well-vascularized (unsuitable: bone, tendon, heavily irradiated, infected wounds, etc.)
    - Contact between graft and recipient bed: fully immobile (decreased shearing and hematoma formation)
    - Staples, sutures, splinting, and appropriate dressings (pressure) are used to prevent movement of graft and hematoma or seroma formation
    - Site: low bacterial count ($<10^5$, to prevent infection)

Classification
1. By species
    - Autograft: from same individual
    - Allograft (homograft): from same species, different individual
    - Xenograft (heterograft): from different species (e.g. porcine)
2. By thickness

Flaps

Definition
• Tissue transferred from one site to another with an intact vascular supply (pedicle)

Classification: According to Various Criteria

	Flap Types
Blood supply	Random pattern, axial, reverse flow
Defect proximity	Local, regional, distant, free
Method of transfer	Advancement, transposition, rotation, interpolation, jumping, waltzing, free
Tissues contained	Cutaneous, fasciocutaneous, musculocutaneous, osteocutaneous, osteomusculocutaneous, omentum

Reconstructive Ladder
• Healing by 2° intension → direct tissue closure → skin graft → local flap → regional flap → distant flap → free flap
• Factors important in flap construction: defect location/size, exposed tissue types, potential donor sites, donor site defects, reconstruction shape, patient's medical history and expectations

Random Pattern Flaps
• Blood supply provided by dermal and subdermal plexus to skin and subdermal tissue with random vascular supply
• Limited length:width ratio to ensure adequate blood supply (2:1)
• Types:advancement, transposition, rotation flaps

Axial Pattern Flaps
• Flap contains well defined artery and vein
• Allowing greater length:width ratio (5-6:1)
• Types: peninsular flap (skin and vessel intact in pedicle) and island flap (well skeletonized vessels in pedicle)

Free Flaps
• Dominant artery and veins supplying a flap are microscopically anastomosed to vessels in the recipient site

Monitoring
• Factors compromising flap integrity: tight dressing/sutures, hematoma, seroma, vascular thrombosis, infection, position pressure, vasoconstrictors (nicotine, caffeine etc), poor flap design

	Normal	Arterial insufficiency	Venous insufficiency
Temperature	Warm	Cool	Warm or cool
Colour	Pink	Pale	Purple/blue
Capillary refill	~2 sec	>2 sec	<2 sec
Point bleed	Slow red bleed	Slow/no bleed	Brisk bleed with dark blood
Turgor	Soft with tissue turgor	Soft	Swollen/tense
Arterial pulse (Doppler)	+	±	±

Breast Surgery

Procedure	Definition	Surgical Details	Other Comments
Implant	Use of synthetic material (silicone or saline implants)	**With expanders** (2 Stages): Use tissue expanders before replacement with implants to help facilitate breast ptosis **Without expanders** (1 Stage): In skin-sparing mastectomy, enough skin is available for immediate placement of implant Reconstruction with implants requires a submuscular placement of devices	Complications: capsular contraction (foreign body reaction unique to implants), rupture or leakage of implant, increased risk of infection, risk of complication increased in previously irradiated breast
Autologous Tissue	Use of patient's own tissue, typically from the abdomen	Many flap options: DIEP (deep inferior epigastric perforator), TRAM (transverse rectus abdominus), Latissimus dorsi, SIEG (superfical inferior epigastric atery), and SGAP (superior gluteal artery perforator)	Offers reduced long-term morbidity and natural consistency
Reduction Mammoplasty	Breast reduction for relief of physical symptoms, and improved breast size and shape	1. Incisions: circular around the areola, vertical from areola incision to infra-mammary fold, along the natural infra-mammary fold 2. Fat, breast tissue, and skin removed 3. May move nipple and areola complex to higher position	Complications: infection, hemorrhage, decreased nipple sensation, inability to breast feed, breast/nipple asymmetry, nipple loss (partial or complete)
Mastopexy	Nipples are raised in ptotic breasts (breast lift)	Many different procedures	
Augmentation	Breast implants	Silicone or saline (subglandular or submuscular)	
Nipple Areola Reconstruction	Final stage of breast reconstruction	Usually require tattooing for areola reconstruction Local vs. distant flap/graft: 1. Local: fish tail or skate flap most common; these flaps allow simultaneous nipple and areola reconstruction 2. Distant: opposite nipple, earlobe, abdominal skin, costal cartilage	

Principles of Breast Surgery

Augmentation Mammoplasty
- Aesthetic procedure designed to increase the volume of the breast
- Other surgical goals include improvements in breast shape, symmetry, and nipple position
- Procedure is accomplished by making an incision, surgically creating a space pocket under the breast, and then inserting an appropriately sized breast implant
- Immediate complications: hematoma, seroma, wound dehiscence, infection
- Late complications: capsular contracture, implant rupture, asymmetry, visible skin wrinkles, palpable implant folds, scarring

Reduction Mammoplasty
- procedure to excise skin, fat and glandular tissue
- Indications are physical complaints including shoulder grooving, neck, back, and shoulder pain, mastodynia, and difficulty finding clothing that fits and is attractive
- Complications: Asymmetry, change in nipple/areolar sensation, infection, partial/total loss of nipple, skin loss/necrosis, fat necrosis, not enough tissue removed, too much tissue removed, poor shape

Mastopexy
- Surgical procedure that attempts to reverse the normal progression of breast ptosis
- Goals are to reposition the nipple–areolar complex, to reposition the breast mound and optimize its contour and volume, to remove redundant skin and tighten the skin, and to provide support for the breast in a lasting manner
- Complications: recurrent ptosis, nipple–areolar complex asymmetry, breast asymmetry, upper pole flattening, poor scarring, and nipple–areolar necrosis

Breast Reconstruction
- Two methods: implants and autologous tissue
- Implants: reconstruction can be performed immediately at the time of mastectomy or on a delayed basis, it can be performed in one or two stages, and it can include implants filled with saline or silicone gel, textured or smooth implants
- Complications: capsular contracture (most common), infection, hematoma, seroma
- Autologous: principal methods include the latissimus dorsi musculocutaneous flap, the transverse rectus abdominis musculocutaneous (TRAM) flap, and the various perforator flaps
- Perforator flaps are the most recent advances; they tend to minimize donor site morbidity by preserving the muscles. Require expertise in microsurgery techniques
- Microvascular complications following free tissue transfers usually are the result of thrombosis of the artery or vein, external pressure or kinking of the vascular pedicle, and poor vessel mismatch

Psychiatry

Essential History and Assessment Tools

History

Psychiatric Assessment
- **ID**: Name, age, marital/relationship status, duration, children: number, where are they, maintain contact?, living situation: who is at home? house/apt/no fixed address, employment: training, if unemployed – last job, how long, why ended, income: public assistance vs. disability (medical or psychiatric reasons), country of origin, date of immigration
- **RFR**
- **CC** (subjective – pts own words):
  - "What has been the problem leading up to your coming here?"
  - "Why is _____ so concerned about you?"
  - "How long has this been going on?"
- **HPI**
  - Time frame
  - Stressors
  - Symptoms
  - Mood:
    - Depression: MSIGECAPS
    - Mania: GST PAID
  - Anxiety:
    - Panic attacks: STUDENTS FEAR the 3 C's
    - Generalized anxiety: BE SKIM
    - Obsessive-compulsive
    - Phobias
    - Post-traumatic stress disorder: TRAUMA
  - Psychosis:
    - Delusions
    - Mind reading/control
    - Command hallucinations
    - Perceptual disturbances: auditory/visual hallucinations
  - Substances
  - Safety: suicidal ideation/homicidal ideation
  - Risk factors
  - Coping strategies
  - Current medications
  - Current supports
- Psychiatric support – next appointment?
- **Past Psychiatric Hx**
  - Most recent admission
  - Number of admissions and which hospitals
  - 1st episode of psychiatric illness
  - 1st psychiatric contact
  - Treatment overview
    - Meds, psychotherapy, ECT

- Suicide attempt history
  - Lethality, outcome, intent
- Legal history
  - Pending charges, incarceration, assault ($\pm$ weapon)
- Smoking
- Alcohol abuse/substance abuse
- Prescription/OTC abuse
- **PMH**
  - General medical condition that may be contributing to psychiatric presentation (e.g. stroke, dementia, cancer, hypothyroidism, lupus, etc.)
  - Hospitalizations
  - Surgeries
- **Medications**
- **Allergies**
- **Social History** (baseline functioning):
  - School – highest level of educational attainment, at what age
  - Relationships
    - Describe current relationship – length, support
    - Intimate relationships in the past, longest relationship
  - Employment history
    - Training
    - Current – type, length, concerns
    - Previous – type, length, why ended
- **Family History**
  - Psychiatric illness in family members

Mental Status Exam

- Appearance: appear (older/younger) stated age, body habitus, attire
- Behavior – tics, mannerisms, movement disorders, psychomotor agitation/retardation
- Attitude – appropriate, hostile, seductive, pleasant, suspicious
- Speech – rate, rhythm, volume, prosody, fluency, spontaneity, quantity, slurring
- Mood – subjective, write in patient's own words
- Affect – objective: quality, range, appropriateness, intensity
- Thought form/process – how ideas are put together internally and how they are expressed: coherence, logic, stream
  - Thought process disorders – tangentiality, circumstantiality, derailing, clang associations, perseveration, flight of ideas
- Thought content – themes, worries, obsessions, preoccupations, ruminations, overvalued ideas
  - Psychosis: ideas of reference, thought insertion/withdrawal/broadcasting, delusions
  - Suicidal ideation: active vs. passive ideation, plan, intent
  - Homicidal ideation: intended victim vs. nonspecific threat
- Perceptions – illusions, hallucinations, depersonalization, derealization
- Cognition – orientation, attention, concentration, memory, intelligence
  - MMSE and clock drawing (ideomotor dyspraxia)
- Insight (be specific)
  - Insight into illness
  - Insight into treatment
- Judgment – recent behaviours and future planning, ability to make socially appropriate judgments that will not lead to trouble, impulse control
- Reliability – compare patient report to chart notes, collaterals

Impression

- Emphasize "why now"
- Risk assessment for SI/HI
- Need for hospitalization, and if not document why not
- Certifiability
  - Past/present test – evidence of risk/harm
  - Future test – evidence (signs and symptoms) of a mental disorder
- Capacity to make treatment decisions

> **Mental Status Exam: ASEPTIC**
> **A**ppearance and behaviour
> **S**peech
> **E**motion (mood and affect)
> **P**erception
> **T**hought content and process
> **I**nsight and judgment
> **C**ognition

Multiaxial Assessment

- Axis I
  - Differential diagnosis of DSM-IV clinical disorders
- Axis II
  - Personality disorders, developmental disability
- Axis III
  - General medical conditions that are potentially relevant to the understanding or management of the mental disorder
- Axis IV
  - Psychosocial and environmental issues
- Axis V
  - Global assessment of functioning (GAF, 0 to 100) incorporating effects of axes I to IV (if suicidal ideation – minimum GAF = 50)

Axis V: Global Assessment of Functioning

91-100	Superior functioning in a wide range of activities
81-90	Absent or minimal symptoms
71-80	If symptoms are present, they are transient and expected reactions to psychosocial stressors; no more than slight impairment in social/occupational/school functioning
61-70	Some mild symptoms or some difficulty in functioning, but generally functioning well
51-60	Moderate symptoms or moderate difficulty in functioning
41-50	Serious symptoms (e.g. suicidal ideation) or serious difficulty in functioning
31-40	Some impairment in reality testing/communication, impairment in several areas
21-30	Behaviour is influenced by delusions/hallucinations or serious impairment in communication/judgement
11-20	Some danger of hurting self or others or occasionally fails to maintain minimal hygiene or gross impairment in communication
1-10	Persistent danger of severely hurting self or others or persistent inability to maintain minimal personal hygiene or serious suicidal act
0	Inadequate information

Screening for the "Big Four"

Mood

- Depression
- Mania
- *Always ask about SI and HI*

Anxiety
- With or without panic attacks
- Social
- Phobias
- Generalized
- Obsessive-compulsive behaviours

Psychosis
- Hallucinations: auditory, visual, tactile, olfactory, gustatory
- Delusions: persecutory, grandiose, religious, somatic, nihilistic, reference
- Negative symptoms: affective flattening, alogia, avolition

Organic
- Endogenous: general medical condition (e.g. stroke, dementia, cancer, hypothyroidism, lupus, etc.)
- Exogenous: prescription medications vs. illicit substances

Depression	Mania
Mood	**G**randiosity
Sleep	**S**leep
Interest	**T**alkative
Guilt	
Energy	**P**leasurable activities, painful consequences
Concentration	
Appetite	**A**ctivity
Psychomotor agitation/ retardation	**I**deas, flight of
Suicidal ideation	**D**istractible

Suicide Screening

Every Patient

"Have you had any thoughts of wanting to hurt/kill yourself?"

Ideation	"Do you have thoughts about ending your life, committing suicide?"
Passive	Would rather not be alive but does not admit to idea that involves act of initiation "I'd rather not wake up" "Life is not worth living" "I wouldn't mind if a car hit me"
Active	"I think about killing myself" "I think about doing ____"
Plan	"Do you have a plan as to how you would end your life?"
Intent	"You talk about wanting to die, but are you planning to do this?" "What has stopped you from ending your life?"
Past attempts	Highest risk if previous attempt in past year

Patient with Suicidal Ideation

Lethality	"Do you want to end your life? Or get relief from your emotional pain?"
Access to means	"What bridge do you think you'll go to/how will you get a gun?"
Time and place	"Have you picked a place? How isolated is it?
Final arrangements	Suicide notes, settling affairs
Protective factors	Family, pets, religion, therapist
Ambivalence	"There must be a part of you that wants to live – you came here tonight for help"

Assessment of Suicide Attempt

Setting – isolated vs. others present	Medical attention – self vs. found
Likelihood of being found	Expectations of dying
Impulsivity vs. premeditation	Time lag from attempt to ER arrival
Intoxication	Feelings about survival: Guilt/remorse vs. disappointment/self-blame

Risk Factors: SAD PERSONS

Sex: male	**P**revious attempt
Age: <19 or >60	**E**thanol
Depression	**R**ational thinking loss (psychosis)
	Social supports lacking
	Organized plan
	No spouse
	Sickness (chronic pain, cancer)

Safety Assessment and Management

Ensure Safety (of self, patient, co-patients)
- Involve security services
- Develop exit strategy
- Decrease stimulation
- Assume non-threatening stance
- Anticipate need for chemical and/or physical restraints

Chemical Restraints
- Benzodiazepines
  - Lorazepam 2 mg PO/SL/IM q1h; reassess after 8 mg
  - Onset typically within 10 min for IM
  - Side effect: drowsiness
  - Can be combined with haloperidol in same syringe
- Antipsychotics
  - Typical
    - Haloperidol 5 mg PO/PO liquid/IM/IV
    - Risperidone 2 mg (M-tab)
    - Side effects:
    1) Extrapyramidal symptoms
       - Tremor, rigidity, akinesia, dystonic reactions
       - Treat with Benztropine (Cogentin®) 2 mg IM/PO
    2) Akathisia
       - Treat with benzodiazepines
  - Atypical
    - Olanzapine 5 mg PO/IM
    - Side effects:
      - Drowsiness
      - Dry mouth
      - Constipation

Physical Restraints
- Restraint policies vary according to each hospital
- Use least restraint possible, ensure appropriate monitoring

Common Conditions

Psychotic Disorders

Differentiating Psychotic Disorders

Disorder	Psychotic Symptoms	Duration	Mood Symptoms
Brief psychotic disorder	≥1 positive symptoms of criterion A	<1 month	None
Schizophreniform disorder	Criterion A	1-6 months	If present, 2°
Schizophrenia	Criterion A	>6 months	If present, 2°
Schizoaffective disorder	≥2 wks (with no mood symptoms)	>1 month	Present
Delusional disorder	Non-bizarre delusions, no hallucinations	>1 month	If present, 2°
2° to substance Intoxication/ withdrawal	Criterion A	During intoxication or ≤1 month after withdrawal	Variable
2° to mood disorder	Delusions/hallucinations (mood congruent)	Unspecified	1°

Differential Diagnosis
- Primary psychotic disorders: schizophrenia, schizophreniform, brief psychotic, schizoaffective, delusional disorder
- Mood disorders: depression with psychotic features, bipolar disorder (manic episode with psychotic features)
- Personality disorders: schizotypal, schizoid, borderline, paranoid, obsessive-compulsive
- General medical conditions: tumour, head trauma, dementia, delirium, metabolic
- Substance-induced psychosis: intoxication or withdrawal

Delusions

Persecutory	Belief that others are trying to cause harm
Delusions of reference	Interpreting publicly known events/celebrities as having direct reference to the patient (e.g. TV/radio has special messages to patient)
Erotomania	Belief that another person is in love with you
Grandiose	Belief of an inflated sense of self-worth or power
Religious	Belief of receiving instructions/powers from a higher being; of being a higher being
Somatic	Belief one has a physical disorder/defect
Nihilistic	Belief that things do not exist; a sense that everything is unreal

Criteria for Schizophrenia
- 2 or more of the following (only one if bizarre delusion or auditory hallucination with ≥2 voices):
  - Delusions
  - Hallucinations
  - Disorganized speech
  - Disorganized behaviour
  - Negative symptoms – alogia, avolition, flat affect
- Social/occupational dysfunction
- Duration at least 6 months

Mood Disorders

Definitions
- Mood disorders are defined by the presence of mood episodes
- Mood episodes represent a combination of symptoms comprising a predominant mood state that is abnormal in quality or duration; examples include: major depressive, manic, mixed, hypomanic
- Types of mood disorders include:
  - Depressive (major depressive disorder, dysthymia)
  - Bipolar (bipolar I/II disorder, cyclothymia)
  - Secondary to GMC, substances, medications

Secondary Causes of Mood Disorders

	Category	Examples
V	Vascular	Cardiomyopathy, CHF, MI, CVA
I	Infectious	Encephalitis/meningitis, hepatitis, pneumonia, TB, syphilis
N	Neoplastic	Pancreatic cancer, carcinoid, pheochromocytoma
D	Degenerative	Huntington's disease, multiple sclerosis, tuberous sclerosis, degenerative (vascular, Alzheimer's)
I	Intoxication/Drugs/Deficiencies	Antihypertensives, antiparkinsonian, hormones, steroids, antituberculous, interferon, antineoplastic medications, vitamin deficiencies (Wernicke's, beriberi, pellagra, pernicious anemia)
C	Congenital	–
A	Autoimmune	SLE, polyarteritis nodosa
T	Traumatic	Traumatic brain injury
E	Endocrine/Metabolic	Hypothyroidism, hyperthyroidism, hypopituitarism, SIADH, porphyria, Wilson's disease, diabetes

Medical Workup of Mood Disorder

- Routine screening:
  - Physical examination, complete blood count, thyroid function test, electrolytes, urinalysis, urine drug screen, vitamin B_{12}
- Additional screening:
  - Neurological consultation, CXR, ECG, CT scan

Criteria for Depression (≥5 x 2 weeks)

MSIGECAPS

Mood (depressed)	**C**oncentration (decreased)
Sleep (increased/decreased)	**A**ppetite (increased/decreased)
Interest (decreased)	**P**sychomotor agitation/retardation
Guilt	**S**uicidal ideation (passive or active)
Energy (decreased)	

Criteria for Mania (≥3, >1 week)

GST PAID

Grandiosity	**P**leasurable activities, painful consequences
Sleep, decreased need	**A**ctivity
Talkative	**I**deas, flight of
	Distractible

Anxiety Disorders

Definition

- Anxiety is a universal human characteristic involving tension, apprehension, or even terror, which serves as an adaptive mechanism to warn about an external threat by activating the sympathetic nervous system (fight or flight)
- Anxiety becomes pathological when
  - Fear is greatly out of proportion to risk/severity of threat
  - Response continues beyond existence of threat or becomes generalized to other similar/dissimilar situations
  - Social or occupational functioning is impaired

Types

- Panic Disorder
- Generalized Anxiety Disorder
- Phobic Disorders
- Obsessive Compulsive Disorders
- Post-traumatic Stress Disorder (PTSD)

Criteria for Panic Disorder (≥4, peaks within 10 minutes)

STUDENTS FEAR the 3 C's

Sweating	**N**ausea
Trembling	**T**ingling
Unsteadiness, dizziness	**S**hortness of breath
Depersonalization, Derealization	**Fear** of dying, losing control, going crazy
Excessive heart rate, palpitations	**3 C's:** Chest pain, Chills, Choking

Criteria for Generalized Anxiety Disorder (most days x 6 months)

BE SKIM

Blank mind	**S**leep disturbance
Easily fatigued	**K**eyed up
	Irritability
	Muscle tension

Differential Diagnosis

Cardiovascular	Post-MI, arrhythmia, congestive heart failure, pulmonary embolus, arrhythmia, mitral valve prolapse
Respiratory	Asthma, COPD, pneumonia, hyperventilation
Endocrine	Hyperthyroidism, pheochromocytoma, hypoglycemia, hyperadrenalism, hyperparathyroidism
Metabolic	Vitamin B_{12} deficiency, porphyria
Neurologic	Neoplasm, vestibular dysfunction, encephalitis
Substance-Induced	Intoxication (caffeine, amphetamines, cocaine, thyroid preparations, OTC for colds/decongestants), withdrawal (benzodiazepines, alcohol)
Other Psychiatric Disorders	Psychotic disorders, mood disorders, personality disorders (OCPD), somatoform disorders

Medical Workup of Anxiety Disorder
- Routine screening: physical examination, CBC, thyroid function test, electrolytes, urinalysis, urine drug screening
- Additional screening: neurological consultation, CXR, ECG, CT scan

Treatment
- CBT – systematic desensitization, relaxation techniques, thought stopping
- Pharmacotherapy
    - SSRIs
    - Benzodiazepines (for acute anxiety)
    - First-line adjunct – atypical antipsychotics (quetiapine, olanzapine, risperidone)

Substance Related Disorders

Types of Substance Disorders
- 47% of those with substance abuse have mental health problems
- 29% of those with a mental health disorder have a substance use disorder (concurrent disorder) – 47% of those with schizophrenia, 25% of those with an anxiety disorder

A. Substance-use Disorders
1. Substance abuse: maladaptive pattern of substance use leading to clinically significant impairment or distress, as manifested by one (or more) of the following occurring within a 12 month period:
    - Recurrent use resulting in failure to fulfill major role obligation
    - Recurrent use in situations in which it is physically hazardous (e.g. driving)
    - Recurrent substance-related legal problems
    - Continued use despite interference with social or interpersonal function

2. Substance dependence: maladaptive pattern of substance use leading to clinically significant impairment or distress as manifested by three (or more) occurring at any time in the same 12 month period:
   - Tolerance (need for increased amount to achieve intoxication or diminished effect with same amount of substance)
   - Withdrawal/use to avoid withdrawal
   - Taken in larger amount or over longer period than intended
   - Persistent desire or unsuccessful efforts to cut down
   - Excessive time to procure, use substance, or recover from its effects
   - Important interests/activities given up or reduced
   - Continued use despite physical/psychological problem caused or exacerbated by substance

B. Substance-induced Disorders
1. Substance intoxication: reversible physiological and behavioural changes due to recent exposure to psychoactive substance
2. Substance withdrawal: substance-specific syndrome that develops following cessation of or reduction in dosage of regularly used substance

CAGE Questionnaire
- Validated screening questionnaire:
   - **C** ever felt the need to **C**ut down on drinking?
   - **A** ever felt **A**nnoyed at criticism of your drinking?
   - **G** ever feel **G**uilty about your drinking?
   - **E** ever need a drink first thing in the morning (**E**ye opener)?
      - For men, a score of 2 out of 4 is a positive screen and for women, a score of 1 out of 4 is a positive screen
      - If positive CAGE, then assess further to determine if problem drinker or alcohol dependence

A "Standard Drink" = 0.5 oz of absolute alcohol = 12 grams of absolute alcohol

Spirit (40%) – 1.5 oz. or 43 mL	1 bottle wine = 5 SD
Table Wine (12%) – 5 oz. or 142 mL	1 "mickey" = 8 SD
Fortified Wine (18%) – 3 oz. or 85 mL	"26-er" = 17 SD
Regular Beer (5%) – 12 oz. or 341 mL	"40 oz" = 27 SD
1 pint beer = 1.5 SD	

Management of Alcohol Withdrawal
- Monitor using the Clinical Institute Withdrawal Assessment for Alcohol (CIWA-A) scoring system
   - Areas of assessment include:
      - Nausea and vomiting, paroxysmal sweats, tactile disturbances, visual disturbances, tremor, anxiety, auditory disturbances, headache, fullness in head, agitation, orientation and clouding of sensorium
   - All categories are scored from 0-7 (except: orientation/sensorium 0-4), maximum score of 67
      - Mild <10
      - Moderate 10-20
      - Severe >20
- Basic treatment protocol using CIWA-A scale
   - Diazepam 20 mg PO q1-2h prn until CIWA-A <10 points; tapering dose not required
   - Observe 1-2 h after last dose and re-assess on CIWA-A scale
   - Thiamine 100 mg IM then 100 mg PO OD for 3 d
   - Supportive care (hydration and nutrition)
- Admit to hospital if:
   - Still in withdrawal after >80 mg of diazepam
   - Delirium tremens, recurrent arrhythmias, or multiple seizures
   - Medically ill or unsafe to discharge home

Other Substances
- Opioids: heroin, morphine, methadone, codeine, oxycontin
- Cannabis: weed, hash
- Cocaine
- Hallucinogens: LSD, mescaline, psilocybin, PCP
- "Club drugs": ecstasy (MDMA), GHB, ketamine, rohypnol, crystal meth

Personality Disorders

General Diagnostic Criteria
- An enduring pattern of inner experience and behaviour that deviates markedly from the expectations of the individual's culture; manifested in two or more of: cognition, affect, interpersonal functioning, impulse control
- Inflexible and pervasive across a range of situations
- Causes distress or impaired functioning not necessarily for the person with the personality disorder, but for those around him/her
- Pattern is stable and well established by adolescence or early adulthood
- Associated with many complications, such as depression, suicide, violence, brief psychotic episodes, drug use and treatment resistance
- Each personality disorder is present in 1% of the population
- Personality disorders are lifelong and chronic
- The mainstay of treatment is psychotherapy with the addition of pharmacotherapy to treat associated axis I disorders (i.e. depression, anxiety, substance abuse)

Cluster A ("mad")
- **Paranoid Personality Disorder** – pervasive distrust and suspiciousness of others, interpret motives as malevolent
- **Schizoid Personality Disorder** – neither desires nor enjoys close relationships including being a part of a family; prefers to be alone, lifelong pattern of social withdrawal, seen as eccentric and reclusive with constricted affect
- **Schizotypal Personality Disorder** – pattern of eccentric behaviours, peculiar thought patterns

Cluster B ("bad")
- **Borderline Personality Disorder** – unstable moods and behaviour, feel alone in the world, problems with self image, istory of repeated suicide attempts, self-harm behaviours
  ****10% suicide rate****
- **Antisocial Personality Disorder** – lack of remorse for actions, manipulative and deceitful, often violate the law, ay appear charming on first impression. (Note: pattern of disregard for others and violation of rights of others must be present before the age of 15, however, for the diagnosis of APD patients must be at least 18.)
- **Narcissistic Personality Disorder** – sense of superiority, needs constant admiration, lacks empathy, but with fragile sense of self, consider themselves "special" and will exploit others for personal gain
- **Histrionic Personality Disorder** – attention-seeking behaviour and excessively emotional, are dramatic, flamboyant and extroverted, cannot form meaningful relationships, often sexually inappropriate

Cluster C ("sad")
- **Avoidant Personality Disorder** – timid and socially awkward with a pervasive sense of inadequacy and fear of criticism, fear of embarrassing or humiliating themselves in social situations; withdrawn and socially inhibited
- **Dependent Personality Disorder** – Pprvasive and excessive need to be taken care of, excessive fear of separation, clinging and submissive behaviours, difficulty making everyday decisions
- **Obsessive-Compulsive Personality Disorder** – preoccupation with orderliness, perfectionism, and mental and interpersonal control, is inflexible, closed off, and inefficient

Common Medications

Common Antipsychotic Agents

	Starting Dose	Maintenance	Maximum	Relative Potency (mg)
TYPICALS				
(In order of potency from high to low)				
Haloperidol (Haldol®)	2-5 mg IM q4-8h 0.5-5 mg PO b/tid 0.2 mg/kg/d PO	Based on clinical effect	20 mg/d PO	2
Perphenazine (Trilafon®)	8-16 mg PO b/tid	4-8 mg PO t/qid	64 mg/d PO	10
Loxapine HCl (Loxitane®)	10 mg PO tid 12.5-50 mg IM q4-6h	60-100 mg/d PO	250 mg/d PO	10
Chlorpromazine (Largactil®)	10-15 mg PO b/t/qid	400 mg/d PO	1000 mg/d PO	100
ATYPICALS				
Risperidone (Risperdal®)	1-2 mg OD/bid	4-8 mg/d PO	8 mg/d PO	High potency
IM long acting preparation (Risperdal Consta®)		25 mg IM q wks		
Olanzapine (Zyprexa®, Zydis®)	5 mg/d PO	10-20 mg/d PO	30 mg/d PO	
Clozapine (Clozaril®)	25 mg PO/bid	300-600 mg/d PO	900 mg/d PO	
Quetiapine (Seroquel®)	25 mg PO/bid	400-800 mg/d PO	800 mg/d PO	Low potency

Side Effects of Antipsychotics

System	Side Effects
Anticholinergic	Dry mouth, difficulty urinating, constipation, blurred vision, toxic-confusional states
Alpha-adrenergic blockade	Orthostatic hypotension, impotence, failure to ejaculate
Dopaminergic blockade	Extrapyramidal syndromes (dystonia, akathisia, pseudo-parkinsonism, dyskinesia), galactorrhea, amenorrhea, impotence, weight gain
Anti-histamine	Sedation
Hematologic	Agranulocytosis (Clozapine)
Hypersensitivity reactions	Liver dysfunction Blood dyscrasias Skin rashes Neuroleptic malignant syndrome Altered temperature regulation (hypothermia or hyperthermia)

Extrapyramidal Side Effects

	Dystonia	Akathisia	Pseudoparkinsonism	Dyskinesia
Acute or tardive	Both	Both	Acute	Tardive
Risk group	Acute: Young Asian and Black males		Elderly females	Elderly females
Presentation	Sustained abnormal posture; torsions, twisting, contraction of muscle groups; muscle spasms (e.g. oculogyric crisis, laryngospasm, torticollis)	Motor restlessness; crawling sensation in legs relieved by walking; very distressing, increased risk of suicide and poor adherence	Tremor Rigidity (cogwheel) Akinesia Postural instability (decreased/absent arm-swing, stooped posture, shuffling gait, difficulty pivoting)	Purposeless, constant movements, involving facial and mouth musculature, or less commonly, the limbs
Onset	Acute: within 5 d	Acute: within 10 d Tardive: >90 d	Acute: within 30 d Tardive: >90 d	Tardive: >90 d
Treatment	Acute: benztropine or diphenhydramine	Acute: lorazepam, propanolol or diphenhydramine; reduce or change neuroleptic to lower potency	Acute: benztropine (or benzodiazepine if side effects); reduce or change neuroleptic to lower potency	Tardive: no good treatment; may try clozapine; discontinue drug or reduce dose

Common Antidepressants

Class	Drug	Daily Starting Dose (mg)	Daily Therapeutic Dose (mg)
SSRI	fluoxetine (Prozac®)	20	20-80
	fluvoxamine (Luvox®)	50-100	150-300
	paroxetine (Paxil®)	10	20-60
	sertraline (Zoloft®)	50	50-200
	citalopram (Celexa®)	20	20-60
	escitalopram (Cipralex®)	10	10-20
SNRI	venlafaxine (Effexor®)	37.5-75	75-225
	duloxetine (Cymbalta®)	40	40-60
NDRI	bupropion (Wellbutrin®)	100	300-450
TCA (3° Amines)	amitriptyline (Elavil®)	75-100	150-300
	imipramine (Tofranil®)	75-100	150-300
TCA (2° Amines)	nortriptyline (Aventyl®)	75-100	75-150
	desipramine (Norpramin®)	100-200	150-300
MAOI	phenelzine (Nardil®)	45	60-90
	tranylcypromine (Parnate®)	30	10-60
RIMA	moclobemide (Manerix®)	300	300-600
NASSA	mirtazapine (Remeron®)	15	15-45

(SSRI=selective serotonin reuptake inhibitors; SNRI=serotonin and norepinephrine reuptake inhibitors; NDRI=norepinephrine and dopamine reuptake inhibitors; TCA=tricyclic antidepressants; MAOI= monoamine oxidase inhibitors; RIMA=reversible inhibition of MAO-A; NASSA=noradrenergic and specific serotonin antagonists)
*Please note dividing dosing is often required with these medications

Treatment Algorithm of Depression

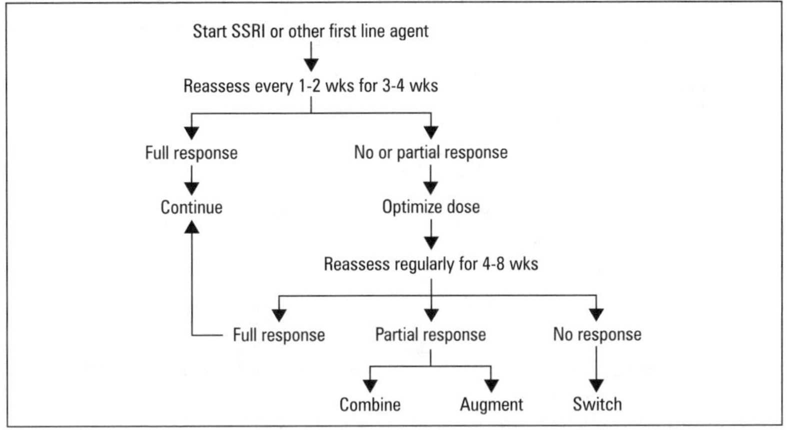

Common Mood Stabilizers

	Dose Range (mg/day)	$T_{1/2}$ (hours)	Appropriate Use
Lithium	600-1500 Therapeutic level: 0.5-1.2 mmol/L	12-24	Maintenance of BAD Treatment of acute mania Augmentation of antidepressants
Divalproex (Epival®)	750-2500 Therapeutic level: 17-50 mmol/L	6-16	Maintenance of BAD Treatment of acute mania Rapid cycling BAD
Carbamazepine (Tegretol®)	400-1600	10-36	Maintenance of BAD Treatment of acute mania Rapid cycling BAD
Lamotrigine (Lamictal®)	15-500	24-34	Maintenance of BAD Treatment of bipolar depression

Common Anxiolytics

Class	Drug	Dose Range (mg/day)	$T_{1/2}$ (hours)	Appropriate Use
Benzodiazepines				
Long-acting	clonazepam (Rivotril®)	0.25-4	18-50	Akathisia, generalized anxiety, seizure prevention, panic disorder
	diazepam (Valium®)	2-40	30-100	Generalized anxiety, seizure prevention, muscle relaxant, alcohol withdrawal
	chlordiazepoxide (Librium®)	5-300	30-100	Sleep, anxiety, alcohol withdrawal
	flurazepam (Dalmane ®)	15-30	50-160	Sleep
Short-acting	alprazolam (Xanax®)	0.25-4.0	6-20	Panic disorder, high dependency rate
	lorazepam (Ativan®)	0.5-6.0	10-20	Sleep, generalized anxiety, akathisia, alcohol withdrawal, sublingual available for very rapid action
	oxazepam (Serax®)	10-120	8-12	Sleep, generalized anxiety, alcohol withdrawal
	temazepam (Restoril®)	7.5-30	8-20	Sleep
	triazolam (Halcion®)	0.125-0.5	1.5-5	Shortest $t_{1/2}$, rapid sleep, but rebound insomnia
Azapirones	buspirone (Buspar®)	20-60	2-11	Generalized anxiety
	zopiclone (Imovane®)	5-7.5	3.8-6.5	Sleep

Respirology

Essential History, Physical Exam and Investigations

History

Symptoms	Risk Factors and Other Key Questions
Cough Sputum (quantify amount, colour) Blood (hemoptysis)	**Smoking**
	Cardiovascular history
	Previous malignancy
Chest pain Pleuritic (knife-like, with breathing) Heavy/ tight	**Recent illness**
	Recent travel/birthplace (TB)
Shortness of breath Exertional Rest Orthopnea (lying flat, how many pillows) PND (waking up at night short of breath)	**Sick contacts**
	Family history of atopy
	Animal exposure/allergies
	Previous CXR or PFTs
Wheezing/stridor	**Occupational exposures**
Constitutional symptoms (fevers, chills, night sweats, unintentional weight loss)	**Environmental exposures**

Physical Exam

Inspection	Percussion
Respiratory distress (rate, pattern of breathing, accessory muscle use, pursed-lip breathing, nasal flaring)	**General** (resonance, dullness)
	Diaphragmatic excursion
Cyanosis (central, peripheral)	
Clubbing	
Chest configuration (kyphosis, scoliosis, barrel chest, pectus excavatum, pectus carinatum)	

Palpation	Auscultation
• Tenderness, deformities • Diaphragmatic excursion • Tactile fremitus • Tracheal position	• Type of breath sounds (tracheal, bronchial, bronchovesicular, vesicular) • Symmetry of air entry • Adventitious sounds (crackles, wheezes, pleural rubs, stridor, rhoncus) **If suspicion of consolidation:** • Egophony: "eeee" sounds like "aaaa" when auscultating over area of consolidation • Whispered pectoriloquy: whispered words (e.g. "one-two-three") sound clearer when auscultating over area of consolidation

DIFFERENTIAL DIAGNOSIS BASED ON PHYSICAL EXAM FINDINGS

Condition	Fremitus	Percussion	Breath Sounds	Adventitious Sounds	Mediastinal Displacement
Consolidation (bronchus open)	Normal/increased	Dull	Bronchial	Crackles	None
Pneumothorax	Absent	Resonant	Absent/decreased	Absent	Tracheal deviation to opposite if under tension
Pleural Effusion	Decreased over affected area	Dull	Absent over fluid Bronchial at upper border	Absent/pleural rub above effusion	Heart displaced to opposite side
Atelectasis (or consolidation with occluded bronchus)	Variable	Dull	Absent/diminished	Crackles	Ipsilateral shift

Taken from *The ASCM I Clinical Skills Handbook*, 2nd Edition. M. Colapinto.

Investigations

Pulmonary Function Tests
- Useful in differentiating the pattern of lung disease (obstructive vs. restrictive)
- Assess lung volumes, flow rates, and diffusion capacity
- Normal values for FEV_1 are approximately $\pm 20\%$ of the predicted values (for age, sex and height); ethnicity may affect predicted values

Subcompartments of Lung Volumes

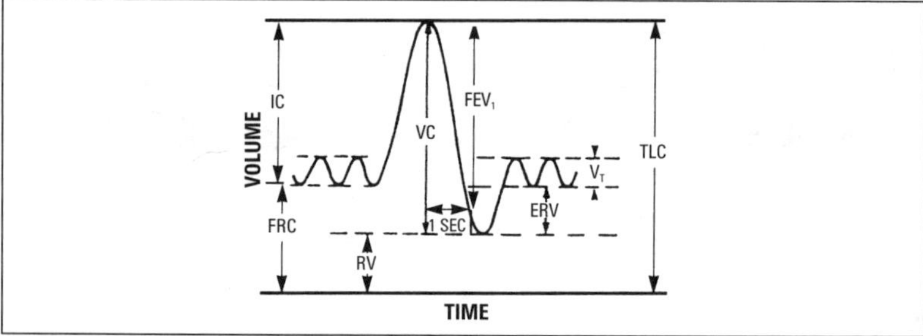

Reprinted from *Principles of Pulmonary Medicine*, 2nd edition, SE Weinberger, Copyright (1992), with permission from Elsevier.

Expiratory Flow Volume Curves

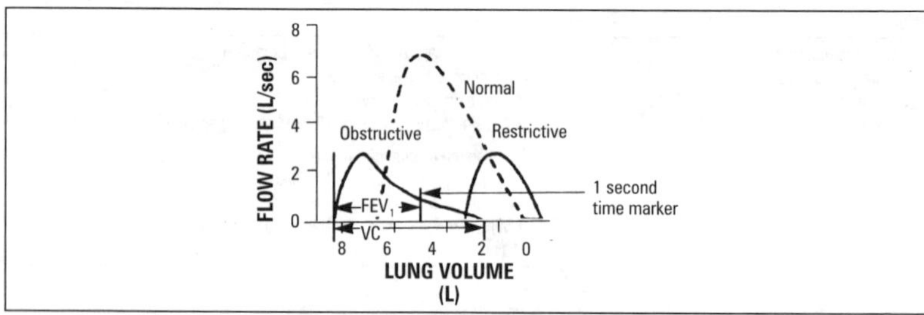

Reprinted from *Principles of Pulmonary Medicine*, 2nd edition, SE Weinberger, Copyright (1992), with permission from Elsevier.

OBSTRUCTIVE LUNG DISEASE
- Characterized by obstructed airflow and decreased flow rates (most marked during expiration)
- May also see air trapping (increased RV/TLC) and hyperinflation (increased FRC, TLC)
- Differential diagnosis includes asthma, chronic obstructive pulmonary disease (COPD), cystic fibrosis (CF), bronchiolitis, and bronchiectasis

RESTRICTIVE LUNG DISEASE
- Characterized by decreased lung compliance and lung volumes
- Differential diagnosis includes interstitial lung disease, neuromuscular disease, chest wall disease, pleural disease, and parenchymal disease (pneumonia)

Comparison of Lung Flow and Volume Parameters in Obstructive vs. Restrictive Lung Disease

		Obstructive	Restrictive
Flow Rates	FEV_1/FVC	↓	↑ or N
Lung Volumes	TLC	↑ or N	↓
	RV	↑ or N	↓
	RV/TLC	↑ or N	N
Diffusion Capacity	DL_{CO}	↓ or N	↓ or N

ARTERIAL BLOOD GASES
- Please see <u>Nephrology</u> for an approach to Acid-Base Disorders

DIFFERENTIAL DIAGNOSIS OF RESPIRATORY ACIDOSIS

Characterized by increased P_aCO_2 secondary to hypoventilation
- **Respiratory centre depression** (decreased RR): drugs (anesthesia, sedatives, narcotics), trauma, increased ICP, encephalitis, stroke, central apnea, supplemental O_2 in chronic CO_2 retainers (e.g. COPD)
- **Neuromuscular disorders** (decreased V_T): myasthenia gravis, Guillain-Barré syndrome, poliomyelitis, muscular dystrophies, ALS, myopathies, chest wall disease (obesity, kyphoscoliosis)
- **Airway obstruction** (decreased FEV): asthma, foreign body
- **Parenchymal disease**: COPD, pulmonary edema, pneumothorax, pneumonia, pneumoconiosis, acute respiratory distress syndrome (ARDS)
- **Mechanical hypoventilation** (inadequate mechanical ventilation)

DIFFERENTIAL DIAGNOSIS OF RESPIRATORY ALKALOSIS

Characterized by decreased P_aCO_2 secondary to hyperventilation
- **Hypoxemia**: pulmonary disease (pneumonia, edema, PE, interstitial fibrosis), severe anemia, heart failure, high altitude
- **Respiratory centre stimulation**: CNS disorders, hepatic failure, Gram-negative sepsis, drugs (ASA, progesterone, theophylline, catecholamines, psychotropics), pregnancy, anxiety, pain
- **Mechanical hyperventilation** (excessive mechanical ventilation)

Common Presentations

Dyspnea

Differential Diagnoses of Dyspnea

* Denotes causes that should be considered for acute dyspnea

Respiratory	Airway disease (wheeze) Asthma*, COPD exacerbation*, upper airway obstruction (anaphylaxis, foreign body, etc.)*, mucus plugging* Parenchymal lung disease (crackles) ARDS*, pneumonia*, interstitial lung disease Pulmonary vascular disease PE, pulmonary HTN, pulmonary vasculitis Pleural disease (pleuritic chest pain) Pneumothorax*, tension pneumothorax*, pleural effusion
Neuromuscular and chest wall disorders (decreased chest expansion)	Polymyositis, myasthenia gravis, Guillain-Barré syndrome, Kyphoscoliosis, C-spine injury*, ALS, diaphragmatic paresis
Cardiovascular (worse with dependency/exertion)	Elevated pulmonary venous pressure LVF with pulmonary edema*, mitral stenosis, decreased cardiac output
Hematological	Severe anemia (pallor)
Psychiatric	Anxiety/psychosomatic*

Hemoptysis

- Investigations: INR/PTT (coagulopathy), sputum culture/stain (infection), cytology (malignancy), ANCA/anti-GBM/U/A (vasculitis), bronchoscopy may be necessary, endoscopy (to rule out GI or ENT source)

Differential Diagnoses of Hemoptysis

Airway Disease	Vascular Disease	Parenchymal Disease	Miscellaneous
Acute or chronic bronchitis	PE	Pneumonia	Impaired coagulation
Bronchiectasis	Increased pulmonary	TB	Pulmonary endometriosis
Bronchogenic CA	venous pressure:	Lung abscess	
Bronchial carcinoid tumour	LVF	Goodpasture's syndrome and	
	Mitral stenosis	other vasculitis	
	Vascular malformation		

Reprinted from Principles of Pulmonary Medicine, 2nd edition, SE Weinberger, Copyright (1992), with permission from Elsevier.

Cough

Differential Diagnoses of Cough

Airway Irritants	Airway Disease
Inhaled smoke, dusts, fumes	URTI including postnasal drip and sinusitis
Aspiration	Acute or chronic bronchitis
Gastric contents (GERD)	Bronchiectasis
Oral secretions	Neoplasm
Foreign body	External compression by node or mass lesion
Postnasal drip	Asthma
	COPD
Parenchymal Disease	
Pneumonia	**CHF**
Lung abscess	
Interstitial lung disease	**Drug-induced (e.g. ACEi)**

Reprinted from Principles of Pulmonary Medicine, 2nd edition, SE Weinberger, Copyright (1992), with permission from Elsevier.

Clubbing

Differential Diagnoses of Clubbing

Pulmonary	Gastrointestinal	Mediastinal
CF	IBD (UC, CD)	Esophageal CA
Pulmonary fibrosis	Chronic infections	Thymoma
Chronic pus in the lung	Laxative abuse	**Other**
(bronchiectasis, abscess,	Polyposis	Graves Disease
infections, etc.)	Malignant tumours	Cirrhosis
Lung CA (primary or mets)	HCC	Thalassemia
Mesothelioma	**Cardiac**	Other malignancies
A-V fistula	Cyanotic congenital heart disease	Primary hypertrophic osteoarthropathy
	Infective endocarditis	

The Solitary Pulmonary Nodule

Definition
• A round or oval, sharply circumscribed radiographic lesion up to 3-4 cm which may or may not be calcified and is surrounded by normal lung – no lymphadenopathy or pleural effusion

Chest X-ray Characteristics of Benign vs. Malignant Solitary Nodule

Parameters	Benign	Malignant
Size	<3 cm, round, regular	>3 cm, irregular, spiculated
Margins	Smooth margin	Ill-defined or notched margin
Features	Calcified pattern: central, "popcorn" pattern if hamartoma, usually no cavitation; if cavitated, wall is smooth and thin, no other lung pathology	Usually not calcified; if calcified, pattern is eccentric, no satellite lesions, cavitation with thick wall, may have pleural effusions, lymphadenopathy
Doubling Time	Doubles in <1 month or >2 yrs	Doubles in >1 month or <2 yrs

Differential Diagnosis for Benign vs. Malignant Solitary Nodule

Benign (70%)	Malignant (30%)
Infectious granuloma (histoplasmosis, coccidiomycosis, TB, atypical mycobacteria)	**Bronchogenic carcinoma** Adenocarcinoma
Other infections (bacterial abscess, PCP, aspergilloma)	Squamous cell carcinoma Large cell carcinoma
Benign neoplasms (hamartoma, lipoma, fibroma)	Small cell carcinoma
Vascular (AV malformation, pulmonary varix)	**Metastatic lesions** Breast
Developmental (bronchogenic cyst)	Head and neck
Inflammatory (Wegener's granulomatosis, rheumatoid nodule, sarcoidosis)	Melanoma Colon Kidney
Other (hematoma, infarct, pseudotumour, rounded atelectasis, lymph nodes, amyloidoma)	Sarcoma Germ cell tumours
	Pulmonary carcinoid

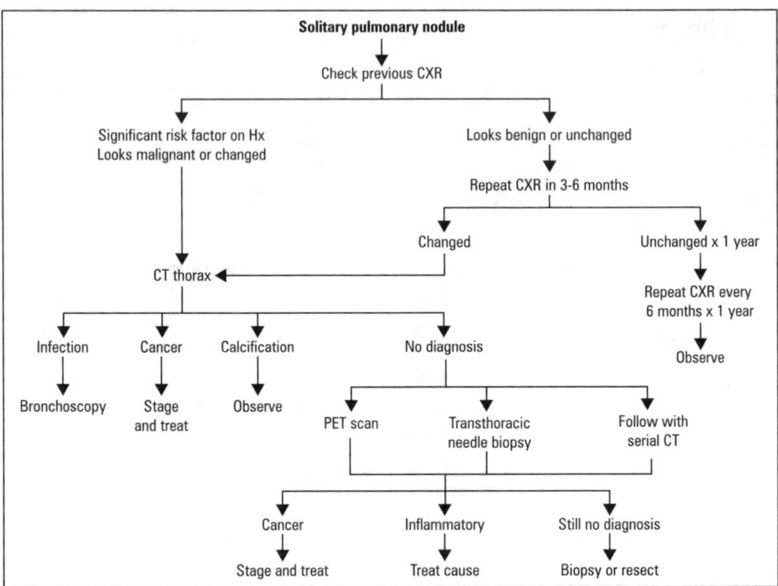

Common Conditions

Asthma

Definition
• Chronic inflammatory disorder characterized by airway hyper-responsiveness and episodic **reversible** airflow obstruction

Triggers
• URTIs, allergens (pet dander, house dust, moulds), irritants (cigarette smoke, air pollution), drugs (NSAIDS, β-blockers), emotion, anxiety, cold air, exercise, GERD

Symptoms and Signs
• Wheezing, cough especially nocturnal, dyspnea + tachypnea, chest tightness, sputum production
• Red flags: fatigue, cyanosis, silent chest, diminished expiratory effort, diminished LOC
• Respiratory distress: nasal flaring, tracheal tug, accessory muscle use, intercostal indrawing, pulsus paradoxus, difficulty speaking

Good Asthma Control
• Daytime symptoms <4 d/wk, night-time symptoms <1 night/wk, normal physical activity, mild and infrequent exacerbations, no asthma-related absences, use of β-agonists <4/wk, FEV_1 or peak flow >90% personal best, peak flow diurnal variation <10%

Investigations
• O_2 saturation
• ABG: decrease PaO_2 during an attack (increased P_aCO_2 ominous), decreased P_aCO_2 in mild asthma due to hyperventilation
• PFT (not conducted during an exacerbation): decrease in FEV_1 >20% with methacholine challenge, increase in FEV_1 >12% with β_2-agonist

Guidelines for Asthma Management

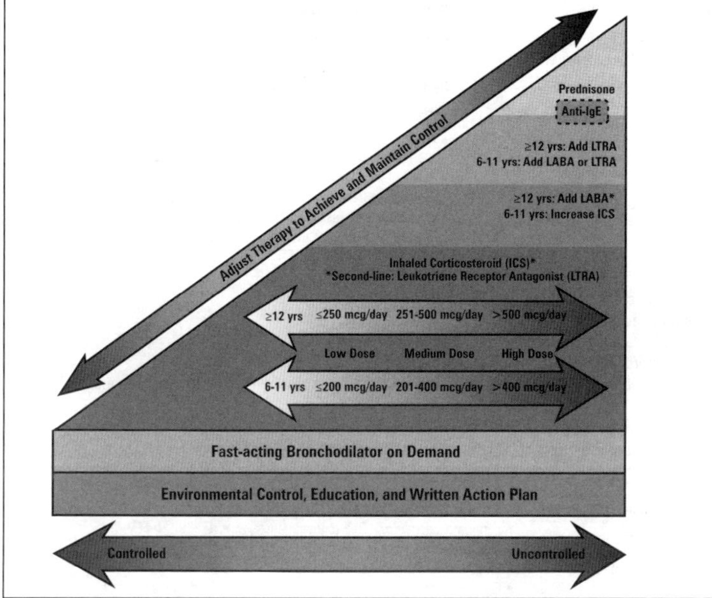

Adapted from Can Respir J 2010; 17(1): 15-24

Emergency Management
1. Inhaled short-acting β_2-agonist nebulized or via MDI with spacer, no role for IV β_2-agonist
2. Add inhaled anticholinergic
3. Ketamine and succinycholine for rapid sequence induction in life-threatening cases requiring intubation
4. SC/IV adrenaline, IV salbutamol if unresponsive
5. Systemic corticosteroid therapy at discharge

Outpatient Management
- Environmental controls: decrease exposure to triggers
- Patient education: disease features, self-monitoring, use of puffers, emergency plan
- Prevention of symptoms: inhaled corticosteroids, long-acting β_2-agonist, methylxanthine, leukotriene receptor antagonists
- Relief of symptoms in acute episodes: short-acting β_2-agonists and anticholinergic bronchodilators, oral steroids, addition of a long-acting β_2-agonist

COPD

Definition
- Characterized by progressive development of fixed or partially reversible airway obstruction, 2 subtypes (usually co-exist)
- Course: gradual decrease in FEV_1 over a period of time with episodes of acute exacerbations

Chronic Bronchitis	Emphysema
Defined clinically as:	**Defined pathologically as:**
Productive cough on most days for at least 3 consecutive months in 2 successive yrs	Dilation and destruction of air spaces distal to the terminal bronchiole without obvious fibrosis
Obstruction is due to narrowing of the airway lumen by mucosal thickening and excess mucus	Decreased elastic recoil of lung parenchyma causes decreased expiratory driving pressure, airway collapse, and air trapping
	2 types: 1) **Centriacinar** (respiratory bronchioles predominantly affected) • Typical form seen in smokers, primarily affects upper lung zones 2) **Panacinar** (respiratory bronchioles, alveolar ducts, and alveolar sacs) • Responsible for less than 1% of emphysema cases, (α-1-antitrypsin deficiency), primary affects lower lobes

Risk Factors
- Smoking is the most important risk factor (likelihood ratio of 8.3)
- Other risk factors include:
  - Environmental factors: air pollution, occupational exposure
  - Treatable factors: increased BMI, a1-antitrypsin deficiency, bronchial hyperactivity
  - Demographic factors: age, family history, male sex, history of childhood respiratory infections, and low SES

Clinical Presentation and Investigations for Chronic Bronchitis and Emphysema

	Symptoms	Signs	Investigations
Bronchitis (Blue Bloater)	• Chronic productive cough • Purulent sputum • Hemoptysis • Mild dyspnea initially	• Cyanotic ($2°$ to hypoxemia and hypercapnia) • Peripheral edema from RVF (cor pulmonale) • Crackles, wheezes • Prolonged expiration if obstructive • Frequently obese	PFT: • $\downarrow$ FEV$_1$, $\downarrow$ FEV$_1$/FVC • N TLC, $\downarrow$ or N DL$_{CO}$ CXR: • AP diameter normal • $\uparrow$ bronchovascular markings • Enlarged heart with cor pulmonale

Clinical Presentation and Investigations for Chronic Bronchitis and Emphysema (continued)

	Symptoms	Signs	Investigations
Emphysema (Pink Puffer)	• Dyspnea ($\pm$ exertion) • Minimal cough • Tachypnea • $\downarrow$ exercise tolerance	• Pink skin • Pursed-lip breathing • Accessory muscle use • Cachectic appearance due to anorexia + increased work of breathing • Hyperinflation/barrel chest, hyperresonant percussion • $\downarrow$ breath sounds • $\downarrow$ diaphragmatic excursion	PFT: • $\downarrow$ FEV$_1$, $\downarrow$ FEV$_1$/FVC • $\uparrow$ TLC (hyperinflation) • $\uparrow$ RV (gas trapping) • $\downarrow$ DL$_{CO}$ CXR: • $\uparrow$ AP diameter • Flat hemidiaphragm (lateral CXR) • $\downarrow$ heart shadow • $\uparrow$ retrosternal space • Bullae • $\downarrow$ peripheral vascular markings

Treatment of Stable COPD
- Prolong survival
  - Smoking cessation: nicotine replacement, bupropion (Zyban®)
  - Vaccination: influenza, pneumovax
  - Home oxygen: to prevent cor pulmonale and decrease mortality if used >15 h/d
    - indications: P$_a$O$_2$ <55 mmHg or <60 mmHg with cor pulmonale or polycythemia

- Symptomatic relief (no mortality benefit)
  - Bronchodilators: mainstay of current drug therapy, used in combination
    - Short-acting anticholinergics (e.g. ipratropium bromide) and short-acting β_2-agonists (e.g. salbutamol, terbutaline)
      - SABAs: rapid onset of action but significant side effects at high doses (e.g. hypokalemia)
      - Short-acting anticholinergics more effective than SABAs with fewer side effects but slower onset of action; take regularly rather than PRN
    - Long acting β_2-agonists (LABAs e.g. salmeterol, formoterol) and long-acting anticholinergics (LAACs e.g. tiotropium bromide)
      - More sustained effects for moderate to severe COPD
    - Inhaled corticosteroid (ICS) + LABA combination (e.g. Advair®: fluticasone + salmeterol, Symbicort®: budesonide + formoterol)
      - ICS/LABA increases effectiveness vs. LABA alone
    - Theophylline: weak bronchodilators; limited evidence to suggest adding to bronchodilator therapy
      - Side effects include nervous tremor, nausea/vomiting/diarrhea, tachycardia, arrhythmias, sleep changes
    - PDE4 inhibitor: roflumilast (DAXAS®) – weak bronchodilator
  - Corticosteroids
    - ICS monotherapy is controversial as effects are inconsistent
    - COPD airways are usually inflamed, but not generally responsive to steroids; therefore avoid chronic use of systemic glucocorticoids
  - Surgical treatment: lung reduction (resection of emphysematous parts of lung, associated with higher mortality if FEV_1 <20%), lung transplant
- Others
  - Patient education, eliminate respiratory irritants/allergens (occupational/environmental), exercise rehabilitation to improve physical endurance

Guidelines for COPD Management

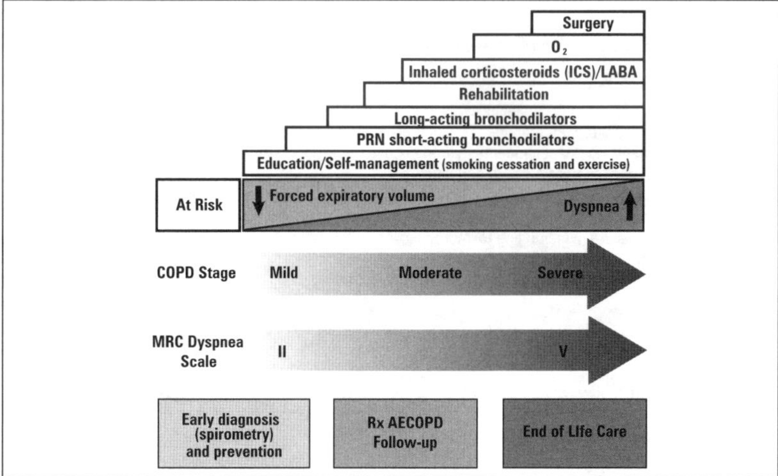

Adapted from Canadian Thoracic Society recommendations for management of chronic obstructive pulmonary disease - 2008 update - highlights for primary care. (2008). Can Respir J 2008; (Suppl A):15

Prognosis in COPD
- Complications
  - $2°$ polycythemia due to hypoxemia
  - Pulmonary hypertension due to reactive vasoconstriction $2°$ to hypoxemia
  - Cor pulmonale from chronic pulmonary HTN
  - Pneumothorax due to formation of bullae in emphysema
- Prognostic factors
  - Severity of airflow limitation (FEV_1) is the single best predictor
  - Development of complicating factors such as hypoxemia or cor pulmonale
- 5-yr survival
  - FEV_1 <1 L = 50%
  - FEV_1 <0.75 L = 33%
- BODE index for risk of death in COPD
  - 10 point index consisting of four factors:
  - **B**ody mass index (BMI): <21 (+1 point)
  - **O**bstruction (FEV_1): 50-64% (+1), 36-49% (+2), <35% (+3)
  - **D**yspnea (MMRC scale): breathless on walking on leveled surface (+1), after 1000 m (+2), with ADLs (+3)
  - **E**xercise capacity (6 min walk distance): 250-349 m (+1), 150-249 m (+2), <149 m (+3)
  - Greater score indicates higher probability that the patient will die from COPD; = score can also be used to predict hospitalization

ACUTE EXACERBATIONS OF COPD

Definition
- Sustained worsening of dyspnea, coughing, increase in sputum volume or purulence

Etiology
- Viral URTI's, bacteria, air pollution, CHF, PE, MI must be considered

Management
1. Assess ABCs, consider assisted ventilation if decreasing LOC or poor ABGs
2. Supplemental O_2 (controlled FiO_2): target 88-92% O_2 saturation for CO_2 retainers
3. Bronchodilators by nebulizer
   - Short acting β_2-agonists used concurrently with anticholinergics
   - Salbutamol and ipratropium bromide via nebulizers x 3 back-to-back
4. Systemic corticosteroids: IV solumedrol, hydrocortisone, methylprednisolone
5. Antibiotics: often used to treat precipitating infection
   - Indications (2 out of 3): increased SOB, increased sputum, or increased sputum purulence (change in colour)
6. Post-exacerbation
   - Rehab with general conditioning to improve exercise tolerance
- ICU admission: for life threatening exacerbations
  - Ventilatory support: non-invasive (NIPPV, CPAP, BiPAP), conventional mechanical ventilation

Bronchiectasis

Definition
- Irreversible dilation of airways (usually medium to small) due to inflammatory destruction of airway walls resulting from persistently infected mucus (*P. aeruginosa* most common once bronchiectasis is established)

Etiology
- Obstruction (tumours, FB, mucus); post-infection (pneumonia, TB, measles, pertussis, *Mycobacterium avium* Complex (MAC), allergic bronchopulmonary aspergillosis); impaired defenses (hypogammaglobulinemia, CF, defective leukocyte function, ciliary dysfunction)

Signs and Symptoms (often difficult to differentiate from chronic bronchitis)
• Chronic cough, purulent sputum, hemoptysis (can be massive), recurrent pneumonia
• Local crackles (inspiratory and expiratory), clubbing

Investigations
• PFTs: obstructive/normal
• CXR: "tram tracking" (specific); nonspecific: increased markings, linear atelectasis, loss of volume in affected areas
• CT Thorax: to define extent and pattern of bronchiectasis

Treatment
• Vaccination (influenza, Pneumovax®), antibiotics (exacerbations)
• Inhaled corticosteroids (oral for major exacerbations)
• Inhaled antibiotics and mucolytics (e.g. hypertonic saline, DNase)
• Chest physiotherapy, breathing exercises, physical exercise
• Pulmonary resection: for focal bronchiectasis in select cases

Sleep Apnea

Definition
• Episodic decreases in airflow during sleep (AHI >15)
  ▪ AHI = Apnea/Hypopnea index = # apneic and hypopneic events per hour of sleep
  ▪ Apnea – no breathing for ≥10 s; Hypopnea – >50% reduction in ventilation for ≥10 s
• Classified as obstructive (OSA), central (CSA), and mixed (MSA)

OBSTRUCTIVE SLEEP APNEA

Etiology
• Transient, episodic obstruction of upper airway in which there is absent/reduced airflow despite persistent respiratory effort
• Usually presents in middle aged obese male snorer

History (obtain history from spouse/partner as well)
• Risk factors: obesity, upper airway abnormality, neuromuscular disease, hypothyroidism, EtOH/sedative use, nasal congestion, sleep deprivation
• Daytime somnolence, personality and cognitive changes, snoring
• Morning headache, CHF symptoms, nocturnal angina

Physical Exam
• Neck thickness, Mallampati score, omo-mental distance
• Signs of polycythemia
• CV: systemic HTN, pulmonary HTN, arrhythmias, cor pulmonale/CHF

Investigations
• Sleep study indicated if: excessive daytime sleepiness, unexplained pulmonary HTN or polycythemia, daytime hypercapnia, titration of optimal nasal CPAP, assessment of objective response to other interventions

Treatment
• Risk factor modification (weight loss, decreased EtOH/sedatives, nasal decongestion, treatment of underlying medical conditions
• CPAP: reduces CV risk and CV related deaths in patients with OSA
• Postural therapy, dental appliance, uvulopalatopharyngoplasty, tonsillectomy

Complications
• Cardiac complications (OSA is an independent risk-factor for HTN): MI, CHF, CAD
• Depression, weight gain, decreased QOL, workplace and vehicular accidents, reduced work/social function

Pulmonary Embolism

Definition
- Clot in the pulmonary arterial tree with subsequent obstruction of the blood supply to the lung parenchyma, may present as a number of clinical syndromes ranging from asymptomatic to massive PE

History
- Risk factors: Virchow's Triad (venous stasis, endothelial cell damage, hypercoagulable state)
- Shortness of breath, pleuritic chest pain, hemoptysis, palpitations and symptoms of DVT

Common Investigations
- CXR: may be normal (most common) or demonstrate atelectasis, pleural effusions, **Hampton's hump** (cone-shaped opacification representing atelectasis/infarction) or **Westermark's sign** (dilated proximal pulmonary artery with decreased distal vascular markings)
- ECG: findings neither sensitive nor specific; sinus tachycardia (most common), nonspecific ST changes, RAD, RBBB, S_1-Q_3-T_3 with large emboli ("classic finding")
- ABG: demonstrating respiratory alkalosis and hypoxemia

Probability of a PE
- Investigations ordered depending on pretest probability
  - Wells criteria

Clinical Prediction Rule for Pulmonary Embolism (Wells Score)

Risk Factors	Points
Clinical signs of DVT	3.0
No more likely alternative diagnosis (using H&P, CXR, ECG)	3.0
Immobilization or surgery in the previous 4 wks	1.5
Previous PE/DVT	1.5
Heart rate >100 beats/min	1.5
Hemoptysis	1.0
Malignancy	1.0
Clinical probability	
Low (<2)	3%
Intermediate (2-6)	28%
High (>6)	78%
Simplified wells: >4 likely; ≤4 unlikely for PE	

Thrombosis and Hemostasis 2000; 83(3):416-20 *JAMA* 2006

Evaluation of a Suspected Pulmonary Embolism

Low clinical probability of embolism:	Intermediate or high probability:
D-dimer (+ve) CT scan (+ve) ruled in	**CT scan (–ve)** ruled out
(–ve) ↓ (–ve) ↓	(+ve) ↓
ruled out ruled out	ruled in

Notes:
Use D-dimers only if low clinical probability, otherwise, go straight to spiral CT
If using V/Q scans (CT contrast allergy or renal failure):
- Negative V/Q scan rules out the diagnosis
- High probability V/Q scan only rules in the diagnosis if have high clinical suspicion
- Inconclusive V/Q scan requires ultrasound, or spiral CT for furthe investigation

- If PE unlikely (i.e. Wells ≤4) a negative D-dimer effectively rules out PE (99.5%); a positive D-dimer is handled as a "likely" pretest probability
- If PE likely (i.e. Wells >4) or D-dimer positive a negative CT thorax rules out PE (98.7%) and a positive CT thorax indicates need to initiate treatment
- If the CT is inconclusive or contraindicated
    - A positive leg Doppler ultrasound or V/Q scan with high probability should initiate treatment
    - A negative leg Doppler ultrasound and a normal V/Q scan effectively rules out a PE
    - A negative leg Doppler ultrasound and a low or intermediate probability V/Q scan prompts serial leg Doppler in 7 d; if positive initiate treatment and if negative stop

Initial Treatment
- Uncomplicated PE: treated with low molecular weight heparin (LMWH)
- If renal failure or increased risk of bleeding: IV unfractionated heparin (UFH)
- If anticoagulation is contraindicated: placement of an inferior vena cava (IVC) filter by interventional radiology
- If massive PE (severe hypoxemia or refractory hypotension): consider thrombolysis
- Start oral anticoagulation with warfarin on the same d as heparin initiated; titrate INR to 2-3 and discontinue heparins when INR therapeutic >24 h

Outpatient Treatment
- If a reversible or treatable risk factor: treat underlying cause and continue anticoagulation for 3-6 months
- If an underlying but untreatable condition: lifelong anticoagulation with a target INR of 2-3 unless there is a significant bleeding risk; with underlying cancer LMWH more effective than warfarin
- If recurrent DVT/PE: lifelong anticoagulation after the second event regardless of cause
- If pregnant: treat with LMWH through pregnancy then warfarin for 4-6 wks post-partum for a minimum total of 3-6 months
- If idiopathic DVT/PE: anticoagulate with warfarin for a minimum of 6 months and then either stop, continue lifelong anticoagulation or complete a hypercoagulable work-up depending on patient risks, pregnancy plans, personal preference and cardiorespiratory reserve
- If patient has cancer – lifelong heparin therapy

VTE Risk Categories and Prophylaxis

Risk Group	Prophylaxis Options
Low thrombosis risk: Medical patients: fully mobile Surgery: <30 min, fully mobile	No specific prophylaxis Frequent ambulation
Moderate thrombosis risk: Most general, gynecologic, urologic surgery Sick medical patients	LMWH Low dose heparin
High thrombosis risk: Arthoplasty, hip fracture surgery Major trauma, spinal cord injury	LMWH Fondaparinux Warfarin (INR 2-3)
High bleeding risk: Neurosurgery, intracranial bleed Active bleeding	TED stockings, pneumatic compression devices LMWH or low dose heparin when bleeding risk decreases

Pneumonia

- See Infectious Diseases

Pleural Effusion

Definition
- An excess amount of fluid in the pleural space

Etiology
- **Transudative**: CHF, cirrhosis, nephrotic syndrome, pulmonary embolism (may cause transudative or exudative effusion), peritoneal dialysis, hypothyroidism, cystic fibrosis
- **Exudative**: **infectious** (parapneumonic associated with bacterial pneumonia and lung abscess, TB, viral infection), **malignancy** (lung cancer, lymphoma, mesothelioma and metastases from breast, ovary and kidney), **vascular** (RA, SLE, PE), **intra-abdominal** (esophageal perforation, pancreatic disease, subphrenic abscess, Meigs' syndrome), **trauma** (chylothorax, hemothorax), **other** (spontaneous, traumatic, tension pneumothorax)

Investigations
- CXR: need >250 cc pleural fluid for visualization, include lateral decubitus with A/P
- Thoracentesis: analysis for colour, protein, LDH, Gram stain, culture, cell count and differential, cytology, glucose, rheumatoid factor, ANA, complement, amylase, pH, blood and triglycerides (see <u>Common Procedures in Clerkship</u>)

Light's Criteria For Pleural Effusion

	Transudate	Exudate
Protein (pleural/serum)	<0.5	>0.5
LDH (pleural/serum)	<0.6	>0.6
Pleural LDH	<2/3 upper limit serum normal	>2/3 upper limit serum normal

*if any one criteria for an exudates is met the effusion is considered an exudate

Simple vs. Complicated Pleural Effusion

	Simple Effusion	Complicated Effusion
pH	>7.2	<7.2
LDH	<1/2 serum	>1/2 serum
Glucose	>2.2	<2.2
Other		Positive Gram stain
Treatment	Treat underlying cause May need drainage	REQUIRES drainage Treat underlying cause

Empyema

Definition
- Pus in pleural space or an effusion with organisms seen on a gram stain or culture (i.e. pleural fluid is grossly purulent) – positive culture NOT required for Dx
- Results from contiguous spread from lung infection (esp. anaerobes), or infection through chest wall (e.g. trauma, surgery)

Signs and Symptoms
- Fever, pleuritic chest pain

Investigations
- CT chest, throacentesis, PMNs (lymphocytes in TB), + visible organisms on Gram stain

Treatment
- Antibiotics (4-6 wks), chest tube, + surgical drainage (loculated/difficult to drain)

Intersitial Lung Disease

Definition
• Inflammatory or fibrotic process in alveolar walls leading to fibrosis of interstitium and characterized by decreased lung compliance, decreased lung volumes, impaired diffusion, hypoxemia without hypercarbia and pulmonary hypertension

Etiology
• >100 known disorders, 65% of cases due to unknown agents
• **Upper lung disease: "FASSTEN"** – **F**armer's lung, **A**nkylosing **S**pondylitis, **S**arcoidosis, silicosis, **T**B (miliary), **E**osinophilic granuloma, **N**eurofibromatosis
• **Lower lung disease: "BADRASH"** – **B**ronchiolitis obliterans with organizing pneumonia (BOOP), **A**sbestosis, **D**rugs (nitrofurantoin, hydralazine, INH, amiodarone), **R**heumatic disease, **A**spiration, **S**cleroderma, **H**amman-Rich syndrome (interstitial pulmonary fibrosis)

Investigations
• CXR: reticulonodular pattern, diffuse ground-glass appearance early with progression to "honeycombing"
• PFT: restrictive pattern, normal or increased flows, decreased DL_{CO}
• ABG: initially may be normal, hypoxemia and decreased $PaCO_2$ may be present
• Other: bronchoscopy, BAL, lung biopsy, c-ANCA, anti-GBM, ESR, ANA, RF, high resolution CT

Malignant Lung Tumours

Characteristics of Bronchogenic Cancer

Cell Type	Incidence	Correlation with smoking	Location	Histology	Metastasis
Adenocarcinoma	M~35% F~40%	Weak	Peripheral	Glandular, mucin producing	Early, distant
Squamous cell carcinoma (SCC)	30%	Strong	Central	Keratin, intercellular bridges	Local invasion and distant spread, may cavitate
SCLC	25%	Strong	Central	Oat cell, neuroendocrine	Disseminated at presentation origin in endobronchial cells
Large cell carcinoma	10-15%	Strong	Peripheral	Anaplastic, undifferentiated	Early, distant

Risk Factors
• Cigarette smoking (85% of lung cancer related to smoking), asbestos (5x increased risk, 80-90x increased risk in smoker), radiation, arsenic, chromium, nickel, genetic damage, parenchymal scarring (granulomatous disease, fibrosis, scleroderma), passive exposure to cigarette smoke, air pollution (exact role uncertain), HIV

Clinical Presentation
• Cough (75%); beware of chronic cough that changes in character
• Dyspnea (60%), chest pain (45%), hemoptysis (35%), other pain (25%), clubbing (21%)
• Constitutional signs: anorexia, weight loss, fever, anemia

RESPIROLOGY

Common Medications

	Drug	Adult dose	Indications	Side Effects
β-2 AGONISTS				
Short-acting	salbutamol/albuterol (Ventolin®) (light blue/navy), terbutaline (Bricanyl®)	1-2 puffs q4-6h prn Max 12 puffs/d	Bronchodilator in acute reversible airway obstruction	CV (angina, flushing, palpitations, tachycardia, can precipitate Afib), CNS (dizziness, headache, insomnia, anxiety), GI (diarrhea, nausea, vomiting), rash, hypokalemia, paroxysmal bronchospasm
Long-acting	salmeterol (Serevent®), formoterol (Oxeze®)	1-2 puffs bid	Maintenance treatment (prevention of bronchospasm) in chronic obstructive lung disease, asthma	
Combination	fluticasone and salmeterol (Advair®) (purple discus)	1 puff bid	COPD and asthma	Common: CNS, headache, dizziness Resp: URTI, GI (N/V, diarrhea, pain/discomfort, oral candidiasis)
Long-acting β-2 agonist and inhaled corticosteroid	Budesonde and formoterol (Symbicort®) (red puffer)			
ANTICHOLINERGICS				
	ipratropium bromide (Atrovent®) (clear/green), tiotropium bromide (Spiriva®)	2-3 puffs qid 1 puff qam	Bronchodilator used in COPD, bronchitis and emphysema	Palpitations, anxiety, dizziness, fatigue, headache, nausea, dry mucous membranes, increased toxicity in combination with other anticholinergic drugs
CORTICOSTEROIDS				
Inhaled	fluticasone (Flovent®) (orange/peach) budesonide (Pulmicort®) ciclesonide (Alvesco®)	2-4 puffs bid 2 puffs bid 1-4 puffs OD	Maintenance treatment of asthma	Headache, fever, N/V, MSK pain, URTI, throat irritation, growth velocity reduction in children/adolescents, HPA axis suppression, increased pneumonia risk in COPD
	beclomethasone (QVAR®, Vanceril®)	1-4 puffs bid (40 µg), 1-2 puffs bid (80 µg)		
Systemic	prednisone (Apo-prednisone®, Deltasone®)	Typically 40-60 mg per day PO 125 mg q8h as initial treatment for	Acute exacerbation of COPD; severe, persistent asthma, PCP	Endocrine (hirsutism, DM/glucose intolerance, Cushing's syndrome, HPA axis suppression), GI (increased appetite, indigestion), ocular (cataracts, glaucoma), edema, AVN, osteoporosis, headache, psych (anxiety, insomnia), easy bruising
	methylprednisolone (Depo-Medrol®, Solu-Medrol®)	IV (sodium succinate) loading dose 2 mg/kg then 0.5-1 mg/kg q6h for 5 d	Status asthmaticus	
ADJUNCT AGENTS	theophylline (Elixophyllin®, Theo-Dur®)	5-13 mg/kg/d PO in divided doses, max 900 mg/d	Treatment of symptoms of reversible airway obstruction due to COPD	GI upset, diarrhea, N/V, anxiety, headache, insomnia, muscle cramp, tremor, tachycardia, PVCs, arrhythmias Toxicity: persistent, repetitive vomiting, seizures
LEUKOTRIENE ANTAGONISTS				
	montelukast (Singular®)	10 mg PO qhs, now only available as once daily slow release	Prophylaxis and chronic treatment of asthma	Headache, dizziness, fatigue, fever, rash, dyspepsia, cough, flu-like symptoms

Rheumatology

Essential History, Physical Exam and Investigations

History	Physical Exam
Pain (OPQRST) Beware: constant pain, night pain (malignancy, infection)	**Inspection (SEADS)** Swelling Erythema Atrophy of muscle
Referred symptoms Shoulder: heart, diaphragm Arm: neck Leg: back Knee, groin: hip	Deformity (changes in shape/bony alignment/posture) Skin changes (bruising, discolouration) **Palpation** Tenderness, warmth, nodules, effusion, crepitus, skin texture, pulses
Inflammatory symptoms Pain, erythema, warmth, swelling, morning stiffness >30 min	**Range of Motion** **Active**: abnormalities due to neurological or mechanical problems –
Mechanical/Degenerative symptoms Pain worse at end of day, better with rest, worse with use	pain, limitation, crepitus **Passive**: abnormalities due to stiffness or pain Hypermobility Note how joint feels at end of ROM
Constitutional symptoms Fever, chills, weight loss, anorexia, fatigue	**Neurologic** Power
Neurological symptoms Bowel and bladder incontinence/complaints, paresthesia, tingling, headaches, weakness	Sensation Gait
Trauma	***GALS Screening: Gait, Arms, Legs, Spine**
Recent Illness	
Travel, birthplace, camping	
Past Medical History Malignancy, vasculitis, IBD, psoriasis, any autoimmune/ rheumatologic conditions	
Presence of EAMs (extra-articular manifestations)	
Impact on ADLs	

Investigations

BLOODWORK
- General: CBC, electrolytes, BUN, creatinine
- ESR (increases with other acute phase reactants, and chronically, with increase in gamma globulins)
  - DDx: RA, PMR, GCA, hypoalbuminemia, anemia, multiple myeloma, bacterial infections, malignancy
  - ESR is insensitive for: PM/DM, AS, PSS, SLE, viral infections
- Acute phase reactants: albumin, C3 and C4 (often decreased in active SLE), fibrinogen, CRP, ferritin

SEROLOGY

Autoantibodies and Their Prevalence in Rheumatic Diseases

Autoantibody	Disease (sensitivity)	Normal Population	Comments
RF	RA 80% Sjögren's 50% SLE 20%	<5%	Autoantibodies (IgM>IgG>IgA) directed against Fc domain of IgG Present in most seropositive diseases Levels correlate with disease severity in RA Non-specific; may be present in IE, TB, hep C, silicosis, sarcoidosis
Anti-CCP	RA 80%		
ANA	SLE 98% MCTD 95% Sjögren's 70-90% CREST 80%	<5% other CTDs	Antibodies against nuclear components (DNA, RNA, histones, centromere) 1:40 dilution found in 5-30% of the normal population Sensitive but not specific for SLE
Anti-dsDNA	SLE 50-70%	0%	Specific for SLE Levels often correlate with disease activity
Anti-Sm	SLE <30%	0%	Specific but not sensitive for SLE
Anti-Ro (SSA)	Sjögren's 40-95% SLE 25%	0.5%	Subacute cutaneous SLE and mothers of babies with neonatal lupus and complete heart block
Anti-La (SSB)	Sjögren's 40% SLE 10%	0%	Usually occurs with anti-Ro
Anti-phospholipid antibodies	APS 100% SLE 31-40%	<5%	By definition present in APS Only small subset of SLE patients develop clinical syndrome of APS (LAC, ACLA)
Anti-histone	Drug-induced SLE >90%	0%	If positive will often get a false positive VDRL/RPR test
	Idiopathic SLE >50%	0%	
Anti-RNP	MCTD		Present in MCTD; present in many other CTD
Anti-centromere	CREST >80%	0%	Specific for CREST variant of PSS
Anti-topoisomerase I (formerly Scl-70)	PSS 26-76%	0%	
c-ANCA	Active Wegener's >90%	0%	Specific and sensitive
p-ANCA	Wegener's 10% other vasculitis	0%	Nonspecific and poor sensitivity
Anti-Jo-1	Dermatomyositis 15-20%		Specific but not sensitive
Antibodies against RBCs, WBCs, or platelets	SLE		Perform direct Coomb's test Test hemoglobin, reticulocyte, leukocyte and platelet count, antiplatelet Abs

URINALYSIS
• See Nephrology

SYNOVIAL FLUID ANALYSIS

Parameter	Normal	Non-Inflammatory	Inflammatory	Infectious	Hemorrhagic
Colour	Clear	Clear	Opaque	Opaque	Sanguinous
Viscosity	High (due to hyaluronic acid)	High	Low	Low	Variable
WBC/mm^3	<200	<2,000	>2,000	>50,000	Variable
% PMN	<25%	<25%	>25%	>50%	Variable
Examples		Trauma Osteoarthritis Neuropathy Hypertrophic osteoarthropathy	Seropositives Seronegatives Crystal arthropathies	Septic arthritis	Trauma Hemophilia

RADIOLOGY
• Plain film, CT, MRI, U/S, bone densitometry, angiography, bone scan depending on initial evaluation

Common Presentations

Back Pain

• See also <u>Family Medicine</u>

Types of Back Pain

Parameter	Mechanical	Inflammatory
Past History	±	++
Family History	–	+
Onset	Acute	Insidious
Age (years)	15-90	<40
Sleep Disturbance	±	++ (worse during 2nd half of night)
Morning Stiffness	<30 min	>1 hour
Involvement of Other Systems	–	+
Exercise	Worse	Better
Rest	Better	Worse
Radiation of Pain	Anatomic (L5-S1)	Diffuse (thoracic, buttock – alternating buttock pain, heel pain)
Sensory Symptoms	+	–
Motor Symptoms	+	–

Joint Pain

History
• Duration: chronic (>6 wks) or acute (<1 wk)
• Articular (vs. non-articular) pain: deep, diffuse pain, limited range of motion on active/passive movement (stress pain), swelling, crepitation, instability, deformity
• Inflammatory: active joint symptoms (erythema, warmth, stress pain, swelling), systemic symptoms, morning stiffness >30 min, pain is worse with rest, improves with activity
• Noninflammatory: absence of active joint symptoms, no systemic symptoms, morning stiffness <30 min, pain is worse with activity, improves with rest, history of trauma

- Extra-articular features: rash, myalgias, weakness, red eyes (reactive), chronic diarrhea (IBD), oral ulcers (seronegative), urethral discharge (reactive/infectious), H/A or neurological symptoms (Lyme disease, vasculitis, entrapment neuropathies)
- Past history of similar complaint
- Family history of rheumatologic diseases
- Medications

Risk Factors/Predisposing/Precipitants
- Reactive: urethritis or gastroenteritis within past 2-4 wks
- Gout: diet, alcohol, diuretics, trauma
- Hemarthrosis: Recent trauma, history of hemophilia
- Arthritis in IBD: active GI disease for peripheral arthropathy but not sacroiliitis

Physical Exam
- Vitals: evidence of systemic infection
- H&N: oral ulcers, red eyes, iritis (on slit lamp examination), conjunctivitis
- CVS: pericardial rub, pericarditis, peripheral pulses
- Resp: inspiratory crackles, pleuritis
- Abdo: masses, tenderness, inspection for evidence of perianal ulcers, genital ulcers
- Derm: local vs. systemic rash
- Nails: ridges, pitting, nail bed capillary telangiectasia
- Neuro: especially if trauma suspected cause
- MSK: must examine all joints. Inspection (erythema, swelling, distribution), palpation (temperature, effusion, tenderness), passive and active range of motion
    - If suspect AS should complete full back exam, including back ROM, Faber test, Schober test, chest wall expansion
    - **FABER** (**F**lexion, **AB**duction, and **E**xternal **R**otation of the hip)
        - With patient supine, place foot ipsilateral to affected side onto opposing knee
            - Pain in the groin area indicates a hip problem, not spine
        - Push down on flexed knee and opposite ASIS
            - Pain in sacroiliac (SI) area indicates a SI joint problem
    - **Schober's Test**
        - With patient standing, mark midline at PSIS and 10 cm above PSIS
        - Ask patient to bend at waist to full forward flexion and measure distance between the 2 lines
        - Decreased lumbar ROM if distance <15 cm

Differential diagnosis = SOFTER TISSUE
- **S**epsis
- **O**A
- **F**racture
- **T**endon/muscle
- **E**piphyseal
- **R**eferred
- **T**umour
- **I**schemia
- **S**eropositive arthritis
- **S**eronegative arthritis
- **U**rate (gout/other crystal athropathies)
- **E**xtra-articular rheumatism (polymyalgia/fibromyalgia)

Arthritis

Clinical Approach To Arthritis

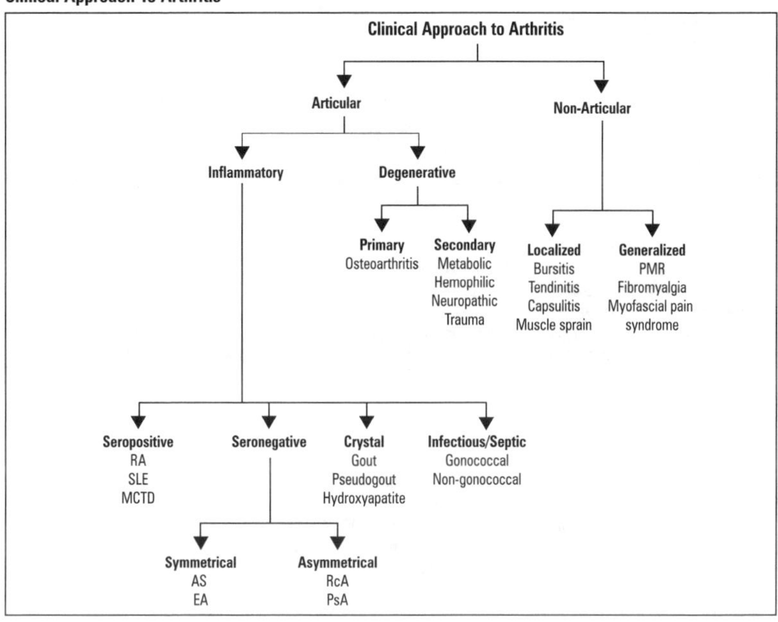

	Seropositive	Seronegative
Demographics	F > M	M > F
Peripheral arthritis	Symmetrical Small and large joint DIP less involved	Usually larger joints, lower extremities (PsA exception), Dactylitis, Enthesitis, DIP in psoriatic arthritis
Pelvic/Axial disease	No (except C-spine)	Yes
Enthesitis	No	Yes
Extra-articular	Nodules Vasculitis Sicca (dry eyes and mouth) Episcleritis Raynaud's phenomenon	Iritis (anterior uveitis) Oral ulcers GI (IBD) GU (urethritis) Dermatological features

Septic Arthritis

Definition
- Non-sterile synovial fluid cultures
- MEDICAL EMERGENCY!

Etiology
- *S. aureus, N. gonorrhoeae* (75% of septic arthritis in young, sexually active adults), streptococci, enteric Gram negatives

Risk Factors
- Extra-articular infection with hematogenous seeding, IVDU, chronic illness (RA, DM, malignancy), prior joint damage (OA, RA, prosthetic joints)

Clinical Features (Gonococcal Arthritis)
- Two syndromes: preceding bacteremia with skin lesions, tenosynovitis, and migrating polyarthritis; or purulent monoarthritis of a large joint (most often the knee)
- Systemic symptoms of infection: fever, malaise
- Local symptoms in involved joint: swelling, warmth, pain, inability to bear weight, marked decrease in ROM
- **Gonococcal triad**: migratory arthritis, tenosynovitis next to inflamed joint, pustular skin rash

Investigations
- Diagnosis with high index of suspicion plus the following:
  - C&S gonococcal (blood, urine, endocervical, urethral, rectal, and orophryngeal cultures), non-gonococcal (blood and urine)
  - Arthrocentesis (synovial fluid analysis): CBC and diff, Gram stain, culture, examine for crystals
    - Infectious = opaque, increased WBC count (inflammatory), PMNs >85%, culture positive
    - Growth of GC from synovial fluid is successful in <50% of cases
  - + plain x-ray: rule out osteomyelitis and baseline to monitor treatment
- Surgical consult, especially in the setting of a prosthetic joint

Gout and Pseudogout

Parameter	Gout	Pseudogout
Definition	Derangement in purine metabolism resulting in hyperuricemia, monosodium urate crystal deposits in tissue (tophi) and synovium	Joint inflammation secondary to phagocytosis of CPPD crystals (microtophi)
Gender	M>F	M=F
Age	Middle-aged males Post-menopausal females	Elderly
Precipitants	Drugs "FACT": **F**urosemide, **A**spirin/Alcohol **C**ytotoxic drugs, **T**hiazide diuretics Foods: shellfish, anchovies, liver and kidney, turkey, sardines	Dehydration, acute illness, surgery, trauma
Onset of Disease	Acute	Acute/insidious
Crystal Type	Negative birefringence, needle-shaped	Positive birefringence, rhomboid-shaped
Distribution	First MTP typical	Knee, wrist, polyarticular
Radiology	"Holes in bones"	Chondrocalcinosis OA (knee, wrist, 2nd and 3rd MCP)
Treatment	Indomethacin, colchicine, allopurinol	NSAIDs

Management

- Symptomatic relief: NSAIDs (indomethacin 25-50 mg TID, diclofenac 50 mg TID), colchicine (0.6 mg q1h until relief, maximum dose, or side effects), joint aspirate
- If above contraindicated, oral glucocorticoids (prednisone 30 mg/d), or intra-articular (7 mg betamethasone)
- Allopurinol is contraindicated in acute gout but may be used to reduce the frequency of attacks in chronic gout
- Chronic pain management

Common Conditions

Seropositive Rheumatic Disorders

- Rheumatoid arthritis (RA)
- Systemic Lupus Erythematosis (SLE)
- Antiphospholipid Antibody Syndrome (APLA)
- Scleroderma
- Polymyositis/Dermatomyositis
- Sjögren's Syndrome (SS)
- Mixed Connective Tissue Disease (MCTD)

Features of Seropositive Arthropathies

	Rheumatoid Arthritis	Systemic Lupus Erythematosus	Scleroderma	Dermatomyositis
Clinical Features				
History	Symmetrical polyarthritis (small joint involvement), AM stiffness (>1 h)	Multi-systemic disease: rash, photosensitivity, Raynaud's, alopecia, cardiac and pulmonary serositis, CNS symptoms, glomerulonephritis	Raynaud's, stiffness of fingers, skin tightness, heartburn/ dysphagia, pulmonary hypertension, renal dysfunction	Heliotrope rash (eyelids), Gottron's papules, macular erythema and poikiloderma (shoulders, neck and chest(, proximal muscle weakness ± pain
Physical Examination	Effused joints Tenosynovitis Nodules Bone-on-bone crepitus Joint deformities	Confirm historical findings (rash, serositis, etc.) ± effused (typically small) joints (can be minimal, look for soft tissue swelling	Skin tightness on dorsum of hand, facial skin tightening, telangiectasia, calcinosis, non-effused joint	Rash, proximal muscle weakness

	Rheumatoid Arthritis	Systemic Lupus Erythematosus	Scleroderma	Dermatomyositis
Laboratory				
Non-specific	Increased ESR in 50-60% Increased platelets Decreased Hb Decreased WBC (Felty's)	Increased ESR Decreased platelets (autoimmune) Decreased Hb (autoimmune) Decreased WBC (leukopenia, lymphopenia)	Increased ESR Increased platelets Decreased Hb Normal WBC	Possible increased ESR Normal platelets Decreased Hb Normal WBC
Specific	RF +ve in ~80%	ANA +ve in 98% Anti-SM +ve in 30% Anti-dsDNA +ve in 50-70% Decreased C3, C4, total hemolytic complement (CH50) False positive VDRL/RPR (in lupus subtypes) Increased PTT (in lupus subtypes; e.g. anti-phospholipid Ab)	ANA +ve in >90% Anti-topoisomerase 1 (diffuse) Anti-centromere (usually in CREST)	CK elevated in 80% ANA +ve in 33% anti-Jo-1, anti-Mi-2 Muscle biopsy – key for diagnosis EMG MRI
Synovial Fluid	Inflammation Leukocytosis (>10,000)	Mild inflammation	Not specific	Not specific
Radiographs	Symmetric/concentric Joint space narrowing Absence of bone repair Periarticular osteopenia Erosions	Non-destructive/ non-erosive ± osteopenia ± soft tissue swelling	± pulmonary fibrosis ± esophageal dysmotility ± calcinosis	± esophageal dysmotility ± interstitial lung disease ± calcification

RHEUMATOID ARTHRITIS

Common Chief Complaints
- Joint pain – chronic, symmetrical, polyarticular
- Systemic symptoms – fever, weight loss, fatigue, myalgias
- If established diagnosis of rheumatoid arthritis, ask about pulmonary symptoms (pulmonary fibrosis), pleural effusions, pericarditis, valvular disease, evidence of other autoimmune diseases

Diagnosis / ARA Classification Criteria
- At least four of the following seven criteria:
  1. Morning stiffness: joint stiffness >1h for >6 wks
  2. Arthritis in 3 or more joint areas: >3 active joints for >6 wks, commonly PIP, MCP, wrist, elbow, knee, ankle, MTP
  3. Arthritis of hand joints: at least 1 active joint in wrist, MCP or PIP for >6 wks
  4. Symmetrical arthritis: bilateral involvement of PIP, MCP, or MTP joints for >6 wks
  5. Rheumatoid nodules: subcutaneous nodules over bony prominences, extensor surfaces or in juxta-articular regions
  6. Serum RF: found in 60-80% of RA patients
  7. Radiographic changes: erosions or periarticular osteopenia, likely to see earliest changes at ulnar styloid, 2nd and 3rd MCP, and PIP joints

Associated Symptoms
- Extra-articular features either vasculitic or associated with lymphocytic infiltrates

Extra-Articular Features of RA Classified by Underlying Pathophysiology

System	Vasculitic	Lymphocytic Infiltrate
Skin and mucus membranes	Periungal infarction, cutaneous ulcers, palpable purpura	Rheumatoid nodules Sjögren's syndrome
Ocular	Episcleritis, scleritis	Keratoconjunctivitis sicca
Head and Neck		Xerostomia, Hashimoto's thyroiditis
Cardiac		Peri-/myocarditis, valvular disease, conduction defects
Pulmonary		Pulmonary fibrosis, pleural effusion, pleuritis, pulmonary nodules
Neurologic	Peripheral neuropathy: sensory stocking-glove, mononeuritis multiplex	
Hematologic		Splenomegaly, neutropenia (Felty's)

Complications
- Joint deformities, chronic pain, reduction in global functioning, anemia of chronic disease

Risk Factors
- Family history of rheumatoid arthritis

Physical Exam
- See physical examination in *Joint Pain*

Investigations
- RF positive in 60-80% of patients – non-specific, seen in other connective tissue diseases (SLE, Sjögren's), chronic inflammation (IE, hepatitis, TB), and 5% healthy population, increases with age
- Anti-CCP (cyclic citrullinated peptide): sensitivity ~80%
- Increased disease activity associated with decreased Hb (anemia of chronic disease), increased platelets, increased ESR/CRP/RF
- X-rays: diagnosing and monitoring disease progression; radiographic damage correlates with disability (see joint erosions 1-2 yrs after dx)

Treatment
- Education about illness, prognosis
- Reduction of inflammation, symptomatic relief: NSAIDs, glucocorticoids, analgesics
- DMARDs – therapy initiated when diagnosis confirmed
- Surgical therapy for treatment of joint degeneration and to improve function (depending on severity)

SYSTEMIC LUPUS ERYTHEMATOSUS

Diagnostic Criteria of SLE: 4 or more of 11 must be present serially or simultaneously "MD SOAP BRAIN"
(American College of Rheumatology, 1997 update)

Criteria	Description
Clinical	
Malar rash	Classic "butterfly rash", sparing of nasolabial folds, no scarring
Discoid rash	May cause scarring due to invasion of basement membrane
Photosensitivity	Skin rash in reaction to sunlight
Oral/nasal ulcers	Usually painless
Arthritis	Symmetric, involving ≥2 small or large peripheral joints, non-erosive
Serositis	Pleuritis or pericarditis
Neurologic disorder	Seizures or psychosis

Criteria	Description
Laboratory	
Renal disorder	Proteinuria (>0.5 g/d or 3+) Cellular casts (RBC, Hb, granular, tubular, mixed)
Hematologic disorder	Hemolytic anemia, leukopenia, lymphopenia, thrombocytopenia
Immunologic disorder	Anti-dsDNA Ab, anti-Sm Ab Antiphospholipid antibodies based on the finding of serum anticardiolipin Ab, lupus anticoagulant, or false positive VDRL C3 and C4 levels used to monitor progression and response to treatment
Antinuclear antibody (ANA)	Most sensitive test (98%)

Note: "4, 7, 11" rule 4 out of 11 criteria (4 lab, 7 clinical) for diagnosis
* These criteria were developed for research purposes. SLE can in some cases be diagnosed in the absence of four of the criteria.

VASCULITIS
Classification of Vasculitis and Characteristic Features

Classification	Characteristic Features
Small vessel	
Non-ANCA-associated	Immune complex mediated (most common mechanism)
Predominantly cutaneous vasculitis	Also known as hypersensitivity/leukocytoclastic vasculitis
Henoch-Schönlein purpura	Vascular deposition of IgA causing systemic vasculitis (skin, GI, renal), seen most frequently in childhood, usually self-limiting condition
Essential cryoglobulinemic vasculitis	Systemic vasculitis caused by circulating cryoproteins
ANCA-associated	
Wegener's granulomatosis (c-ANCA > p-ANCA)	Granulomatous inflammation of vessels of respiratory tract and kidneys, most common in middle age, most present initially with symptoms of URTI
Churg-Strauss syndrome (50% ANCA positive)	Granulomatous inflammation of vessels with hyper-eosinophilia and eosinophilic tissue infiltration, sometimes associated with p-ANCA or c-ANCA Other manifestations may include myocarditis and neuropathy
Microscopic polyangiitis (70% ANCA positive, usually p-ANCA)	Pauci-immune necrotizing vasculitis, affecting kidneys (necrotizing glomerulonephritis), lungs (capillaritis and alveolar hemorrhage), and skin, most common in middle age
Medium vessel	
Polyarteritis nodosa	Segmental non-granulomatous necrotizing inflammation Any age (average 40-50s), unknown etiology in most cases, M>F
Kawasaki's	T lymphocyte response and granuloma formation, most common in children
Large vessel	
Giant cell arteritis (GCA)/ Temporal arteritis	Over 50 yrs of age, F>M, inflammation of large vessels, often the temporal artery; can result in blindness if not treated urgently
Takayasu's arteritis	"Pulseless disease", chronic inflammation, most often the aorta and its branches, usually young adults of Asian descent, F>M
Other Vasculitides	
Buerger's disease	Also known as "thromboangiitis obliterans"; inflammation secondary to pathological clotting, affects small and medium-sized vessels of distal extremities, most important etiologic factor is cigarette smoking, most common in Asian males, may lead to distal claudication and gangrene
Behçet's disease	Pathology: leukocytoclastic vasculitis, multi-system disorder presenting with uveitis, recurrent oral and genital ulceration, venous thrombosis, skin and joint involvement, more common in Mediterranean and Asia, average age 30, M>F
Mimickers of vasculitis	Cholesterol emboli, atrial myxoma

GIANT CELL ARTERITIS/TEMPORAL ARTERITIS

Definition: large vessel vasculitis

Signs and Symptoms
* New onset temporal headaches ± scalp tenderness due to inflammation of involved portion of the temporal or occipital arteries
* Sudden, painless loss of vision and/or diplopia due to narrowing of the ophthalmic or posterior ciliary arteries
* Tongue and jaw claudication (pain in muscles of mastication on chewing)
* Polymyalgia rheumatica (proximal myalgia, constitutional symptoms, elevated ESR) occurs in 30% of patients
* Aortic arch syndrome (involvement of subclavian and brachial branches of aorta result in pulseless disease), aortic aneurysm ± rupture

Diagnosis
* GCA Criteria: (Presence of 3+ criteria yields sensitivity of 94%, specificity of 91%)
    * Age >50, new headache, temporal artery tenderness or decreased pulse, ESR>50, abnormal artery biopsy

Investigations
* Diagnosis made by clinical suspicion, increased ESR, increased CRP, temporal artery biopsy within 14 d of starting steroids, angiography

Treatment – untreated GCA can lead to permanent blindness in 20-25%
* If suspect GCA, immediately start high dose prednisone 1 mg/kg in divided doses, tapering prednisone as symptoms resolve (do NOT wait for biopsy); highly effective in treatment and in prevention of blindness and other vascular complications
* ASA 81 mg OD + PPI (for GI protection)
* IV methylprednisolone if visual loss has already occurred

Seronegative Arthropathies

A COMPARISON OF THE SPONDYLOARTHROPATHIES

Feature	AS	PsA	ReA	EA
M:F	5:1	1:1	8:1	1:1
Age onset	20s	35-45	20s	any
Peripheral arthritis	25%	96%	90%	Common
Distribution	Axial, LE	Any	LE	LE
Sacroiliitis	100%	40%	80%	20%
Dactylitis	Uncommon	35%	Common	Uncommon
Enthesitis	Common	Common	Common	Less Common
Skin lesions	Rare	100% Psoriasis	Common Keratoderma	Occasional Pyoderma, Erythema nodosum
Uveitis	30%	Occasional	20%	Rare
Urethritis	Rare	Occasional	Common	Rare
Aortic Regurgitation	Occasional	Rare	Occasional	Occasional
HLA-B27	90%	40%	80%	30%

AS = Ankylosing Spondylitis, PsA = Psoriatic Arthritis, ReA = Reactive Arthritis, EA = Enteropathic Arthritis

Polymyalgia Rheumatica

PMR Criteria
1. Age over 50
2. Bilateral aching/morning stiffness >1 month (esp in muscles of neck, shoulder girdle and pelvic girdle)
3. ESR over 40 mm/h (normal is <12)
4. Prompt response to low-dose corticosteroids (15-20 mg/d)

*Must screen for Giant Cell Arteritis (GCA)
* May also have signs of systemic inflammation with malaise, weight loss, sweats, and low grade fever

Raynaud's Phenomenon

Investigations
- Reversible digital ischemia in response to stress or cold; affects fingers, toes, ears, and nose
- Classically see blanching » cyanosis » rubor; may also get associated cold, numbness and paresthesias

Differential Diagnosis
- Primary (50%) = Raynaud's disease; treatment is non-pharmacologic or nifedipine if severe
- Secondary (50%)
  - Rheumatic disease: SLE, RA, scleroderma, Sjogren's syndrome
  - Arterial disease: peripheral atherosclerosis, thromboangiitis obliterans
  - Hematologic: cryoglobulinemia, antiphospholipid antibody syndrome
  - Trauma (frostbite, vibrating tools)
  - Drugs (propranolol, ergotamine, estrogen, certain chemotherapy agents)

Osteoarthritis

Definition
- Progressive deterioration of articular cartilage resulting from failed repair of joint damage from repetitive stresses on the joint (breakdown of cartilage and bone)
- Primary (idiopathic, most common)
- Secondary
  - Post-traumatic or mechanical, post-inflammatory (e.g. RA) or post-infectious, heritable skeletal disorders (e.g. scoliosis), endocrine disorders (e.g. acromegaly, hyperparathyroidism, hypothyroidism), metabolic disorders (e.g. gout, pseudogout, hemochromatosis, Wilson's disease, ochronosis), neuropathic (also known as Charcot joints – atypical joint trauma due to loss of proprioceptive senses e.g. diabetes, syphilis), avascular necrosis (e.g. steroids, alcohol, sickle cell), other (e.g. congenital malformation)

Epidemiology
- Most common arthropathy (12% of people aged 25-74)
- Increased prevalence with increasing age (35% of 30 yr olds, 85% of 80 yr olds)

Risk Factors
- Genetic predisposition, advanced age, obesity (for knee OA), female, trauma

Signs and Symptoms of OA

Symptoms	Signs
Joint pain with motion; relieved with rest	Joint line tenderness; stress pain
Short duration of stiffness ($<1/2$ h) after immobility	Bony enlargement at affected joints
Joint instability/buckling	Malalignment/deformity (angulation)
Loss of function	Limited ROM
Joint locking	Periarticular muscle atrophy
Insidious, gradually progressive	Crepitus on passive ROM
	Inflammation mild if present

Joint Involvement
- Any joint can be affected especially knee, hip, hand, spine (shoulder, elbow, wrist and ankle are less common)
- Hand: DIP (Heberden's nodes), PIP (Bouchard's nodes), CMC (usually thumb squaring), MCP is usually spared (except the 1st MCP)
- Hip: dull or sharp pain in trochanter, groin, anterior thigh, or knee; internal rotation and abduction are lost first
- Knee: narrowing of one compartment of knee (medial > lateral)
- Foot: common in first MTP
- Lumbar spine: common, may have neurological impingement
- Cervical spine: neck pain, in lower cervical area

Investigations
- Blood work: normal CBC, ESR, RF and ANA
- Synovial fluid non-inflammatory
- Radiology – x-ray:
  - **4 Hallmarks of OA**: 1) Joint space narrowing 2) Subchondral sclerosis 3) Subchondral cyst formation 4) osteophytes

Treatment
- Presently, no treatment alters the natural history of OA
- Non-pharmacological therapy
  - Weight loss if overweight, rest/low-impact exercise, physiotherapy with heat, massage, exercise programs, occupational therapy (aids, splints, cane, walker, bracing)
- Medical therapy
  - NSAIDs, acetaminophen
  - Joint injections: hyaluronan, corticosteroids
- Surgical treatment
  - Joint replacement

Osteoporosis

- See also Endocrinology

Definition
- Skeletal disorder characterized by compromised bone strength and increased risk of fracture
- T-score <-2.5 = osteoporosis, -2.5 to -1.0 = osteopenia, >-1.0 = normal
- Major risk factors: age >65, vertebral compression fracture, fragility fracture after age 40, FHx of osteoporotic fracture, systemic glucocorticoid therapy, malabsorption syndrome, primary hyperparathyroidism, propensity to fall, osteopenia apparent on x-ray film, hypogonadism, early menopause (before age 45)
- Physical exam: gait, height, kyphosis, rib-pelvis ≤ 2 finger breadths, occiput-wall distance >5 cm (for kyphosis)

Treatment
- Non-pharmacologic (exercise, smoking cessation), calcium, vitamin D supplements, bisphosphonate, PTH, SERM (raloxifene)

Fibromyalgia

Definition
• Chronic, widespread pain with characteristic tender points

Diagnosis
• History of widespread pain for at least 3 months in all 4 quadrants of body ("hurts all over")
  ▪ Associated symptoms: sleep disturbances, feeling of joint swelling but normal joint exam, fatigue, neurologic symptoms (hyperalgesia, paresthesias), GI symptoms (irritable bowel or bladder syndrome), headaches, depression, anxiety
• Pain in 11 of 18 tender points by digital palpation
• Diagnosis of exclusion:
  ▪ Rule out PMR, polymyositis, thyroid disorders, sleep apnea, etc.
  ▪ Presence of second disorder does not exclude diagnosis of fibromyalgia

Treatment
• Patient education and reassurance
• Exercise program (walking, aquatic exercises), physical therapy (stretching, muscle strengthening, massive), stress reduction, CBT
• Biofeedback, meditation, acupuncture may be helpful
• NSAIDs, SNRIs, low-dose TCAs, anti-convulsants; not narcotics

Common Medications

Genetic Drug Name	Trade Name	Dosing	Mechanism of Action
DMARDs (Biologics)			
etanercept $$$	Enbrel®	25 mg biweekly or 50 mg weekly SC injections	Fusion protein of TNF receptor and Fc portion of IgG
infliximab $$$	Remicade®	3-5 mg/kg IV q8wks	Chimeric mouse/human monoclonal anti-TNF-α
anakinra $$$	Kineret®	100 mg SC OD	Interleukin-1 receptor antagonist
adalimumab $$$	Humira®	40 mg SC q2wks	Monoclonal anti-TNF-α
abatacept $$$	Orencia®	IV infusion	Co-stimulation modulator of T-cell activation
rituximab $$$	Rituxan®	2 IV infusions, 2 wks apart	Causes B-cell depletion, binds to CD20
certolizumab $$$	Cimzia®	400 mg SC q2wks x3 then 200 mg SC q4wks	PEGylated monoclonal anti-TNF-α
golimumab $$$	Simponi®	50 mg SC q month	Monoclonal anti-TNF-α
tocilizumab $$$	Actemra®	4-8 mg/kg IV q4wks	Interleukin-6 receptor antagonist

Common Medications for Osteoarthritis

Class	Generic Drug Name	Trade Name	Dosing	Indications	Contraindications
	acetaminophen	Tylenol®	500 mg tid	1st line	
NSAIDs	ECASA		325-975 mg qid	2nd line	GI bleed
	ibuprofen	Advil,® Motrin®	200-600 mg tid		Renal impairment
	diclofenac	Voltaren®	25-50 mg tid		Allergy to ASA, NSAIDs
	diclofenac/misoprostol	Arthrotec®	50-75/200 mg tid		Pregnancy (T3)
	naproxen	Naprosyn®, Aleve®	125-500 mg bid		
	meloxicam	Mobicox®	7.5-15 mg OD		
COX-2 Inhibitors	celecoxib	Celebrex®	200 mg OD	High risk for GI bleed: age >65 hx of GI bleed, PUD	Renal impairment Sulfa allergy (celecoxib) Cardiovascular disease

Other treatments	Comments
Combination analgesics (acetaminophen + codeine)	Enhanced short term effect compared to acetaminophen alone More adverse effects: sedation, constipation, nausea, GI upset
Intra-articular corticosteroid injection	Short-term (weeks-months) decrease in pain and improvement in function
Intra-articular hyaluronan q6months	Modest decrease in pain Used for mild-moderate OA of the knees Precaution with chicken/egg allergy
Topical NSAIDs	1.5% wt/wt topical diclofenac (Pennsaid®) May use for patients who fail acetaminophen treatment and who wish to avoid systemic therapy
Capsaicin cream	Mild decrease in pain
Glucosamine sulfate/chondroitin	Limited clinical studies No regulation by Health Canada

DMARDs Used in Rheumatoid Arthritis

Generic Drug Name	Trade Name	Dosing	Contraindications	Adverse Effects
COMMONLY USED				
hydroxychloroquine $	Plaquenil®	400 mg OD initially 200-400 mg OD maintenance	Retinal disease, G6PD deficiency	GI symptoms, macular damage, neuromyopathy, skin rash
sulfasalazine $	Salazopyrim® Azulfidine® (US)	1000 mg bid-tid	Sulfa/ASA allergy, kidney disease, G6PD deficiency	GI symptoms, headache, leukopenia, rash
methotrexate $	Rheumatrex® Folex/Mexate®	qweekly 7.5-25 mg PO/IM/SC	Bone marrow suppression, liver disease, significant lung disease, immunodeficiency, pregnancy, EtOH abuse	Urticaria, GI symptoms, tubular necrosis, myelosuppression, cirrhosis, pneumonitis, oral ulcers
leflunomide $$	Arava®	10-20 mg PO OD	Liver disease	Alopecia, GI symptoms, pulmonary infiltrates, liver dysfunction
NOT COMMONLY USED				
cyclosporine $$	Neoral®	3 mg/kg in divided dose	Kidney/liver disease, infection, hypertension	Bleeding, hypertension, decreased renal function, hair growth, tremors
gold (injectable) $	Solganal® Myocrysine®	50 mg weekly initially, followed monthly	IBD, kidney/liver disease	Rash, mouth soreness/ulcers, proteinuria, marrow suppression
azathioprine $	Imuran®	1-2 mg/kg	Kidney/liver disease TPMT deficiency	Pancytopenia, biliary stasis, rash, hair loss, vomiting, diarrhea
cyclophosphamide $	Cytoxan®	1-2 mg/kg PO pulse IV as per protocol	Kidney/liver disease	Cardiotoxicity, GI symptoms, hemorrhagic cystitis, nephrotoxicity, bone marrow suppression, sterility

Urology

Anatomy

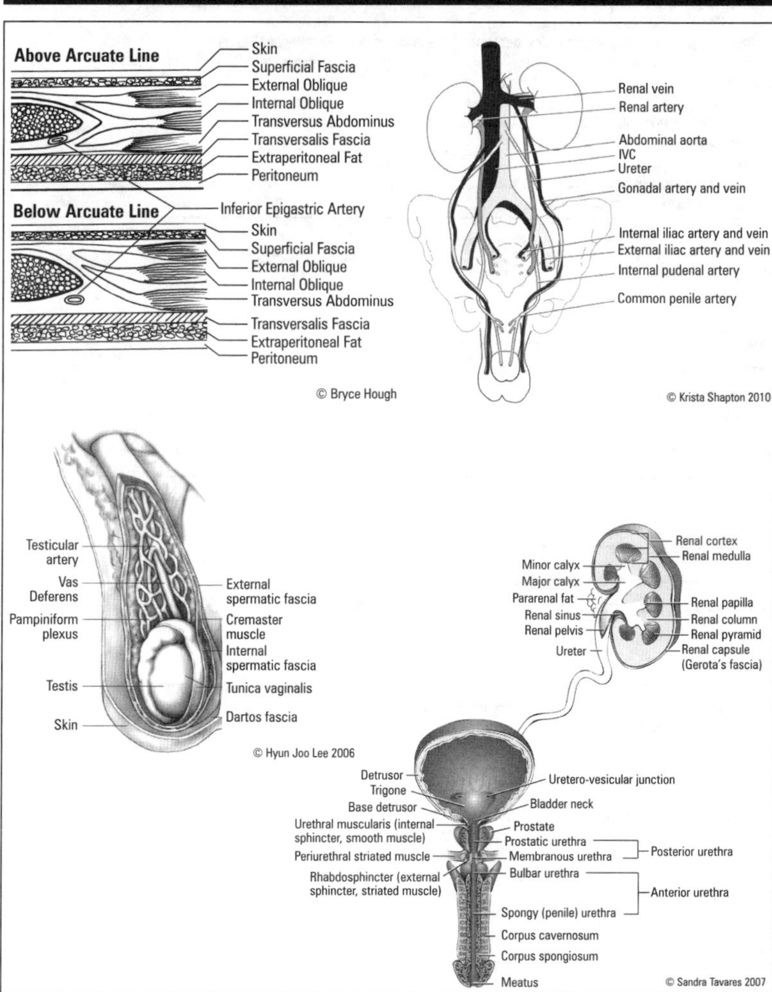

Essential History, Physical Exam and Investigations

History

Symptoms and Signs	Risk Factors
Pain (OPPQRSTUVW)	**Smoking**
Hematuria (see table below)	**Alcohol, other substance use**
Storage (frequency, urgency, nocturia, dysuria)	**Medications**
Voiding (straining, hesitancy, intermittency, decreased force or caliber of stream, prolonged voiding, post-void dribbling, incomplete emptying)	**Past medical history**
	Family history
Incontinence (stress, urge, overflow)	**Ethnicity**
Urethral discharge (blood, pus, constant vs. intermittent)	**Occupational exposures**
Scrotal Swelling/Testicular Masses (painful vs. painless)	**Surgical history**
Erectile Dysfunction	
Infertility	
Systemic Symptoms (fevers, chills, weight loss, nausea, vomiting)	
Confusion (beware of UTI in the elderly)	

Physical Exam

Inspection

Abdomen: suprapubic distension or tenderness, CVA tenderness, masses, scars

Penis: inflammation and deformities of shaft, foreskin, glans and urethral opening

Scrotum: size, rashes, ulcers, varicoceles, masses, transillumination

Inguinal region: hernias

Palpation

Kidney: very difficult to palpate even when enlarged

Abdomen: bladder not palpable unless >150 cc

Pelvic Exam: in females presenting with urinary complaints

Penis: lesions, discharge, scars, fibrosis (Peyronie's disease), position of urethral meatus

Scrotum: size of testes, masses (painful vs. painless), nodularity, varicocele

Hernias: inguinal (done standing with cough), femoral

Lymph nodes:
Inguinal/subinguinal: inflammation (penis, scrotum, vulva), malignancy (penis, glans, scrotal skin, distal urethra)
Left supraclavicular lymphadenopathy: testicular, prostate cancer
Iliac: metastases (bladder and prostate)

DRE: always do after urinalysis

DRE: PROSTATIC CHARACTERISTICS

Feature	Normal	Pathologic
Size, Symmetry	4 cm length and width (chestnut size)	Enlarged: BPH, advanced prostatic carcinoma
Consistency	Rubbery	Hard nodular: prostatic carcinoma
Mobility	Variable	Fixed: advanced prostatic carcinoma
Sensitivity	No pain (even on palpation)	Painful: prostatitis

Source: *Essentials of Clinical Exam*, 5th Ed.

Investigations

URINALYSIS – see Nephrology

PSA
- No consistent evidence that PSA screening decreases mortality
- Routine screening not currently recommended; patients should make informed decisions about whether to undergo PSA test
- DRE and PSA can be used to monitor progression of disease or response to therapy
- Causes of increased PSA: BPH, prostatitis, prostatic ischemia/infarction, acute urinary retention, prostate biopsy/surgery, prostatic massage, urethral catheterization, TRUS, strenuous exercise, ejaculation, acute renal failure, coronary bypass graft, radiation therapy

Normal PSA Value by Age Group

Age Range (years)	Serum PSA Concentration (μg/L)		
	Asian men	Caucasian men	Men of African descent
40-49	≤ 2.0	≤ 2.5	≤ 2.0
50-59	≤ 3.0	≤ 3.5	≤ 4.0
60-69	≤ 4.0	≤ 4.5	≤ 4.5
70-80	≤ 5.0	≤ 6.5	≤ 5.5

Source: Prostate Cancer Canada

CYSTOSCOPY
- Endoscopic inspection of the lower urinary tract
- Indications: hematuria, LUTS (storage or voiding), urethral and bladder neck strictures, stones, bladder tumour surveillance, evaluation of upper tracts with retrograde pyelography (ureteral stents, catheters)

Common Presentations

Hematuria

- Initial (anterior urethra), terminal (bladder, neck and prostatic urethra), total (bladder and above)

Differential Diagnosis

Pseudohematuria	Pre-renal	Renal	Post-renal
Per vaginal bleeding (menses, endometriosis)	Anticoagulants	Stone	Stone
Dyes (beets, rhodamine B in candy and juices)	Thromboembolism	Trauma	Neoplasms
Hemoglobin (hemolytic anemia)	Sickle cell disease	Renal cell carcinoma	Cystitis
Myoglobin (rhabdomyolysis)	Neoplasms	Transitional cell carcinoma	Urethritis
Drugs (rifampin, phenazopyridine, pyridium, phenytoin)	Leukemia	Wilms' tumour	BPH
Porphyria		Pyelonephritis	Foreign body
Laxatives (phenolphthalein)		Glomerulonephritis	Urethral stricture
		Interstitial nephritis	Trauma
		Tuberculosis	Tuberculosis
		Infarct	Polyps
		Polycystic kidneys	Exercise-induced
		Arteriovenous malformation	
		Exercise-induced	

Investigations

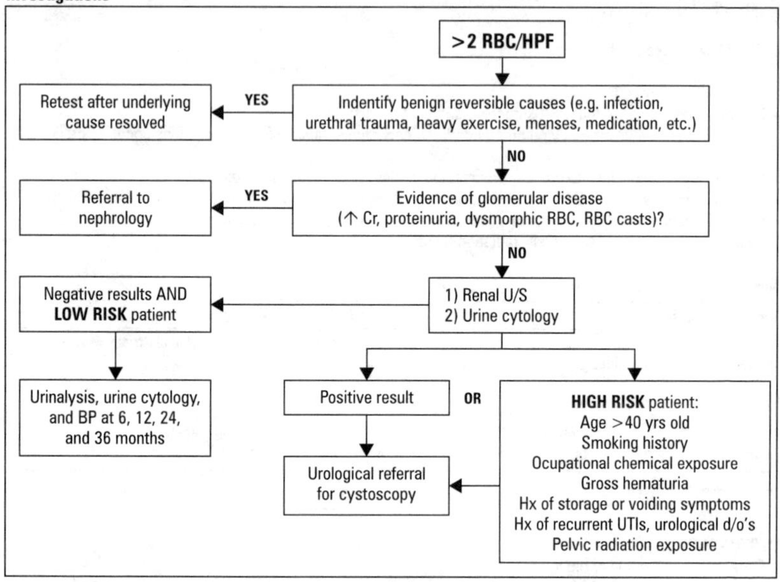

Hydronephrosis

- Dilation of kidney caused by backward pressure of trapped urine
- Mechanical (congenital, acquired) vs. functional (neurogenic, pharmacologic, pregnancy) etiologies
- Investigations: history (pain especially flank; urine output; medications; pregnancy; trauma; fever; history of UTIs, calculi and PID), labs (CBC, electrolytes, Cr, BUN, urine R&M, C&S), imaging (U/S is best modality)
- Treatment aims to relieve the cause of obstruction/stasis
- Urgent treatment (percutaneous nephrostomy or ureteral stenting) required if associated with infection, acute renal failure, or severe pain

Urinary Incontinence

- **Stress incontinence:** involuntary leaking with sudden increases in intra-abdominal pressure
  - Due to urethral/sphincter problem
  - Diagnose by history and stress test (Valsalva or cough with full bladder)
- **Urge incontinence:** involuntary leaking preceded by strong, sudden urge to void
  - Due to inappropriate bladder contractions (e.g. detrusor overactivity)
  - Diagnose by urodynamics: small capacity (if bladder is irritable), uninhibited contractions
- **Mixed incontinence:** urinary leakage associated with urgency and also with increased intrabdominal pressure
  - Due to a combination of bladder and sphincter problems
  - Diagnosis by history of both stress and urge incontinence
- **Overflow incontinence:** involuntary leakage when intravesical pressure exceeds urethral pressure
  - Due to obstruction (e.g. BPH, stricture) or weak bladder (e.g. autonomic neuropathy from DM, multiple sclerosis, anticholinergic medications)
  - Primarily a clinical diagnosis

- **Functional incontinence:** urinary loss caused by inability to reach toilet in time
  - Physical immobility, confusion

Urinary Retention

Etiology
- Outflow obstruction: bladder neck or urethra (calculus, clot, foreign body, neoplasm), urethra (stricture, valve, diverticuli, phimosis, trauma), prostate (neoplasm, BPH)
- Bladder innervation: spinal cord (injury, disc herniation, multiple sclerosis), stroke, DM, pelvic surgery
- Pharmacologic: anticholinergics, antihypertensives, antihistamines, narcotics, ephedrine/pseudoephedrine, psychosomatic substances (e.g. ecstasy)
- Infection: UTJ, prostatitis, abscess, herpes, infected foreign body

Physical Exam
- General inspection, including urethral discharge
- Palpable and/or percussible bladder
- DRE to assess size of prostate and anal sphincter tone
- Neurological exam: deep tendon reflexes, anal wink, saddle sensation

Management

ER	Ward	Discharge/Outpatient
ABCs	Admit if: acute renal failure, abnormal DRE, signs of septicemia, significant hematuria post bladder decompression	Investigations: consider PSA
Lines (indwelling Foley, nephrostomy or retrograde ureteral catheter if upper urinary tract obstruction)	Investigations: voiding cystourethrogram, retrograde urethrography, urodynamic testing	Tx: etiology dependent; management of stones and BPH (e.g. tamsulosin 0.4-0.8 mg PO or TURP)
Monitor ins and outs	Tx: etiology dependent; manage stones and BPH, and treat infections if present	Follow-up with urology (if Foley in place for acute urinary retention, catheter to be removed by home care nurse or during outpatient visit with a trial of void)
Investigations: CBC; electrolytes; Cr; BUN; urine R&M, C&S; abdominal/pelvic ultrasound, KUB x-ray	Consult/refer to nephrology if renal dysfunction is evident	Follow-up with nephrology if indicated
Tx: etiology dependent; goal in ER is to evacuate retained urine		
Consult/refer to urology and nephrology if obstructive nephropathy evident		

Acute Scrotum

DIFFERENTIAL DIAGNOSIS OF SCROTAL SWELLING

Painless	Painful
Hydrocele	Epididymitis
Spermatocele	Orchitis
Varicocele	Torsion
Tumour	Tumour (hemorrhagic)
Indirect inguinal hernia	Hernia (strangulated)
	Hematocele
	Granulomatous orchitis

APPROACH TO A SCROTAL MASS/SCROTAL SWELLING

Condition	Pain	Palpation	Additional Findings
Torsion (EMERGENCY)	+	Diffuse tenderness	Negative cremaster reflex, negative Prehn's sign
Epididymitis	+	Epididymal tenderness	Positive cremaster reflex, positive Prehn's sign
Orchitis	+	Diffuse tenderness	Positive cremaster reflex, positive Prehn's sign
Hematocele	+	Diffuse tenderness	No transillumination
Hydrocele	−	Testis not separable from hydrocele	Transillumination
Spermatocele	−	Testis separable from spermatocele	Transillumination
Varicocele	±	"Bag of worms"	No transillumination
Indirect inguinal hernia	+ if strangulated	Testis separable from hernia, cord not palpable, cough impulse may transmit, may be reducible	No transillumination
Tumour	+ if hemorrhagic	Hard lump/nodule	
Generalized/ dependent edema	−	Diffuse swelling	Often post-op or immobilized
Idiopathic	−		

Management
- Torsion: scrotal exploration and surgical detorsion with bilateral orchiopexy
- Tumour: orchiectomy ± retroperitoneal lymph node dissection, chemotherapy, radiation
- Hematocele/spermatocele/hydrocele/varicocele: monitor vs. surgery

Renal Mass

APPROACH TO THE RENAL MASS

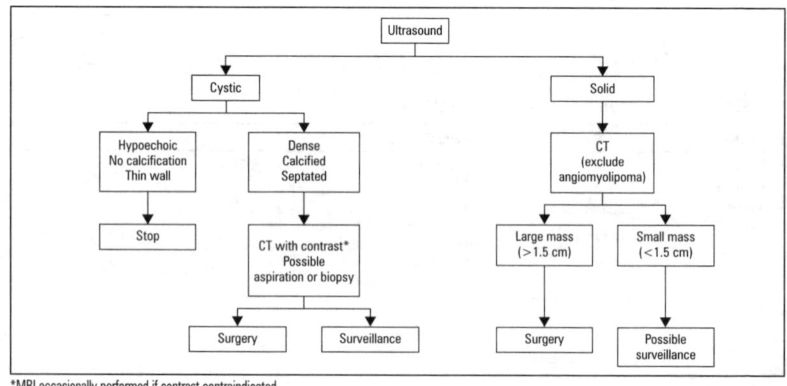

*MRI occasionally performed if contrast contraindicated

Dysuria

Differential Diagnosis

Infectious	Cystitis, urethritis, prostatitis, epididymitis and orchitis (if associated with lower tract inflammation), cervicitis, vulvovaginitis, perineal inflammation/infection, TB, vestibulitis
Neoplasm	Renal cell, bladder, prostate, penis, vagina/vulva, BPH
Calculi	Bladder stone, ureteral stone, kidney stone
Inflammatory	Seronegative arthropathies (reactive arthritis: arthritis, uveitis, urethritis), drug side effects, autoimmune disorders, chronic pelvic pain syndrome (CPPS), interstitial cystitis
Hormonal	Endometriosis, hypoestrogenism
Trauma	Catheter insertion, post-coital cystitis (honeymoon cystitis)
Psychogenic	Somatization disorder, depression, stress/anxiety disorder
Other	Contact sensitivity, foreign body, radiation/chemical cystitis

Common Conditions

Benign Prostatic Hyperplasia (BPH)

Clinical Features
- Voiding and storage symptoms
- DRE: smooth, rubbery, symmetrically enlarged prostate
  - Size of prostate does not correlate well with symptoms

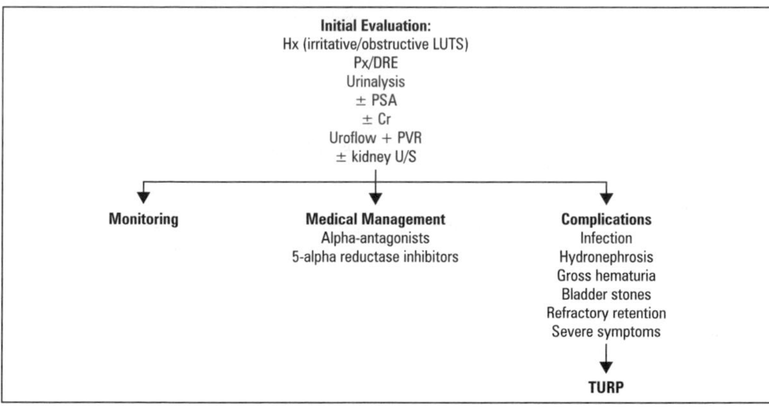

Complications
- Retention, overflow incontinence, hydronephrosis and renal compromise, infection, gross hematuria, urolithiasis

Treatment
- Conservative treatment (watchful waiting and lifestyle changes) for those with mild symptoms
- For those with greater symptoms, consider:
  - Medications (α-adrenergic antagonists, 5-α reductase inhibitors)
  - Minimally invasive therapy, TURP, or open prostatectomy

Urolithiasis

Differential Diagnosis

Renal colic, acute ureteral obstruction, ureteropelvic junction (UPJ) obstruction, acute abdominal crisis (biliary, bowel obstruction, pancreatitis, AAA), gynecological (ectopic pregnancy, torsion/rupture of ovarian cyst, endometriosis), pyelonephritis (fever, chills, pyuria), radiculitis (L1; herpes zoster, nerve root compression), Munchausen's syndrome
- If presenting with hematuria, consider UTI, tumour

Classification
- Calcium stones (75-85%), struvite stones (infectious), uric acid stones, cystine stones, other (very rare)

Location
- Calyx: may cause flank discomfort, recurrent infection or persistent hematuria; may remain asymptomatic for years and not require treatment
- Pelvis: tend to cause obstruction at UPJ; staghorn calculi are branched stones that fill the renal pelvis and branch into the calyces; often associated with infection
- Ureter: stones <5 mm will pass spontaneously in 75% of patients

Clinical Features
- Pain is secondary to upstream distention
    - Non-colicky flank pain due to renal capsular distention
    - Severe colicky pain radiating from flank to groin region due to stretching of collecting system or ureter (ureteral colic)
- Pain is often accompanied by nausea, vomiting, urinary frequency, dysuria, oliguria, hematuria (90% microscopic), diaphoresis, tachycardia, tachypnea, and B symptoms

Risk Factors/Precipitants
- Family or personal history of stone disease
- History of gout, DM, IBD, hypercalcemia disorders (hyperparathyroidism, sarcoidosis, histoplasmosis), myeloproliferative disorders
- Dehydration
- Nutrition (low citrate, magnesium; excess vitamin C, calcium, oxalate, purines)
- Lithogenic medications: indinavir, thiazides, chemotherapy or cytotoxic drugs, steroid use
- Sedentary lifestyle and obesity

Investigations
- Minimum evaluation: CBC, electrolytes, Cr, BUN, urinalysis (R&M, C&S), stone analysis
- Imaging: kidneys, ureters, and bladder (KUB) x-ray, CT scan, abdominal U/S, IVP (rarely used)
- Cystoscopy for suspected bladder stone
- Metabolic studies if recurrent Ca^{2+} stone formers
    - PTH (if hypercalcemic)
    - 24h urine x2 for volume, Cr, Na^+, Ca^{2+}, PO_4^{3-}, uric acid, Mg^{2+}, oxalate, citrate

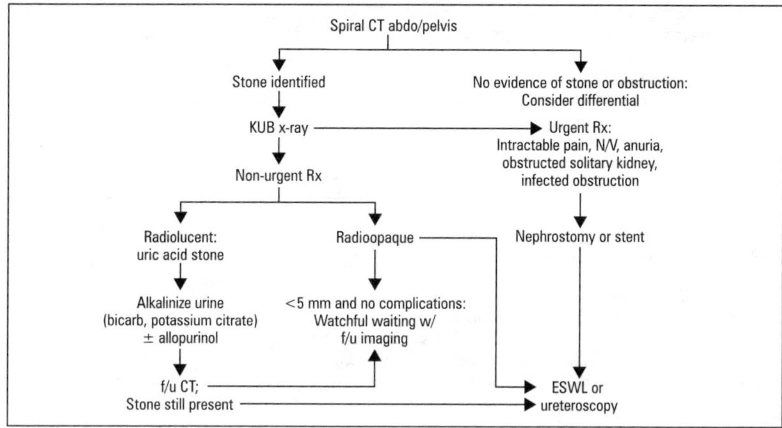

Management

Acute
- Analgesics (codeine, meperidine, morphine)
- NSAIDs (decrease intra-ureteral pressure)
- α-blockers (increase rate of spontaneous passage in distal ureteral stones)
- Antibiotics (for UTI)
- If vomiting, IV fluids and antiemetics
- Indications for admission to hospital: intractable pain, intractable vomiting, fever (suggests infection), compromised renal function, single kidney with ureteral obstruction/bilateral obstructing stones
- Interventional care indicated if obstruction endangers patient: ureteric stent via cystoscopy, image-guided percutaneous nephrostomy

Discharge/Outpatient (Elective)
- Medical
  - Conservative if stone <5 mm and no complications
  - Fluids to increase urine volume to >2 L/d (3-4 L if cystine)
  - Medical therapy for prevention or treatment (uric acid, cystine) specific to stone type
    - Calcium: cellulose phosphate, orthophosphate for absorptive causes
    - Calcium oxalate: thiazides, ± potassium citrate, ± allopurinol, calcium
    - Uric acid: alkalinize urine (bicarbonate, potassium citrate), ± allopurinol
    - Struvite: antibiotics (stone must be removed to treat infection)
    - Cystine: alkalinize urine, penicillamine/MPG (complex cystine), captopril
    - Alkalinization of urine (bicarbonate, potassium citrate)
- Interventional
  - Kidney: stent if stone is >2 cm, ESWL if stone <2 cm (unless cystine stone)
  - Percutaneous nephrolithotomy (extraction or fragmentation) if:
    - Stone >2 cm
    - Staghorn
    - UPJ obstruction
    - Calyceal diverticulum
    - Cystine stones (poorly fragmented with ESWL)
    - Failure of less invasive modalities

- Ureter: ESWL and ureteroscopy are the primary modalities of treatment
  - Ureteroscopy (extraction or fragmentation) if: failed ESWL, ureteric stricture, reasonable alternative for distal 1/3 of ureter
  - Open ureterolithotomy (very rare)
- Bladder: transurethral cystolitholapaxy, remove outflow obstruction (TURP or stricture dilatation)

Clinical Pearl
Uric acid stones are radiolucent on plain KUB x-ray and radio-opaque on spiral CT

Pyelonephritis/UTI

Risk Factors/Precipitants
- Stasis and obstruction: residual urine in poorly flushing system
- Foreign body: introduce pathogen or acts as nidus of infection, history of instrumentation
- Decreased resistance to organisms (immunosuppression, DM, etc.)
- Other factors (trauma, anatomic variance, female, previous UTI, sexual activity)

Etiology
- Ascending infection with GI organisms (most common), hematogenous (TB, perinephric abscess), lymphatic, direct (IBD, diverticulitis)
- Common organisms (**KEEPPS**): *K*lebsiella, *E*. coli, *E*nterococci, *P*roteus, *P*seudomonas, *S*. saprophyticus

UTI

Definition
- >100 000 bacteria/mL (mid stream urine) or if symptomatic, 100 bacteria/mL may be significant

Classification
- **Uncomplicated**: lower urinary tract infection in a setting of functionally and structurally normal urinary tract
- **Complicated**: pyelonephritis and/or structural/functional abnormality
- **Unresolved bacteriuria**: urinary tract is not sterilized during therapy; resistance, non-compliance, or wrong antibiotic coverage
- **Recurrent UTI**: reinfection (80%), bacterial persistence (urine cultures become sterile during therapy but resultant reinfection of the urine by the same organisms)

Clinical Features
- **Storage symptoms** (frequency, nocturia, dysuria, urgency), **voiding symptoms** (hesitancy, incomplete emptying, prolonged voiding, decreased force/caliber of stream), **hematuria**
- Malodourous urine
- Confusion in the elderly

Investigation
- Indication: persistence of pyuria/symptoms after adequate therapy; severe infection with an increase in creatinine; hematuria; recurrent/persistent infections; male; child
- Midstream urine R&M, C&S
  - Dipstick: leukocytes + nitrites + hematuria
  - Microscopy: >5 WBC/HPF in un-spun urine of >10 WBC/HPF in spun urine, bacteria, + WBC casts
  - Gram stain: GN bacilli, CP cocci, >1 bacterium/oil immersion field
  - C&S: midstream, catheterized or suprapubic aspirate
  - Routine cultures: *Klebsiella* sp., *E.coli* (90%), other Gram negatives, *Enterococci*, *Proteus mirabilis*, *Pseudomonas*, *S. saprophyticus*
  - Non-routine cultures: TB, *Chlamydia trachomatis*, *Ureaplasma urealyticum*, fungi (*Candida*)

Management
- Identify organism and treat:
  - TMP/SMX 1 DS tab PO bid x 3 d (7-10d for males)
  - Ciprofloxacin 500 mg PO bid x 3 d
  - Nitrofurantoin 100 mg PO qid x 7 d
- Acute cystitis in pregnancy:
  - Cephalexin 250-500 mg PO qid x 7 d
  - Nitrofurantoin 100 mg PO qid x 7 d
- Identify cause and correct predisposing cause
- Consider long term, low dose prophylaxis in recurrent UTI
- Indications for admission include those with complicated UTI (discussed above), as well as:
  - Concern regarding poor compliance or follow-up, severe disease or suspected urosepsis, comorbid illness, known abnormal urinary tract anatomy, indwelling catheter

---

Clinical Pearl
In the elderly, the only sign of UTI may be confusion
Males with UTI should be worked up for a specific cause of infection
Febrile UTI in women – rule out acute pyelonephrits; febrile UTI in men rule out acute prostatitis

---

PYELONEPHRITIS

Definition
- Inflammation of kidney and its pelvis usually due to bacterial contamination

Etiology
- Stones, structures, prostatic obstruction, vesicoureteric reflux, neurogenic bladder, catheters, DM, sickle-cell disease, polycystic kidney disease, immunosuppression, post-renal transplant, pregnancy

Clinical Features
- Rapid onset (hours to days)
- LUTS (frequency, urgency, dysuria, hematuria)
- Consitutional symptoms: fever, chills, rigors, nausea, vomiting, myalgia, malaise
- CVA tenderness or exquisite flank pain
- Note: dysuria is not a symptom of pyelonephritis without concurrent cystitis

Investigations
- CBC + differential: leukocytosis, high % neutrophils, left shift
- Imaging (if complicated pyelonephritis or symptoms do not improve within 72 h of treatment: abdominal/pelvic U/S or CT)
- Blood cultures, electrolytes, BUN/Cr, urine R&M and C&S

Management
- May treat as outpatient if hemodynamically stable
- For acute uncomplicated pyelonephritis:
  - Ciprofloxacin 500 mg PO bid x 7 d
  - TMP/SMX 1 DS tab PO bid x 14 d
  - Amoxicillin/clavulanic acid 875/125 mg PO bid x 14 d
- Indication for admission include those with moderate to severe illness, including:
  - + + temperature, leukocytosis, vomiting and dehydration, sepsis, failure to improve after 48 h of PO therapy
  - Admit, hydrate and treat with Ampicillin IV and Gentamycin IV
- Acute pyelonephritis in pregnancy:
  - Ceftriaxone 1 to 2 g IV qid until afebrile for 48 h, then switch to po antibiotics to complete 14 d of treatment
- Emphysematous pyelonephritis: emergency nephrectomy
- Stone obstruction: admit and emergency stenting or percutaneous nephrostomy tube

Common Medications

	Class	Drug	Adverse Effects
Erectile dysfunction	Phosphodiesterase 5 inhibitor	sildenafil (Viagra®) tadalafil (Cialis®) vardenafil (Levitra®)	Severe hypotension (very rare) Contraindicated if history of priapism, or in conditions predisposing to priapism (leukemia, myelofibrosis, polycythemia, sickle cell disease) Contraindicated with nitrates
	Prostaglandin E_1	alprostadil (MUSE, Caverject®) PGE_1 + phentolamine + papaverine mixture	Penile pain Presyncope
Benign prostatic hyperplasia	α_1 blockers	terazosin (Hytrin®) doxazosin (Cardura®)	Presyncope Leg edema
	α_{1A} selective	tamsulosin (Flomax®) alfuzosin (Xatral®)	Retrograde ejaculation Headache Asthenia Nasal congestion
	5α-reductase inhibitor	finasteride (Proscar®) dutasteride (Avodart®)	Sexual dysfunction PSA reduction
Prostatic carcinoma	GnRH agonist	leuprolide (Lupron®, Eligard®) goserelin (Zoladex®)	Hot flashes Headache Decreased libido
	Non-steroidal antiandrogen	flutamide (Eulexin®) bicalutamide (Casodex®)	Hepatotoxic: AST/ALT monitoring
	Steroidogenesis inhibitors	ketoconazole spironolactone	GI symptoms Hyperkalemia Gynecomastia
Continence and overactive bladder	Antispasmotic	oxybutynin (Uromax®, Ditropan XL®)	Dry mouth Blurred vision Constipation Supraventricular tachycardia
	Anticholinergic	oxybutynin (Ditropan®) tolterodine (Detrol®) trospium (Trosec®) solifenacin (Vesicare®) darifenacin (Enablex®)	As above
	Tricyclic antidepressant	imipramine (Tofranil®)	As above Weight gain Orthostatic hypotension Prolonged PR interval

References

The following are sample references for each chapter in the handbook. For a full list of references, please refer to the Toronto Notes Textbook 2012.

Antibiotic Quick Reference and Common Medications
Compendium of Pharmaceuticals and Specialties. www.e-therapeutics.ca
Hardman JG and Limbird LR, editors. Goodman and Gilman's the Pharmacological Basis of Therapeutics. 9th ed. New York: McGraw-Hill; 1996.
Kalant H, Grant DM, Mitchell J, editors. Principles of Medical Pharmacology. 7th ed.Toronto: Elsevier Canada; 2007.
Katzung BG, editor. Basic and Clinical Pharmacology. 8th ed. New York: McGraw-Hill Companies; 2001.
Micromedex health care series. www.micromedex.com

Medical Imaging
American College of Radiology (ACR) Breast Imaging Reporting and Data System Atlas (BI-RADS Atlas). Reston, Va: American College of Radiology; 2003
Brant WE, Helms CA (1999). Fundamentals of diagnostic radiology. Philadelphia. Lippincott Williams and Wilkins.
Chen MYM, Pope, TL, Ott DJ. (2004) Basic Radiology. New York. Lange Medical Books/McGraw Hill.
Daffner RH (1993). Clinical radiology: the essentials. Baltimore: Williams & Wilkins.
Erkonen WE, Smith WL. (2005). Radiology 101. Philadelphia: Lippincott Williams & Wilkins.
Fleckenstein P, Tranun-Jensen J (2001). Anatomy in Diagnostic Imaging. 2nd ed. Copenhagen: Blackwell Publishing.
Gay S, Woodcock Jr RJ (2000). Radiology Recall. Baltimore: Lippincott Williams & Wilkins.
Goodman LR (2007). Felson's Principles of Chest Roentgenology: A Programmed Text. 3rd ed. Philadelphia: Saunders.
Novelline RA (2004). Squire's Fundamentals of Radiology. 6th ed. Cambridge:Harvard.
Ouellette H, Tetreault P. (2002). Clinical Radiology made ridiculously simple. Miami: MedMaster.

Ethical and Legal Aspects of Medicine
Baile WF, Buckman R, Lenzi R, et al. (2000). SPIKES - A six-step protocol for delivering bad news: application to the patient with cancer. Oncologist. 5(4): 302-11.
CMA Code of Ethics, Canadian Medical Association www.cma.ca.
CPSO Policy Statements, College of Physicians and Surgeons of Ontario www.cpso.on.ca/policies/mandatory.htm.
Downie J, Caulfield T, Flood C. Canadian Health Law and Policy, Markham, LexisNexis, 2007.
Etchells E, Sharpe G, Elliott C and Singer PA. Bioethics for clinicians: 3. Capacity. CMAJ 1996,155(6):657-661.
Ferris LE, Barkun H, Carlisle J, Hoffman B, Katz C, and Silverman M. Defining the physician's duty to warn: consensus statement of Ontario's Medical Expert Panel on Duty to Inform. CMAJ 1998;158:1473-1479.
Health Care Consent Act, 1996. S.O. 1996, c. 2, Sched. A.

Hébert P. Doing Right: A Practical Guide to Ethics for Physicians and Medical Trainees, 2nd ed. Toronto, Oxford University Press; 2009.
Hébert PC, Hoffmaster B, Glass KC, Singer PA. Bioethics for clinicians: 7. Truth telling. CMAJ 1997;156:225-8.
Medical Council of Canada. Objectives of the considerations of the legal, ethical and organizational aspects of the practice of medicine. 1999. Online at the Medical Council of Canada website (www.mcc.ca).
Shah CP. Public health and preventive medicine in Canada. 5th ed. Toronto: Elsevier Canada; 2003. p 357-360, 426. Reprinted by permission of Elsevier Canada, 2006.

Anesthesia
Allain RM. Alston TA, Dunn PF, Kwo J, Rosow CE (Eds.) (2010). Clinical Anesthesia Procedures of the Massachusetts General Hospital, 8th ed. Philadelphia: Lippincott.
Barash PG, Cullen BF, Stoelting RK, Calahan M, Stock MC (Eds.) (2009). Clinical Anesthesia, 6th ed. Philadelphia: Lippincott.
Collins VJ. (Ed.)(1996). Physiologic and pharmacologic bases of anesthesia. Philadelphia: Lippincott Williams and Wilkins.
Hurford WE, et al. (Eds). (2002). Clinical anesthesia procedures of the Massachusetts General Hospital, 6th edition. Philadelphia: Lippincott Williams and Wilkins.
Kalant H, Roschlau WH (Eds). (1998). Principles of medical pharmacology. New York: Oxford University Press.
Lawrence PF. (2000). Anesthesiology. In Essentials of Surgical Specialties RM Bell, MT Dayton (Eds.)(pgs 1-67). Philadelphia: Lippincott Williams and Wilkins.
Malignant Hyperthermia Association of the United States Website. Last accessed on September 26th 2010. Retrieved from <http://www.mhaus.org>.
Miller RD. (Ed.). (2000). Anesthesia, 5th edition. Philadelphia: Churchill Livingstone, Inc.
Yaphe, J. (2008.) Circulation. In: A Helman (Ed.) The ABCs of Emergency Medicine, 11th edition. Toronto: University of Toronto.

Cardiology and CVS Surgery
Anderson JL, Adams CD, Antman EM, et al.2011 ACCF/AHA Focused Update Incorporated Into the ACC/AHA 2007 Guidelines for the Management of Patients With Unstable Angina/Non-ST-Elevation Myocardial Infarction. Circulation. 2011 May 10;123(18):e426-579.
Antman EM, Anbe DT, Armstrong PW, et al. ACC/AHA guidelines for the management of patients with ST-elevation myocardial infarction--executive summary.Circulation. 2004 Aug 3;110(5):588-636.
Bonow RO, Carabello BA, Chatterjee K, et al. 2008 Focused update incorporated into the ACC/AHA 2006 guidelines for the management of patients with valvular heart disease.Circulation. 2008 Oct 7;118(15):e523-661.
Gibbons RJ, Balady GJ, Bricker JT, et al. Committee to Update the 1997 Exercise Testing Guidelines. ACC/AHA 2002 guideline update for exercise testing: summary article. J Am CollCardiol. 2002 Oct 16;40(8):1531-40.
Hiratzka LF, Bakris GL, Beckman JA, et al.2010 ACCF/AHA/AATS/ACR/ASA/SCA/SCAI/SIR/STS/SVM guidelines for the diagnosis and management of patients with thoracic aortic disease: executive summary. Catheter CardiovascInterv. 2010 Aug 1;76(2):E43-86.
Wann LS, Curtis AB, January CT, et al. 2011 ACCF/AHA/HRS focused update on the management of patients with atrial fibrillation (updating the 2006 guideline).Circulation. 2011 Jan 4;123(1):104-23.
Weitz JI, Byrne J, Clagett GP, et al. Diagnosis and treatment of chronic arterial insufficiency of the lower extremities: a critical review.Circulation. 1996 Dec 1;94(11):3026-49.

Dermatology

Bolognia JL, Jorizzo JL, Rapini RP, editors. Textbook of Dermatology. Vol. 1 and 2. Toronto: Mosby, 2003.

Cummings SR et al. Approaches to the prevention and control of skin cancer. Cancer Metastatis Rev. 1997;16:309.

DeShazo RD et al. Allergic reactions to drugs and biologic agents. JAMA. 1997;278:1895.

Ellis C, et al. ICCAD II Faculty. International Consensus Conference on Atopic Dermatitis II (ICCAD II): Clinical update and current treatment strategies. Br J Dermatol. 2003; 148 (suppl 63):3-10.

Goodheart H, Goodheart's Photoguide to Common Skin Disorders: Diagnosis and management. 3rd Edition. Philadelphia: Lippincott, Williams and Wilkins, 2008

Johnson RA, Suurmond D, Wolff K, editors. Colour atlas and synopsis of clinical dermatology. 5th ed. New York: McGraw Hill, 2005.

Kraft J, Ng C, Bertucci V. University of Toronto Pharmacology Handbook: Dermatology Chapter. Toronto: publication pending.

Lebwohl MG, Heymann WR, Berth-Jones J, Coulson I, editors. Treatment of skin disease: Comprehensive therapeutic strategies. 2nd ed. Philadelphia: Mosby, 2006.

Paller AS, Mancini AJ. Hurwitz clinical pediatric dermatology: A textbook of skin disorders of childhood and adolescence. 3rd ed. China: Elsevier, 2006.

Sterry W, Paus W, Burgdorf W editors. Thieme Clinical Companions: Dermatology. 5th ed, New York: Thieme, 2005.

Wolff K, and Johnson RA, Fitzpatrick's Colour Atlas and Synopsis of Clinical Dermatology. 6th Edition. New York: McGraw Hill, 2009

Emergency Medicine

Cecil's Essentials of Medicine 8th ed. Andreoli TE, Carpenter CJ, Griggs RC, Benjamin IJ.Saunders, 2010.

Chu, P. Blunt Abdominal Trauma: current concepts. Current Orthopedics 2003; 17, 254-259.

Clinical procedures in emergency medicine. 5rd ed. Roberts JR and Hedges JR (ed). WB Saunders Co, 2009.

Elliott WJ. Hypertensive emergencies. Crit Care Clin. 2001; 17(2):435-51.

Emergency medicine: A comprehensive study guide, 7th ed. Tintinalli JE and Kelen GE (ed). McGraw-Hill Professional Publishing, 2004.

Emergency Medicine On Call.Keim, Setal. McGraw Hill. 2004.

Principles of Medical Pharmacology, 7th ed. Kalant H, Roschlau WH New York: Oxford University Press, 2006.

Stiell IG et al. The Canadian CT Head Rule for patients with minor head injury. Lancet 2001; 357(9266):1391-6.

Stiell IG et al. The Canadian C-spine rule for radiography in alert and stable trauma patients. JAMA 2001; 286(15):1841-8.

Varon J, Marik P. The Diagnosis and management of hypertensive crises. Chest. 2000; 118(1):214-27.

Warden C et al. Evaluation and management of febrile seizures in the out-of-hospital and emergency department settings. Ann Emerg Med. 2003; 41;215-222

Wells PS, Anderson DR, Rodger M, et al. Derivation of a simple clinical model to categorize patients probability of pulmonary embolism: increasing the models utility with the simpliRED d-dimer. ThrombHaemost. 2000; 83: 416-20.

Endocrinology

Agus AZ. Etiology of hypercalcemia. Uptodate Online 2010; Version 10.2. www.uptodate.com

American Diabetes Association. Management of dyslipidemia in adults with diabetes (Position Statement). Diabetes Care 2002; 25(S1):S74-77.

Braunwald E, Fauci AS, Kasper DL, Hauser SL et al. Diabetes Mellitus in Harrison's Principles of Internal Medicine Volume 2. New York: The McGraw Hill Companies, 2001. pp 2109-2135.

Burman KD. Overview of thyroiditis. Uptodate Online 2002; Version 10.2. www.uptodate.com

Canadian Diabetes Association Clinical Practice Guidelines Expert Committee. Canadian Diabetes Association 2008 clinical practice guidelines for the prevention and management of diabetes in Canada. Canadian Journal of Diabetes 2008; 32(Supplement 1): S1-S201.

Canadian Task Force on Preventive Health Care. Prevention of osteoporosis and osteoporotic fractures in post-menopausal women. Canadian Medical Association Journal 2004; 170(11):1665-1667.

Greenspan FS, Garber DG. Basic and Clinical Endocrinology. New York: Lange Medical Books/ McGraw Hill, 2001. pp 100-163, 201-272, 623-761.

Kronenberg HM, Larsen PR, Melmed S, Polonsky, K. Williams Textbook of Endocrinology Ninth Edition. Philadelphia: W.B. Saunders Company, 1998.

NIH Consensus Development Panel on Osteoporosis Prevention, Diagnosis and Therapy. Osteoporosis prevention, diagnosis, and therapy. Journal of the American Medical Association 2001; 285(6):785-795.

Tsui E, Barnie A, Ross S, Parkes R et al. Intensive insulin therapy with insulin lispro: a randomized trial of continuous subcutaneous insulin infusion versus multiple daily insulin injection. Diabetes Care 2001; 24(10):1722-1727.

Family Medicine

Assendelft WJJ et al. Spinal manipulative therapy for low-back pain. Cochrane Database of Systematic Reviews 2004, Issue 1.

Bent S et al. Does this woman have an acute uncomplicated urinary tract infection? JAMA. 2002;287(20):2701-10.

Canada's Food Guide to Healthy Eating. Health Canada. Last updated 2007.

Canadian Hypertension Education Program. 2009 Canadian Hypertension Education Program recommendations - an annual update. Can Fam Physician 2009; 55(7):697-700.

Canadian Task Force on Preventive Health Care. The Canadian Guide to Clinical Preventive Health Care. Ottawa: Minister of Supply and Services Canada and http://www.ctfphc.org.

Centor RM et al. (1981). The diagnosis of strep throat in adults in the emergency room. Med Decis Making. 1: 239-46.

Comuz J, Guessous I, Farrat B. Fatigue: a practical approach to diagnosis in primary care. CMAJ 2006; 174(6): 765-7.

David AK, et al. Family Medicine: Principles and Practice, 6th ed. New York: Springer-Verlag Inc. 2003.

Derby CA et al. Modifiable risk factors and erectile dysfunction: can lifestyle changes modify risk? Urology 2000;56(2):302-6.

Domino FJ et al. The 5-Minute Clinical Consult 2010, 18th Ed. Lippincott Williams & Wilkins. 2009.

Fogarty CT, Burge S, McCord E. Communicating with patients about intimate partner violence: screening and interviewing approaches. Fam Med 2002; 34(5): 369-75.

Gilbert DN et al. The Sanford Guide to Antimicrobial Therapy, 39th Ed.. Sperryville, VA: Antimicrobial Therapy, Inc. 2009.

Hughes JR et al. Antidepressants for smoking cessation. Cochrane Database of Systematic Reviews 2007; Issue1.

Hunt P (2001). Motivating Change. Nursing Standard, 16(2): 45-52, 54-55.

Pampallona S et al. Combined pharmacotherapy and psychological treatment for depression: a systematic review. Arch Gen Psychiatry. 2004;61(7):714-9.

Rambout L et al. Prophylactic vaccination against human papillomavirus infection and disease in women: a systematic review of randomized controlled trials. CMAJ. 2007;177(5):469-79.

Toward Optimized Practice Program. Guideline for the diagnosis and management of community acquired pneumonia: adult. 2002 (2008 update).

Wong T & Latham-Carmanico C. Canadian guidelines on sexually transmitted infections. Ottawa; Public Health Agency of Canada 2006 (reviewed 2008).

Zink T, Chaffin J. Herbal "health"products: What family physicians need to know, American Family Physician. 1998. 58(5):1133-1140.

Gastroenterology

Abraham C, Cho JH. Inflammatory Bowel Disease. NEJM. 361(21): 2066-2078.

American Gastroenterological Association Position statement: Evaluation of dyspepsia. Gastroenterology. 129(5):1753-1755, 2005.

Aranda-Michel J, Giannella R. Acute Diarrhea: A Practical Review. American Journal of Medicine. 10(6): 670:676, 1999.

Colorectal cancer screening: Recommendation statement from the Canadian Task Force on Preventative Health Care. CMAJ. 165(2): 206-8, 2001.

Donowitz M, Kokke FT, Saidi R. Evaluation of Patients with Chronic Diarrhea. NEJM. 332 (11): 725:729, 1995.

Howden CW, Hunt RH. Guidelines for the management of Helicobacter Pylori infection. Am J Gastroenterology. 93:2330-2338, 1998.

Jennings JSR, Howdle, PD. Celiac Disease. Current Opinion in Gastroenterology. 17(2): 118:126, 2001.

Laine, L, Peterson WL. Bleeding peptic ulcer. NEJM. 331:717-727, 1994.

Reynolds, T. Ascites. Clinics in Liver Disease. 4(1): 151-168, 2000.

Sandowski SA. Cirrhosis. Clin Fam Pract. 2(1): 59-77, Mar 2000.

Whytcomb DC. Acute pancreatitis. NEJM. 2142-2150, 2006.

General Surgery

Bland KI et al. The Practice of General Surgery. First Edition. W.B. Saunders Co, Toronto. 2002.

Canadian Task Force on Preventive Health Care. Colorectal cancer screening. CMAJ. 165(2):206-208. 2001

Applegate KE. Intussusception in children: evidence-based diagnosis and treatment. Pediatr Radiol. 2009 Apr;39 Suppl 2:S140-3.

Doherty GM. Current Surgical Diagnosis and Treatment, 12th ed. McGraw-Hill, New York, 2006.

Ferzoco LB et al. Acute diverticulitis. NEJM. 338(21):1521-26. 1998.

Hong Z, Wu J, Smart G, Kaita K, Wen SW, Paton S, Dawood M. Survival analysis of liver transplant patients in Canada 1997-2002. Transplant Proc. 38(9):2951-6. 2006.

Hortobagyi GN. Treatment of breast cancer. NEJM. 339(14):974-984. 1998

Olsen O, Gøtzsche PC. Screening for breast cancer with mammography (Cochrane review) In: the Cochrane Library, Issue 3, 2003. Oxford: Update Software.

The University of Cincinnati Residents. The Mont Reid Surgical Handbook. Mosby Inc., St. Louis, 1997.

Geriatric Medicine

British Geriatrics Society and Royal College of Physicians. (2006). Guidelines for prevention, diagnosis and management of delirium in older people. Concise guidance to good practice series. No. 6.

Fick DM, Cooper JW, Wade WE, Waller JL, Maclean R, Beers MH. Updating the Beers Criteria for potentially inappropriate medication use in older adults. Arch Intern Med. 2003; 163: 2716-24.

Fuller G. Falls in the elderly. Am Fam Phys. 2001; 61(7): 2159-72.

Ganz DA, Bao Y, Shekelle PE, Rubenstein LZ. Will my patient fall? JAMA. 2007; 297: 77-86.

Hartikainen S, Lönnroos E, Louhivuori K. Medication as a risk factor for falls: critical systematic review. J Gerontol A Biol Sci. 2007; 62(10): 1172-81.

Inouye, SK. (2007). The Hospital Elder Life Program. Retrieved May 4, 2010 from http://elderlife.med.yale.edu/public/lifestyle.php?pageid=01.01.02.

Young J, Murthy L, Westby M, Akunne A, O'Mahony R. Diagnosis, prevention, and management of delirium: summary of NICE guidance. BMJ. 2010; 341:c3704.

Lachs M, Pillemer K. Elder Abuse. Lancet. 2004; 364:1192-1263.

Robertson RG, Montagnini M. Geriatric failure to thrive. Am Fam Phys. 2004; 70(2): 343-8.

Sarkisian CA, Laches MS. "Failure to thrive" in older adults. Ann Intern Med. 1996; 124: 1072-8.

Verdery RB. Clinical evaluation of failure to thrive in older people. Clin Geriatr Med. 1997; 13:769-78.

Gynecology

Bélisle S, Blake J, Basson R, Desindes S, Graves G, Grigoriadis S, et al. Canadian Consensus Conference on Menopause, 2006 update. J Obstet Gynaecol Can 2006;28(2 Suppl 1):S1-S94.

Cunningham FG, McDonald PC, and Gant NF (eds.), Williams Obstetrics, 14th ed, Appleton and Lange, 1993.

Davis V and Dunn S. Emergency Postcoital Contraception. SOGC Clinical Practice Guidelines. No. 82 July 2000.

Dickey R. Managing Contraceptive Pill Patients 9th edition. EMIS Inc. Medical Publishers., USA 1998.

Erdman JN. Human Rights in Health Equity: Cervical cancer and Hpv vaccines. American journal of law & medicine 2009; 35: 365-387.

Luciano AA, Solima RG. Ectopic Pregnancy: From Surgical Emergency to Medical Management. Ann NY Acad Sci 2001; 943: 235-254.

Lujan ME, Chizen DR, Pierson RA. Diagnostic criteria for polycystic ovary syndrome: Pitfalls and controversies. J Obstet Gynaecol Can. 2008.

Tingulstad S, Hagen B, Skjeldestad FE, et al. The risk of malignancy index to evaluate potential ovarian cancers in local hospitals. BR J Obstet Gynecol. 1999;93(3):448-52.

Hematology

Bates SM and Ginsberg JS. Treatment of deep-vein thrombosis. NEJM, 2004;351:268-277.

Bazemore AW, Smucker DR. Lymphadenopathy and Malignancy. American Family Physician. 2002:66;2103-2110.

Callum JL, Pinkerton PH. Bloody Easy 3rd edition: Blood Transfusions, Blood Alternatives and Transfusion Reactions. Sunnybrook and Women's College Health Sciences Centre: Toronto, 2011.

Canadian Pediatric Society. Transfusion and risk of infection in Canada: Update 2006. Pediatrics and Child Health. 2005;11(3):158-162.

Driscoll MC. Sickle Cell Disease. Pediatrics in Review. 28:7 259 – 286

Habermann TM, Steensma DP. Lymphadenopathy. Mayo Clinic Proc, 2000: 75(7);723-732.

Landaw, SA. Approach to the adult patient with thrombocytopenia. In: Up To Date, Rose, BD (Ed), Up To date, Waltham, MA 2005.

Liesner RJ and Machin SJ. ABC of clinical haematology: Platelet disorders. BMJ. 1997;314:809.

Liesner RJ and Goldstone AH. ABC of clinical haematology: The acute leukaemias. BMJ. 1997;314:733.

Valentine KA and Hull RD. Clinical use of heparin and low molecular weight heparin. UpToDate, Rose BD (Ed), UpToDate, Waltham MA 2006.

Infectious Disease

2009 Guidelines for Antimicrobial Use. Antibiotic Subcommittee of the Pharmacy & Therapeutics Committee. University Health Network

American Academy of Pediatrics. Pickering LK, Baker CJ, Long SS, McMillan JA, eds. Red Book: 2006 Report of the Committee on Infectious Diseases. 27th ed. Elk Grove Village, IL: American Academy of Pediatrics; 2006.

Croft MA and Jacquerioz FA. Drugs for preventing malaria in travelers. Cochrane Database Syst Rev 2009; (4): CD006491.

Kncokaert DC, et a.l. Fever of Unknown Origin in adults: 40 years on. Journal of Internal Medicine. 2003; 253: 263-275.

Lai CL, et al. Viral Hepatitis B. Lancet. 2003; 362:2089-94

Levinson, Warren and Ernest Jawetz. Medical Microbiology and Immunology: Examination and Board Review. 7th Edition. McGraw Hill 2003.

Li JS, et al. Proposed modifications to the Duke Criteria for the Diagnosis of Infective Endocarditis. Clin Infect Dis. 2000;30(4)633-638.

Schaechter M, Engleberg N, Eisenstein B, Medoff G. Mechanisms of Microbial Disease. Lippincott Williams & Wilkins; 1998.

Schlossberg, D, Ed. Current Therapy of Infectious Disease.2nd Edition. Mosby Inc, St Louis, Missouri, 2001.

Nephrology

Androgue HJ, Madias NM. (1999). Management of life threatening acid-base disorders part I. NEJM, Vol. 338 (1): 26-33.

Androgue HJ, Madias NM. (1999). Management of life threatening acid-base disorders part II. NEJM, Vol. 338 (2): 107-11.

Halperin M, Kamel K. (1998). Potassium. The Lancet, Vol 352: 135-40.

Thadhani R, Pascual M, Bonventre JV. (1996). Acute renal failure. NEJM, Vol. 334(22):1448-1460.

Neurology

Adams HP Jr., Bendixen BH, Kappelle LJ, Biller J, Love BB, Gordon DL, et al. Classification of subtype of acute ischemic stroke. Definitions for use in a multicenter clinical trial. Stroke. 1993;24(1):35-41.

Aminoff MJ, Greenberg DA, Simon RP. Lange: Clinical Neurology, 6th edition. Toronto: McGraw-Hill Companies.

Cecil Essentials of Medicine 7th Edition Andreoli, Carpenter, Griggs, Benjamin. Saunders Elsevier.

Chronicle EP, Mulleners WM. Anticonvulsant drugs for migraine prophylaxis. Cochrane Database of Systematic Reviews. 2004, Issue 3.

The ESPRIT Study Group. Aspirin plus dipyridamole versus aspirin alone after cerebral ischaemia of arterial origin (ESPRIT): randomised controlled trial. Lancet 2006; 367:1665-1673.

Francis GJ et al. Acute and preventive pharmacologic treatment of cluster headache. Neurology. 2010; 75:463-473.

Frontera W, Silver J. (2002) Essentials of Physical Medicine and Rehabilitation. Philadelphia: Hanley and Belfus Inc., pp. 778-782.

Gage BF, Waterman AD, Shannon W, Boechler M, Rich MW, Radford MJ.Validation of clinical classification schemes for predicting stroke: results from the National Registry of Atrial Fibrillation. JAMA. 2001;285(22): 2864–70.

Headache Classification Subcommittee of the International Headache Society. The International Classification of Headache Disorders, 2nd edition. Cepahalagia. 2004; 24(S1):9-160.

Johnston SC, Rothwell PM, Nguyen-Huynh MN, Giles MF, Elkins JS, Bernstein AL, et al. Validation and refinement of scores to predict very early stroke risk after transient ischaemic attack. Lancet. 2007;369:283-92.

Lindsay K, Bone I (2003). Neurology and Neurosurgery Illustrated. Philadelphia: Churchill Livingstone pp. 244.
Lowenstein DH, Alldredge BK. Status epilepticus. NEJM. 1998;338(14):970-6.
Mumenthaler M, Mattle H. Fundamentals of Neurology. Thieme: Stuttgart and New York, 2006.
Scherokman B, Selwa L and Alguire PC. Approach to Common Neurological Symptoms in Internal Medicine:
AAN Core Curricula 2011.

Neurosurgery

Brott TG, Hobson RW, George H et al. Stenting versus endarterectomy for treatment of carotid stenosis. New
Engl J Med. 2010;363(1):11-23.
Carpenter CCJ, Griggs RC, Loscalzo J, eds (2001). Cecil Essentials of medicine, 5th edition. Philadelphia: WB
Chronicle EP, Mulleners WM. Anticonvulsant drugs for migraine prophylaxis. Cochrane Database of
Systematic Reviews. 2004, Issue 3.
Coen PG, Scott F, Leedham-Green M et al. European Journal of Pain 2006;10:695-700.
Common Presenting Complaints.
Lindsay K, Bone I (2003). Neurology and Neurosurgery Illustrated. Philadelphia: Churchill Livingstone pp. 244.
Lowenstein DH, Alldredge BK. Status epilepticus. NEJM. 1998;338(14):970-6.
Noseworthy JH, Lucchinetti C, Rodriguez M, Weinshenker BG. Multiple sclerosis. NEJM. 2000; 343(13):938-
52.
Zerr et al. Analysis of EEG and CSF 14-3-3 proteins as aids to the diagnosis of Creutzfeldt-Jakob disease.
Neurology. 2000. 55(6): 811-815.

Obstetrics

American College of Obstetricians and Gynecologists www.acog.org
The Society of Obstetricians and Gynaecologists of Canada www.sogc.org
ABC of labour care: Unusual presentations and positions and multiple pregnancy. BMJ 1999; 318: 1192-1194.
Carol, Blenning. An Approach to the Postpartum Office Visit. American Family Physician. Dec 2005, 72(12);
2491 – 2496.
Chodirker et al. Canadian Guidelines for Prenatal Diagnosis Part 1 & Part 2. SOGC Clinical Practice Guidelines.
July 2001 and June 2000. No 105.
Hod M, Bar J, Peled Y, Fried S, Katz I, Itzhak M, Ashkenazi S, Schindel B, Ben-Rafael Z. Antepartum
management protocol. Timing and mode of delivery in gestational diabetes. Obstet Gynecol. 2009
Jan;113(1):206-17.
North York General Hospital Genetics Program. Integrated Prenatal Screening. 1999.

Ophthalmology

Bradford C. Basic Ophthalmology for Medical Students and Primary Care Residents. 7th ed. San Francisco:
American Academy of Ophthalmology; 1999.
Wilson FM. Practical Ophthalmology: A Manual for Beginning Residents. 4th ed. American Academy of
Ophthalmology; 2005.
Friedman N, Pineda R, Kaiser P. The Massachusetts Eye and Ear Infirmary Illustrated Manual of
Ophthalmology. Toronto: W.B. Saunders Company; 1998.
Kanski JJ. Clinical Ophthalmology: A Systematic Approach. 6th ed. Oxford: Butterworth-Heinemann; 2007.
Stein R, Stein H. Management of Ocular Emergencies. 4th ed. Montreal: Mediconcept; 2006.
Tasman W, Jaegar EA. Duane's Ophthalmology: 2011 ed. Philadelphia: Lippincott Wiliams & Wilkins; 2010.

Orthopedics

AAOS. The treatment of distal radius fractures: Summary of recommendations, 2009

Adams JC, Hamblen DL. Outline of fractures: including joint injuries. 11th ed. Toronto (ON): Churchill Livingstone, 1999.

Brinker M, Miller M. Fundamentals of orthopedics. Philadelphia (PA): W.B. Saunders, 1999.

Dee R, Hurst LC, Gruber MA, Kottmeier SA, editors. Principles of orthopedic practice. 2nd ed. Toronto (ON): McGraw-Hill, 1997.

Hamilton H, McIntosh G, Boyle C. Effectiveness of a low back classification system. Spine J. 2009; 9(8): 648-657.

Miller SL. Malignant and benign bone tumours. Radiol Clin North Am. 2000; 39(4): 673-699.

Murrell GA, Walton JR. Diagnosis of rotator cuff tears. Lancet. 2001: 357. 769.

Ochiai DH. The orthopedic intern pocket survival guide. McLean (VA): International Medical Publishing, 2007.

Otolaryngology

Bailey BJ. Head and Neck Surgery-Otolaryngology. 2nd ed. Philadelphia. Lippincott Williams and Wilkins. 1998.

Fakhry C, Westra WH, Li S, et al. Improved Survival of Patients with Human Papillomavirus-Positive Head and Neck Squamous Cell Carcinoma in a Prospective Clinical Trial. J Natl Cancer Inst. 2008; 100:261-9.

Jafek BW, Murrow BW. ENT Secrets. 2nd ed. Philadelphia. Hanley & Belfus. 2001. p608.

McIsaac WJ, Coyte PC, Croxford R, et al. Otolaryngologists' perceptions of the indications for typanostomy tube insertion in children. CMAJ. 2000; 162:1285-1288.

Pasha R. Otolaryngology Head and Neck Surgery Clinical Reference Guide. 2nd ed. San Diego. Plural Publishing. 2006.

Pediatrics

2009-2010 Drug Handbook and Formulary. In: Lau E, ed. Toronto: The Hospital for Sick Children Department of Pharmacy; 2009.

Advisory Committee Statement National Advisory Committee on Immunization. Volume 28. ACS-2.

Albright EK. Current Clinical Strategies. Pediatric History and Physical Examination. 4th Edition. Current Clinical Strategies Publishing 2003.

Amato RSS. Human Genetics and Dysmorphology. Nelson's Essentials of Pediatrics. 3rd Edition. W.B. Saunders co. pp 129-146, 2002.

Apparent Life-Threatning Events. Pediatric Emergency Medicine. Saunders Elsevier. pp269-272, 2008.

Corrigan J, Boineau F. Hemolytic-Uremic Syndrome. Pediatrics in Review. 2001 Nov; 22(11).

D'Augustine S, Flosi T. Tarascon Pediatric Outpatient Pocketbook. 1st Ed. Tarascon Publishing; 2008.

Jain L and Douglas E. Physiology of Fetal Lung Fluid Clearance and the Effect of Labor. Seminars in Perinatology 2006.

Nelson essentials of pediatrics. 5th ed. Philadelphia, PA.: Elsevier Saunders; 2006.

Newburger JW, Takahashi M, Gerber MA, et al. Diagnosis, treatment, and long-term management of Kawasaki disease: a statement for health professionals from the Committee on Rheumatic Fever, Endocarditis and Kawasaki Disease, Council on Cardiovascular Disease in the Young, American Heart Association. Circulation. 2004;110(17):2747.

Niermeyer S. et al. International Guidelines for Neonatal Resuscitation: An excerpt from the Guidelines 2000 for Cardiopulmonary Resuscitation and Emergency Cardiovascular Care: International Consensus on Science. Contributors and Reviews for the Neonatal Resuscitation. Guidelines. Pediatrics. 2000; 106(3):E29.

Treatment of acute otitis media in an era of increasing microbial resistance. Pediatric Infectious Diseases Journal. 1998; 17:576-579.

Wubbel L, McCracken D, McCracken GH. Management of Bacterial Meningitis. Pediatrics in Review. 1998 Mar; 19(3).

Zorc JJ, Kiddoo DA, Shaw KN. Diagnosis and management of pediatric urinary tract infections. Clin Microbiol Rev. 2005; 18(2):417.

Plastic Surgery

American Society for Surgery of the Hand. The hand: examination and diagnosis third edition. Philadelphia: Churchill-Livingston, 1990.

Georgiade GS, Riefkohl R, Levin LS. Georgiade plastic, maxillofacial and reconstructive surgery third edition. Baltimore: Williams and Wilkins, 1997.

Janis JE. Essentials of Plastic Surgery: A UT Southwestern Medical Center Handbook. St. Louis, MO: Quality Medical, 2007.

Vasconez HC, Ferguson REH, Vasconez LO. Plastic & reconstructive surgery. In: Doherty GM, Way LW, eds. Current surgical diagnosis & treatment twelfth edition. Norwalk, CT: McGraw-Hill, 2006.

Weinzweig J. Plastic surgery secrets. Philadelphia: Hanley and Belfus Inc, 1999.

Psychiatry

American Psychiatric Association. Diagnostic and Statistical Manual of Mental Disorders-4th ed. Text Revision. Washington, (DC): American Psychiatric Publishing Inc., 2000.

Folstein MF, Folstein SE and McHugh PR. Mini-Mental State: A practical method for grading the state of patients for the clinician. Journal of Psychiatr Res. 1975; 12:189-198.

Koch T. A Tour of the Psychotropics. 4th ed. Mental Health Service, St Michael's Hospital. Toronto (Canada).

MTA Cooperative Group. A 14-month randomized clinical trial of treatment strategies for attention-deficit/ hyperactivity disorder. Arch Gen Psychiat. 1999; 56(12):1073-86.

Zimmerman, M. Interview Guide for Evaluating DSM-IV Psychiatric Disorders and the Mental Status Examination. East Greenwich (RI). Psych Products Press. 1994.

Respirology

Bach PB, Brown C, Gelfand SE. Management of acute exacerbations of chronic obstructive pulmonary disease: a summary and apprasial of published evidence. Annals of Internal Medicine 2001;134:600-620.

Bartlett JG, Dowell SF, Mandell LA et al. Practice guidelines for the management of community-acquired pneumonia in adults. Clin Infect Dis 2000;3 1:347-82.

Ferri F. Practical guide to the care of the medical patient. 5th ed. St.Louis: Mosby/Elsevier Sciences. 2001.

File TM. The epidemiology of respiratory tract infections. Semin Respir Infect 2000 Sep;15(3):184-94. Review.

Fine MJ, Auble TE, Yealy DM, et al. A prediction rule to identify low-risk patients with community-acquired pneumonia. NEJM. 1997 Jan 23; 336(4):243-50.

Holleman D, Simel D. Does the clinical examination predict airflow limitation? JAMA. 1995; 273:313-319.

Light RW, Macgregor MI, Luchsinger PC, et al. Pleural effusions: the diagnostic separation of transudates and exudates. Ann Intern Med. 1972; 77(4): 507-13.

Rheumatology

ACR Subcommittee on Rheumatoid Arthritis Guidelines, 2002. Guidelines for the Management of Rheumatoid Arthritis: 2002 Update.

CMAJ Clinical Basics Rheumatology Series.

Klippel JH, Weyand CM, and Wortmann RL. Primer on Rheumatic Diseases, 11th ed. Arthritis Foundation, 1997.

Van der Linden. A proposal for modification of the New York criteria. Arthritis Rheum, 1984; 27:361.

Vitali C, Bombardieri S, Jonsson R, et al. Classification criteria for Sjögren's syndrome: a revised version of the European criteria proposed by the American-European Consensus Group. Ann Rheum Dis 2002;61:554-8.

Wade, J.P. 15. Osteoporosis. CMAJ 2001;165(1):45-50.

Wolfe F, Smythe HA, Yunus MB, et al. The American College of Rheumatology 1990 criteria for the classification of fibromyalgia: report of the multicenter criteria committee. Arthritis Rheum 1990; 33:160-72.

Wolfe F, Clauw DJ, Fitzcharles M-A, et al. The American College of Rheumatology Preliminary Diagnostic Criteria for Fibromyalgia and Measurement of Symptom Severity. Arthritis Care & Research 2010; 62:600-610.

Urology

American Urological Association. http://www.auanet.org/guidelines/

Bremnor JD, Sadovsky R. Evaluation of dysuria in adults. American Family Physician. 2002; 65(8): 1589-1597.

Canadian Urological Association. http://www.cua.org/guidelines_e.asp

Cohen RA, Brown RS. Microscopic hematuria. New England Journal of Medicine. 2003; 348: 2330-2338

Ferri F. Practical Guide to the Care of the Medical Patient (6th ed.) 2006. St. Louis: Mosby.

Galejs LE. Diagnosis and treatment of the acute scrotum. American Family Physician. 1999; 59(4): 817-24

Goldman L, Ausiello D. Cecil Textbook of Medicine (23rd ed.) 2007. Philadelphia: Saunders.

Israel GM, Bosniak MA. An update of Bosniak renal cyst classification system, Urology. 2005; 66(3): 484-8

Macfarlane MT. House Officer Series: Urology (3rd ed.) 2001. Philadelphia: Lippincott.

Morton AR, Iliescu EA, Wilson JWL. Nephrology: 1. Investigation and treatment of recurrent kidney stones. CMAJ. 2002; 166(2): 213-218.

Tanagho EA, McAninch JW. Smith's General Urology (17th ed.) 2007. New York: McGraw-Hill.

Teichman JMH. Acute renal colic from ureteral calculus. NEJM. 2004; 350(7): 684-693

Wein AJ, Kavoussi LR, Novick AC, Partin AW, Peters CA. Campbell's Urology (10th ed.) 2011. Philadelphia: Saunders.

Wieder JA. Pocket Guide to Urology (4th ed.) 2010. Oakland: Wieder.

Index

E

ECF Volume; 272
ECG; 69
Ectopic Pregnancy; 331
Emphysema; 448
Empyema; 454
Endometrial Carcinoma; 225
Endometriosis; 223
Endophthalmitis; 343
Epidural Abscess; 306
Epidural Anesthesia; 60
Epistaxis; 382
ERCP; 178
Erysipelas; 421
Erythema Infectiosum; 101
Esophagogastroduodenoscopy; 177
Exercise (Stress) Testing; 71
Extradural Hematoma; 307

F

Facial Fractures; 417
Facial Pain; 290
Failure to Thrive (FTT)
    Frailty; 211
    Pediatric; 400
Falls; 210
Fatigue; 161
Febrile Neutropenia; 262
Femoral Hernia; 202
Fever
    Of Unknown Origin; 263
    Pediatric; 401
Fibroids; 224
Fibromyalgia; 470
First and Second Trimester Bleeding; 318
Flail Chest; 112
Floaters; 340
Fluid Balance; 60
Fluid Resuscitation; 286
Framingham Data; 169

G

Gastroesophageal Reflux Disease (GERD); 184
Generalized Anxiety Disorder; 434

Genital Lesions; 219
Geriatric Giants; 207
Gestational Diabetes; 333
Gianotti-Crosti Syndrome; 101
Giant Cell Arteritis; 467
GI Bleed
    Lower; 183
    Upper; 182
Glasgow Coma Scale; 109
Glaucoma
    Acute Angle Closure; 343
Gonococcal triad; 462
Gonorrhea; 223
Gout; 462
Graves' Disease; 135
Group A β-hemolytic Streptococcus (GABHS); 174

H

HAART; 262
Hiatus Hernia; 203
Hampton's Hump; 452
Hand, Foot and Mouth Disease; 102
Hand Pain; 415
Headache; 119, 162, 297
Head and Neck Malignancies; 384
Head Injury; 303
    Minor; 303
Hearing Loss; 377
Heinz Bodies; 238
Hematuria; 270, 475
Hemochromatosis; 177
Hemodialysis; 285
Hemoglobin (Hb); 237
Hemolytic Uremic Syndrome (HUS); 243
Hemoptysis; 444
Hemorrhagic Shock; 108
Hemothorax; 112
Heparin; 246
Heparin Induced Thrombocytopenia (HIT); 243
Hepatitis; 188
Hernia; 202
Herpes Simplex Virus of Vulva; 222
Hip Fracture; 370
HIV/AIDS; 261
Hoarseness; 380
Hormone Replacement Therapy (HRT); 229
Howell-Jolly bodies; 238
Human Papillomavirus (HPV); 221